Synopsis of Pathophysiology in Nuclear Medicine

Abdelhamid H. Elgazzar

Synopsis of Pathophysiology in Nuclear Medicine

Second Edition

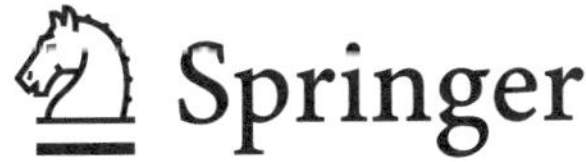
Springer

Abdelhamid H. Elgazzar
Dept. of Nuclear Medicine
Kuwait University
Safat, Kuwait

ISBN 978-3-031-20648-1   ISBN 978-3-031-20646-7   (eBook)
https://doi.org/10.1007/978-3-031-20646-7

This Springer imprint is published by the registered company Springer Nature Switzerland AG
The registered company address is: Gewerbestrasse 11, 6330 Cham, Switzerland

Preface to First Edition

In the last two decades, there have been a revolutionary expansion of nuclear medicine which is due to the dynamic nature of the field which is creativity and innovation conducting. This expansion and continuing development require up-to-date knowledge in the field and relevant disciplines. For the imaging professionals as well as for the users from different clinical specialties to effectively utilize the modern diagnostic and therapeutic applications of nuclear medicine, it is a must to understand the basis of these applications. Nuclear medicine is a unique field which requires diverse knowledge which includes many basic science components such as physics, chemistry, radiation biology, dosimetry, and others. Knowledge of the pathophysiological features of diseases is of crucial importance to the understanding, effective practice and utilization of nuclear medicine. This concept has an increasing importance given the rapid advancement of the field and the change to study molecular changes of normal and diseased organs. This was behind the book on pathophysiological basis of nuclear medicine, and its fourth edition. The idea of the synopsis came from the readers and colleagues who demanded a simplified text of the subject to help students, including in-training technology students, technologists, residents, and practicing physicians, while the other text remains as a comprehensive reference with more details.

In this volume, simple presentation of the basic understanding of the principles of pathophysiology, normal and abnormal cells, essential cell biology, and basis of radiopharmaceutical uptake and distribution in physiological and different pathological processes are included. Since clinical nuclear medicine is simply the application of such basic principle in the study of many conditions of virtually every organ in the body, the pathophysiological features of relevant disease processes are discussed in several chapters of organ systems along with essentials in imaging and its clinical significance.

The book starts by an introductory chapter defining and explaining basic pathophysiology, followed by a chapter on effects of ionizing radiation and essential of cell biology including the features of different cells and tissues with their biological features. The mechanisms of radiopharmaceutical uptake by different tissues and effects of pathophysiological changes on its distribution are included in a separate chapter. These basic parts are followed by chapters for organ systems in addition to chapters on inflammation, oncology, and basis of the therapeutic effects of radionuclides and applications in treating relevant diseases.

I am looking from this work to provide a brief, simple, readable, easy-to-use, yet comprehensive and informative enough text to help the students, and professionals understand nuclear medicine in depth which will be reflected on practice and patient care for those in imaging fields as well as in other clinical disciplines.

Safat, Kuwait   Abdelhamid H. Elgazzar, MD, FCAP, ABNM

Acknowledgment

My thanks and gratitude go to all who supported and helped to make this work a reality, particularly Dr. Jehan Alshammari, Mrs. Heba Issam, Dr. Israa Alqasabi, Mrs. Jehan Ghoneim, Dr. Khalid Khattab and Dr. Mohammed Sakr.

My appreciation is extended to all the contributors for Edition 1, 2, 3 and 4 of the *Pathophysiological Basis of Nuclear Medicine* for which the fourth edition is coming with their valuable prior and current contribution and cooperation.

Contents

Pathophysiology: General Principles

1

1.1 Introduction

Understanding the pathophysiology of disease is essential for all who study and work in any field of medicine. Since nuclear medicine deals with functional and molecular changes, it becomes crucial to understand the pathophysiological changes of relevant diseases and disease-like conditions to properly study and practice the field.

Pathophysiology has been changing and expanding with added new knowledge. Since the late 1970s, tremendous developments in molecular biology and genetics have provided medical science with an unprecedented chance to understand the molecular basis of disease. Disease can now be defined on the basis of abnormal deviation from normal regional biochemistry. Since pathophysiology is a bridge between pathology and physiology, it is imperative to understand the principles of both disciplines.

1.2 Pathology

Pathology is concerned with the study of the nature of disease, including its causes, development, and consequences with emphasis on the structural changes of diseases. Specifically, pathology describes the origin of disease, its etiologies, and how it progresses and manifests clinically in individuals in order to determine its treatment. Pathology plays a vital role across all facets of medicine throughout life, and currently it extends to the examination of molecules within organs, tissues, or body fluids.

1.3 Definition of Disease

The precise definition of disease is as complex as an exact definition of life. It may be relatively easier to define disease at a cellular and molecular level than at the level of an individual. Throughout the history of medicine, two main concepts of disease have predominated: ontological and physiological [1, 2].

The ontological concept views a disease as an entity that is independent and self-sufficient and runs a regular course with a natural history of its own. The physiological concept, on the other hand, defines disease as a deviation from normal physiology or biochemistry; the disease is a statistically defined deviation of one or more functions from those of healthy people under circumstances as close as possible to those of a person of the same sex and age of the patient. Most diseases begin with cell injury, which occurs if the cell is unable to maintain homeostasis.

A. H. Elgazzar, *Synopsis of Pathophysiology in Nuclear Medicine*,
https://doi.org/10.1007/978-3-031-20646-7_1

1.3.1 Homeostasis

The term homeostasis is used by physiologists to mean maintenance of static, or constant, conditions in the internal environment by means of positive and negative feedback of information. About 56% of the adult human body is fluid. Most of the fluid is intracellular, and about one-third is extracellular fluid that is in constant motion throughout the body and contains the ions (sodium, chloride, and bicarbonate) and nutrients (oxygen, glucose, fatty acids, and amino acids) needed by cells to maintain life. Extracellular fluid was described as the internal environment of the body, and it was hypothesized that the same biological processes that make life possible are also involved in disease [1]. As long as all the organs and tissues of the body perform functions that help to maintain homeostasis, the cells of the body continue to live and function properly [1].

1.3.2 The Genome

At birth, molecular blueprints collectively make up a person's genome or genotype that will be translated into cellular structure and function. A single-gene defect can lead to biochemical abnormalities that produce many different clinical manifestations of disease, or phenotypes, a process called pleiotropism. Many different gene abnormalities can result in the same clinical manifestations of disease—a process called genetic heterogeneity. Thus, diseases can be defined as abnormal processes as well as abnormalities in molecular concentrations of different biological markers, signaling molecules, and receptors.

1.4 Physiology

Physiology is the study of normal, healthy bodily function. It is concerned with the science of the mechanical, physical, bioelectrical, and biochemical functions of humans in good health, their organs, and the cells of which they are composed. It is a broad science which aims to understand the mechanisms of living, from the molecular basis of cell function to the integrated behavior of the whole body.

1.5 Pathophysiology

Pathophysiology is a convergence of pathology and physiology. It deals with the disruption of normal mechanical, physical, and biochemical functions, either caused by a disease or resulting from a disease or abnormal syndrome or condition that may not qualify to be called a disease and now includes the molecular mechanisms of disease. In the year 1839, Theodor Schwann discovered that all living organisms are made up of discrete cells [3]. In 1858, Rudolf Virchow observed that a disease could not be understood unless it were realized that the ultimate abnormality must lie in the cell. He correlated disease with cellular abnormalities as revealed by chemical stains, thereby founding the field of cellular pathology. He defined pathology as physiology with obstacles [3].

Since the time of Virchow, gross pathology and histopathology have been a foundation of the diagnostic process and the classification of disease. Traditionally, the four aspects of a disease process that form the core of pathology are etiology, pathogenesis, morphological changes, and clinical significance [4]. The altered cellular and tissue biology and all forms of loss of function of tissues and organs are ultimately the result of cell injury and cell death. Therefore, knowledge of the structural and functional reactions of cells and tissues to injurious agents, including genetic defects, is the key to understanding the disease process. Currently, diseases are defined and interpreted in molecular terms and not just as general descriptions of altered structure. Accordingly, pathology is evolving into a bridging discipline that involves both basic science and clinical practice and is devoted to the study of the structural and functional changes in cells, tissues, and organs that underlie disease [4]. The use of molecular, genetic, microbiological, immunological, and morphological techniques is helping us understand both ontological and physiological causes of disease.

1.6 Basic Major Principles of Pathophysiology

1.6.1 Cell Injury

Cellular injury occurs if the cell is unable to maintain homeostasis. The causes of cellular injury may be hypoxia (oxygen deprivation), inflammation/infection, or exposure to toxic chemicals. In addition, immunological reactions, genetic derangements, and nutritional imbalances may also cause cellular injury (Table 1.1). In hypoxia, glycolytic energy production may continue, but ischemia (loss of blood supply) compromises the availability of metabolic substrates and may injure tissues faster than hypoxia. Various types of cellular injury and their responses are summarized here.

1.6.1.1 Biochemical Cell Injury Mechanisms

Regardless of the nature of injurious agents, there are a number of common biochemical themes or mechanisms responsible for cell injury [5]:

1. ATP depletion: Depletion of ATP is one of the most common consequences of ischemic and toxic injury. ATP depletion induces cell swelling, decreases protein synthesis, decreases membrane transport, and increases membrane permeability.
2. Oxygen and oxygen-derived free radicals: Ischemia causes cell injury by reducing blood supply and cellular oxygen. Radiation, chemicals, and inflammation generate oxygen-free radicals that cause destruction of the cell membrane and cell structure.

Table 1.1 Mechanisms of cellular injury

Hypoxic: Most common
Chemical
Structural trauma
Inflammation/Infectious
Immunological
Genetic derangement
Nutritional imbalance

3. Loss of calcium homeostasis: Most intracellular calcium is in the mitochondria and endoplasmic reticulum. Ischemia and certain toxins increase the concentration of Ca2+ in cytoplasm, which activates a number of enzymes, causes intracellular damage, and increases membrane permeability.
4. Mitochondrial dysfunction: A variety of stimuli (free Ca2+ levels in cytosol, oxidative stress) cause mitochondrial permeability transition (MPT) in the inner mitochondrial membrane, resulting in the leakage of cytochrome c into the cytoplasm.
5. Defects in membrane permeability: All forms of cell injury and many bacterial toxins and viral proteins damage the plasma membrane. The result is an early loss of selective membrane permeability.

1.6.1.2 Intracellular Accumulations

Normal cells generally accumulate certain substances such as electrolytes, lipids, glycogen, proteins, calcium, uric acid, and bilirubin that are involved in normal metabolic processes. As a manifestation of injury and metabolic derangements in cells, abnormal amounts of various substances, either normal cellular constituents or exogenous substances, may accumulate within the cytoplasm or in the nucleus, either transiently or permanently. Abnormal accumulations of organic substances such as triglycerides, cholesterol and cholesterol esters, glycogen, proteins, pigments, and melanin may be caused by disorders in which the cellular capacity exceeds the synthesis or catabolism of these substances. Dystrophic calcification occurs mainly in injured or dead cells, while metastatic calcification may occur in normal tissues due to hypercalcemia that may be a consequence of increased parathyroid hormone, destruction of bone tissue, renal failure, and vitamin D-related disorders.

All these accumulations harm cells by "crowding" the organelles and by causing excessive and harmful metabolites that may be retained within the cell or expelled into extracellular fluid and circulation.

Table 1.2 General response to injury

Cellular adaptation
Atrophy
Hypertrophy
Hyperplasia
Metaplasia
Dysplasia
Cell death
Apoptosis
Necrosis

1.6.2 Cell and Tissue Response to Injury

The normal cell is able to handle normal physiological and functional demands, the so-called normal homeostasis. However, physiological and morphological cellular adaptations normally occur in response to excessive physiological conditions or to some adverse or pathological stimuli [4]. The cells adapt in order to escape and protect themselves from injury. An adapted cell is neither normal nor injured but has an altered steady state, and its viability is preserved. If a cell cannot adapt to severe stress or pathological stimuli, the consequence may be cellular injury that disrupts cell structures or deprives the cell of oxygen and nutrients. Cell injury is reversible up to a certain point, but irreversible (lethal) cell injury ultimately leads to cell death, generally known as necrosis. By contrast, an internally controlled suicide program, resulting in cell death, is called apoptosis (Table 1.2).

1.6.2.1 Cell Adaptation

Some of the most significant physiological and pathological adaptations of cells involve changes in cellular size, growth, or differentiation [4, 5]. These include (a) atrophy, a decrease in size and function of the cell (Fig. 1.1); (b) hypertrophy, an increase in cell size (Fig. 1.2); (c) hyperplasia, an increase in cell number (Fig. 1.3); (d) metaplasia, an alteration of cell differentiation (Fig. 1.4); and dysplasia, an abnormal growth or development of cells (Fig. 1.5). The adaptive response may also include the intracellular accumulation of normal endogenous substances (lipids, protein, glycogen, bilirubin, and pigments) or abnormal exog-

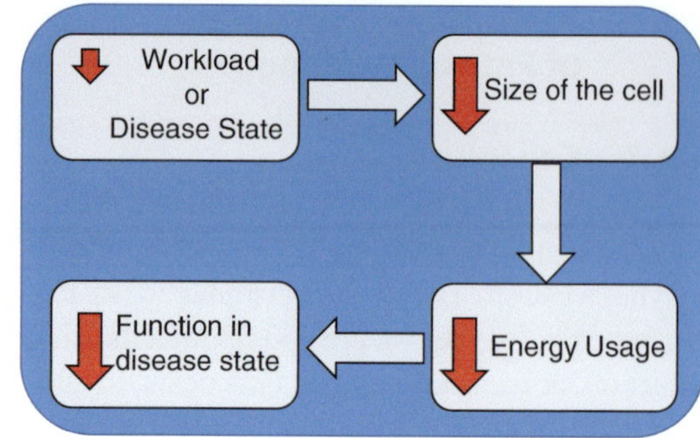

Fig. 1.1 Atrophy

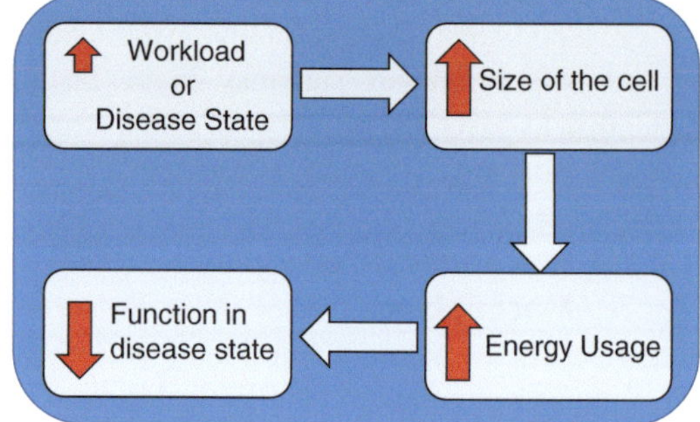

Fig. 1.2 Hypertrophy

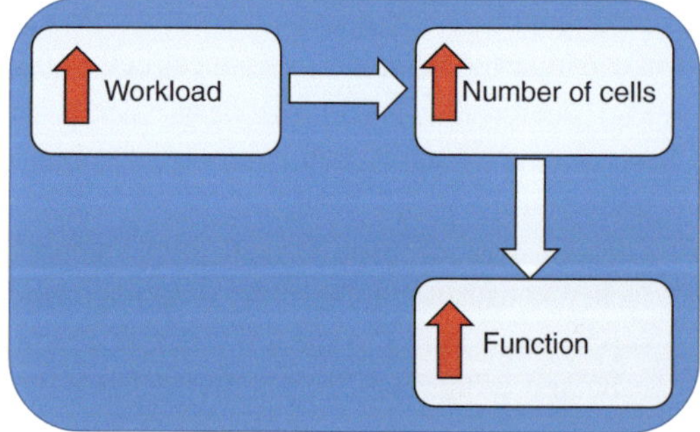

Fig. 1.3 Hyperplasia

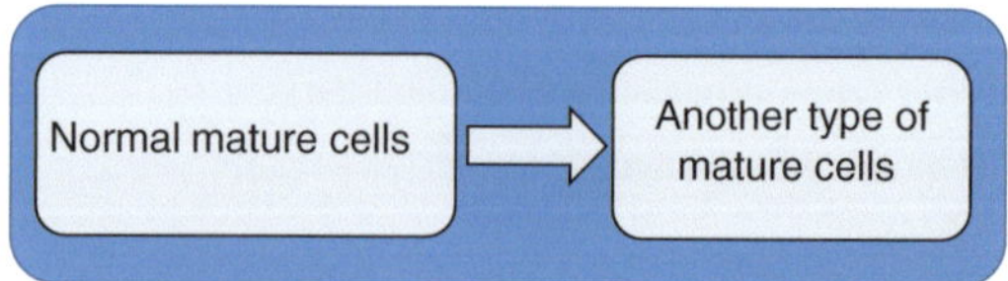

Fig. 1.4 Metaplasia

enous products. Cellular adaptations are a common and central part of many disease states. The molecular mechanisms leading to cellular adaptation may involve a wide variety of stimuli

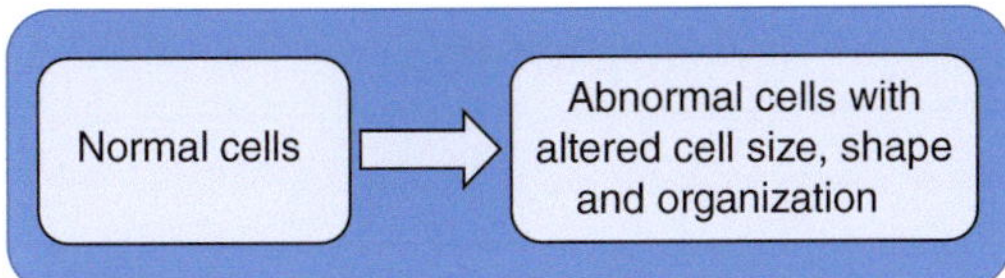

Fig. 1.5 Dysplasia

and various steps in cellular metabolism. Increased production of cell signaling molecules, alterations in the expression of cell surface receptors, and overexpression of intracellular proteins are typical examples.

1.6.2.1.1 Atrophy

Atrophy is a decrease in the size of cells, which may lead to decrease in the size of a body part, organ, or tissue which was normal in size for the individual, considering age and circumstance, prior to the diminution. Examples include muscle atrophy from lack of use (most common) or disease.

1.6.2.1.2 Hypertrophy

Hypertrophy is a non-tumorous enlargement of a tissue or organ as a result of an increase in the size rather than the number of constituent cells. Examples include myocardial muscle hypertrophy due to prolonged strain secondary to hypertension.

1.6.2.1.3 Hyperplasia

Hyperplasia is the abnormal multiplication or increase in the number of normal cells in a normal arrangement in an organ or a tissue. Typical hyperplasia is a physiological response to a specific stimulus, and the cells remain subject to normal regulatory control mechanisms. Examples include endometrial hyperplasia resulting from high levels of estrogen.

1.6.2.1.4 Metaplasia

Metaplasia is the transformation of one mature differentiated cell type into another mature differentiated cell type, as an adaptive response to some insult or injury. By this change in differentiation, and hence patterns of gene expression, the cells should be more resistant to the effects of the insult.

It is usually a reversible phenomenon. Examples include transformation of columnar epithelial cells of salivary gland ducts to squamous epithelial cells when stones are present. Development of glandular epithelium (glandular metaplasia) in the esophagus in patients with gastric acid reflux is another example (Barrett's esophagus) where normal squamous epithelial cells change to columnar cells.

1.6.2.1.5 Dysplasia

Dysplasia is an abnormality resulting in alteration in size, shape, and organization of adult cells or organs. It is characterized by a decreased amount of mature cells and an increased amount of immature cells, leading to an abnormal arrangement of tissue. Such cells could return to proper formation, but in some cases, the cells worsen and become carcinogens. In dysplasia, cell maturation and differentiation are delayed, in contrast to metaplasia, in which cells of one mature, differentiated type are replaced by cells of another mature cell [6].

1.6.2.2 Cell Death

Cell death is extremely important in the maintenance of tissue homeostasis, embryonic development, immune self-tolerance, and regulation of cell viability by hormones and growth factors.

1.6.2.2.1 Necrosis (Nonregulated, Inflammatory Accidental Cell Death)

Necrosis is cellular death resulting from the progressive derivative action of enzymes on the lethally injured cells, ultimately leading to the processes of cellular swelling, dissolution, and rupture. Cell membranes swell and become permeable. Lytic enzymes destroy the cellular contents, which then leak out into the intercellular space, leading to the mounting of an inflammatory response (Fig. 1.6a). The morphological appearance of necrosis is the result of denaturation of proteins and enzymatic digestion (autolysis or heterolysis) of the cell. Different types of necrosis occur in different organs or tissues. The most common type is coagulative necrosis, result-

a   Accidental Cell Death

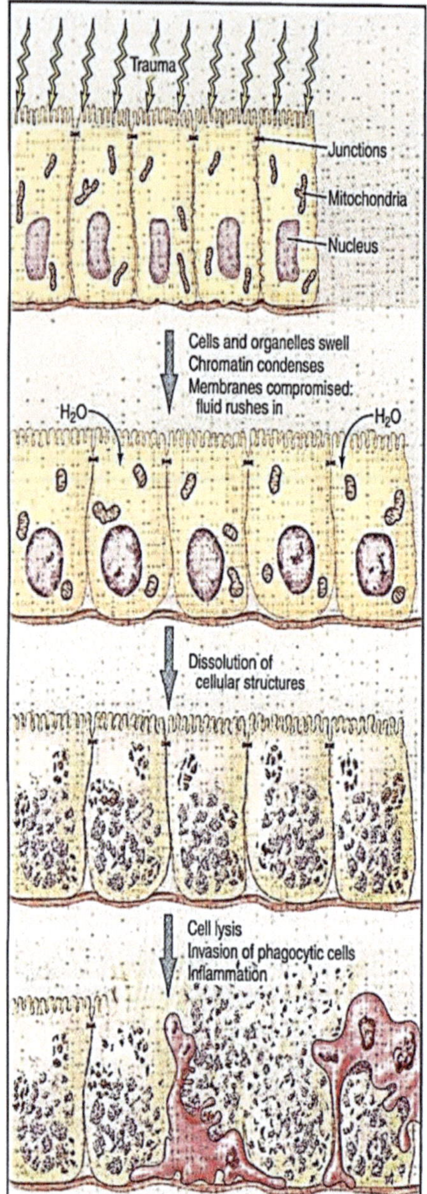

b   Apoptosis

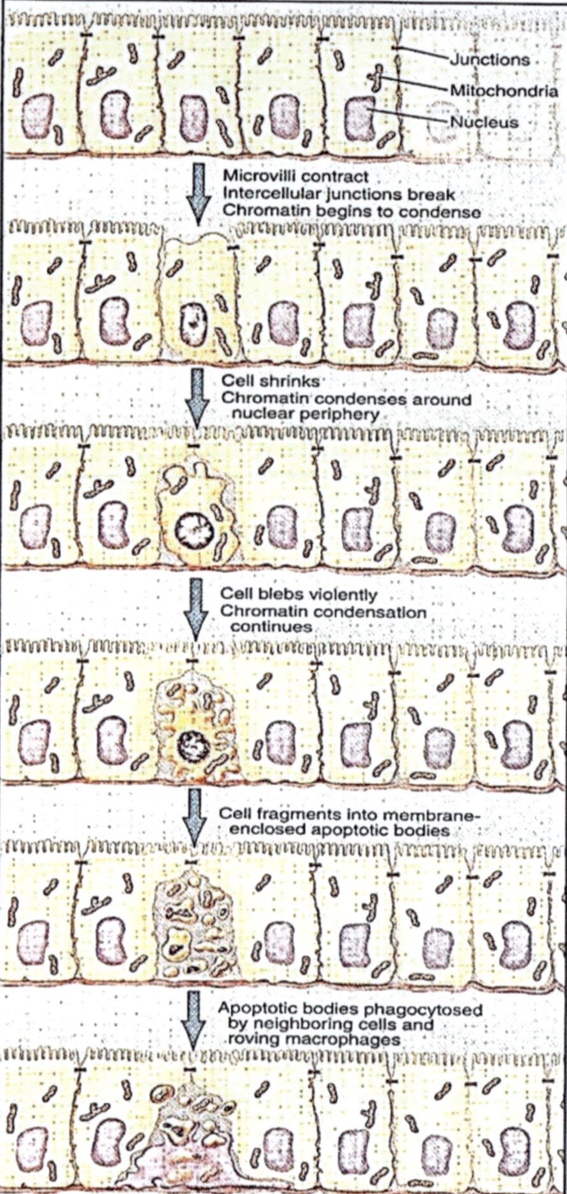

Fig. 1.6 (**a**, **b**) Diagram illustrating cell death. Accidental cell death (**a**) where necrosis occurs as a result of injury to cells. Typically, groups of cells are affected. In most cases, necrotic cell death leads to an inflammatory response (red "angry" macrophages). (**b**) Illustrates apoptosis or active cell suicide, which typically affects single cells. Neighboring cells remain healthy. Apoptotic cell death does not lead to an inflammatory response (From Pollard and Earnshaw [7] with permission)

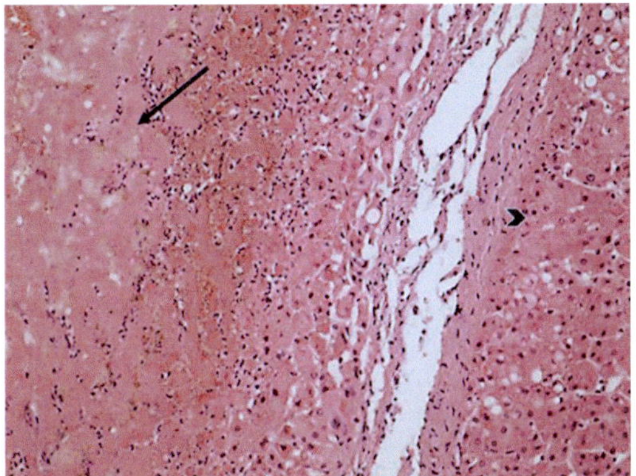

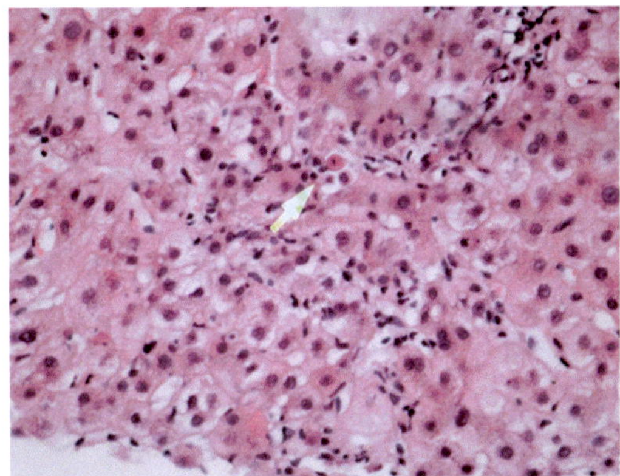

Fig. 1.7 Coagulative necrosis in a case of myocardial infarction. Note the necrotic area on the left side (*arrow*) with no cellular details and loss of nuclei compared to normal myocardial cells on the right side (*arrowhead*)

Fig. 1.8 A photomicrograph of a liver biopsy for a patient with hepatitis C and cirrhosis owing to an apoptosis body (*arrow*), which is a small sealed membrane vesicle formed to prevent the leak of potentially toxic or immunogenic contents of the dying cell and hence prevent inflammation, autoimmune reactions, and tissue destruction

ing from hypoxia and ischemia. It is characterized by denaturation of cytoplasmic proteins, breakdown of organelles, and cell swelling (Fig. 1.7), and it occurs primarily in the kidneys, heart, and adrenal glands. Liquefactive necrosis may result from ischemia or bacterial infections. The cells are digested by hydrolases, and the tissue becomes soft and liquefies. As a result of ischemia, the brain tissue liquefies and forms cysts. In infected tissue, hydrolases are released from the lysosomes of neutrophils; they kill bacterial cells and the surrounding tissue cells, resulting in the accumulation of pus. Caseous necrosis, present in the foci of tuberculous infection, is a combination of coagulative and liquefactive necrosis. In fat necrosis, the lipase enzymes break down triglycerides and form opaque, chalky necrotic tissue as a result of saponification of free fatty acids with alkali metal ions. The necrotic tissue and the debris usually disappear by a combined process of enzymatic digestion and fragmentation or they become calcified.

1.6.2.2.2 Apoptosis (Regulated, Noninflammatory Cell Death)

Apoptosis, a type of cell death implicated in both normal and pathological tissue, is designed to eliminate unwanted host cells in an active process of cellular self-destruction effected by a dedicated set of gene products. Apoptosis occurs during normal embryonic development and is a homeostatic mechanism to maintain cell populations in tissues. It also occurs as a defense mechanism in immune reactions and during cell damage by disease or noxious agents. Various kinds of stimuli may activate apoptosis. These include injurious agents (radiation, toxins, free radicals), specific death signals (TNF and Fas ligands), and withdrawal of growth factors and hormones. Within the cytoplasm, a number of protein regulators (Bcl-2 family of proteins) either promote or inhibit cell death. In the final phase, the execution caspases activate the proteolytic cascade that eventually leads to intracellular degradation, fragmentation of nuclear chromatin, and breakdown of cytoskeleton (Fig. 1.6b).

The most important morphological characteristics are cell shrinkage, chromatin condensation, and formation of cytoplasmic blebs and apoptotic bodies (Fig. 1.8) that are subsequently phagocytosed by adjacent healthy cells and macrophages. Unlike necrosis, apoptosis is characterized by nuclear and cytoplasmic shrinkage and affects scattered single cells. Two major apoptotic pathways have been defined in mammalian cells: death receptor pathway and mitochondrial pathway.

Cells undergo programmed death in response to both internal surveillance mechanisms and signals sent by other cells (Fig. 1.6b). Thus, some cells effectively volunteer to die, whereas other cells are nominated for death by others [7–9].

References

1. McCormick F (2010) The molecular pathology of cancer. Nat Rev Clin Oncol 7:251–265
2. Harris TJ, McCormick F (2010) The molecular pathology of cancer. Nat Rev Clin Oncol 7:251–265
3. Pentimalli A, Giordano A (2017) Cell biology and genetics. Reference Module Life Sci. https://doi.org/10.1016/B978-0-12-809633-8.12390-8
4. Wagner HN Jr (1995) Nuclear medicine: what it is and what it does. In: Wagner HN Jr, Szabo Z, Buchanan JW (eds) Principles of nuclear medicine. W.B. Saunders, Philadelphia, pp 1–8
5. Virchow R (1958) Disease, life and man. Stanford University Press, Stanford
6. McCance KL, Huether SE (2005) Pathophysiology. The biologic basis for disease in adults and children, 4th edn. Mosby-Year Book, St. Louis
7. Kumar V, Abbas A, Aster JC (2020) Robbins and Cotzan, pathologic basis of disease, 10th edn. Saunders, Philadelphia
8. Gallizzi I, Vitale I, Abrams HM et al (2012) Molecular definition of cell death subroutines: recommendations of the nomenclature committee on cell death. Cell Death Differ 19:107–120
9. Pollard TD, Earnshaw WC (2002) Cell biology. Saunders, Philadelphia

Ionizing Radiation: Biologic Effects and Essential Cell and Tissue Biology

2.1 Essential Cell and Tissue Biology

2.1.1 Cell Structure and Function

The different substances that make up the cell are collectively called protoplasm, which is composed mainly of water, electrolytes, proteins, lipids, and carbohydrates. The two major parts of the cell are the nucleus and cytoplasm. The cytoplasm is separated from the extracellular fluid by a cell membrane, while the nucleus is separated from the cytoplasm by a nuclear membrane (Fig. 2.1). The major organelles in the cell are organelles derived from membranes, organelles involved in gene expression, and organelles involved in energy production [1]. The important subcellular structures of the cell and their functions are summarized in Table 2.1.

2.1.1.1 Plasma Membrane

The plasma membrane encloses the cell, defines its boundaries, and maintains the essential difference between the cytoplasm and the extracellular environment. The cell membranes are assembled from four major components: a lipid bilayer, membrane proteins, sugar residues, and a network of supporting fibers. The lipid bilayer is a major barrier, impermeable to water-soluble molecules such as ions, glucose, and urea. The major classes of membrane lipid molecules are phospholipids, cholesterol, and glycolipids. The membrane proteins are responsible for most membrane functions such as transport, cell identity, and cell adhesion and constitute transport channels, transport molecules, specific receptors, and enzymes. The cell surface often has a loose carbohydrate coat called glycocalyx. The sugar residues generally occur in combination with proteins (glycoproteins, proteoglycans) or lipids (glycolipids).

2.1.1.2 Cytoplasm and its Organelles

Cytoplasm is an aqueous solution (cytosol) that fills the cytoplasmic matrix, the space between the nuclear envelope and the cell membrane. The cytosol contains many dissolved proteins, electrolytes, glucose, certain lipid compounds, and thousands of enzymes. In addition, glycogen granules, neutral fat globules, ribosomes, and secretory granules are dispersed throughout the cytosol. Many chemical reactions of metabolism occur in the cytosol, where substrates and cofactors interact with various enzymes. The various organelles suspended in the cytosol are either surrounded by membranes (nucleus, mitochondria, and lysosomes) or derived from membranous structures (endoplasmic reticulum, Golgi apparatus). All biological membranes are phospholipid bilayers with embedded proteins.

© The Author(s), under exclusive license to Springer Nature Switzerland AG 2023

A. H. Elgazzar, *Synopsis of Pathophysiology in Nuclear Medicine*,

https://doi.org/10.1007/978-3-031-20646-7_2

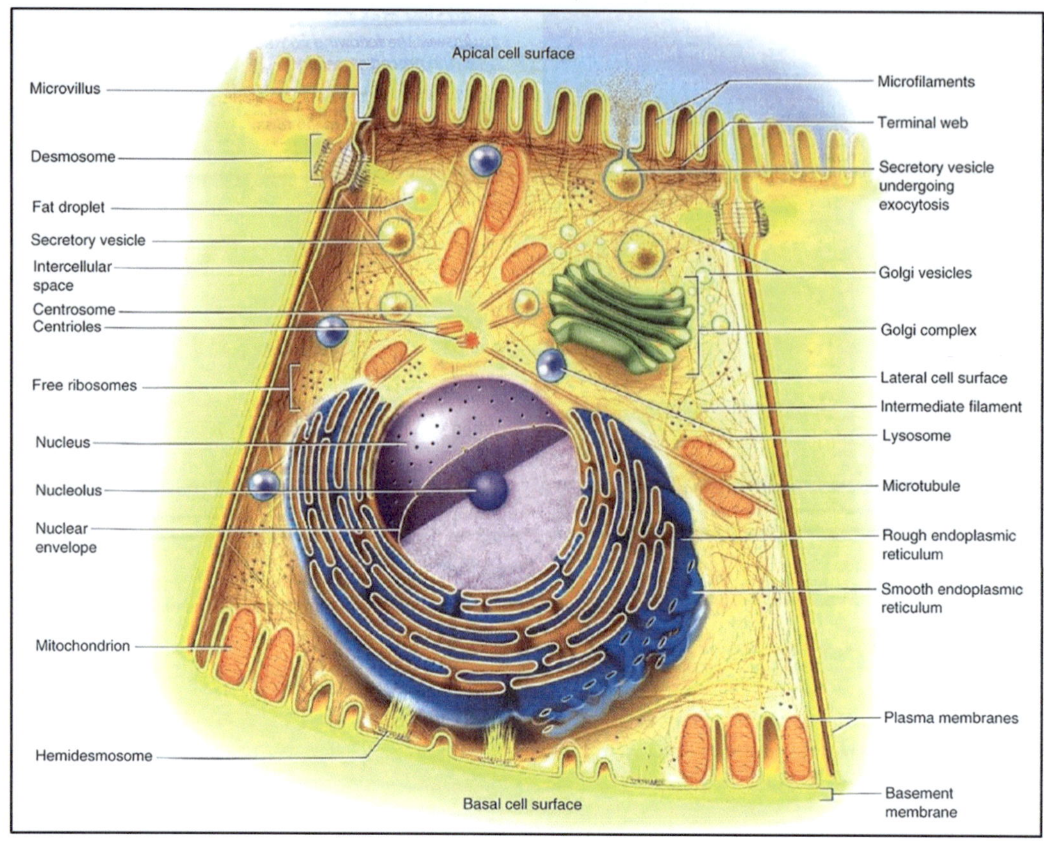

Fig. 2.1 Schematic drawing of the cell clearly depicting the intricate network of interconnecting intracellular structures such as the endoplasmic reticulum (rough and smooth), mitochondria, lysosomes, and nucleus (Reprinted with permission from Saladin [1])

Table 2.1 Cell structures (components) and their function [1–5]

Cell structure	Major functions
Plasma membrane	Cell morphology and movement, transport of ions and molecules, cell-to-cell recognition, cell surface receptors
Endoplasmic reticulum	Formation of compartments and vesicles, membrane synthesis, synthesis of proteins and lipids, detoxification reactions
Lysosomes	Digestion of worn-out mitochondria and cell debris, hydrolysis of proteins, carbohydrates, lipids, nucleic acids
Peroxisomes	Oxidative reactions involving molecular oxygen, utilization of hydrogen peroxide (H_2O_2)
Golgi complex	Modification and sorting of proteins for incorporation into organelles and for export; formation of secretory vesicles
Microbodies	Isolation of particular chemical activities from the rest of the cell body
Mitochondria	Cellular respiration; oxidation of carbohydrates, proteins, and lipids; urea and heme synthesis
Nucleus	DNA synthesis and repair; RNA synthesis and control; center of the cell; directs protein synthesis and reproduction
Chromosomes	Contain hereditary information in the form of genes
Nucleolus	RNA processing, assembles ribosomes
Ribosomes	Sites of protein synthesis in cytoplasm
Cytoplasm	Metabolism of carbohydrates, lipids, amino acids, nucleotides
Cytoskeleton	Structural support, cell movement, cell morphology

2.1.1.2.1 The Endoplasmic Reticulum

An interconnecting network of tubular and flat membranous vesicular structures is called the endoplasmic reticulum (ER). Like the cell membrane, the walls of the ER are composed of a lipid bilayer containing many proteins and enzymes. The regions of ER rich in ribosomes are termed rough or granular ER, while the regions of ER with relatively few ribosomes are called smooth or agranular ER. Ribosomes are large molecular aggregates of protein and ribonucleic acid (RNA) that are involved in the manufacture of various proteins by translating messenger RNA (mRNA) copies of genes.

2.1.1.2.2 The Golgi Complex

The Golgi complex or apparatus is a network of flattened smooth membranes and vesicles. It is the delivery system of the cell. It collects, packages, modifies, and distributes molecules within the cell or secretes the molecules to the external environment. Within the Golgi bodies, the proteins and lipids synthesized by the ER are converted to glycoproteins and glycolipids and collected in membranous folds or vesicles called cisternae, which subsequently move to various locations within the cell. In a highly secretory cell, the vesicles diffuse to the cell membrane and then fuse with it and empty their contents to the exterior by a mechanism called exocytosis. The Golgi apparatus is also involved in the formation of intracellular organelles such as lysosomes and peroxisomes.

2.1.1.2.3 Lysosomes

Lysosomes are small vesicles formed by the Golgi complex and have a single limiting membrane. Lysosomes maintain an acidic matrix (pH 5 and below) and contain a group of glycoprotein digestive enzymes (hydrolases) that catalyze the rapid breakdown of proteins, nucleic acids, lipids, and carbohydrates into small basic building molecules. In white blood cells, lysosome contents are released into the vacuole around the bacteria and serve to kill and digest those bacteria. Lysosomes also release hydrolytic enzymes into the cytoplasm to digest the entire cell. This is termed programmed cell death (apoptosis) or selective cell death, which is one of the principal mechanisms involved in the removal of unwanted cells and tissues in the body.

2.1.1.2.4 Peroxisomes

Peroxisomes are small membrane-bound vesicles or microbodies derived from the ER or Golgi apparatus. Many of the enzymes within the peroxisomes are oxidative enzymes that generate or utilize hydrogen peroxide (H_2O_2). Peroxisomes protect the cell from its own production of toxic hydrogen peroxide. White blood cells, for example, produce hydrogen peroxide to kill bacteria. The oxidative enzymes in peroxisomes breakdown the hydrogen peroxide into water and oxygen. Peroxisomes are also involved in the oxidative metabolism of long-chain fatty acids.

2.1.1.3 Mitochondria

Mitochondria are tubular or sausage-shaped organelles (1–3 µm). They are composed mainly of two lipid bilayer-protein membranes. The outer membrane is smooth and derived from the ER. The inner membrane contains many infoldings or shelves called cristae which partition the mitochondrion into an inner matrix called mitosol and an outer compartment. The outer membrane is relatively permeable but the inner membrane is highly selective and contains different transporters. The inner membrane contains various proteins and enzymes necessary for oxidative metabolism, while the matrix contains dissolved enzymes necessary to extract energy from nutrients. The total number of mitochondria per cell depends on the specific energy requirements of the cell and may vary from less than a hundred to up to several thousand. Mitochondria are the "powerhouses" of the cell. The cell derives energy from glucose, amino acids, and fatty acids. In a process called glycolysis, glucose is converted to pyruvic acid, which subsequently enters mitochondria where it begins a sequence of chemical reactions called the citric acid or Krebs cycle. Various enzymes present in the inner membrane oxidize the pyruvic acid to carbon dioxide and water. The oxidative metabolism of the glucose molecule generates 36 molecules of

ATP. The amino acids and fatty acids are converted to acetyl coenzyme A (in the cytoplasm) which also enters the citric acid cycle and gets oxidized with the generation of ATP molecules.

2.1.1.4 Ribosomes

Ribosomes are large complexes of RNA and protein molecules and are normally attached to the outer surfaces of the ER. The major function of ribosomes is to synthesize proteins. Each ribosome is composed of one large and one small subunit with a mass of several million daltons.

2.1.1.5 Cytoskeleton

The cytoplasm contains a network of protein fibers, called the cytoskeleton, that provides a shape to the cell and anchors various organelles suspended in the cytosol. The fibers of the cytoskeleton are made up of different proteins of different sizes and shapes such as actin (actin filaments), tubulin (microtubules), and vimentin and keratin (intermediate filaments).

2.1.1.6 Nucleus

The nucleus is the largest membrane-bound organelle in the cell, occupying about 10% of the total cell volume. The nucleus is composed of a double membrane, called the nuclear envelope, that encloses the fluid-filled interior, called nucleoplasm. The outer membrane is contiguous with the ER. The nuclear envelope has numerous nuclear pores, permitting certain molecules to pass into and out of the nucleus. The primary functions of the nucleus are the control of cell division and the phenotypic expression of genetic information that directs all of the activities of a living cell. The cellular deoxyribonucleic acid (DNA) is located in the nucleus as a DNA histone protein complex known as chromatin that is organized into chromosomes. The total genetic information stored in the chromosomes of an organism is said to constitute its genome. The human genome consists of 24 chromosomes(22 different chromosomes and two sex chromosomes). The smallest unit of DNA that encodes a protein product is called a gene and consists of an ordered sequence of nucleotides located in a particular position on a particular chromosome. There are approximately 100,000 genes per human genome, and only a small fraction(15%) of the genome is actively expressed in any specific cell type. The genetic information is transcribed into ribonucleic acid (RNA), which subsequently is translated into a specific protein on the ribosome. The nucleus contains a subcompartment called the nucleolus that contains large amounts of RNA and protein. The main function of the nucleolus is to form granular subunits of ribosomes, which are transported into the cytoplasm where they play an essential role in the formation of cellular proteins.

2.1.2   The Genetic Material and Gene Expression

2.1.2.1 The Genetic Material: DNA

The ability of cells to maintain a high degree of order depends on the hereditary or genetic information that is stored in the DNA [5–9]. Within the nucleus of all mammalian cells, a full complement of genetic information is stored, and the entire DNA is packaged into chromosomes.

2.1.2.1.1   DNA Structure

DNA was first discovered in 1869 as a white substance from the cell nuclei of human pus and was called "nuclein." Since nuclein was slightly acidic, it was known as nucleic acid. In the 1920s, two sorts of nucleic acids (DNA and RNA) were identified. The structure of DNA molecule as a polynucleotide was later shown to be formed by the polymerization of nucleotides. Each nucleotide subunit of DNA molecule is composed of three basic elements: a phosphate group, a five-carbon sugar (deoxyribose), and one of the four types of nitrogen-containing organic bases. Two of the bases, thymine and cytosine, are called pyrimidines, while the other two, adenine and guanine, are called purines. Although some forms of cellular DNA exist as single-stranded structures, the most widespread DNA structure represents DNA as a double helix containing two polynucleotide strands that are mirror images of each other (Fig. 2.2).

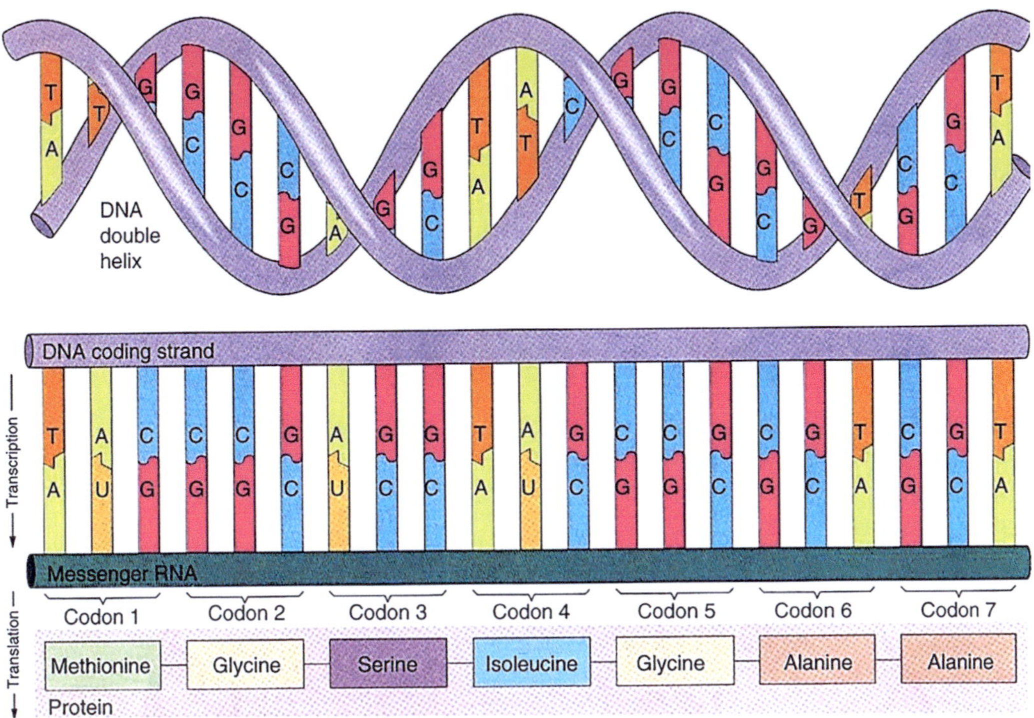

Fig. 2.2 The double-stranded DNA molecule consists of bases, deoxyribose sugar, and phosphate. Note the hydrogen bonds between the two strands of DNA molecules (Reprinted with permission from Saladin [1])

The "backbone" of the DNA molecule is composed of the deoxyribose sugars joined by phosphodiester bonds to a phosphate group, while the bases are linked in the middle of the molecule by hydrogen bonds. The relationship between the bases in a double helix is described as complementarity, since adenine always bonds with thymine and guanine always bonds with cytosine. As a consequence, the double-stranded DNA contains equal amounts of purines and pyrimidines.

2.1.2.1.2   DNA Replication

All the chromosomes in the nucleus duplicate their DNA prior to every cell division in order to serve as genetic material. When a DNA molecule replicates, the double-stranded DNA separates or unzips at one end, forming a replication fork(Fig. 2.3). The process of replication proceeds by a mechanism in which a new DNA strand is synthesized that matches each of the original strands serving as a template. At the end of each round of replication, one of the parental strands is maintained intact, and it combines with one newly synthesized complementary strand.

2.1.2.1.3   DNA Mutation

A mutation is any inherited change in the genetic material involving irreversible alterations in the sequence of DNA nucleotides. These mutations may be phenotypically silent (hidden) or expressed (visible). Mutational damage to DNA is generally caused by one of three events: (a) Ionizing radiation causes double-stranded breaks in DNA due to the action of free radicals on phosphodiester bonds. (b) Ultraviolet radiation creates DNA cross-links due to the absorption of UV energy by pyrimidines.(c) Chemical mutagens modify DNA bases and alter base-pairing behavior. Mutations in germ line tissue are of enormous biological significance, while somatic mutations may cause cancer.

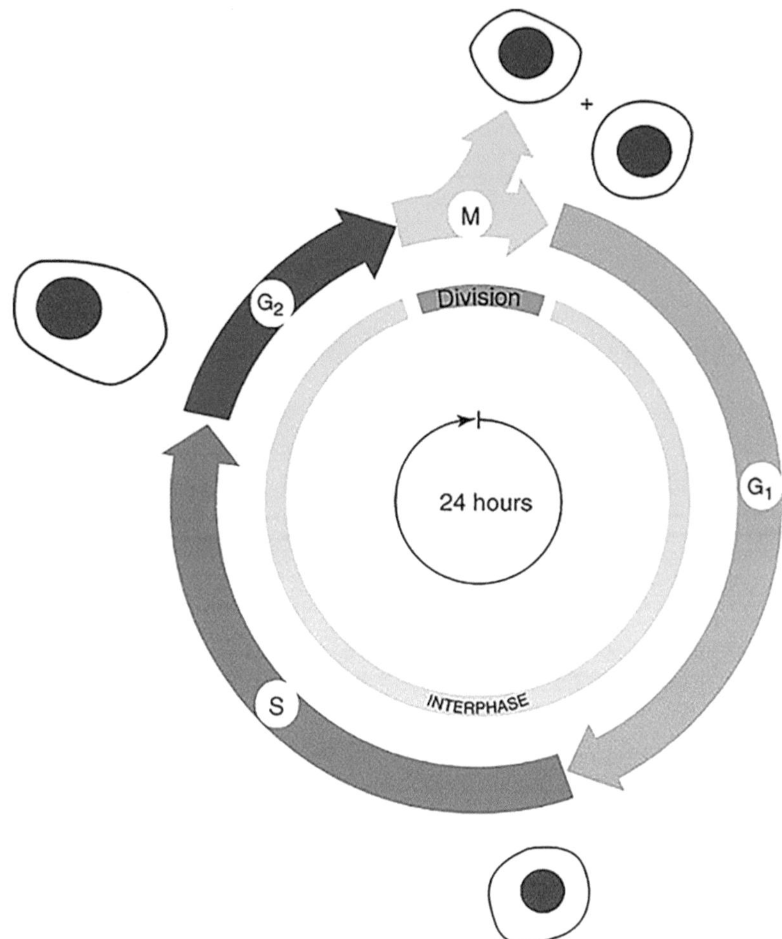

Fig. 2.3 The cell division cycle is generally represented by four successive phases. During the interphase, the cell grows continuously, and only during M phase does it undergo division. DNA replication occurs during S phase, while G1 and G2 are the gaps during which cells normally show additional growth such as protein and enzyme synthesis. Cells in G1, if they are not committed to DNA replication (that is, entering S phase), may enter into a resting state, often called G0, where they can remain for days, or even years, before resuming proliferation (Reprinted with permission from Alberts et al.) [13]

2.1.2.1.4 DNA Recombination

DNA can undergo exchange events through recombination leading to genetic material rearrangement. Recombination is defined as the creation of new gene combinations and may include exchange of an entire chromosome or rearranging the position of a gene or a segment of a gene on a chromosome.

2.1.2.2 Gene Expression and Protein Synthesis

Heredity is the ability of the cell to use the information in its DNA to control and direct the synthesis of all proteins in the body, as proteins are the tools of heredity. The production of RNA is called transcription and is the first stage of gene expression. The result is the formation of messenger RNA (mRNA) from the base sequence specified by the DNA template. All types of RNA molecules are transcribed from the DNA. The mRNA molecules are finally transported to the ER in the cytoplasm, where proteins are synthesized. RNA is chemically similar to DNA, the main difference being that the RNA molecule contains ribose sugar and another pyrimidine, uracil, in place of thymine. RNAs are classified according to the different roles they play in the course of protein synthesis. mRNA molecules carry the genetic code to the ribosomes, where they serve as templates for the synthesis of proteins. The transfer RNA (tRNA) molecule transfers specific amino acids from the soluble amino acid pool to the ribosomes and ensures the alignment of these amino acids in a proper sequence. Ribosomal RNA (rRNA) forms the structural framework of ribosomes, where most proteins are synthesized. All RNA molecules are synthesized in the nucleus.

2.1.2.3 Genetic Code

The genetic code in a DNA sense strand consists of a specific nucleotide sequence coded in successive "triplets" that will eventually control the sequence of amino acids in a protein molecule. An important feature of the genetic code is that it is universal; all living organisms use precisely the same DNA codes to specify proteins.

2.1.2.4 DNA Translation: Protein Synthesis

More than half of the total dry mass of a cell is made up of proteins. The second stage of gene expression after transcription is the synthesis of proteins, which requires complex catalytic machinery. The process of mRNA-directed protein synthesis by ribosomes is called translation and is dependent on two other RNA molecules, rRNA and tRNA as described earlier. Some proteins emerging from the ribosome are ready to function, while others undergo a variety of post-translational modifications in order to convert the protein to a functional form.

2.1.3   Cell Reproduction

The human body consists of some 200 trillion cells, all of them derived from a single cell, the fertilized egg, which undergoes millions of cell divisions. Cells reproduce by duplicating their contents and then dividing in two. The reproduction of a somatic cell involves two sequential phases: *mitosis* (the process of nuclear division) and *cytokinesis* (cell division). In gametes, the nuclear division occurs through a process called *meiosis*. Meiosis introduces genetic variation into the daughter cells while mitosis cannot. Mitosis is normally for growth and maintenance and meiosis is for sexual reproduction. The life cycle of the cell is the period of time from cell division to the next cell division. The duration of the cell cycle, however, varies greatly from one cell type to another and is controlled by the DNA-genetic system.

2.1.3.1 The Cell Cycle

In all somatic cells, the cell cycle (Fig. 2.4) is broadly divided into M phase (or mitosis) and interphase (growth phase). In most cells, M phase takes only a small fraction of the total cycle when

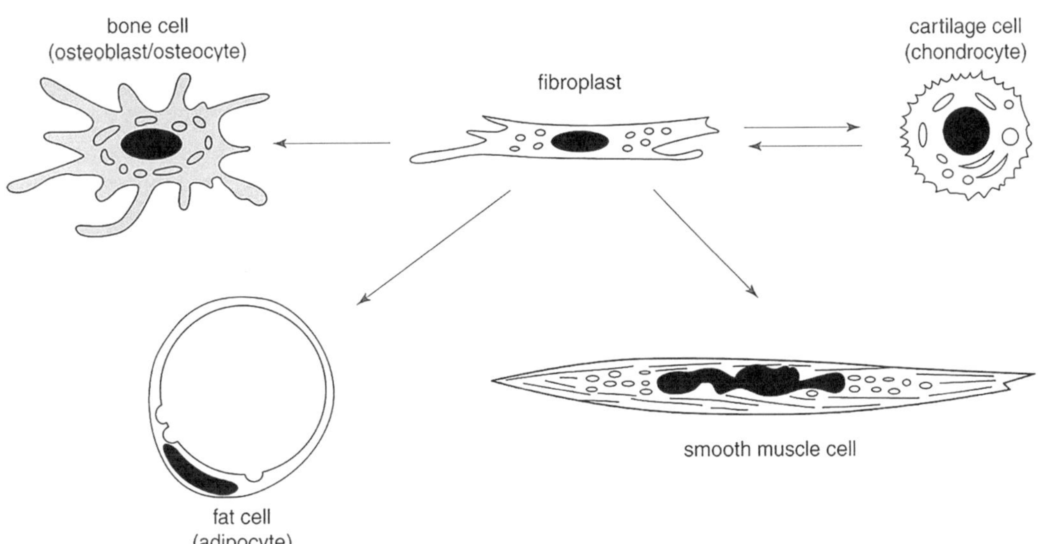

Fig. 2.4 The family of connective tissue cells includes fibroblasts, cartilage cells, and bone cells, as well as fat cells and smooth muscle cells, which appear to have a common origin. *Arrows* show the possible interconversions. Many types of fibroblasts may exist, with differences in their differentiation potential (Reprinted with permission from Alberts et al. [13])

the cell actually divides. The rest of the time the cell is in interphase, subcategorized into three phases: G1, S, and G2. During the G1 phase, most cells continue to grow until they are committed to divide. If they are not ready to go into S phase, they may remain for a long time in a resting state known as G0 before they are ready to resume proliferation. During G2 phase, cells synthesize RNA and proteins and continue to grow, until they enter into M phase.

2.1.3.2 Mitosis and Cytokinesis

One of the first events of mitosis takes place in the cytoplasm. A pair of centrioles is duplicated just prior to DNA replication. Toward the end of interphase, the two pairs of centrioles move to the opposite poles of the cell. The complex of microtubules (spindle) pushes the centrioles farther apart, creating the so-called mitotic apparatus. It is very important to note that mitochondria in the cytoplasm are also replicated before mitosis starts, since they have their own DNA. Based on specific events during nuclear division, mitosis is subcategorized into four phases(prophase, metaphase, anaphase, and telophase).During *prophase*, the nuclear envelope breaks down, chromosome condensation continues, and the centromere of the chromatids is attached to opposite poles of the spindle. During *early metaphase*, the spindle fibers pull the centromeres to the center, forming an equatorial plate. At the end of metaphase, the centromeres divide the chromatids into equal halves. During *anaphase*, the sister chromatids are pulled apart and physically separated and drawn to opposite poles, thus completing the accurate division of the replicated genome. By the end of anaphase, 23 identical pairs of chromosomes are on the opposite sides of the cell. During telophase, the mitotic apparatus is disassembled, the nuclear envelope is reestablished around each group of 23 chromosomes, the nucleolus reappears, and finally chromosomes begin to uncoil into a more extended form to permit expression of rRNA genes. Cytokinesis is the physical division of the cytoplasm and the cell into two daughter cells, which inherit the genome as well as the mitochondria.

2.1.3.3 Rates of Cell Division

For many mammalian cells, the standard cell cycle is generally long but may be few hours for fast-growing tissues. Many adult cells such as nerve cells, cells of the lens of the eye, and muscle cells lose their ability to reproduce. Certain epithelial cells of the intestine, lungs, and skin divide continuously and rapidly in less than 10 h. The early embryonic cells do not grow but divide very rapidly with a cell cycle time of less than 1 h. In general, mitosis requires less than an hour, while most of the cell cycle time is spent during G1 or G0 phase. It is possible to estimate the duration of S phase by using tracers such as 3H-thymidine or bromodeoxyuridine (BrdU).

2.1.3.4 Chromosomes and Diseases

Many of the processes involved in maintaining the organization and equal division of chromosomes between daughter cells such as DNA replication and repair, or mitosis and meiosis, are very complicated and can go wrong from time to time. A chromosomal disease or syndrome is found in situations where defects in some aspect of chromosome organization or behavior lead to a disease state.

2.1.4 Cell Transformation and Differentiation

The zygote and blastomeres resulting from the first few cleavage divisions are totipotent, capable of forming any cell in the body. As the development progresses, the developmental options of cells narrow and become omitted. The fate of the cell becomes fixed and is said to be determined. The determined cell may pass through many developmental stages but cannot move into another developmental track. For example, a muscle cell cannot become a nerve cell. Restriction and determination signify the progressive limitation of the development capacities in the embryo. Differentiation refers to the actual morphological or functional expression of the portion of genome that remains available to a determined cell or group of cells and characterizes the phenotypic specialization of cells. Thus, differentiation is the process of acquiring specific new characteristics resulting in observable changes in cellular function. Cells within a developing embryo display the least amount of differentiation. On the other hand, in the adult, undifferentiated cells are known as pluripotent cells, precursor cells, or stem cells that are not totally committed to a specific function. The three germ layers, ectoderm, mesoderm, and endoderm, have different fates. The endoderm forms a tube, the primordium of the digestive tract. It gives rise to the pharynx, esophagus, stomach, intestines, and several other associated organs such as liver, pancreas, and lungs. While the endoderm forms the epithelial components of these structures, the supporting muscular and fibrous elements arise from the mesoderm. In general, the mesoderm gives rise to the muscles and connective tissues of the body, first in the form of mesenchyme and ultimately cartilage, bone and fibrous tissue, and the dermis (the inner layer of the skin). In addition, the tubules of the urogenital system, vascular system, and the cells of the blood also develop from the mesoderm. The ectoderm forms the epidermis and the entire nervous system. In a process known as neurulation, the central portion of the ectoderm creates a neural tube that pinches off from the rest of ectoderm and will form the brain and spinal cord. Some of the ectodermal cells develop into the neural crest and form all of the peripheral nervous system as well as the pigment cells of the skin.

2.1.5 Normal and Malignant Growth

2.1.5.1 Normal Growth

2.1.5.1.1 Types of Cells and Tissue

In the human body, specialized cells of one or more types are organized into cooperative assemblies, the tissues that perform one or more unique functions. Different types of tissue compose organs, and organs in turn are integrated to perform complex functions. The four major tissue types are epithelial, muscle, connective, and nervous. There are also tissues that do not exist as isolated units but rather in association with one another and in variable proportions, forming different organs and systems in the body such as blood and lymphoid tissues. Such tissue cells are in contact with a network of extracellular macromolecules known as extracellular matrix, which holds cells and tissues together, that provides an organized latticework within which cells can migrate and interact with one another. All tissues are further divided into many subtypes (Table 2.2).

2.1.5.1.2 Muscle Tissue

There are three types of specialized contractile cells that contain actin and myosin. These are smooth muscle, skeletal muscle, and cardiac muscle cells. Muscular tissue is composed of elongated cells that have the specialized function of contraction. Muscles are similar in many aspects but differ in their activation mechanisms, energy supplies, and arrangement of contractile filaments.

Skeletal Muscle
Skeletal muscle is composed of bundles of very long, cylindrical, multinucleated cells.

Cardiac Muscle
Cardiac muscle is specialized for repetitive, fatigue-free contractions to maintain the circulation of blood. The muscle contracts at regular intervals by action potentials from specialized pacemaking cells. Cardiac muscle cells are short and branched. Extracellular calcium is required for cardiac and smooth muscles but not for skeletal muscle.

Smooth Muscle
Smooth muscle cells are generally confined to internal organs, such as blood vessels to regulate blood pressure, the gastrointestinal tract to control food movement, and the respiratory system to facilitate breathing.

2.1.5.1.3 Nerve Tissue

Nerve cells, or neurons, are independent anatomical and functional units with complex morpho-

Table 2.2 Tissue types [3–6]

Tissue	Tissue type	Location	Function
Epithelial	Simple squamous	Lines major organs	Absorption, filtration, secretion
	Simple cuboidal	Lines tubules and ducts of glands	Absorption and secretion
	Simple columnar	Lines the GI tract	Secretion and absorption
	Stratified squamous	Lines interior of mouth, tongue, vagina	Protection
	Transitional	Lines the urinary bladder	Permits stretching
Connective	Loose connective	Deep layers of the skin, blood vessels, organs	Support, elasticity
	Dense connective	Tendons, ligaments	Attaches structures together, provides strength
	Elastic connective	Lungs, arteries, trachea, vocal cords	Provides elasticity
	Reticular connective	Spleen, liver, lymph nodes	Provides internal scaffold for soft organs
	Cartilage	Ends of long bones, trachea, tip of nose	Provides flexibility and support
	Bone	Bones	Protection, support, muscle attachment
	Vascular connective tissue	Within blood vessels	Transport of gases, blood clotting
	Adipose tissue	Deep layers of the skin, surrounds heart, kidney	Support, protection, heat conservation
Muscle	Smooth muscle	GI tract, uterus, blood vessels, and bladder	Propulsion of materials
	Cardiac muscle	Heart	Contraction
	Skeletal muscle	Attached to bones	Movement
Neural	Different types of neurons	Brain and spinal cord	Conduction of electrical impulse, neurotransmission

logical characteristics. They are responsible for the reception, transmission, and processing of stimuli and the release of neurotransmitters and other formational molecules. Most neurons consist of three parts, dendrites, cell body, and axon. The dendrites are multiple elongated processes specialized in receiving stimuli from the environment, sensory epithelial cells, or other neurons. The cell body or perikaryon represents the trophic center for the whole nerve cell and is also receptive to stimuli. The axon is a single process specialized in generating or conducting nerve impulses to other cells.

2.1.5.1.4 Epithelial Tissue

Epithelial tissues are composed of closely aggregated polyhedral cells with very little intracellular substance. Adhesion between these cells is strong, forming cellular sheets that cover the sur-face of the body and line its cavities. The principal osteoblasts, which synthesize the organic components of the matrix; and osteoclasts, which are multinucleated cells involved in the resorption and remodeling of bone tissue functions of epithelial tissues are covering and lining surfaces, absorption, secretion, and contractility. Benign and malignant tumors can arise from most types of epithelial cells. A carcinoma is a malignant tumor of epithelial cell origin. Malignant tumors derived from glandular epithelial tissue are usually adenocarcinomas.

2.1.5.1.5 Matrix

These connective tissues are responsible for providing and maintaining organ and tissue form in the body. They provide a matrix that serves to connect and bind the cells and organs and give support to the body. Unlike other tissue types that are formed mainly by cells, the major constituent of connective tissue is its extracellular matrix, composed of protein fibers, an amorphous ground substance, and tissue fluid in addition to cells.

2.1.5.2 Indigenous Connective Tissue

These cells arise in connective tissue and remain there. They include fibroblasts, fat cells, mast cells, osteoblasts, and chondrocytes and arise from primitive mesenchymal cells.

2.1.5.2.1 Fibroblasts

These are spindle shaped, with oval flattened nuclei. They synthesize and secrete most of the macromolecules of the extracellular matrix. In response to tissue damage, fibroblasts proliferate and migrate into the wound, where they synthesize new matrix to restore the integrity of the tissue.

2.1.5.2.2 Mast Cells

These are secretory cells that mediate immediate hypersensitivity reactions. Mast cells are distributed along the blood vessels within the connective tissue. A variety of stimuli such as mechanical trauma, heat, X-rays, toxins, and other stimuli can induce secretion of the contents of their granules, mainly histamine.

2.1.5.2.3 Fat Cells

Fat cells (adipocytes) are round cells of different sizes. These cells take up fatty acids and glycerol from the blood after a meal and synthesize triglycerides for storage in the lipid droplet. During fasting, these triglycerides are hydrolyzed and the fatty acids are released back into the blood to provide energy for organs. Fat cells also secrete a hormone leptin, which binds to receptors in the brain and modulates appetite to avoid obesity. There are two types of fat cells which have different locations, structures, and colors. White fat cell, which is common, contains one large central droplet of white or yellow fat in the cytoplasm. Brown fat is less abundant than white fat and contains numerous lipid droplets, vascular blood vessels, and abundant brown mitochondria, giving it its color, and is used to generate heat in response to cold. In cold weather, the sympathetic nervous system stimulates brown fat to generate heat by fatty acid oxidation. Anaerobic glycolysis therefore becomes the main source of ATP production instead of lipid metabolism and then glucose turn over within brown fat increases. This is behind the prominent FDG uptake by brown fat that mimics tumors uptake (Fig. 2.5). Unlike white fat tissue, which is present throughout the body, brown adipose tissue has a more limited distribution. In animals ending their hibernation period, or in newborn mammals(including humans) who are exposed to a cold environment, nerve impulses liberate norepinephrine into the tissue. This neurotransmitter activates the hormone lipase, promoting hydrolysis of triglycerides to fatty acids and glycerol. Liberated fatty acids are metabo-

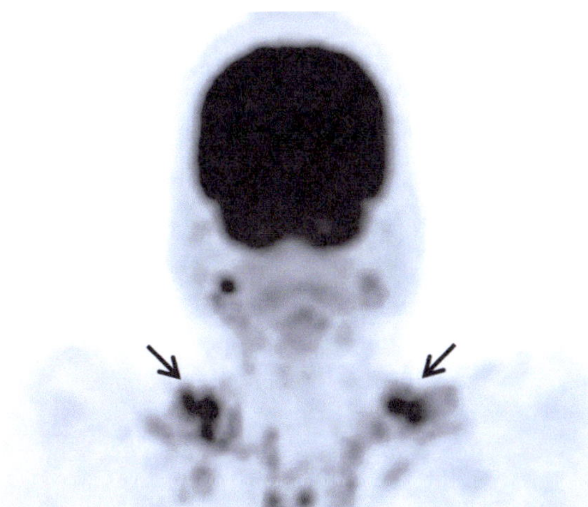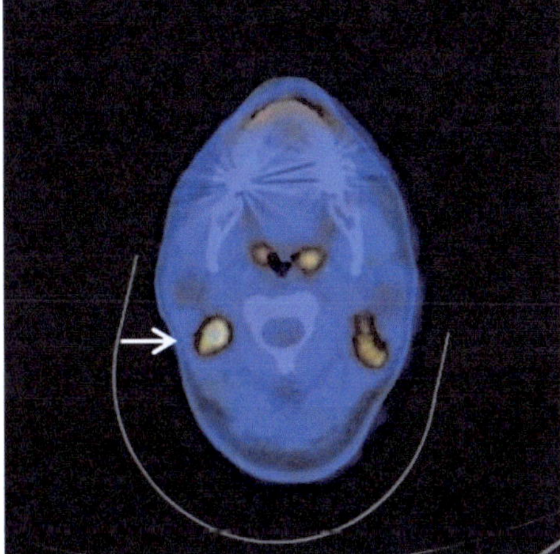

Fig. 2.5 Representative sections of [F-18]FDG PET/CT illustrating increased tracer uptake in brown fat (*arrows*)

lized, producing heat, elevating the temperature of the tissue, and warming the blood passing through it. Heat production is increased, because the mitochondria in the cell have a transmembrane protein called thermogenin in their inner membrane. White fat cells can generate very common benign tumors called lipomas. Malignant adipocyte-derived tumors (liposarcomas) are among the more common tumors of connective tissue. Tumors of the brown adipose cells (hibernomas) are relatively rare.

2.1.5.2.4 Bone Cells

The bone is a specialized connective tissue composed of intracellular calcified material, the bone matrix, and three cell types. These are osteocytes, which are found in cavities within the matrix, osteoblasts, which synthesize the organic components of the matrix; and osteoclasts, which are multinucleated cells involved in the resorption and remodeling of bone tissue.

2.1.5.2.5 Cartilage Cells

Cartilage consists of cells, chondrocytes, and an extensive extracellular matrix composed of fibers and ground substance. Chondrocytes synthesize and secrete the extracellular matrix, and cells themselves are located in matrix cavities called lacunae. Collagen, hyaluronic acid, proteoglycans, and small amounts of several glycoproteins are the principal macromolecules present in all types of cartilage matrix. Cartilage supports soft tissues. Since it is smooth surfaced and resilient, cartilage is a shock-absorbing and sliding area for joints. Cartilage is also essential for the development and growth of long bones.

2.1.5.2.6 Immigrant Cells

These cells travel transiently through the blood or lymph and enter the connective tissue as needed. The blood contains many cells with a specialized function. All blood cells derive from pluripotent stem cells. These stem cells are also responsible for restoring blood cell production. Destruction of stem cells, for example, by chloramphenicol leads to aplastic anemia. These cells include erythrocytes (red blood cells), granulocytes, monocytes, lymphocytes, plasma cells, and platelets.

2.1.5.3 Neoplastic Growth

Cellular reproduction is normally a tightly controlled process. Social control genes regulate cell division, proliferation, and differentiation under normal conditions. Certain stimuli and growth factors, both physiological and pathological, can influence a cell's rate of reproduction. Uncontrolled cellular division that serves no purpose is called neoplasia. The uncontrolled growth of an abnormal cell that serves no purpose will give rise to a tumor or neoplasm that can be either benign or malignant. Transformation is the process by which a normal cell becomes a cancer cell. The common characteristics of cancerous tissue include local increase in cell population, loss of normal arrangement of cells, variation of cell shape and size, increase in nuclear size and density of staining, increase in mitotic activity, and abnormal mitoses and chromosomes. Cancer cells produce a number of substances referred toas tumor cell markers. These can be hormones, enzymes, gene products, or antigens that are found on tumor cell plasma membrane or in the blood, spinal fluid, or urine. Regarding the tissue origin of cancer, in children up to 10 years of age, most tumors develop from hematopoietic organs, nerve tissues, connective tissues, and epithelial tissues (in decreasing order). This proportion gradually changes with age, so that after 45 years of age, more than 90% of all tumors are of epithelial origin [10].

2.1.6 Cellular Metabolism

2.1.6.1 Role of ATP

The chemical reactions involved in maintaining essential cellular functions are referred to together as cellular metabolism. The life processes are driven by energy; anabolism requires energy while catabolism releases energy. Atoms can store potential energy by means of electrons at higher energy levels. Energy is stored in chemical bonds when atoms combine to form molecules. Cells extract the chemical energy from nutrients and transfer the energy to a molecule known as adenosine triphosphate (ATP). Oxidative cellular metabolism and oxidative phosphorylation reactions result in the formation of ATP that is used throughout the cell to energize all the intracellular metabolic reactions. ATP is used to promote three major categories of cellular function: membrane transport of ions such as Na+, K+, Ca2+, Mg2+, and Cl–; synthesis of biochemicals such as proteins, enzymes, and nucleotides; and mechanical work such as muscle contraction.

2.1.6.2 Production of ATP

The catabolism of nutrients can be divided into three different phases. Phase 1 represents the process of digestion that happens outside the cells where proteins, polysaccharides, and fats are broken down into their corresponding smaller subunits: amino acids, glucose, and fatty acid. In phase 2, the small molecules are transported into the cell, where the major catabolic processes take place with the formation of acetyl coenzyme A (acetyl-CoA) and a limited amount of ATP and NADH. Finally, in phase 3, the acetyl-CoA molecules are degraded in mitochondria to CO_2 and H_2O with the generation of ATP.

2.1.6.2.1 Glycolysis

The most important process in phase 2 of catabolism is the degradation of glucose in a sequence often biochemical reactions known as glycolysis or oxidative cellular metabolism. Glycolysis can produce ATP in the absence of oxygen. Each glucose molecule is converted into two pyruvate molecules with a net generation of six ATP molecules. If oxygen is absent, or significantly reduced within the cell, the pyruvate is converted to lactic acid, which then diffuses into extracellular fluid. In many of the normal cells, glycolysis accounts for less than 5% of the overall ATP generation within the cell.

2.1.6.2.2 Oxidative Phosphorylation

Phase 3 begins in the mitochondria with a series of reactions called the citric acid cycle (also known as the tricarboxylic acid cycle or the Krebs cycle) and ends with oxidative phosphorylation. Oxidative phosphorylation is the last step in catabolism, releasing a great deal of chemical energy that is used to make the major portion of cellular ATP.

2.1.7 Transport through the Cell Membrane

The cellular intake or output of different molecules occurs by different transport mechanisms of the plasma membrane, depending on the chemical and biochemical characteristics of the solute molecule. The cell membrane is a barrier for the transport of water molecules and water-soluble substances across the cell membrane. The major transport systems in mammalian cells are summarized in Table 2.3.

2.1.7.1 Transport of Water and Solutes

2.1.7.1.1 Diffusion

Body fluids are composed of two types of solutes: electrolytes, which ionize in solution and exhibit polarity (cations and anions), and non-electrolytes. The continual movement of solute molecules among each other in liquids or in gases is called diffusion. The solute molecules in the extracellular fluid or in the cytoplasm can diffuse across the plasma membrane. Diffusion through the cell membrane is divided into two separate subtypes known as simple diffusion and facilitated diffusion (Fig. 2.6a). Simple diffusion can occur through the cell membrane, either through the intermolecular interstices of the lipid bilayer or through transport proteins (watery channels). Facilitated diffusion (carrier-mediated diffusion) involves translocating a solute through a cell membrane down its concentration gradient as in the case of simple diffusion, without expenditure of metabolic energy. However, facilitated diffusion requires the interaction of a carrier protein (transporter) with the solute molecules. Upon entering the protein channel, the solute chemically binds to the transporter and induces a con

Table 2.3 Transport mechanisms across plasma cell membrane

Mechanism	Transport process	Examples
Nonspecific processes		
Simple diffusion	Direct through the membrane and dependent on concentration gradient	Oxygen movement into cells
Osmosis	Direct and via diffusion of water molecules across a semipermeable membrane	Movement of water into cells when placed in hypotonic solution
Endocytosis		
Phagocytosis	Particles are engulfed by membrane through vesicle formation	Ingestion of bacteria or particles by leukocytes
Pinocytosis	Fluid is engulfed by membrane through vesicle formation	Transport of nutrients by human egg cells
Exocytosis	Extrusion of material from a cell involves membrane vesicles	Secretion of proteins by cells via small membrane vesicles
Specific processes		
Facilitated diffusion (passive diffusion)	Transport of molecules into the cells involves protein channels or transporters and is dependent on concentration gradient	Movement of glucose into most cells
Primary active transport	Transport of molecules against concentration gradient involves carrier protein and requires energy derived from hydrolysis of ATP	Na^+, K^+, Ca^{2+}, H^+, and cl^-ions
Secondary active transport	As a consequence of primary active transport, diffusion energy sodium ions can pull other solutes into the cell (co-transport)	Glucose and amino acids
Receptor-mediated endocytosis	Endocytosis is triggered by the binding of a molecule to a specific receptor on the cell surface, followed by internalization of vesicles	Cholesterol (LDL)and transferrin uptake by cells

formational change in the carrier protein, so that the channel is open in the intracellular side and releases the molecule (Fig. 2.6a).

2.1.7.1.2 Active-Mediated Transport

Active transport systems, or pumps, move the solute molecules through a cell membrane against its concentration gradient, and this requires the expenditure of some form of energy(Fig. 2.6a). As a result, the concentration of solute molecules on either side of the plasma membrane is not equal. For example, the concentration of Na + ions in the extracellular fluid is ten times more than the concentration of Na + ions in the cytoplasm, while the converse is true with K+ ions. In active transport, the transporters are very specific for a solute and exhibit saturation kinetics. In addition, the carrier protein imparts energy to the solute to move against electrochemical or concentration gradient. If the energy source is removed or inhibited, active transport mechanism is abolished. Most of the ions, amino acids, and certain sugars are actively transported across the plasma membrane. In primary active transport, the energy is derived directly from the hydrolysis of ATP to ADP. The best-known active transport system is the Na+/K + -dependent ATPase pump, found in virtually all mammalian cells. The transporter protein is an enzyme ATPase. Secondary active transport represents a phenomenon called co-transport, in which molecules are transported through the plasma membrane from the energy obtained not directly from the hydrolysis of ATP, but from the electrochemical gradient across the membrane.

2.1.7.1.3 Transport by Vesicle Formation

The transport of macromolecules such as large proteins, polysaccharides, nucleotides, and even other cells across the plasma membrane is accomplished by a unique process called endocytosis, which involves special membrane-bound vesicles. The material to be ingested is progressively enclosed by a small portion of the plasma

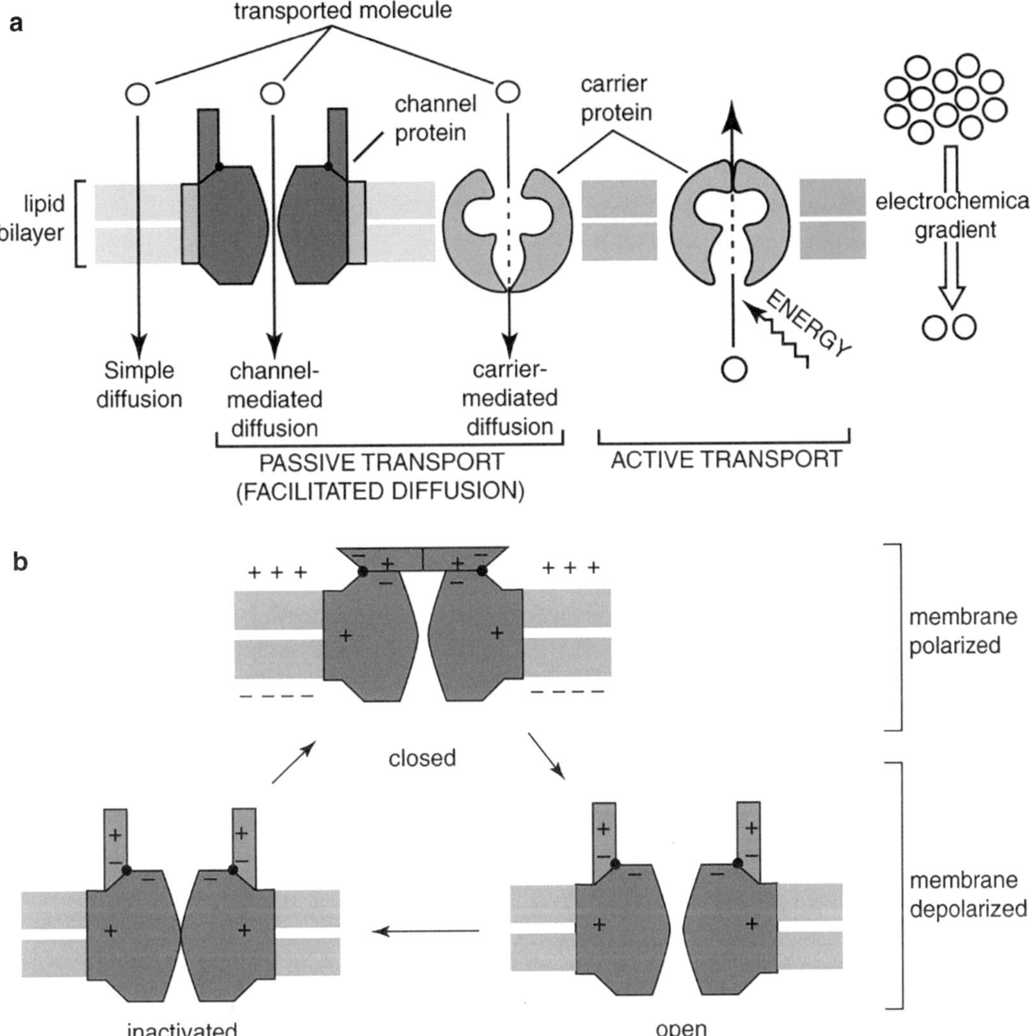

Fig. 2.6 (a) Membrane transport mechanisms of small molecules. Simple diffusion is dependent purely on concentration gradient. Facilitated diffusion involves either channel proteins or carrier proteins within the plasma membrane. While diffusion of molecules occurs spontaneously, active transport also requires an input of metabolic. (b) Voltage-gated cation channels are present on the plasma membrane of all electrically excitable cells. An action potential is triggered by a depolarization of the plasma membrane. When the membrane is at rest (highly polarized), the channel is closed, but when the membrane is depolarized, the channel may exist in an open state (sodium ions move into the cell) or in an inactivated state (Reprinted with permission from Albertset al [13].)

membrane, which first invaginates and then pinches off to form an intracellular vesicle. Many of the endocytosed vesicles end up in lysosomes, where they are degraded. Endocytosis is subcategorized into two types: pinocytosis involves ingestion of fluid and solutes via small vesicles, while phagocytosis involves ingestion of large particles such as microorganisms via large vesicles called phagosomes. Specialized cells that are professional phagocytes, such as macrophages and neutrophils, mainly carry out phagocytosis. For example, more than 1011 senescent red blood cells are phagocytosed by macrophages every day in a human body. The reverse of endocytosis is exocytosis, which involves transport of macromolecules within vesicles from the interior of the cell to a cell surface or into the extracellular fluid.

2.1.7.1.4 Transport by Transmission of Electrical Impulses

Nerve and muscle cells are "excitable"; this implies that they are capable of self-generation of electrochemical impulses at their cell membranes. There is a difference in the ionic composition of extracellular fluid (ECF) and intracellular fluid (ICF). When a cell such as a neuron is stimulated through voltage-regulated channels in sensory receptors or at synapses, ion channels for sodium open, and as a result, there is a net movement of Na + into the cell and the membrane potential decreases, making the cell more positively charged (Fig. 2.6b). The decrease in resting membrane potential is known as depolarization. At the point where the rapid change in the resting membrane potential reverses the polarity of the cell, it is referred to as an action potential or simply a nerve impulse. Immediately following an action potential, the membrane potential returns to the resting membrane potential. The increase in membrane potential is known as repolarization, which results in the negative polarity of the cell as the voltage-gated sodium channels close and potassium channels open. The Na+/K + -ATPase pump moves K+ back into the cell and Na + out of it.

2.1.8 Cell Death (See also Chaps. 1 and 12)

Cell death is extremely important in maintenance of tissue homeostasis, embryonic development, immune self-tolerance, killing by immune effector cells, and regulation of cell viability by hormones and growth factors [11–15]. Deregulation of cell death, however, is a feature of disease including cancer, myocardial infarction, cerebral stroke, and autoimmunity [14]. Based on the new recommendations of the nomenclature committee for cell death, it is classified into regulated and non-regulated. Regulated form is represented predominantly by apoptosis but also includes other forms (Table 2.4).

Table 2.4 Cell death classification

1. Regulated (programmed, noninflammatory)
Apoptosis
Autophagy
Necroptosis
Mitotic catastrophe
Lysosomal-mediated programmed cell death
2. Nonregulated (inflammatory, accidental)
Necrosis

2.1.8.1 Imaging Cell Death

Detection of cell death is an important as it can be valuable in clinical developments particularly in cancer therapy. This can be achieved by molecular imaging including MRI and by several molecular probes for SPECT and PET imaging. These probes include Annex-v which can detect phosphatidylserine which is exposed within few hours of apoptotic stimulus [15].Annex-v is now in clinical trials. Phosphatidylserine targeted peptides have been used for detecting response of melanoma and lymphoma therapy in murine models for example. Other molecular probes detect mitochondrial and plasma membrane depolarization as features of cell death [15].

2.2 Biologic Effects of Ionizing Radiation

2.2.1 Ionizing Radiation

Ionization is the process of ion production by ejection of electrons from atoms and molecules after exposure to high temperature, electrical discharges, or electromagnetic and nuclear radiation. Ionizing radiation is subdivided into electromagnetic radiation (X-rays and gamma rays) and particulate radiation including neutrons and charged particles (alpha and beta particles).

Exposure to ionizing radiation comes from several natural and man-made sources (Table 2.5). The nuclear medicine professional should be able to provide information to the patient and the public about the radiation risks from these sources and to provide a comparison of exposure from medical procedures to natural sources. Biological effects of ionizing radiation depend on several factors that make them variable and inconsistent. The effects are classified based on their nature and timing after exposure into early or delayed, somatic or hereditary, and stochastic or deterministic (Fig. 2.7). Stochastic effects refer to random and unpredictable effects usually following chronic exposure to low-dose radiation. Hereditary effects and carcinogenesis following diagnostic imaging is of a stochastic nature.

The effects can be classified into early or deterministic, which have a threshold, and delayed or stochastic, with no threshold. Effects are also classified into somatic and hereditary. The somatic include early and delayed effects (cancer). Deterministic (non-stochastic) effects are nonrandom and have a highly predictable response to radiation. There is a threshold of radiation dose after which the response is dose related. Some of the known deterministic effects are radiation-induced lung fibrosis and cataract.

Table 2.5 Sources of ionizing radiation

Natural sources	Man-made sources
External radiation	Medical
Cosmic rays	Occupational
Terrestrial radiation (radioactive material in rocks, such as potassium-40)	Nuclear power
	Nuclear explosions
	Nuclear accidents
Internal radiation	
Inhalation (radon gas)	
Ingestion	

2.2.2   Mechanisms of Radiation Effects

Ionizing radiation exerts its effects on biological targets through two major mechanisms [10, 16], direct and indirect (Fig. 2.8).

2.2.2.1 Direct Effect
The direct effect theory or target theory proposes that ionizing radiation acts by direct hits on target atoms. All atoms or molecules within the cells, such as enzymatic and structural proteins and RNA, are vulnerable to radiation injury. DNA, however, is the principal target, in which ionizing radiation produces single- or double-stranded chromosomal breaks.

2.2.2.2 Indirect Effect
The direct mechanism theory was found to be inadequate in explaining cellular radiation injuries. The indirect theory proposes that ionizing radiation exerts its effect via radiolysis of cellular water, forming free radicals. These free radicals interact with atoms and molecules within the cells, particularly DNA, to produce chemical modifications and consequently harmful effects. When X-rays interact with water, two types of free radicals are formed:

$$H^{\circ} \rightarrow H^{\circ}\left(hydrogen\right) + OH^{\circ}\left(hydroxy\right)$$

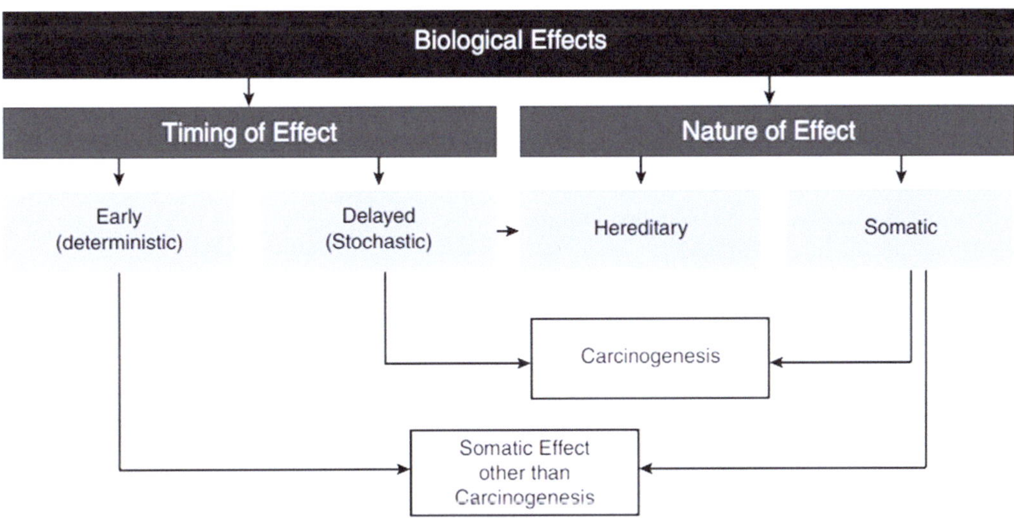

Fig. 2.7 The various biological effects of ionizing radiation

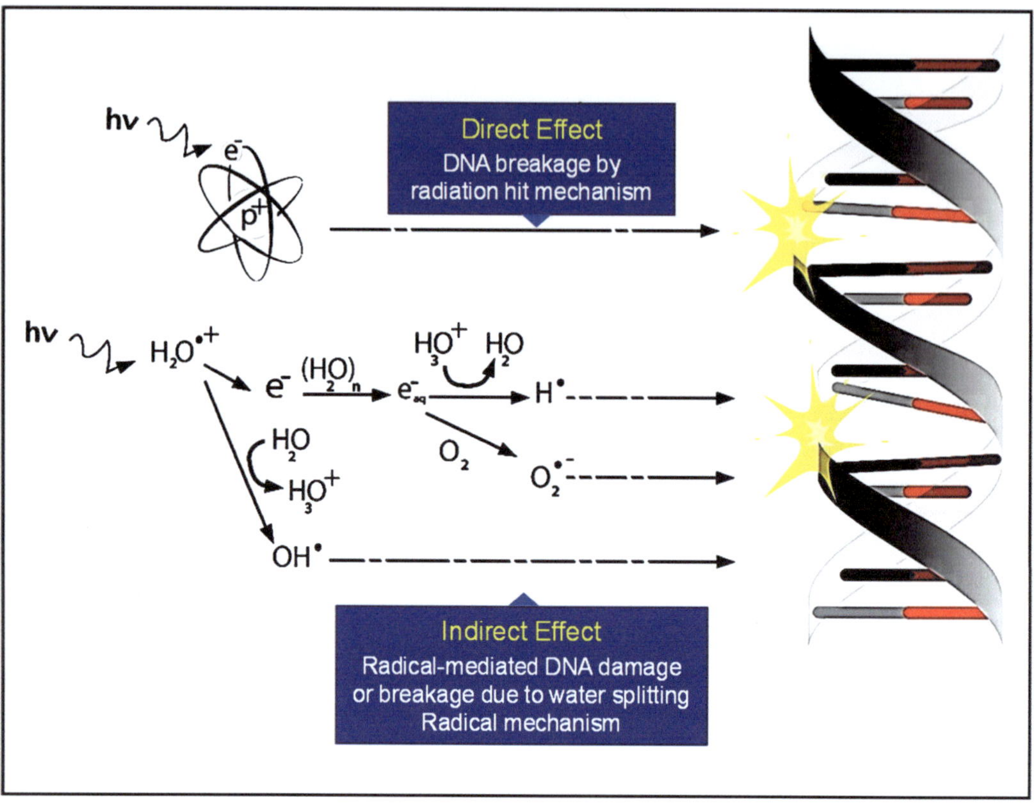

Fig. 2.8 The two mechanisms of ionizing radiation effects on biological tissue, the direct, or target, mechanism and the indirect, through production of free radicals that consequently cause damage

The presence of an excess of oxygen during irradiation of cells allows the formation of additional free radicals:

$$H^{\circ} + O_2 \rightarrow HO_2^{\circ} \, (\text{hydroxyperoxy free radicals})$$

$$HO_2^{\circ} + HO_2^{\circ} \rightarrow H_2O_2^{\circ} + O_2$$

It is worth noting that antioxidants block hydroxyperoxy free radical combination into the highly unstable hydrogen peroxide.

It has been estimated that about two thirds of biological damage caused by low linear energy transfer (LET) radiation is due to indirect action [17]. Biological damage by high LET is primarily by direct ionization action. Figure 2.9 illustrates how radiation leads to tissue damage.

Radiation effects have been observed in extents beyond that explained by effects exerted on directly irradiated cells. Cells in temporal or spatial distance from the initial radiation insult have been shown to have delayed effects of radiation. Two phenomenon are described: the bystander effect and genomic instability.

2.2.2.2.1 Bystander Effect

The cells in the vicinity of irradiated cells show effects that cannot be attributed to targeting by ionizing radiation tracks. Additionally, when cells are irradiated and later transferred to another medium, the cells in proximity in the new medium exhibit DNA damage, mutation, and car-

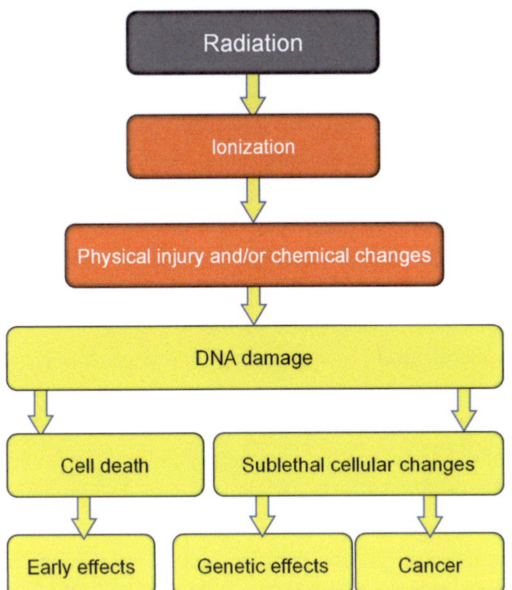

Fig. 2.9 Intracellular changes induced by ionizing radiation that lead to cell damage

cinogenesis. Through cell-to-cell interaction, the directly irradiated cells communicate with adjacent cells and spread the effect of radiation to a larger number of cells. The mechanism is not clearly understood; however, gap junctional intercellular communication [18] or release of soluble factors (such as cytokines) from irradiated cells is proposed. The bystander effect has been mainly described for densely ionizing radiation (such as alpha particles) but also is seen in low LET radiation (such as gamma or X-rays).

2.2.2.2.2   Genomic Instability

Maximal radiation-induced genetic damage is formed shortly (minutes to hours) after radiation exposure. Nevertheless, it has been observed that not only the irradiated cells but also descendents may show delayed effects. Cells that sustain nonlethal DNA damage show increased mutation rate in descendent cells several generations after the initial exposure. Delayed effects include delayed reproductive death up to six generations following the primary insult.

2.2.3   Factors Affecting Radiation Hazards

Radiation injury can be modified by factors related to the ionizing radiation and the target tissue.

2.2.3.1   Factors Related to Ionizing Radiation

Certain factors related to radiation itself determine the various effects for the same radiation dose to biological organs.

2.2.3.1.1   Types of Radiation

Various types of radiation differ in penetrability based on LET, which expresses energy loss per unit distance traveled (kiloelectron volts per micrometer). This value is high for alpha particles, lower for beta particles, and even less for gamma rays and X-rays. Thus, alpha particles penetrate a short distance but induce heavy damage, and beta particles travel a longer distance but much shorter than gamma rays.

2.2.3.1.2   Mode of Administration

The radiation dose is obviously an important factor. In addition, a single dose of radiation causes more damage than the same dose being divided (fractionated). Collectively these two factors are expressed as dose per fraction.

2.2.3.1.3   Dose Rate

Dose rate expresses the time for which dose is administered. The longer the duration for the same total dose, the better the chance of cellular repair and the smaller the damage.

2.2.3.2   Factors Related to Biological Target

Certain properties of tissues and cells can significantly modify the biological effects of ionizing radiation.

2.2.3.2.1   Radiosensitivity

Although all cells can be affected by ionizing radiation, normal cells and their tumors vary in their sensitivity to radiation. Slowly and rapidly growing cells have different radiosensitivity in relation to their movement through the cell cycle. Radiosensitivity varies with the rate of mitosis and cellular maturity. Blood-forming cells are very sensitive to radiation, while neurons, muscle, and parathyroid cells are highly radioresistant. Within a given cell, the nucleus in general is relatively more radiosensitive than the cytoplasm.

2.2.3.2.2 Repair Capacity of Cells

Some cells are known to have a higher capacity than others to repair the damage caused by ionizing radiation; consequently, the biological effects of the same radiation dose are different. Significant repair is known to occur quickly, within 3 h.

2.2.3.2.3 Cell Cycle Phase

All phases of the cell cycle can be affected by ionizing radiation. The radiosensitivity of a given cell varies from one cell cycle phase to another. Overall, sensitivity appears to be greatest in G_2 phase; irradiation during this phase retards the onset of cell division. Irradiation during mitosis induces chromosomal aberrations, i.e., breaks, deletions, translocations, and others. The sensitivity of a given cell cycle phase also differs from one cell type to another and by alteration of radiation injury [17]. For example, the reproductive cells are most sensitive during the M phase, while damage to DNA synthesis and chromosomes occurs mostly when the cell is in the G_2 phase. Recovery from sublethal damage occurs in all phases of the cell cycle. However, this is most pronounced in the S phase, which is also the most radioresistant phase [17].

2.2.3.2.4 Degree of Tissue Oxygenation

Molecular oxygen is known to have the ability to potentiate the response to radiation; this is known as the oxygen effect. The amount of molecular oxygen rather than the rate of oxygen utilization by the cells is the most important factor for increasing the sensitivity of cells to radiation. The probable mechanism is the allowance of additional free radicals, which enhance the damage of cells [19].

2.2.4 Radiation-Induced Cell Injury

In general, an injury which has a high chance of repair is sublethal, that which can be repaired with treatment is potentially lethal, and that which is permanent is lethal. The nucleus is relatively more radiosensitive than the cytoplasmic structures. Nuclear changes after radiation include swelling of the nuclear membrane and disruption of chromatin materials. Cytoplasmic changes include swelling, vacuolization, disintegration of mitochondria and endoplasmic reticulum, and reduction in the number of polysomes [10, 19]. Depending on the dose of radiation and the subcellular changes, along with the previously described factors, the potential effects on the cell vary (Table 2.6). After ionizing radiation exposure, cellular injury occurs in one of the following forms [20]:

1. Division delay: After exposure to radiation in the range of 0.5–3 Gy, delayed mitosis is observed.
2. Reproductive failure: The failed mitotic activity is permanent and eventually cell death ensues. This is observed in a linear fashion

Table 2.6 Types of cellular damage in relation to approximate radiation dose (modified from [3] with permission)

Dose [grays (rads)]	Types of damage	Comments
0.01–0.05 (1–5)	Mutation (chromosomal aberration, gene damage)	Irreversible chromosome breaks, may repair
1 (100)	Mitotic delay, impaired cell function	Reversible
3 (300)	Permanent mitotic inhibition, impaired cell function, activation and deactivation of cellular genes and oncogenes	Certain functions may repair; one or more divisions may occur
>4–10 (>400–1000)	Interphase death	No division
500 (50,000)	Instant death	No division
		Proteins coagulate

after exposure to more than 1.5 Gy. Below this level, the reproductive failure is random in nature and nonlinear.

3. Interphase death: Apoptosis, or programmed cell death, is defined as a particular set of microscopic changes associated with cell death. Radiation-induced apoptosis is highly related to the type of involved cell. Lymphocytes, for example, are highly susceptible to radiation by this mechanism.

2.2.5 Various Effects of Radiation

The biological effect of low-level radiation is extremely difficult to study in a controlled environment. The effects of high radiation exposure to populations during accidents or nuclear war have been the main source of information.

At low doses, radiation can trigger only partially understood effects that can lead to cancer or genetic damage. These effects take years or generations to appear. At high doses, the effect may become evident within minutes, hours, or days. It is important for physicians to be familiar with the early effects of high radiation doses (1 Gy or more to the whole body), since the possibility that people may be exposed to such doses is increasing.

2.2.5.1 Early Radiation Effects

2.2.5.1.1 Acute Whole-Body Exposure Syndromes

Following exposure to a large, single, short-term whole-body dose of ionizing radiation, the resulting injury is expressed as a series of clinical symptoms. The sequence of events can be generally divided into four clinical periods:

1. The prodromal period, up to 48 h, when the symptoms include anorexia, nausea, vomiting, and diarrhea.
2. The latent period, from 48 h to 2–3 weeks after exposure, when the patient becomes asymptomatic.
3. The manifest phase, from week 6 to week 8 after exposure, when variable symptoms appear based on the radiation dose.
4. The recovery period: If the patient survives, recovery occurs from 6 weeks to several months after exposure.

The presentation of these periods and their duration depend on the amount of radiation exposure [10, 17]. In general, about half of those who receive doses of 2 Gy suffer vomiting within 3 h, and symptoms are rare after doses below 1 Gy. With a sufficiently high radiation dose, acute radiation sickness may result. Additional symptoms related to specific organ injury may occur, based on the dose, and can be divided according to the known acute radiation syndromes:

Radiation Sickness
The symptoms can be mild, such as loss of appetite and mild fatigue, or evident only on laboratory tests with mild lymphopenia (subclinical), or may be severe, appearing as early as 5 min after exposure to very high doses of 10 Gy or more and also include fatigue, sweating, fever, apathy, and low blood pressure. Lower doses delay the onset of symptoms and produce less severe symptoms or a subclinical syndrome that can occur with doses of less than 2 Gy to the whole body, and recovery is complete with 100% survival.

Hematopoietic (Bone Marrow) Syndrome
This occurs at higher doses of more than 1.5–2 Gy to the whole body. With doses up to 4 Gy, a radiation prodrome is seen, followed by a latent period of up to 3 weeks. The clinical effects are not seen for several weeks after the radiation dose, when anemia, petechiae, increased blood pressure, fatigue, ulceration in the mouth, epilation, purpura, and/or infection appear. At doses on the order of 4–8 Gy, a modified bone marrow syndrome occurs. The initial problem is more severe, the latest period is shortened, and the manifest illness is more severe. Death is possible due to bleeding with exposure in this dose range.

Gastrointestinal Syndrome

This syndrome occurs with still higher doses of 6–10 Gy which cause manifestations related to the gastrointestinal tract in addition to those of the bone marrow syndrome. Initially, loss of appetite, apathy, nausea, and vomiting occur for 2–8 h. These effects may subside rapidly. Several days later, malaise, anorexia, nausea, vomiting, high fever, persistent diarrhea, abdominal distention, and infections appear. During the second week of irradiation, severe dehydration, hemoconcentration, and circulatory collapse may be seen, eventually leading to death.

Central Nervous System Syndrome

The central nervous system is generally resistant to radiation effects. A dose higher than 10 Gy is required to cause substantial effects on the brain and the nervous system. Symptoms include intractable nausea and vomiting, confusion, convulsions, coma, and absent lymphocytes. The prognosis is poor, with death in a few days.

2.2.5.1.2 Acute Regional Effects

When enough radiation is delivered locally to a certain part of the body, as in the case of radiation therapy, which focuses on a certain field, acute effects can appear in the exposed area. Examples include skin erythema and gastrointestinal edema and ulceration.

2.2.5.2 Delayed Radiation Effects

There is considerable debate over the effects of low-level radiation. At one end, there are several theories and reports describing the harmful effects of low-level radiation and how underestimated the risks are. At the other extreme, there are theories and reports of harmless and even potentially useful effects of exposure to such levels of radiation.

The theories describing the effects of low-level radiation and the projected risk estimates of cancer development or genetic effects in human are purely mathematical and not actual observations. The data from populations exposed to high-level radiation were extrapolated to determine the likelihood of these events at low-level radiation exposure. Such events in any given population occur at extremely low rates and to further complicate the issue after long latency periods; therefore, solid epidemiological data are difficult to obtain.

2.2.5.2.1 Cancer

Cancer is the most important concern of radiation. It has been recognized for more than 90 years that ionizing radiation causes cancers. Tissues with a high rate of cell proliferation are more prone to radiation tumor induction. Cancer becomes evident only long after the first damage is done, following a period of latency. Leukemia first appears at least 2–5 years after exposure, while solid tumors appear after at least 10 years, often several decades. The tumors reported to be associated with radiation include leukemia, multiple myeloma, and cancers of the breast, colon, thyroid, ovary, lung, urinary bladder, stomach, CNS (other than brain), and esophagus.

There is no clear evidence that low-level radiation causes cancer. Holm et al. [21] studied 6000 patients given a diagnostic dose of ^{131}I. There was no increase in the incidence of thyroid cancer in this population, including a subset of 2000 children. Saenger et al. [22] also studied 2000 patients treated with ^{131}I in doses of up to several hundreds of MBq with 20 years follow-up. The incidences of thyroid cancer and leukemia were identical to those among patients treated surgically for the same conditions.

To complicate the issue further, recently acquired data minimize the effects of low-level radiation in the induction of cancer and even suggest that such levels of radiation exposure may be useful [23, 24]. DNA mutations unrelated to radiation are produced continuously. It is estimated that each day, the intrinsic human metabolism produces 240, 000 DNA mutations in each cell of the body [25]. During youth, these are repaired and, in general, cancer occurs infrequently. With old age, the capability to repair may decrease and cancer appears more frequently. A high dose of 2 Gy adds 4000 (20 mutations/cGy) to the daily 240,000 mutations. Ward [19, 26] determined that a low radiation dose of 0.2 Gy stimulates repair by 50%–100% and adds only 400 mutations to the intrinsic 240,000 mutations. It is the reduced ability of our repair mechanism to correct the very high background of intrinsic mutations that increases the risk of developing cancer. Genetic impairment of DNA repair capacity results in death from cancer at an early age. Loss of DNA repair capacity with age increases the risk of cancer. Exposure to high doses of radiation similarly reduces the repair capacity of cellular DNA and increases the risk of cancer [27, 28].

2.2.5.2.2 Genetic Effects

Genetic effects may include changes in the number and structure of chromosomes and gene mutations, dominant or recessive. They depend on the following factors:

1. The stage of germ cell development: Immature germ cells appear to be capable of repair, while in mature germ cells there is little or no repair (Table 2.7).
2. Dose rate: The repair process starts simultaneously with radiation damage. The damage with a high-dose rate is greater; lower dose rates produce fewer mutations. At a low-intermediate dose rate, the time period is an important factor as far as the final outcome of the radiation injuries is concerned. However, this does not hold true in the case of a high radiation rate, where the repair process is minimal due to the direct action of injury.
3. Dose fractionation: The time interval between fractions is very important for the frequency

of mutations. The number of translocations will be reduced by dose fractionation; however, the incidence of mutations will not be affected by increasing the time interval between fractions.
4. Interval between exposure and conception: The frequency of mutation is very low if conception occurs after 7 weeks, but it is high when the interval between radiation exposure and conception is 7 weeks or less.

2.2.5.2.3 Effects on the Unborn Child

The embryonic stage is one of the most radio-sensitive stages in the life of any organism. The classical triad of effects of radiation on the embryo is growth retardation; embryonic, fetal, or neonatal death; and congenital malformation. The probability of finding one or more of these effects is dependent upon radiation dose, the dose rate, and the stage of gestation at exposure. Stage of development is particularly important, since the organ which is differentiated at that time will be most vulnerable; this determines the type of abnormality or malformation that will be observed. During the first two weeks of conception, the effect of radiation is an all-or-none effect, where the embryo is aborted. Following this period and up to 8 weeks, the embryo is very vulnerable to congenital malformations. Organogenesis starting then after might lead to mental retardation, congenital malformation as well as organ-specific effects. For example, radioactive iodine administered to a pregnant mother who passed 10–13 weeks of gestation will cross the placenta and accumulate in the already formed fetal thyroid. A summary of the possible effects from irradiation at various stages of gestation is shown in Table 2.7. Development of cancer at an early age is controversial. Studies have suggested an increased risk of hematopoietic and solid tumors at an early age [29, 30]. However, a comparison between individuals whose parents were exposed to radiation during the atomic bombing of Hiroshima and Nagasaki and those whose parents were not showed no significant differences in a large number of variables including congenital effects, still births, and cancer at an early age.

Table 2.7 Effects of radiation on the unborn child

Stage of gestation (days)	Possible effects
1–9	Death of embryo is most likely, with little chance of malformation
10–12	Reduced lethal effect with still little chance of malformation
13–56	Production of congenital malformation and retarded growth
57–112	Extreme mental retardation (time of most severe effect on CNS)
113–175	Less frequent effect on CNS
After 175	Very low frequency of CNS effects (no reported case of severe retardation)

2.2.5.2.4 Other Delayed Somatic Effects

Cataract
Chronic and acute exposure of the eyes can lead to cataracts secondary to inducing lens fiber disorganization. Not all radiation is equally effective in producing cataracts; neutrons are much more efficient than other types of radiation. In man, the cataractogenic threshold is estimated at 2–5 Gy as a single dose or 10 Gy as a fractionated dose. The period between exposure and the appearance of the lens opacities averages 2–3 years, ranging from 10 months to more than 30 years [31, 32].

Hypothyroidism
The thyroid gland is exposed to irradiation during radiation therapy of malignant head and neck tumors or the treatment of hyperthyroidism with ^{131}I. Patients who received doses 10–40 Gy to the thyroid for the treatment of other malignant diseases developed hypothyroidism a few months to many years after exposure. A lower moderate dose of (10–20 Gy) can result in hypothyroidism, while 500 Gy or more is required to destroy the thyroid completely.

Aplastic Anemia
Human exposure to radiation can cause aplastic anemia, depending upon the dose and fractionation. Death may be the end result of aplastic anemia. It has been suggested that permanent anemia is caused by a reduced capability of cellular proliferation due to accumulation of residual injury in stem cells. It is important to realize that when part of the body is irradiated, bone marrow that survives unimpaired will replace what is damaged. If only 10% of active bone marrow escapes irradiation, mortality can be decreased from 50% to zero, based on animal studies.

2.2.6 Psychological and Psychiatric Effects of Ionizing Radiation Exposure

In addition to noticeable CNS effects discussed earlier, exposure to radiation has other vital side effects that cannot be ignored; the psychological effects. Exposure to ionizing radiation whether due to environmental contamination such as radiation accidents, radiotherapy and diagnostics, occupational roles and space travel is a possible risk-factor for cognitive dysfunction [33]. Which can be early or late effect. This effect is not only due to high-level exposure but also low levels [34]. Molecular studies described the various inflammatory and signaling mechanisms involved in cellular damage and repair which consequently drive physiological alterations that may lead to functional alterations [35].

Studies researched these topics decades ago till the present. Perceptions and memories were explored in atomic veterans and patients treated for brain tumors. Findings suggest that side effects involve emotional and cognitive processing of a new perspective that contradicts prior beliefs, trouble with memories, and memory loss [36]. Cognitive deficits are related to certain factors that must be considered, including the human life span, as effects might differ with age at exposure and outcome assessment. Family members' health conditions, which may exacerbate distress, is another factor to be considered.

A case study of men who were exposed to non-background ionizing radiation while participating in atmospheric nuclear tests showed that the subjects have developed a virtually identical complex of debilitating psychiatric symptoms resulted from almost entirely focused upon the health effects of the radiation to which the subjects were exposed to. This symptom complex appears to comprise a syndrome [37].

Another recent study recently published, researched the potential psychological issues faced by British nuclear weapons testing program veterans. The study assessed the prevalence of clinically relevant anxiety and aimed to explore experiences of worry and the broader potential psychological impact and effects. The results of this qualitative study showed the following: More than third (33.7%) of the participants met the criteria for clinically relevant anxiety, the interviewers generated from (21.3%) of the participants three interconnected themes giving a rich description of the verbal data in relation to the psychological impact, namely "worry, responsibility, and guilt" and "change across the life course." Frustration and anger toward authorities resulting from perceived negligence and deception were also there. In addition, the participants showed some instances of worry regarding their family members' health [35]. Data suggest that guilt toward family members' health must be considered in potentially exposed individuals and transparency from authorities of medical personnel when dealing with any radiological exposure are of importance to reduce potential distress and anxiety [35].

2.2.7 Exposure from Medical Procedures

For medical radiation, the chest X-ray delivers 0.1–0.2 mSv to the chest wall and the gall bladder series approximately 0.25 rem. The average nuclear medicine procedure delivers 3 mSv to the whole body. The absorbed dose from the C-14 urea breath test is equivalent to that received during a 1 h flight. When these values are compared with those of natural sources of radiation, particularly cosmic rays, which deliver an average of 3.6 mSv per year in the United States and are higher in certain areas, the real magnitude of the low level of radiation can be appreciated. These levels of exposure from diagnostic medical procedures have no detectable biological effects. It is estimated that less than 0.006% of those undergoing nuclear medicine procedures in the United States might be affected annually. PET studies deliver higher doses to the patient to compensate for the short half-life of positron-emitting radioisotopes. Because these radioisotopes are of high energy and prepared in high initial dosing to account for the rapid decay, PET technologist, radiopharmacists, and workers at cyclotrons are usually exposed to higher doses than other workers in the nuclear medicine field. Table 2.8 summarizes the updated radiation doses from the common medical imaging procedures with the doses from natural sources.

Therapeutic applications of radioisotopes involve not only malignant but also benign conditions, such as hyperthyroidism and arthroplasty, and are widely expanding. In the treatment of thyroid cancer, large doses of ^{131}I may cause depression of the bone marrow. For example, 3.7 GBq of ^{131}I delivers 0.5 to 1 Gy to hematopoietic system simulating an effect of external whole-body radiation. It is essential to mention that the level of exposure from medical exposure has globally increased according to recent surveys [39]. The global exposure per capita has increased from 0.4 mSv in 2000 to 0.62 mSv in 2008 (Table 2.9).

Medical exposure has grown rapidly over recent years; hence, the medical exposure is near comparable to that of exposure from natural background sources in the United States. This has been attributed mainly to the use of CT scanning [40].

Although globally the exposure of medical exposure is still around 20% of the total exposure per caput since the exposure from natural sources contributes to slightly less than 80%, the exposure from medical exposure in certain groups of countries with high physician-to-population ratios has dramatically increased to be almost equal to the dose from natural exposure as illustrated in the United States. This increase has been attributed mainly to the increase in the utilization of CT scans.

Positive health effects have also been noted [6–47], i.e., decreased mortality and decreased cancer rates, in human populations exposed to low-level radiation and reported in large studies [41]. Several studies were carried out to compare areas of high background to those with low radiation. Lower cancer incidence and/or mortality rates in the former were the finding in many such studies in China [43], India [44], Iran [45], and the United States [46]. It has to be noted, however, that this form of epidemiological studies does not compare individual's radiation exposure to cancer rate; therefore, strong conclusion cannot be solely based on such studies. On the other hand, none of these studies has found a higher

Table 2.8 Radiation dose from common natural and medical sources

Diagnostic X-ray procedures	Effective Dose Per Scan Dose Based on ICRP 103* (mSv)
X-ray CT of the head and neck	1.2
X-ray CT of the chest	6.2
Panoramic dental radiography	0.026
Intravenous urography (IVU)	3
Barium enema (lower GI X-ray)	6
Chest X-ray	0.1
Mammography	0.36
Diagnostic nuclear medicine Procedures	**Effective Dose Per Scan Based Dose Based on ICRP 103 (mSv)**
Tc-99 m-MAA lung perfusion study.	0.017 (mSv/MBq)
Tc-99 m-DTPA lung ventilation study (ventilation can be evaluated with the 99mTc-labeled aerosols, DTPA and Technegas).	0.015 (mSv/MBq)
Tc-99 m-MDP bone scan (20 mCi)	4
Effective doses from CT component of PET/CT (diagnostic).	2.60–21.45
Effective doses from FDG-PET/CT (total)	8–26.85
Effective doses from FDG-PET (5–15 mCi)	3.515–10.545
CT component of PET/CT (attenuation only)	0.5–1.0
One-day Tl-201 stress (3.5 mCi)/ redistribution protocol	15.3
Tl-201 stress (3.0 mCi) / redistribution with optional additional imaging protocols (re-injection of Tl-201 (1.5 mCi) after redistribution imaging).	19.7
Exposure from "natural radiation"	**Effective Dose Per Scan Based Dose Based on ICRP 103 (mSv)**
Two-hour flight at altitude of approximately 6100 m	0.004
World Health Organization recommended reference level per year for intake of radionuclides in water (IAEA, 2001).	0.1
Ingestion (food and drinking-water)	0.3
Terrestrial sources	0.5
Inhalation of natural gas at home (mainly radon)	1.2
Cosmic radiation (at sea level)	0.4
Total background radiation level	2.4

[38]

Table 2.9 Changes in exposure from medical sources

Year	Annual per caput dose (mSv)
1988	0.35
1993	0.30
2000	0.40
2008	0.62

UNSCEAR 2008 Report [39]

cancer incidence in high background radiation zones. An epidemiological study [47] comparing cancer mortality in Canada's nuclear industry workers to that in non-radiation workers has found similar favorable effects for low-radiation exposure. The former group of workers had cancer mortality of 58% of the national average as compared to 97% of that in the latter. Cohen [20] studied the relationship between lung cancer death rates and residential radon gas in the United States. He found that lung cancer decreased for increments in radon levels. These findings were consistent even after reanalysis and correcting for confounding factors such as smoking. To date, there is considerable debate regarding this study.

References

1. Saladin K (2010) Anatomy and physiology. The unity of form and function, 5th edn. McGraw hill, Boston
2. Devin TM (2010) Textbook of biochemistry with clinical correlates, 7th edn. Wiley-Liss, New York
3. Guyton AC, Hall JE (2020) Textbook of human physiology, 14th edn. Elsevier Saunders Elsevier, Philadelphia
4. Junqueira LC, Carneiro J, Kelley R (1995) Basic histology, 8th edn. Prentice-Hall
5. Huether SE, McCance KL (2021) Pathophysiology. The biologic basis for disease in adults and children, 8th edn. Mosby Elsevier, St. Louis
6. Li L, Xie T (2005) Stem cell niche: structure and function. Annu Rev Cell Dev Biol 21:605–631
7. Pollard TD, Earnshaw WC (2002) Cell biology, 1st edn. Saunders, Philadelphia
8. Raven PH, Johnson GB (2013) Biology, 10th edn. Mosby Year Book, St. Louis
9. Sumner AT (2003) Chromosomes organization and function, 1st edn. Blackwell, Oxford
10. Kumar V, Abbas A, Aster J (2020) Robbins and Cotran pathologic basis of disease, 10th edn. W.B. Saunders, Philadelphia
11. Yin XM, Dong Z (2003) Essentials of apoptosis: a guide for basic and clinical research, 1st edn. Humana Press, Totowa
12. Widmaier E, Raff H, Strang K (2010) Vander's human physiology: the mechanisms of body function with ARIS, 12th edn. Mc-Graw Hill, Boston
13. Alberts B, Johnson A, Lewis J et al (2002) Molecular biology of the cell, 4th edn. Garland Science, New York
14. Galluzzi I, Vitale I, Abrams JM et al (2012) Molecular definition of cell death subroutines: recommendations of the Nomenclature Committee on cell death. Cell Death Differ 19:107–120
15. Neves AA, Brindle KM (2014) Imaging cell death. J Nucl Med 55:1–4
16. United Nations Environment Program (1988) Radiation: doses, effects, risks. Blackwell, Oxford, pp 65–84
17. Prasad KN (1995) Handbook of radiobiology, 2nd edn. CRC Press, Boca Raton
18. Bolus NE (2001) Basic review of radiation biology and terminology. J Nucl Med Technol 29:67–73
19. Ward JF (1988) DNA damage produced by ionizing radiation in mammalian cells: identities, mechanisms of formation, and reparability. Prog Nucleic Acid Res Mol Biol 35:95
20. Cohen BL (1995) Test of the linear-no threshold theory of radiation carcinogenesis in the low dose rate region. Health Phys 68:157
21. Holm I, Hall P, Wiklund K et al (1991) Cancer risk after iodine-131 therapy for hyperthyroidism. J Natl Cancer Inst 83:1072
22. Saenger EL, Thomas GE, Tompkins EA (1968) Incidence of leukemia following treatment of hyperthyroidism. Preliminary report of the cooperative thyrotoxicosis therapy follow-up study. JAMA 205:855
23. Matanoski GM, Tonascia JA, Correa-Villasenor A et al (2008) Cancer risks and low-level radiation in U.S. shipyard workers. J Radiat Res 49:83–91
24. Cameron J (1992) The good news about low-level radiation exposure: health effects of low-level radiation in shipyard workers. Health Phys Soc Newslett 20:9
25. Billen D (1990) Spontaneous DNA damage and its significance for the "negligible dose" controversy in radiation protection. Radiat Res 124:242
26. Ward JF (1987) Radiation chemical methods of cell death. In: Fielden EM, Fowler JF, Hendry JH, Scott D (eds) Proceedings of the 8th international congress of radiation research, vol II. Taylor and Francis, London, pp 162–168
27. Quingyi W (1993) DNA repair and aging in basal cell carcinoma: a molecular epidemiology study. Proc Natl Acad Sci U S A 90:1614
28. Koshland DE, Sancar A, Hanawalt PC, Modrich P (1994) DNA repair enzymes and mechanisms. Science 266:1925–1927
29. Kneala GW, Stewart AM (1976) Mantel-Haenszel analysis of Oxford data. II. Independent effects of fetal irradiation subfactors. J Natl Cancer Inst 57:1009
30. Committee on the Biological Effects of Ionizing Radiations (1980) The effects on population of exposure to low levels of ionizing radiation. National Academic Press, Washington DC
31. International Commission on Radiological Protection (1969) Radiosensitivity and spatial distribution of dose, publication no 14. Pergamon, Oxford
32. Dodo T (1975) Cataract. J Radiat Res 16(Suppl):132
33. Narasimhamurthy RK, Mumbrekar KD, Rao BSS (2022) Effects of low dose ionizing radiation on the brain- a functional, cellular, and molecular perspective. Toxicology 465:153030. (n progress)
34. Pasqual E, Boussin F, Bazyka D, Nordenskjold A, Yamada M et al (2021) Cognitive effects of low dose of ionizing radiation—lessons learned and research gaps from epidemiological and biological studies. Environ Int 147:106295
35. Collett G, Young WR, Martin W, Anderson RM (2021) Exposure worry: the psychological impact of perceived ionizing radiation exposure in British nuclear test veterans. Int J Environ Res Public Health 18:12188
36. Garcia B (1994) Social-psychological dilemmas and coping of atomic veterans. Am J Orthopsychiatry 64:651–655
37. Vyner HM (1983) The psychological effects of ionizing radiation. Cult Med Psychiatry 7:241–261
38. Valentin A (ed) (2007) The 2007 recommendation of the international commission on radiation protection. Ann ICRP 37:1–339
39. UNSCEAR 2008 Report. *Sources and effects of ionizing radiation,* United Nations Scientific Committee on the effects of atomic radiation, New York, 2010

40. United Nations Scientific Committee on the effects of atomic radiation (UNSCEAR 2008) (2010) Sources and effects of atomic radiation, vol 1. United Nations publication, Vienna
41. UNSCEAR (United Nations Scientific Committee on the Effects of Atomic Radiation) (1994) Annex B: adaptive responses to radiation in cells and organisms. Document A/Ac. 82/R.542, approved 11 March 1994
42. Johansson L (2003) Hormesis, an update of the present position. Eur J Nucl Med Mol Imaging 30:921–933
43. Feinendegen LE (2005) Low doses of ionizing radiation: relationship between biological benefit and damage induction. A synopsis. World J Nucl Med 4:21–34
44. High Background radiation research group (1980) Health survey in high background radiation areas in China. Science 209:877–880
45. Nambi KS, Soman SD (1987) Environmental radiation and cancer in India. Health Phys 52:653–657
46. Ghiassi-nejad M, Mortazavi SMJ, Cameron JR, Niroomand-Rad A, Karam PA (2002) Very high background radiation areas of Ramsar, Iran: preliminary biological studies. Health Phys 82:87–93
47. Jagger J (1998) Natural background radiation and cancer death in Rocky Mountain states and Gulf Coast states. Health Phys 75:428–430

Basis of Radiopharmaceutical Localization

3

3.1 Radiopharmaceuticals

A disease is defined in terms of the failure of a normal physiological or biochemical process. Nuclear medicine utilizes these processes. Its diagnostic procedures measure (a) regional blood flow, transport, and cellular localization of various molecules; (b) metabolism and bioenergetics of tissues; (c) physiological function of organs; and (d) intracellular and intercellular communication. A number of radiopharmaceuticals are used for imaging the function and structure of many organs and tissues. Others are available for the treatment of different malignancies, joint diseases, palliation of pain due to bony metastases, and other conditions.

3.2 Mechanism(s) of Radiopharmaceutical Localization

The uptake and retention of radiopharmaceuticals by different tissues and organs involve many different mechanisms, summarized in Table 3.1. Many radiopharmaceuticals were designed to take advantage of the pathophysiology in order to increase the specificity of nuclear medicine imaging techniques. Some radiopharmaceuticals are not specific for a particular disease. Hence, the cellular uptake might include a combination of different mechanisms, as in the case of 67Ga citrate. The unique chemistry of each radiopharmaceutical may determine the manner in which it is transported and retained within a specific tissue or organ. The different mechanisms of localization are discussed below, using specific examples of the more common radiopharmaceuticals.

3.2.1 Isotope Dilution

The dilution principle is based on the concept of "diluting" a radiotracer (or tracer) of known activity (or mass) in an unknown volume. By measuring the degree to which the radiotracer was diluted by the unknown volume, one can determine the total volume (or mass) of the unknown volume. The dilution principle is currently used for a quantitative determination of RBC volume (mass), plasma volume, and total blood volume. It is very important that the radiotracer remains only in the blood volume to be measured. Nondiffusible intravascular agents such as 51Cr-RBCs are used to measure RBC mass, while 125I-HSA is used to measure plasma volume. The use of 99mTc-RBCs for the measurement of cardiac ejection fraction and gastrointestinal bleeding studies is another application of the dilution principle.

© The Author(s), under exclusive license to Springer Nature Switzerland AG 2023
A. H. Elgazzar, *Synopsis of Pathophysiology in Nuclear Medicine*,
https://doi.org/10.1007/978-3-031-20646-7_3

Table 3.1 Mechanisms of radiopharmaceutical localization

Localization mechanism	Radiopharmaceuticals
Compartmentalized localization	^{125}I-HAS, ^{125}Cr-RBC, ^{99m}Tc-RBC, Xe-133, ^{111}In-DTPA, ^{99m}Tc-DTPA, ^{99m}Tc-sulfur-colloid
Passive diffusion	^{99m}Tc-DTPA (brain), ^{99m}Tc-HMPAO, ^{99m}Tc-ECD, ^{99m}Tc-sestamibi, ^{99m}Tc-tetrofosmin, [^{13}N]NH$_3$, ^{67}Ga-citrate, [^{18}F]FDOPA, [^{18}F]FMISO
Facilitated diffusion	[^{18}F]FDG, ^{99m}Tc-disofenin and mebrofenin, ^{99m}Tc (V) DMSA (MTC)
Active transport	^{123}I$^-$ and ^{131}I$^-$, ^{99m}TcO$_4^-$ (thyroid), ^{201}Tl$^+$, ^{82}Rb$^+$, ^{123}I-MIBG, ^{99m}Tc (III) DMSA (renal), [^{18}F]FACBC, [^{18}F]FLT, [^{18}F]FET, [^{18}F]choline and [^{11}C]choline
Filtration	^{99m}Tc-DTPA (renal), ^{99m}Tc-MAG$_3$, ^{125}I-iothalamate, and ^{51}Cr-EDTA
Secretion	^{99m}TcO$_4^-$ (stomach), ^{99m}Tc-MAG$_3$
Phagocytosis	^{99m}Tc-sulfur colloid
Cell sequestration	Denatured ^{99m}Tc-RBC
Capillary blockade	^{99m}Tc-MAA
Ion exchange	^{89}Sr^{2+}, ^{18}F$^-$
Chemisorption	^{99m}Tc-MDP, ^{99m}Tc-HDP, ^{153}Sm-EDTMP
Cellular migration	^{111}In-oxine-WBC, ^{99m}Tc-HMPAO-WBC
Receptor binding	^{68}Ga-DOTA-PSMA, ^{18}F-PSMA, ^{131}I-tositumomab and ^{111}In/^{90}Y-ibritumomab tiuxetan, ^{111}In-octreoscan, ^{68}Ga-DOTA-octreotide, ^{64}Cu-DOTA-tyr^3-octreotate, [^{18}F]florbetapir, [^{18}F]florbetapir, [^{18}F]flutemetamol, [^{18}F]FES, [^{123}I]ioflupane (DaTscan)

3.2.2 Capillary Blockade

The technique most commonly used to determine the perfusion to an organ depends on trapping the radiolabeled particles (microembolization) in the capillary bed of an organ such as lung, heart, or brain. Following intravenous injection, 99mTc-MAA particles are physically trapped in the arteriocapillary beds of the lung and block the blood flow to the distal regions. Therefore, the mechanism of localization of particles in the lungs is purely a mechanical process, called capillary blockade.

3.2.3 Physicochemical Adsorption

The 99mTc-phosphonates accumulate in hydroxyapatite crystal (containing Ca2+ and phosphate ions) matrix or in the amorphous (noncrystalline) calcium phosphate. The uptake mechanism of sodium fluoride [18F] resembles that of 99mTc-labeled diphosphonates in which the OH$^-$ ions in hydroxyapatite are exchanged for F-18$^-$ ions. However, it has faster blood clearance and a twofold higher uptake in bone. The principal uptake mechanism of the radiotracer appears to be simply "physicochemical adsorp-

tion." However, the exact mechanisms involved in the extraction of the radiotracer from the blood through the endothelial cells, extracellular fluid, and finally hydroxyapatite crystal are not known. Primary bone tumors such as osteogenic sarcomas avidly accumulate bone agents because of the production of bone matrix in extraosseous tissue. Metastatic deposits that produce a vigorous osteoblastic response will appear as hot spots in a bone scan, while the lesions that generate osteolytic reactions may not accumulate the bone agent [1].

The localization of bone-seeking radiotracers in increased amounts at the tumor-bone interface provides the basis for the use of radionuclides in the treatment of bone pain. Several radiopharmaceuticals (see Chap. 13) are used for the relief of bone pain in patients with confirmed osteoblastic bone lesions.

3.2.4 Cellular Migration and Sequestration

111In-oxine- or 99mTc-HMPAO-labeled autologous mixed leukocytes (predominantly neutrophilic polymorphonuclear leukocytes, PMNs) are routinely used to image various inflammatory diseases and infectious processes. The inflammatory reaction is a well-described sequence of events in response to an infection (see Chap. 4). Following intravenous administration of radiolabeled leukocytes, the labeled cells migrate to the site of infection, similar to the circulating leukocytes, because they are attracted by the immediately generated chemotactic factors, such as complement subcomponents. In a similar manner, 111In-platelet localization at the site of active thrombus formation also involves simple cellular migration, since platelets play a major role in thrombus formation. Accessory splenic tissue can develop after splenectomy. Heat-damaged 99mTc-RBCs are more specific for the detection of accessory splenic tissue.

Following intravenous administration, the spleen sequesters heat-damaged RBCs in the same way that old and damaged circulating RBCs are normally removed.

3.2.5   Membrane Transport

Transport through the lipid bilayer or through the transport proteins may involve simple diffusion, passive transport (facilitated diffusion), or active transport mechanisms. Certain macromolecules may also be transported by vesicle formation, involving either endocytosis or exocytosis mechanisms.

3.2.5.1   Simple Diffusion

Many radiopharmaceuticals localize in target organs, which involve a simple diffusion process. The direction of movement of the radiotracers by diffusion is always from a higher to a lower concentration, and the initial rate of diffusion is directly proportional to the concentration of the radiotracer. A net movement of molecules from one side to another will continue until the concentration on each side is at chemical equilibrium. Following the administration of gases used for ventilation studies, such as 133Xe, 127Xe, and 81mKr, through inhalation, gases are distributed within the lung air spaces by diffusion, proportional to ventilation. The gases pass from the

lungs into the pulmonary venous circulation and are released through the lungs by the mechanism of alveolar capillary diffusion. Similarly, distribution of 99mTc-Technegas within the lung also involves diffusion. On the other hand, the irregular distribution of 99mTc-DTPA aerosol preparation within the lung is due mostly to gravity sedimentation depending on particle size.

3.2.5.1.1   Simple Diffusion and Intracellular Metabolism/ Binding

The blood-brain barrier (BBB) plays an important role in the mechanism of localization of many radiopharmaceuticals in the brain. The endothelial cells of the cerebral vessels form a continuous layer without gap junctions, preventing diffusion of water-soluble molecules. In certain pathological conditions, the BBB is disrupted, allowing water-soluble molecules to diffuse from the blood into brain tissue.

Brain perfusion imaging agents such as 99mTc-HMPAO and 99mTc-ECD are lipophilic radiotracers that cross the BBB via passive diffusion. The extraction of these tracers by the brain tissue is proportional to regional cerebral blood flow (rCBF). The retention of these tracers within the neuronal tissue following diffusion and extraction is assumed to be due to intracellular binding or metabolic degradation to polar metabolites or charged complexes that cannot be washed out of the cell by back diffusion as exemplified by the cellular retention of 99mTc-ECD and 99mTc-pertechnetate in labeled RBC. With 99mTC-ECD, the radiotracer freely diffuses into the brain tissue, where it is hydrolyzed by the action of esterase to an acid which is trapped in the brain tissue. For 99mTcO4, the tracer is reduced intracellularly by the circulating stannous ion, and the reduced 99mTc binds to Hgb to form 99mTcHgb that does not diffuse out of the brain tissue.

3.2.5.1.2   Simple Diffusion and Mitochondrial Binding

A number of 99mTc radiopharmaceuticals such as sestamibi and tetrofosmin have been developed for imaging myocardial perfusion. Although 99mTc-sestamibi is cationic, similar to 201Tl+, the transport of this agent through the cell membrane involves only passive diffusion [2]. The myocardial cell uptake of 99mTc-sestamibi is due to intracellular binding of 99mTc-sestamibi associated mainly with the mitochondria.

Mitochondrial retention of 99mTc-sestamibi, however, is not organ or tumor specific, but appears to be a mechanism common to most types of tissue.

The intracellular levels of Ca2+ in normal cells are significantly low. However, with irreversible ischemia, extracellular calcium enters the cell and is sequestered in the mitochondria, resulting in mitochondrial destruction. The increased calcium concentration in the mitochondria blocks 99mTc-sestamibi binding to the mitochondria. These 99mTc lipophilic cationic complexes are also used for imaging of parathyroid localization, and tumor imaging and mechanism of uptake again are associated with the mitochondria. There are significant differences between sestamibi and tetrofosmin regarding intracellular localization based on in vitro studies. While 90% of total sestamibi was associated with mitochondria, most of the tetrofosmin accumulated in the cytosolic fraction [3].

The transport of the tracer out of the tumor cell is mediated by P-glycoprotein (Pgp), a 17 kd plasma membrane lipoprotein encoded by the human multidrug resistance (MDR) gene, and accordingly 99mTc sestamibi is useful for imaging Pgp expression.

3.2.5.1.3　Simple Diffusion and Increased Permeability

This mechanism is illustrated with 67Ga-citrate localization in a variety of tumors and inflammatory lesions. Following intravenous administration of carrier-free 67Ga as gallium citrate, 67Ga is bound to the iron transport glycoprotein, transferring in normal plasma, and is transported to normal tissues and tumor sites predominantly as 67Ga-transferrin complex [4]. The initial entry of 67Ga into tumor tissue involves simple diffusion of the unbound or loosely bound form of 67Ga, whereas its uptake

by normal soft tissues is strongly promoted by its binding to transferrin [5]. There is increased transferrin concentration within the interstitial fluid of the tumors. The increased permeability of the tumor cell membrane compared with normal cells also accounts for increased diffusion of non-transferrin-bound gallium species into cells. The accumulation of 67Ga within tumor cells is very much dependent upon the intracellular binding of 67Ga to iron-binding proteins such as lactoferrin and ferritin or other higher molecular weight molecules, which can chelate gallium with greater affinity, thereby preventing back diffusion of free gallium [6]. 68Ga-citrate is similar to 67Ga-citrate but is a positron-emitting radiopharmaceutical and shares the same uptake pathway. 68Ga is produced by a 68Ge/68Ga generator (t ½68 min.) and is not dependent on a cyclotron.

3.2.5.2　Facilitated Diffusion

3.2.5.2.1　18F-Fluorodeoxyglucose (FDG)

All cells use glucose to generate metabolic energy. For brain tissue, glucose is the primary source of energy, but in the heart, glucose becomes the primary source of energy for ischemic myocardium.

Glucose is transported into the cell across the plasma membrane by facilitated diffusion, mediated by members of the glucose transporter (Glut) protein family (Glut 1–6) [7]. Similar to glucose, FDG is also transported into normal and malignant cells by facilitated diffusion.

3.2.5.2.2　Hepatobiliary Agents

Evaluation of hepatocyte function using radiopharmaceuticals that are excreted via biliary secretion is another example of a carrier-mediated transport mechanism. Following intravenous administration, 99mTc-disofenin (Hepatolite) and 99mTc-mebrofenin (Choletec) diffuse through pores in the endothelial lining of the sinusoids and bind to the anionic membrane-bound carriers on the hepatocyte. The hepatic uptake is facilitated by carrier-mediated, non-sodium-dependent, organic anionic pathways similar to those of bilirubin. Subsequent biliary excretion of the radiotracer is relatively passive following the flow of bile through the biliary tree. The bile may be stored and concentrated temporarily in the gallbladder or excreted directly into the intestine. Since bilirubin is excreted by the same hepatocyte transport system, higher serum bilirubin levels may have a significant effect on the biodistribution and hepatic excretion of radiopharmaceuticals.

3.2.5.3 Active Transport

Active transport involves translocating a solute molecule through a cell membrane against its concentration gradient and requires the expenditure of some form of energy. Active transport is driven by either hydrolysis of ATP to ADP (primary active transporters) or utilization of an electrochemical gradient of Na + or H+ (secondary active transporters) across the membrane. If the energy source is inhibited or removed, the transport system will not function.

3.2.5.3.1 Radioiodide and 99mTc-Pertechnetate Anions

Thyroid tissue selectively traps certain anions, such as I–, TcO4–, and ClO4–, by an active transport mechanism using the same pathway; hence, they are the competitive inhibitors of each other. The clinical implication is that iodinated contrast agents or iodine-containing medications may interfere with the accumulation of 99mTcO4 in the thyroid, thereby leading to poor image quality. However, only iodide is used by the thyroid gland to synthesize thyroid hormones, while the other anions diffuse out of the gland. *In addition to thyroid tissue, the salivary glands, stomach, bowel, and genitourinary tract show significant uptake (secretion) of radioiodide and pertechnetate.*

3.2.5.3.2 201Thallous Chloride

Since the thallous ion (Tl (OH)2+) acts as an analog of the K+ ion, 201Tl has been used to image myocardial perfusion in order to evaluate the extent of myocardial ischemia and/or infarction. Positron emitter 82Rb—a monocation, like potassium—is also used for imaging myocardial perfusion.

The myocardial uptake of thallium and rubidium involves active cation transport mechanisms including both passive diffusion and ATP or energy-dependent pathways [8].

201Tl has also been used for tumors such as brain tumors, osteosarcomas, low-grade lymphomas, Kaposi's sarcomas, and parathyroid tumors. Accumulation of 201Tl in the tumor is a function of tumor blood flow, increased cell membrane permeability, and an active transport system involving the Na+/K+ ATPase pump within cell membranes. It has been demonstrated that the cellular uptake of 201Tl is inhibited by ouabain, digitalis, and furosemide, which block the Na+/K+ pump [9].

3.2.5.3.3 Renal Agents

Glomerular filtration rate (GFR) provides the best estimate of functioning renal tissue. The measurement of GFR requires a molecule such as inulin that has a stable plasma concentration and is freely filtered in the glomerulus and not secreted or reabsorbed by the tubule. The radiotracers most commonly used for measurement include 125I-iothalamate, 99mTc-DTPA, or 51Cr-EDTA, since they meet the necessary requirements for glomerular filtration. No specific transport mechanisms are involved in the filtration process, and the GFR is determined by the sum of hydrostatic and colloid osmotic forces across the glomerular membrane. Radiopharmaceuticals such as radioiodinated hippuran and 99mTc-mercaptoacetyltriglycine (MAG3) are partly filtered in the glomerulus but mostly excreted by tubular secretion. Compared with radioiodinated hippuran (30% by glomerular filtration), most of 99mTc-MAG3 is bound to plasma proteins and only about 10% may undergo glomerular filtration [10].

3.2.5.4 Phagocytosis

Most of the 99mTc-sulfur colloid (SC) particles are in the range of 0.1–1.0 μm. The cells of the reticuloendothelial system (RES) engulf the colloid particles and remove them from circulation. Kupffer's cells (macrophages in liver sinusoids) and reticular cells (macrophages in spleen) accumulate the particles by phagocytosis. Cold lesions identified on a liver scan with 99mTc-SC may be due to an intrahepatic tumor displacing the usual distribution of RES cells. Similarly, radiation damage in the liver and bone marrow is seen as cold areas due to decreased RES function. 99mTc-SC has been used extensively in lymphoscintigraphy in order to identify a "sentinel node" (the first lymph node to receive lymphatic drainage from a tumor site) in patients with many tumors such as breast cancer and melanoma [11]. If radiocolloid is introduced into the interstitial fluid, it drains into the lymphatic vessels and then into regional lymph nodes. Colloid particles smaller than 0.1 μm show rapid clearance from the interstitial space into lymphatic vessels and significant retention in lymph nodes. Because of their small particle size, 99mTc-antimony sulfide colloid (0.002–0.015 μm) and 99mTc-human serum albumin or nanocolloid (0.01–0.02 μm) are ideal for lymphoscintigraphy studies. Since these agents are not available in the United States and other countries, filtered 99mTc-SC preparation (using a 0.2 μm filter) is being used for sentinel node detection [11].

3.2.5.5 Receptor-Mediated Endocytosis

There are three main types of endocytosis that are distinguished by the size of the vesicle formed and the cellular machinery involved. *Phagocytosis* is the process by which cells ingest large objects, such as bacteria, viruses, or remnants of cells, which have undergone apoptosis. The membrane invaginates enclosing the wanted particles in a pocket and then engulfs the object by pinching it off, and the object is sealed off into a large vacuole known as a phagosome. *Pinocytosis*: This process is concerned with the uptake of solutes and single molecules such as proteins. Both phagocytosis and pinocytosis are nonreceptor-mediated forms of endocytosis and may result in the cell engulfing nonspecific or unwanted particles. *Receptor-mediated endocytosis* is a more specific active event where the cytoplasm membrane folds inward to form coated pits. In this case, proteins or other trigger particles lock into receptors/ligands in the cell's plasma membrane. It is then and only then that the particles are engulfed. These inward budding vesicles bud to form cytoplasmic vesicles. This process may also result in engulfing of unwanted particles, but not to the extent of pino/phagocytosis.

Receptor-mediated endocytosis depends on the interaction of that molecule with a specific binding protein in the cell membrane called a receptor. It allows cells to take up specific macromolecules called ligands, such as proteins that bind insulin (a hormone), transferrin (an iron-binding protein), or low-density lipoprotein cholesterol carriers. This mechanism is involved in neval uptake of 99mTc-DMSA and 111In-DTPA octreotide for example.

3.2.6 Metabolic Substrates and Precursors

Cancer cells have an altered metabolism compared with normal cells. As a result, cancer cells use more glucose than normal cells. Due to the increased rate of cell proliferation, the protein and DNA synthesis is augmented, and the cancer cells need to transport increased amounts of precursors such as amino acids and nucleotides. A number of radiopharmaceuticals were developed based on the increased demand of metabolic substrates of tumor cells.

3.2.6.1 Metabolic Trapping of FDG

The glucose analog deoxyglucose, which has one oxygen atom less than the glucose molecule (Fig. 3.1), is transported into the cell in the same way as glucose. 18F-2-deoxy-2-fluoro-d-glucose (FDG) similar to d-glucose is transported into the cell by facilitated diffusion and is phosphorylated by hexokinase to FDG-6-phosphate. In the next step of glycolysis, the enzyme glucose-6-phosphate isomerase does not react with FDG-6-phosphate due to very strict structural and geometric demands. Accordingly, the very polar FDG-6-phosphate is trapped in the cytoplasm [12]. FDG-6-phosphate may be converted back to FDG, but the enzyme glucose-6-phosphatase, which is responsible for this reaction, is either at very low levels or absent in cancer tissue (Fig. 3.2). FDG-PET is

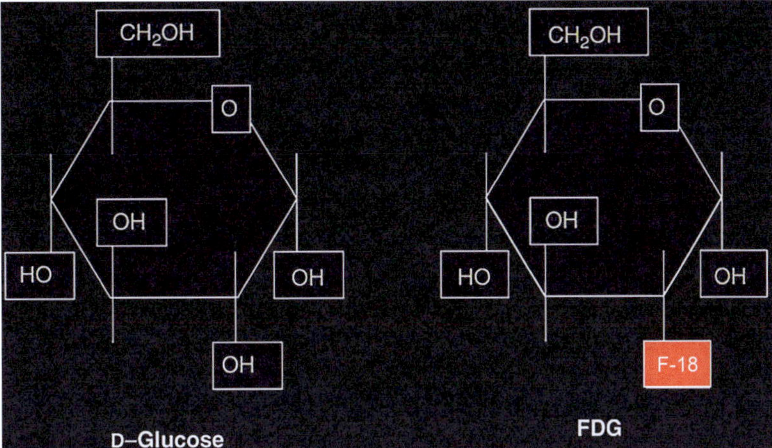

Fig. 3.1 [^{18}F]2-deoxy-2-fluoro-D-glucose (FDG). In FDG the hydroxyl group in the 2-position of D-glucose is replaced by ^{18}F

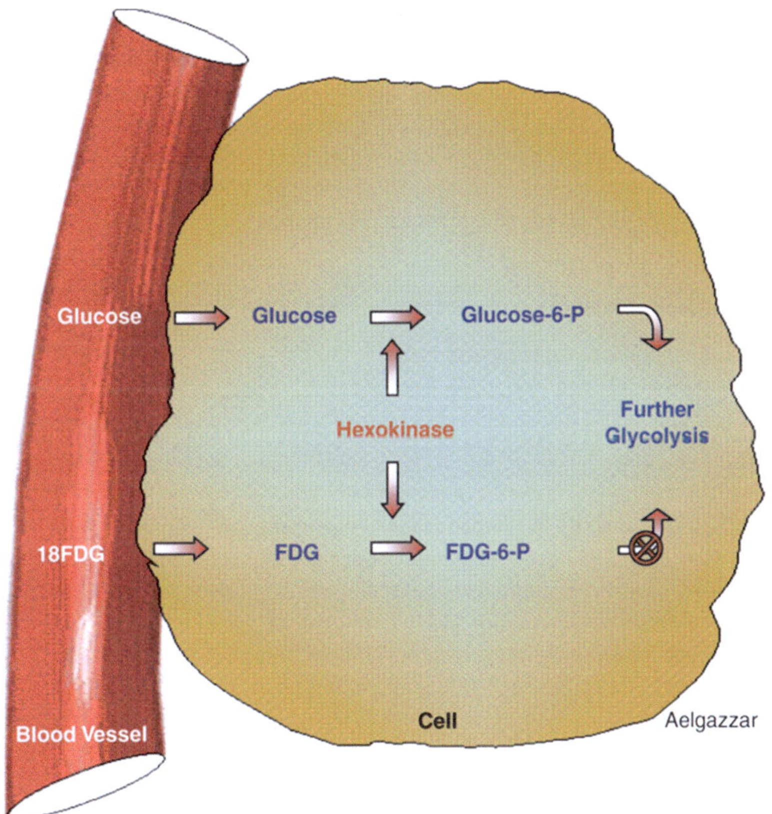

Fig. 3.2 Glucose and FDG are transported into the cell and phosphorylated, but FDG does not undergo further metabolism and accumulates in proportion to glucose utilization (increased in tumors, macrophages, and ischemic myocytes)

now being extensively used for an increasing number of clinical indications at different stages of cancer, e.g., diagnosis, staging, monitoring of response to therapy, prediction of prognosis, and finally detection of recurrence. In addition, FDG accumulates in granulomatous tissue and macrophages infiltrating the areas surrounding necrotic tumor tissue [13] and has a role to play in imaging certain conditions of infection/inflammation.

3.2.6.2 Radiolabeled Amino Acids

Since amino acids are the biological building blocks of proteins, radiolabeled amino acid uptake within tumors may reflect the increased protein synthesis rate of proliferating tumor cells or simply an increased rate of amino acid transport across the tumor cell membrane [14]. Methionine has been the most widely used amino acid tracer, in the form of l-[methyl-11C] methionine. The predominant mechanism of methionine tumor uptake reflects the increased rate of active membrane transport process rather than the rate of protein synthesis [15]. Since tyrosine reflects the protein synthesis rate, radiolabeled tyrosine and a number of tyrosine analogs have been introduced including l-[1-11C]tyrosine, l-[2-18F] fluorotyrosine, l-4-[18F]fluoro-m-tyrosine, and l-[3-18F]-a-methyltyrosine (FMT) [16]. Among these tracers, more recently, the tyrosine analog l-*O*-[2-18F]fluoroethyltyrosine (FET), which is not incorporated into proteins but nevertheless transported by an active transport mechanism, was developed. FET is stable in vivo with fast brain and tumor uptake kinetics [17].

3.2.7 Radiopharmaceuticals for Tissue Hypoxia Imaging

Hypoxia may result from either insufficient regional perfusion (acute or transient hypoxia), as in myocardium, or insufficient oxygen diffusion (chronic hypoxia), as in tumors. Since hypoxia cannot be predicted, noninvasive techniques for identifying hypoxic regions in tumor, myocardium, and brain tissue are being developed. The compound 2-nitro misonidazole (MISO) is transported into the cell by diffusion. In the cytoplasm, the nitro group (NO2) undergoes one electron enzymatic reduction to the free radical anion [18]. In normoxic cells, this reaction step is reversed by intracellular oxygen and the oxidized molecule diffuses out of the cell. In hypoxic tissue, the free radical is further reduced to a reactive species, hydroxylamine, and then to an amine [18]. Free radicals are attached irreversibly to cellular macromolecules and are retained within the cell. Reduction of these molecules occurs in all tissue with viable enzymatic processes, but retention occurs only in those tissues with low oxygen tension. A number of radiolabeled compounds incorporating a 2-nitroimidazole moiety to image tumor hypoxia have been developed. 18F-fluoromisonidazole (FMISO) is probably the most extensively studied hypoxia-selective radiopharmaceutical [19]. Radiolabeled agents of copper have been investigated to develop PET tracers for hypoxia imaging, since copper has an amenable coordination and electrochemistry that would lend itself to redox-mediated trapping in cells. One of these compounds, 64Cu-ATSM (Cu-diacetyl-*bis*-(N4-methylthiosemicarbazone), has been shown to be selectively trapped in hypoxic tissue but rapidly washed out of normoxic cells [20]. Among the iodinated compounds, successful imaging of tumor hypoxia has been reported using a sugar containing the MISO derivative 123I-iodoazomycin arabinoside (IAZA) [21]. Significant in vivo deiodination, however, limits the clinical usefulness of this compound. A 99mTc-labeled hypoxic imaging agent, a propylene amine oxime (PnAO) derivative of 2-nitroimidazole, showed hypoxia selectivity in tumor models but has slow clearance due to high lipophilicity [22]. It was recently reported that a complex of core legends without the nitroimidazole group labeled with 99mTc also showed very high tumor hypoxia selectivity. A prototype formulation of one of these compounds, 99mTc-HL91 (4,9-diaza-3,3,10,10-tetramethyldodecane-2,11-dione dioxime), has demonstrated uptake in a variety of tumors [23].

3.2.8 Cell Proliferation Radiopharmaceuticals

In normal tissue, there is a balance between cell growth and cell death. Within a tumor, growth is favored. Most benign tumors grow slowly over a period of years, but most malignant tumors grow rapidly, sometimes at an erratic pace. The number of cells in the S-phase of cell cycle is also higher compared with normal cells. As a result, there is an increased requirement of substrates (nucleotides) for DNA synthesis. Nucleotide incorporation into DNA in tumor tissue determined in vitro using [3H]-thymidine (thymidine labeling index) is a measure of tumor proliferation [24]. 11C-thymidine has been used for many years as a PET tracer to image tumors [25]. Due to the rapid metabolism of this tracer in blood, however, the tumor uptake of 11C-thymidine is not optimal for imaging studies and quantitation is difficult. 125I-5-iodo-2′-deoxyuridine (IudR), an analog of thymidine (TdR), has recently been developed by replacing the 5-methyl group with an iodine atom [26]. Within the tumor cell, IudR is phosphorylated and incorporated in DNA [27].

18F-fluoro-3′-deoxy-3′-l-fluorothymidine (FLT) was developed for imaging cell proliferation [28]. Similar to thymidine, 18F-FLT is transported into the cell by both passive diffusion and facilitated transport by Na+− dependent carriers, where it is phosphorylated by thymidine kinase 1 (TK1) into 18F-FLT-monophosphate that is trapped in the cell. 18F-FLT can be useful in the evaluation and measurement of the response of anticancer therapy (see also Chap. 12).

3.2.9 Specific Receptor Binding

The term receptor is generally used to describe a specific cellular binding site for a small ligand, such as peptide hormones and neurotransmitters. In the case of antigen-antibody interactions, antigen expressed on a cell may be regarded as a receptor for a specific antibody. Antigen molecules may be present either in or on cells but may also be secreted into the extracellular fluid and circulation. The mechanism of localization of receptor-binding radiopharmaceuticals is specific and depends on receptor or antigen expression of the tumor tissue. Examples include the binding of an antibody or antibody fragment to an antigen and peptides, hormones, or neurotransmitter binding to their receptors. Many tumor cells express antigens or receptors that are expressed in small amounts in normal cells. But tumor cells have higher expression of these antigens and receptors. The radionuclide of use should match the pharmacokinetics of the biological molecule.

For example, antibodies should be labeled with long half-life radionuclides such as ^{111}In and ^{131}I, while peptides can be labeled with shorter lived radionuclides such as ^{99m}Tc, ^{18}F, or ^{123}I for imaging studies. Iodine-131 is the most used radionuclide for both diagnostic and therapeutic studies. Radioiodide can be labeled on tyrosine residue in the antibody or peptide. However, the other radionuclides are indirectly labeled in which they are coordinated to a chelate such as DTPA or DOTA that is covalently attached to the biological molecule.

^{131}I-tositumomab and ^{111}In/^{90}Y-ibritumomab tiuxetan are monoclonal murine IgG that bind to CD20 receptors on B cells and non-Hodgkin's lymphoma tumor cells. These labeled antibodies are used for diagnosis, monitoring, and treatment of non-Hodgkin's lymphoma [29]. Many neuroendocrine tumors have an overexpression of somatostatin receptors (SSTRs) and there are five SSTR subtypes. The two naturally occurring SST peptides, 14 and 28 amino acids long, are known to have short biological half-life due to enzymatic degradation. A number of biologically stable SST analogs were synthesized. Octreotide analog is an 8-amino acid-long analog that has a high affinity to 2 and 5 SSTR subtypes. ^{111}In-pentetreotide (octreoscan), a radiolabeled form of octreotide, is used to detect, localize, and evaluate such somatostatin-expressing tumors by binding to these receptors. When octreotide is labeled with ^{90}Y or ^{177}Lu, it is used for therapeutic purposes. Recently, ^{68}Ga-DOTA-octreotide has been approved for PET studies of neuroendocrine tumors [30]. In addition, ^{64}Cu-DOTA-tyr^3-octreotate has been approved as a PET diagnostic agent for neuroendocrine tumors, but Cu-64 emits β^- so it can be used for therapeutic purposes as well [31].

F-18-florbetapir (Amyvid, Eli Lilly), F-18-florbetaben (Neuraceq, Piramal Imaging), and F-18-flutemetamol (GE Healthcare, Vizamyl™) are radiopharmaceuticals used for patients who are being evaluated for Alzheimer's disease (AD) and other causes of cognitive impairment in the cortical regions and hippocampus. After injection, the tracers diffuse through the blood-brain barrier and bind with high affinity and specificity to β-amyloid neuritic plaques (Aβ aggregates) in the brain of adult patients with cognitive impairment. They rapidly enter the brain and quickly wash out from the brain if not bound to β-amyloid neuritic plaques [32]. These radiotracers share a common imaging target and similar imaging characteristics (Aβ tracers). They can differ in their tracer kinetics, specific binding ratios, and optimal imaging parameters; therefore, they will have different recommended injected doses, time to initiate imaging postinjection, and scan duration [33].

F-18-fluoroestradiol (F-18-FES) is an analog of estrogen and is used to detect estrogen receptor-positive breast cancer lesions. It has a high overall sensitivity and specificity in assessing the ER status in breast cancers. F-18-FES uptake has been approved to guide in therapy selection and to predict endocrine treatment response [34].

I-123-ioflupane (DaTscan) is a chemical derivative of cocaine. It binds to presynaptic dopamine transporters, which are primarily located in the striatum. Loss of dopamine transporter density, as occurs in Parkinson's disease, results in reduced uptake of the radiopharmaceutical. The radiotracer localizes to the dopamine transporters in the basal ganglia [35].

3.2.9.1 Radiolabeled Peptides

3.2.9.1.1 Somatostatin Receptors

There are two naturally occurring bioactive somatostatin (SST) products, a 14-amino-acid (SST14) and a 28-amino-acid (SST28) form. SST is secreted throughout the body and has multiple physiological functions including the inhibition of secretion of growth hormone, glucagon, insulin, gastrin, and other hormones by the pituitary and gastrointestinal tract. The diverse biological effects of SST are mediated through a family of G-protein-coupled receptors, of which five subtypes have been identified by molecular cloning [28]. Human SST receptors (SSTRs) have been identified on many cells of neuroendocrine origin as well as on lymphocytes. In addition, most neuroendocrine tumors, small-cell lung cancers, and medullary thyroid carcinomas express SSTRs in high density [36, 37]. The expression of SSTR subtypes in human tumor tissues, however, seems to vary with tumor type [38]. A number of somatostatin analogs (seglitide, octreotide, somatuline, or lanreotide) with greater biological stability than SST14 have been synthesized. These derivatives consist of hexapeptide and octapeptide molecules, which incorporate the biologically active core of SST14 [28]. It is important to recognize that SST14 binds to all five SSTR subtypes with comparable affinity. By contrast, octreotide binds with higher affinity to SSTR 2, 3, and 5, while lanreotide and RC-160 bind to SSTRs 1–4 with comparable affinity. None of the synthetic peptides show high-affinity binding to SSTR 1.

3.2.9.1.2 Radiolabeled SST Analogs

Selective receptor-targeting radiopeptides have emerged as an important class of radiopharmaceuticals for molecular imaging and therapy of tumors that overexpress peptide receptors on the cell membrane. Peptides labeled with γ-emitting radionuclides bind to their receptors, allowing clinicians to visualize receptor-expressing tumors noninvasively. Peptides labeled with β-particle emitters could also eradicate receptor-expressing tumors [39]. 111In-DTPA-d-Phe1-pentetreotide or octreoscan (Mallinckrodt Inc., St. Louis), with a high specific activity (5–6 mCi of 111In/10 μg octreotide), was developed. *It binds to SSTR 2 and 5 subtypes with greater affinity than the unlabeled octreotide.* 99mTc-radiolabeled somatostatin analogs have also been used to evaluate patients with neuroendocrine tumors as well as with thyroid cancer recurrences [16]. Due to the very specific localization of octreotide analogs in neuroendocrine tumors, radiolabeled SST analogs were also developed for the therapy of neuroendocrine tumors. 90Y-DOTATyr3-octreotide (DOTATOC) was developed. 90Y-DOTATOC has been evaluated for the treatment of gastroenteropancreatic neuroendocrine tumors (GEPNET); however, 90Y radionuclide does not emit accompanying gamma ray(s) for imaging therapeutic efficacy [40–43]. 177LuDOTA TOC has also been evaluated for treating GEPNET, and 177Lu emits gamma ray that can be used for post-therapeutic monitoring [43–49]. 68GaDOTA/TOC may be the radiopharmaceutical of choice for peptide receptor radionuclide therapy (PRRT) principally due to the fact that 68Ga is a positron-emitting radionuclide that can be used in PET/CT imaging [44, 45].

3.2.9.1.3 Vasoactive Intestinal Peptide (VIP) Receptors

VIP is a 28-amino-acid neuroendocrine mediator with a broad range of biological activity in diverse cells and tissues. In addition to being a vasodilator, VIP promotes the growth and proliferation of normal and malignant cells. Cell membrane VIP receptors are widely distributed throughout the gastrointestinal tract, but they are also found on various other cell types. Increased VIP receptor expression has been seen on adenocarcinomas, breast cancers, melanomas, neuroblastomas, and pancreatic carcinomas [46].

High-specific-activity 123I-VIP (150–200 MBq/μg) was prepared by Virgolini et al. [47]. In clinical studies, they were able to demonstrate specific uptake in primary tumors as well as in liver, lung, and lymph node metastases of pancreatic adenocarcinoma, colon adenocarcinoma, or gastrointestinal neuroendocrine tumors. In vitro receptor studies with cloned VIP receptors clearly demonstrated that 123I-VIP bound to VIP receptors as well as unlabeled VIP [47]. In addition, they observed interaction between VIP and SST on various cell types, including primary tumor cells.

3.2.9.2 Steroid Hormone Receptors

Sex steroid hormones—estrogen, progesterone, and testosterone—bind with high affinity to intracellular receptors. The majority of breast cancers are hormone dependent, as indicated by increased expression of intracellular estrogen or progesterone receptors. Noninvasive quantitative imaging of estrogen or progesterone receptor content in breast cancer may be useful for predicting the responsiveness of hormonal therapy. Various steroid and nonsteroidal estrogen analogs have been radiolabeled with positron-emitting radionuclides, 77Br and 18F. Among these tracers, 16α-[−[18F]fluoro-17β-estradiol (FES) showed high affinity and selectivity to estrogen receptors and has shown a potential for detecting estrogen receptor-positive metastatic foci [48]. Similarly, 21-[18F]fluoro-16a-ethyl-19-norprogesterone (FENP) has shown a potential for imaging progesterone receptors. Recently, 123I-labeled *cis*-11-β-methoxy-17a-iodovinylestradiol (Z-[123I]MIVE) was introduced as a radioligand to image estrogen receptor expression in breast cancers [49]. These radiotracers are transported into the cell by passive diffusion and bind to steroid receptors within the nucleus.

3.2.9.3 Adrenergic Presynaptic Receptors

Tumors arising from the neural crest share the characteristic of amine precursor uptake and decarboxylation (APUD) and contain large amounts of adrenaline, dopamine, and serotonin within the secretory granules in the cytoplasm. Tumors of the adrenergic system include pheochromocytomas (arise in adrenal medulla) or paragangliomas (extra-adrenal tissue). Metaiodobenzylguanidine (MIBG) is an analog of noradrenaline, originally developed by Wieland et al. [50]. 131I-MIBG was initially used to image pheochromocytoma. It has since been used for imaging neuroblastoma, medullary thyroid carcinoma, retinoblastoma, melanoma, and bronchial carcinoma. Wieland et al. [51] observed that 131I-MIBG accumulated in the chromaffin cells of the adrenal medulla. Since MIBG is structurally similar to noradrenaline, MIBG is believed to be transported into the cell by the reuptake pathways of the adrenergic presynaptic neurons [51]. Within the cells, MIBG is transported into the catecholamine-storing granules by means of the ATPase-dependent proton pump. The major difference between MIBG and noradrenaline is that MIBG does not bind to postsynaptic adrenergic receptors. Reduced 131I-MIBG uptake by the tumors is seen in patients using drugs such as labetalol, calcium channel blockers, and antipsychotic and sympathomimetic agents.

3.2.9.4 LDL Receptors

Plasma low-density lipoprotein (LDL) carries cholesterol to the adrenal glands. Cholesterol is the substrate for adrenal steroid hormone (cortisol and aldosterone) synthesis. 131I-6-β-iodomethyl-19-norcholesterol (NP-59) is the agent of choice for imaging patients with adrenal cortical diseases [52]. Two other analogs, 131I-6-iodocholesterol and 75Se-β-iodomethyl-19-norcholesterol (Scintadren), have also been proven to be clinically useful for imaging the adrenal glands. NP-59 and other radioiodinated cholesterol analogs are transported by plasma LDL and are accumulated in the adrenal cortex via LDL receptors.

Subsequently, NP-59 is esterified like cholesterol and stored intracellularly without further metabolism or incorporation into adrenocortical steroid hormones.

3.2.9.5 Radiolabeled Antibodies

Antibodies (Ab), also called immunoglobulins (Ig), are a group of glycoprotein molecules produced by B-lymphocytes in response to antigenic stimulation. Each antibody binds to a restricted part of the antigen called an epitope. A particular antigen can have several different epitopes. However, a monoclonal antibody (MAb) is specific for a particular epitope rather than the whole antigen molecule. The antibody structure is made of two F(ab') regions and one Fc' region. The enzyme pepsin cleaves the IgG molecule to yield the F(ab')2 and Fc' fragments, while the enzyme papain splits the IgG molecule into two Fab fragments and the Fc' fragment. The Fab region binds to the antigen, while the Fc' region mediates effector functions such as complement fixation and monocyte binding. Almost all MAbs used in nuclear medicine for diagnosis and therapy belong to the IgG class. MAbs derived from mice are called murine MAbs. Since the Fc' portion of the murine antibody is antigenic in human beings and induces the formation of human anti-mouse antibody (HAMA), chimeric antibodies are being developed in which murine variable regions of Fab' are attached to constant regions of human IgG.

Most tumor cells synthesize many proteins or glycoproteins that are antigenic in nature. These tumor-associated antigens (TAA) such as CEA, TAG-72, PSA, and PSMA may also be expressed in small amounts in normal cells, but tumor cells typically produce them in large amounts [53–55].

^{131}I-tositumomab and ^{111}In/^{90}Y-ibritumomab tiuxetan are monoclonal murine IgG that bind to CD20 receptors on B cells and non-Hodgkin's lymphoma tumor cells. These labeled antibodies are used for diagnosis, monitoring, and treatment of non-Hodgkin's lymphoma [29, 56].

3.2.10 Imaging Gene Expression Mechanism

Following the completion of human genome sequencing, the discovery of molecular mechanisms of carcinogenesis, and the significant advances in gene therapy, it may be possible to assess gene function and regulation by radionuclide imaging of gene expression. Radionuclide imaging of gene expression involves two main general methods: (a) using antisense oligonucleotides targeted toward the mRNA of a particular gene or (b) using reporter genes to track the expression of endogenous or exogenous genes. The antisense oligonucleotides have emerged as highly selective inhibitors or modulators of gene expression. When labeled to an appropriate radionuclide, the antisense oligonucleotide can be used for imaging or therapy [57].

References

1. Krasnow AZ, Hellman RS, Timins ME et al (1997) Diagnostic bone scanning in oncology. Semin Nucl Med 27:107–141
2. Delmon-Moingeon LI, Piwinca-Wormas D, Van den Abbeele AD, Holman BL, Davison A, Jones AG (1990) Uptake of the cation hexakis (2-methoxyisobutylisonitrile)-technetium-99 m by human carcinoma cell lines in vitro. Cancer Res 50:2198–2202
3. Arbab AS, Koizumi K, Toyama K, Araki T (1996) Uptake of technetium-99 m-tetrofosmin, technetium-

99 m-MIBI and thallium-201 in tumor cell lines. J Nucl Med 37:1551–1556

4. Vallabhajosula SR, Harwig JF, Siemsen JK et al (1980) Radiogallium localization in tumors: blood binding and transport and the role of transferrin. J Nucl Med 21:650–656

5. Hayes RL, Rafter JJ, Byrd BL, Carlton JE (1981) Studies of the in vivo entry of ga-67 into normal and malignant tissue. J Nucl Med 22:325–332

6. Weiner RE (1996) The mechanism of 67 ga localization in malignant disease. Nucl Med Biol 23:745–751

7. Mueckler M (1994) Facilitative glucose transporters. Eur J Biochem 219:713–725

8. Weich HF, Strauss HW, Pitt B (1977) The extraction of thallium-201 by the myocardium. Circulation 56:188

9. Sessler MJ, Geck P, Maul FD et al (1986) New aspects of cellular Tl-201 uptake: co-transport is the central mechanism of ion uptake. Nucl Med 25:24–27

10. Eshima D, Taylor A (1992) Tc-99 m mercaptoacetyltriglycine (Tc-99mMAG3): update on the new Tc-99 m renal tubular function agent. Semin Nucl Med 22:61–73

11. Alazraki NP, Eshima D, Eshima LA et al (1997) Lymphoscintigraphy, the sentinel node concept, and the intraoperative gamma probe in melanoma, breast cancer, and other potential cancers. Semin Nucl Med 27:55–67

12. Gallagher BM, Fowler JS, Gutterson NI et al (1978) Metabolic trapping as a principle of radiopharmaceutical design: some factors responsible for the biodistribution of [18F]2-deoxy-2-fl uoro-D-glucose. J Nucl Med 19:1154–1161

13. Kubota R, Yamada S, Kubota K et al (1992) Intratumoral distribution of fl uorine-18- fluorodeoxyglucose in vivo: high accumulation in macrophages and granulation tissues studied by microautora-diographic comparison with FDG. J Nucl Med 33:1872–1980

14. Vaalburg W, Coenen HH, Crouzel C et al (1992) Amino acids for the measurement of protein synthesis in vivo by PET. Nucl Med Biol 19:227–237

15. Ishiwata K, Kubota K, Murakami M, Kubota R, Senda M (1993) A comparative study on protein incorporation of L-[methyl-3H]methionine, L-[1-14C]leucine and L-[2-18F]fluorotyrosine in tumor bearing mice. Nucl Med Biol 20:895–899

16. Gambini JP, Quagliata A, Finozzi R, Serra P, Lago G, Gaudiano J, Engler H, Alonso O (2011) Tc-99 m- and Ga-68-labeled somatostatin analogues in the evaluation of Hurthle cell thyroid cancer. Clin Nucl Med 36:803–804

17. Wester HJ, Herz M, Weber W (1999) Synthesis and radiopharmacology of O -[2-18F]fluorethyltyrosine for tumor imaging. J Nucl Med 40:205–212

18. Nunn A, Linder K, Strauss HW (1995) Nitroimidazoles and imaging hypoxia. Eur J Nucl Med 22:265–280

19. Rasey JS, Koh WJ, Evans ML et al (1996) Quantifying regional hypoxia in tumors with positron emission tomography: a pretherapy study of 37 patients. Int J Radiat Oncol Biol Phys 36:417–428

20. Lewis JS, McCarthy DW, McCarthy TJ, Fugibayashi Y, Welch MJ (1999) Evaluation of 64Cu-ATSM in vitro and in vivo in a hypoxic tumor model. J Nucl Med 40:177–183

21. Parliament MB, Chapman JD, Urtasunn RC et al (1992) Noninvasive assessment of human tumor hypoxia with 123I-iodoazomycin arabinoside: preliminary report of a clinical study. Br J Cancer 65:90–95

22. Ballinger JR, Kee JWM, Rauth AM (1996) In vitro and in vivo evaluation of a technetium-99 m-labeled 2-nitroimidazole (BMS181321) as a marker of tumor hypoxia. J Nucl Med 37:1023–1031

23. Cook GJR, Houston S, Barrington SF, Fogelman I (1998) Technetium-99 m-labeled HL91 to identify tumor hypoxia: correlation with fl uorine-18-FDG. J Nucl Med 39:99–103

24. Livingston RB, Ambus U, George SL, Freireich EJ, Hart JS (1974) In vitro determination of thymidine-[3H] labeling index in human solid tumors. Cancer Res 34:1376–1380

25. Goethals P, Lameire N, van Eijkeren M (1996) Methylcarbon-11 thymidine for in vivo measurement of cell proliferation. J Nucl Med 37:1048–1052

26. Kassis AI, Adelstein SJ (1996) Preclinical animal studies with radioiododeoxyuridine. J Nucl Med 37(Suppl):10s–12s

27. O'Donoghue JA (1996) Strategies for selective targeting of auger electron emitters to tumor cells. J Nucl Med 37(Suppl):3s–6s

28. Patel YC, Greenwood MT, Panetta R, Demchyshyn L, Niznik H, Srikant CB (1995) Minireview: the somatostatin receptor family. Life Sci 57:1249–1265

29. Davies A (2007) Radioimmunotherapy for B-cell lymphoma: Y^{90} ibritumomab tiuxctan and I^{131} tositumomab. Oncogene 26:3614–3628

30. Deppen SA, Blume J, Bobbey AJ, Shah C, Graham MM, Lee P, Delbeke D, Walker RC (2016) 68Ga-DOTATATE compared with 111In-DTPA-octreotide and conventional imaging for pulmonary and Gastroenteropancreatic neuroendocrine Tumors: a systematic review and meta-analysis. J Nucl Med 57:872–878

31. Ullrich M, Bergmann R, Peitzsch M, Zenker EF, Cartellieri M et al (2016) Multimodal somatostatin receptor theranostics using [(64)Cu]Cu−/[(177)Lu]Lu-DOTA-(Tyr(3))octreotate and AN-238 in a mouse pheochromocytoma model. Theranostics 6:650–665

32. Auvity S, Tonietto M, Caillé F et al (2020) Repurposing radiotracers for myelin imaging: a study comparing 18F-florbetaben, 18F-florbetapir, 18F-flutemetamol,11C-MeDAS, and 11C-PiB. Eur J Nucl Med Mol Imaging 47:490–501

33. Yeo JM, Waddell B, Khan Z, Pal S (2015) A systematic review and meta-analysis of (18)F-labeled amyloid imaging in Alzheimer's disease. Alzheimer's Dement (Amst, Netherlands) 1:5–13

34. Liao GJ, Clark AS, Schubert EK, Mankoff DA (2016) 18F-Fluoroestradiol PET: Current Status and Potential Future Clinical Applications. J Nucl Med 57:1269–1275

35. Roussakis AA, Piccini P, Politis M (2013) Clinical utility of DaTscan™ (123I-Ioflupane injection) in the diagnosis of parkinsonian syndromes. Degener Neurol Neuromuscul Dis 3:33–39

36. Reubi JC, Laissue J, Krenning EP, Lamberts SWJ (1992) Somatostatin receptors in human cancer:incidence, characteristics, functional correlates and clinical implication. J Steroid Biochem Mol Biol 43:27–35

37. Krenning EP, Kwekkeboom DJ, Bakker WH, Breeman WA, Kooij PP, Oei HY, van Hagen M, Postema PT, de Jong M, Reubi JC (1993) Somatostatin receptor scintigraphy with [111In-DTPA-D-Phe1]- and [123I-Tyr3]-octreotide: the Rotterdam experience with more than 1000 patients. Eur J Nucl Med 20:716–731

38. Virgolini I, Pangerl T, Bischof C, Smith-Jones P, Peck-Radosavljevic M (1997) Somatostatin receptor subtype expression in human tissues: a prediction for diagnosis and treatment of cancer? Eur J Clin Investig 27:645–647

39. de Jong M, Breeman WAP, Kwekkeboom DJ, Valkema R, Krenning EP (2009) Tumor imaging and therapy using radiolabeled somatostatin analogues. Acc Chem Res 42:873–880

40. Kunikowska J, Krolick L, Hubalewska-Dydejczyk A et al (2011) Clinical results of radionuclide therapy of neuroendocrine tumors with 90Y-DOTA-TATE and tandem90Y/177Lu-DOTA-TATE: which is a better therapy option? Eur J Nucl Med Mol Imaging 38:1788–1797

41. de Jong M, Breeman WA, Valkema R et al (2005) Combination radionuclide therapy using 177Lu and 90Y-labeled somatostatin analogs. J Nucl Med 46(Suppl 1):13S–17S

42. Bodei L, Cremonesi M, Grana CM et al (2011) Peptide receptor radionuclide therapy with 177LuDOTATATE:the IEO phase I-II study. Eur J Nucl Med Mol Imaging 38:2125–2155

43. Felce A, Fraternali A, Frasoldati A et al (2012) Radiolabeled somatostatin analogues therapy in advanced neuroendocrine tumors: a single center experience. J Oncol 2012:320198

44. Oberg K (2012) Molecular imaging radiotherapy: theranostics for personalized patient management of neuroendocrine tumors (NETs). Theranostics 2:448–458

45. Baum RP, Virgolini I, Ambrosin V et al (2010) Procedure guidelines for PET/CT tumor imaging with 68Ga-DOTA-conjugated peptides: 68Ga-DOTATOC, 68Ga-DOTA-NOC, 68Ga_DOTA-TATE. Eur J Nucl Med Mol Imaging 37:2004–2010

46. Reubi JC (1995) In vitro identifi cation of vasoactive intestinal peptide receptors in human tumors: implications for tumor imaging. J Nucl Med 36:1846–1853

47. Virgolini I, Raderer M, Kurtaran A et al (1994) Vasoactive intestinal peptide-receptor imaging for the localization of intestinal adenocarcinomas and endocrine tumors. N Engl J Med 331:1116–1121

48. Katzenellenbogen JA (1995) Designing steroid receptor-based radiotracers to image breast and prostate tumors. J Nucl Med 36(Suppl):8s–13s

49. Rijks LJM, Boer GJ, Endert E et al (1996) The stereoisomers of 17 −[123I]iodovinyloestradiol and its 11 q −methoxy derivative evaluated for their estrogen receptor binding in human MCF-7 cells and rat uterus. Med 23:295–307

50. Wieland DM, Swanson DP, Brown LE, Beierwalters WH (1979) Imaging the adrenal medulla with an I-131-labeled anti-adrenergic agent. J Nucl Med 20:155–158

51. Jaques S Jr, Tobes MC, Sisson JC, Baker JA, Wieland DM (1984) Comparison of sodium dependency of uptake of metaiodobenzylguanidine and norepinephrine into cultured bovine adrenomedullary cells. Mol Pharmacol 26:539–546

52. Beierwalters WH, Weiland DM, Yu T, Swanson D, Mosley S (1978) Adrenal imaging agents. Rationale, synthesis, formulation and metabolism. Semin Nucl Med 8:5–21

53. Wester HJ, Schottelius M (2019) PSMA-targeted radiopharmaceuticals for imaging and therapy. Semin Nucl Med 49:302–312

54. Lin M, Ta RT, Kairemo K, Le DB, Ravizzini GC (2021) Cancer Biother Radiopharm 36:237–225

55. Okarvi SM (2019) Recent developments of prostate-specific membrane antigen (PSMA)-specific radiopharmaceuticals for precise imaging and therapy of prostate cancer: an overview. Clin Transl Imaging 7:189–208

56. Jacene HA, Filice R, Kasecamp W, Wahl RL (2007) Comparison of 90Y-ibritumomab Tiuxetan and 131I-Tositumomab in clinical practice. J Nucl Med 48:1767–1776

57. Gambhir SS, Barrio JR, Herschman HR et al (1996) Imaging gene expression: principles and assays. J Nucl Cardiol 6:219–233

Inflammation

4

4.1 Definitions

Inflammation was described as early as 3000 BC in an Egyptian papyrus [1] and is still a common problem despite continuous advancements in prevention and treatment methods. The recent outbreak of the new viral infection Covid-19 [2] is an evidence of how infection is still a common problem, and new types can emerge. Infection can be serious and life threatening. It can cost more than other diseases such as cancer and diabetes. The proper and timely diagnosis, knowledge of comorbidities and delineation of the site, and extent of inflammation are crucial to the clinical management of infection and for monitoring the response to therapy [3].

This issue is relevant to nuclear medicine, since physiological along with morphological imaging has an important role in achieving this goal.

Inflammation is a complex tissue reaction to injury. Injury may be caused not only by living microbes, i.e., bacteria, viruses, or fungi, leading to infection, but also by injurious chemical, physical, immunological, or radiation agents (Fig. 4.1). Inflammation is fundamentally a protective reaction against the cause of cell injury as well as the consequence of such injury. However, inflammation is potentially harmful and may even be life threatening. Since most of the essential components of the inflammatory process are found in the circulation, inflammation occurs only in vascularized tissue. Inflammation is generally considered a nonspecific response, because it happens in the same way regardless of the stimulus and the number of exposures to the stimulus [3, 4]. About inflammation and infection. This is different from the immune system, which has memory, and the antigens are specific and induce a specific response. If infection is the initial event causing tissue injury, the challenge for the host is to react as quickly as possible to terminate the spread of infection, even at the cost of further tissue damage [5].

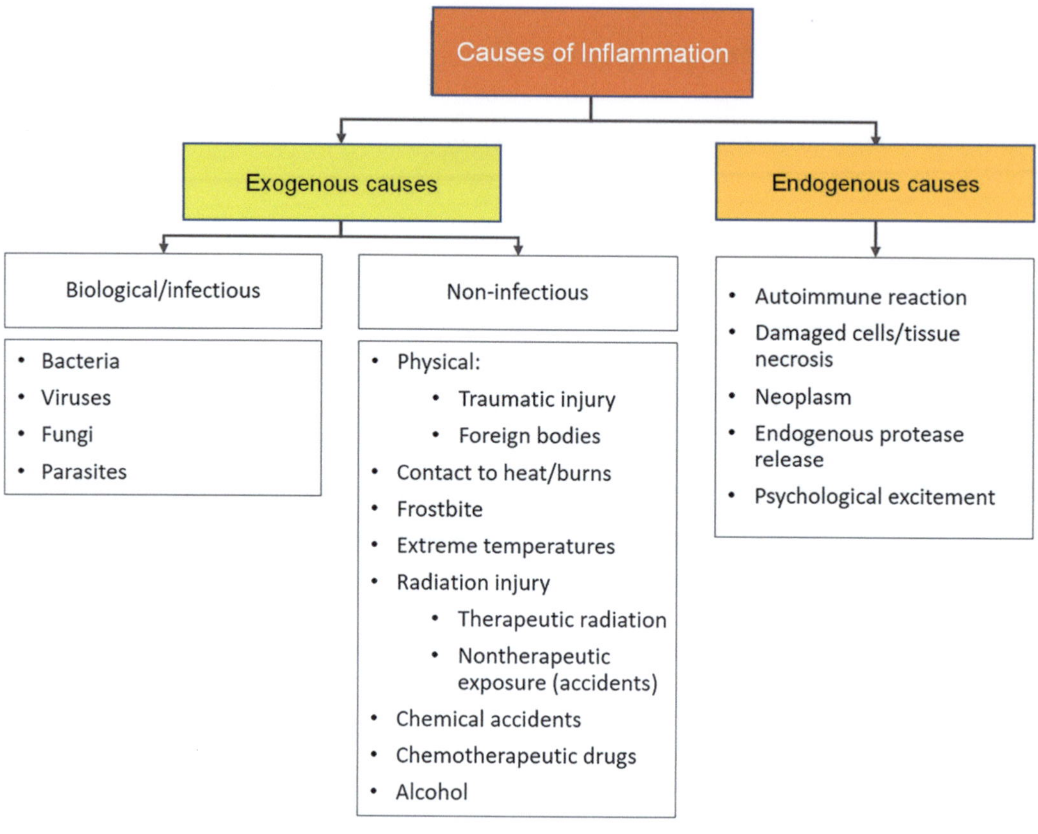

Fig. 4.1 Summary of the causes of inflammation

4.2 Classification of Inflammation

Inflammation may be classified as acute or chronic. Acute inflammation is the immediate or early response to injury and is of relatively short duration. It lasts for minutes, hours, or at most few days. Chronic inflammation, on the other hand, is of longer duration and may last from weeks to years [63]. The distinction between acute and chronic inflammation, however, depends not only on the duration of the process but also on other pathological and clinical features.

4.3 General Pathophysiological Changes of Inflammation

Inflammation causes biologic and tissue changes that may be systemic and/or regional at the site of injury and surrounding tissue (Fig. 4.2).

4.3.1 Local Pathophysiological Changes of Inflammation

4.3.1.1 Acute Inflammation

Acute inflammation continues only until the threat to the host has been eliminated, which usually takes 8–10 days, although this is variable. Inflammation is generally considered to be chronic when it persists for longer than 2 weeks [72]. Many regional and systemic changes accompanying acute inflammation are mediated by certain chemicals produced endogenously called chemical mediators and are behind the spread of the acute inflammatory response following injury to a small area of tissue into uninjured sites. These chemical mediators include mediators released from cells such as histamine and prostaglandins and others in plasma which are released by the systems contained in the plasma. These are the four enzymatic cascade systems, namely the complement system, the kinins, the coagulation factors, and the fibrino-

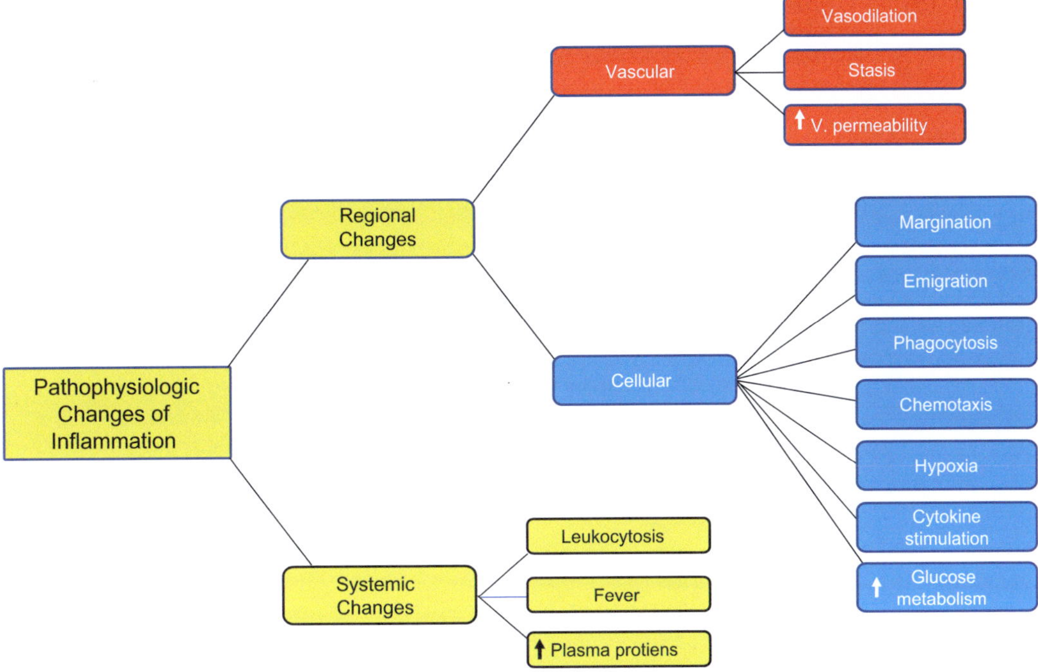

Modified from; Elgazzar, Inflammation/Infection. Multimodality Imaging with Essential Pathophysiology. Kuwait University Press, 2022

Fig. 4.2 Regional and general pathophysiologic changes of inflammation

lytic system, which produce several inflammatory mediators [8–10]. Table 4.1 summarizes the main chemical mediators of inflammation. Acute inflammation is characterized by the following major regional components.

4.3.1.1.1   Local Vascular Changes

1. Vasodilation following transient vasoconstriction is one of the most important changes that accompany acute inflammation, and it persists until the end of the process. It involves first the arterioles and then results in the opening of new capillary beds in the area.
2. Increased vascular permeability due to:
   - Contraction of endothelial cells with widening of intercellular gaps.
   - Direct endothelial injury, resulting in endothelial cell necrosis and detachment.
   - Leukocyte-mediated endothelial injury: Leukocytes adhere to the endothelium, which becomes activated, thereby releasing toxic oxygen species and proteolytic enzymes and causing endothelial injury.

   - Angiogenesis: Endothelial cells may proliferate and form new capillaries and venular beds. These capillary sprouts remain leaky until endothelial cells differentiate.
3. Stasis (slowing of circulation) resulting from increased permeability with extravasation of fluid into the extravascular spaces causing the concentration of red blood cells in the small vessels and increased viscosity of blood and slowing of circulation in the local vessels

Figures 4.3 and 4.4 illustrate the main vascular changes.

4.3.1.1.2   Formation of Exudate

Increased permeability of the microvasculature, along with the other changes described, leads to leakage of "exudate," an inflammatory extravascular fluid with a high protein content and cellular debris with a specific gravity of above 1.020. This is the hallmark of acute inflammation, which may also be called exudative inflammation. Exudate varies in composition. In early or mild

Table 4.1 Chemical mediators of inflammation

Mediator	Characteristics and role in inflammation
A. *Cell factors*	
Histamine	Stored in mast cells, basophil and eosinophil leukocytes, and platelets
Release from sites of storage is stimulated by complement components C3a and C5a and by lysosomal proteins released from neutrophils	
Responsible for vasodilation and the immediate phase of increased vascular permeability	
Lysosomal compound	Released from neutrophils and includes cationic proteins, which may increase vascular permeability, and neutral proteases, which may activate complement
Prostaglandins	Long-chain fatty acids derived from arachidonic acid and synthesized by many cell types. Some prostaglandins potentiate the increase in vascular permeability caused by other compounds
Leukotrienes	Synthesized from arachidonic acid, especially in neutrophils, and have vasoactive properties
5-Hydroxytryptamine (serotonin)	A potent vasoconstrictor present in high concentrations in mast cells and platelets
Lymphokines	Released by lymphocytes and may have vasoactive or chemotactic effects
B. *Plasma factors*	
Products of complement activation	
C5a	Chemotactic for neutrophils, increases vascular permeability, releases histamine from mast cells
C3a	Similar to but less active than C5a
C567	Chemotactic for neutrophils
C56789	Cytolytic activity
C4b, 2a, 3b	Facilitates phagocytosis of bacteria by macrophages (opsonization of bacteria)
Kinin system	Bradykinin included in the system is the most important vascular permeability factor, also a mediator for pain which is a major feature of acute inflammation
Coagulation factors	Responsible for the conversion of soluble fibrinogen into fibrin, a major component of the acute inflammatory exudate
Fibrinolytic system	Plasmin included in the fibrinolytic system is responsible for the lysis of fibrin into fibrin degradation products, which have a local effect on vascular permeability

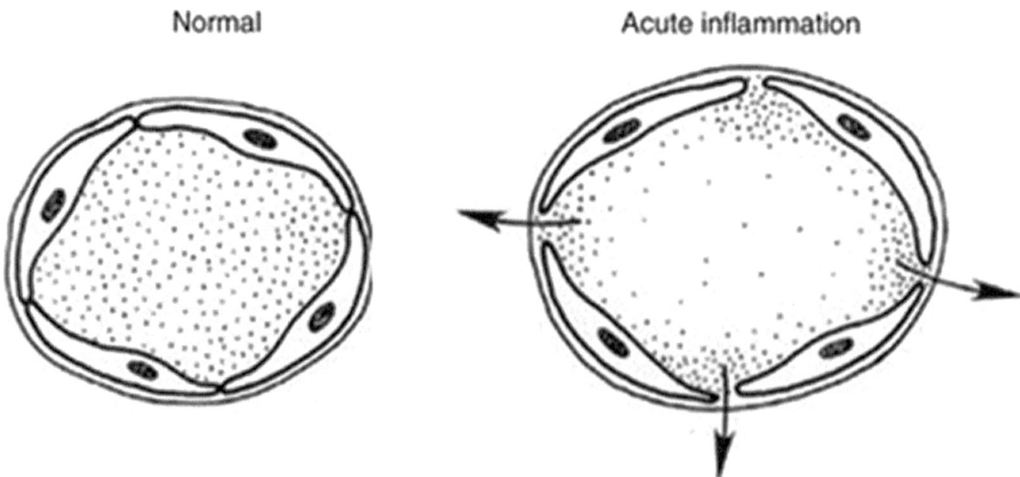

Fig. 4.3 Diagram illustrating the vasodilation of vessels and opening of the intercellular gaps in infammation

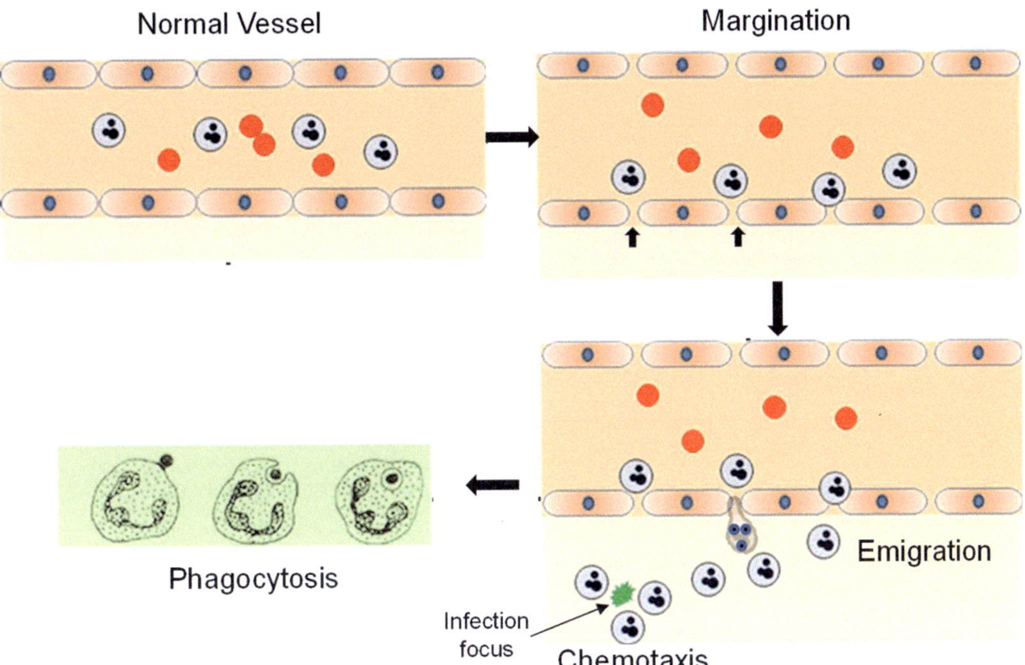

Fig. 4.4 Sequence of cellular changes that accompany inflammation

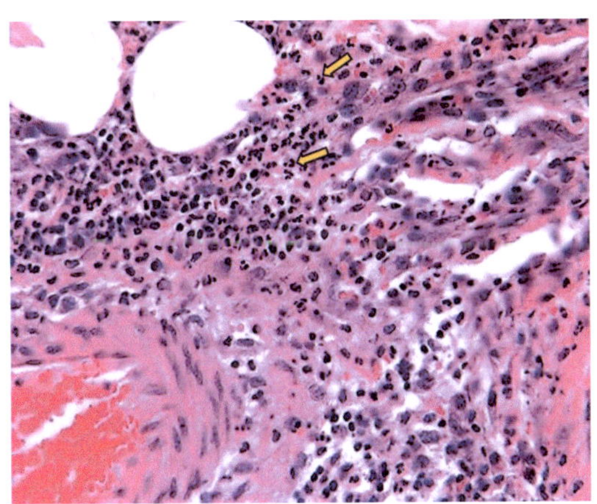

Fig. 4.5 Microphotograph of acute inflammation showing numerous inflammatory cells particularly polymorphonuclear leukocytes (arrows)

inflammation, it may be watery (serous exudate) with low plasma protein content and few leukocytes. In more advanced inflammation, the exudate becomes thick and clotted (fibrinous exudate). When large numbers of leukocytes accumulate (Fig. 4.5), the exudate consists of pus and is called suppurative, while if it contains erythrocytes due to bleeding, it is referred to as hemorrhagic. Pus, accordingly, is a variant of exudate that is particularly rich in leukocytes, mostly neutrophils and parenchymal cell debris. Exudate should be differentiated from "transudate," which is a fluid with low protein concentration and a specific gravity of less than 1.012. Transudation is associated with normal endothelial permeability [7, 8].

4.3.1.1.3   Local Cellular Events

1. Margination: After stasis develops, leukocytes will be peripherally oriented along the vascular endothelium, a process called leukocytic margination (Fig. 4.4).
2. Emigration (diapedesis): Leukocytes emigrate from the microcirculation and accumulate at the site of injury.
3. Chemotaxis: Once outside the blood vessel, the cells migrate at varying rates of speed in interstitial tissue toward a chemotactic stimulus in the inflammatory focus. Granulocytes, including the eosinophils,

basophils, and some lymphocytes, respond to such stimuli and aggregate at the site of inflammation. The primary chemotactic factors include bacterial products, complement components C5a and C3a, kallikrein and plasminogen activators, products of fibrin degradation, prostaglandins, and fibrinopeptides. Histamine is not a chemotactic factor but facilitates the process. Some bacterial toxins, particularly from gram-negative bacteria and streptococcal streptolysins, inhibit neutrophil chemotaxis [6–8].

4. Phagocytosis: This defense mechanism is particularly important in bacterial infections. The polymorphonuclear leukocytes and macrophages ingest debris and foreign particles.

4.3.1.2 Local Sequelae of Acute Inflammation

Acute inflammation has several possible local sequelae. These include resolution, suppuration (formation of pus), organization, and progression to chronic inflammation. Resolution means complete restoration of tissues to normal. Organization of tissues is their replacement by granulation tissue with formation of large amounts of fibrin, new capillaries growing into fibrin, macrophages migrating into the zone, and proliferation of fibroblasts resulting in fibrosis and the consequent organization of exudate.

4.3.1.3 Chronic Inflammation

Acute inflammation may progress to a chronic form characterized by reduction of the number of polymorphonuclear leukocytes and proliferation of fibroblasts with collagen production. Chronic inflammation may be primary with no preceding acute inflammatory reaction. Chronic inflammation, whether following acute inflammation or not, is characterized by a proliferative (fibroblastic) rather than an exudative response with predominantly mononuclear cell infiltration (macrophages, lymphocytes, and plasma cells) (Fig. 4.6). Abnormal vascular permeability is also common, but to a lesser extent than in acute inflammation with formation of new capillaries.

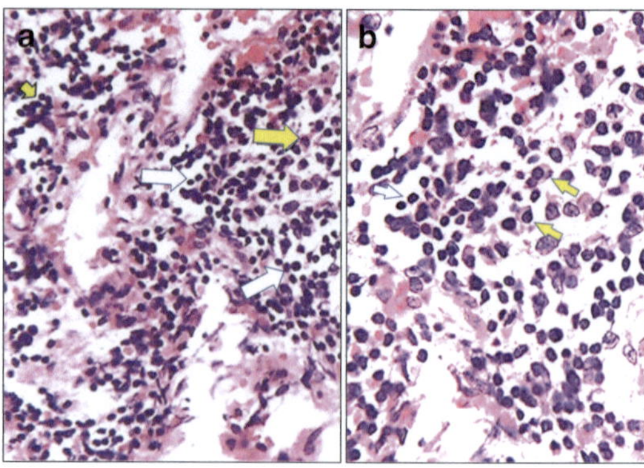

Fig. 4.6 Low power (**a**) and (**b**) Higher power microphotograph of chronic inflammation illustrating the different types of inflammatory cells, the mononuclear cells including lymphocytes (yellow *arrows*) and plasma cells (white *arrows*)

4.3.1.4 Abscess Formation

Abscess is defined as a collection of pus in tissues, organs, or confined spaces and usually caused by bacterial infection. The abscess formation starts by a phase of cellulitis, characterized by hyperemia, leukocytosis, and edema, without cellular necrosis or suppuration. This stage is also called phlegmon. It may be followed by necrosis, liquefaction, and formation of pyogenic membrane surrounding the pus, which results in abscess formation that can be present with both acute and chronic inflammation.

4.3.2 Systemic Pathophysiological Changes of Inflammation

Three major systemic changes are associated with inflammation: leukocytosis, fever, and an increase in plasma proteins. Leukocytosis is an increased production of leukocytes due to stimulation by several products of inflammation such as complement C3a and colony-stimulating factors. A febrile response is due to the pyrogens. The increase in plasma proteins is due to stimulation of the liver by some products of inflammation, leading to increased synthesis of certain proteins referred to as acute-phase reactants which include C-reactive protein, fibrinogen, and haptoglobin as anti-inflammatory [7].

4.3.3 Pathophysiological Changes of Healing

Healing of tissue after injury is closely linked to inflammation since it starts by acute inflammation. Healing may lead to restoration of normal structure and function of the injured tissue (resolution) or to the formation of a scar consisting of collagen (repair) when resolution is not achieved because the tissue is severely injured or cannot regenerate.

In either case, acute inflammation occurs first and for this reason is considered the defensive phase of healing. Healing (resolution and repair) occurs in two overlapping phases, reconstruction and maturation. The reconstructive phase starts 3–4 days after injury, continues for approximately 2 weeks, and is characterized by fibroblasts followed by collagen synthesis. The maturation phase is characterized by cell differentiation, scar formation, and remodeling of the scar; it begins several weeks after injury and may take up to 2 years to complete.

4.4 Pathophysiology of Major Soft Tissue Inflammation

4.4.1 Abdominal Inflammation

There are several types of abdominal infection: abscess, cellulitis (phlegmon), i.e., early inflammation of the soft tissue prior to or without formation of an abscess, and peritonitis. Abscesses can fall into three categories:

1. Intraperitoneal abscess.
2. Retroperitoneal abscess.
3. Visceral abscess (hepatic, pancreatic, splenic).

The organisms causing abscesses may reach the tissue by direct implantation such as penetrating trauma and may spread from contiguous infection through hematogenous or lymphatic routes from a distant site or through migration of resistant flora into an adjacent, normally sterile area such as in perforation of an abdominal viscus. Factors predisposing to abscess formation include impaired host defense mechanisms, trauma/surgery, obstruction of urinary, biliary, or respiratory passages, foreign bodies, chemical or immunological irritation, and ischemia. Abdominal surgery (particularly of the colon, appendix, and biliary tree) and trauma are the most common; less common are appendicitis, diverticulitis, and pelvic inflammatory disease. Management of these infections requires prompt recognition, early localization, and effective drainage, as well as appropriate antimicrobial use. Once the diagnosis is made and the abscess is localized, treatment should begin promptly. Localization is crucial since, for example, percutaneous drainage is inappropriate for abscesses in certain locations such as the posterior subphrenic space or in the porta hepatis [9]. Accumulation of leukocytes in the abscess is the pathophysiological basis for using labeled white blood cells for abscess imaging. In the acute phase, migration of leukocytes is vigorous. Later, the migration rate slows down and the cell type changes from predominantly neutrophils to mononuclear cells (lymphocytes, plasma cells, and macrophages). This pathophysiological change associated with the chronic state explains the better diagnostic accuracy of labeled leukocyte scans in acute as opposed to chronic abscesses. *Inflammatory Bowel Disease (IBD):* IBD is an idiopathic disease, probably involving an immune reaction of the body to its own intestinal tract tissue. The two major types of IBD are ulcerative colitis (UC) and Crohn's disease (CD) [10–12].

In UC, inflammation always begins in the rectum, extends proximally a certain distance, and then abruptly stops. A clear demarcation exists between involved and uninvolved mucosa. The rectum is always involved in UC and may remain confined to the rectum in approximately 25% of cases. Pancolitis occurs in 10% of patients. UC primarily involves the mucosa and the submucosa, with formation of crypt abscesses and mucosal ulceration. In severe UC, inflammation and necrosis can in rare cases extend below the lamina propria to involve the submucosa and the circular and longitudinal muscles. Crohn's disease, on the other hand, consists of segmental involvement by a nonspecific granulomatous inflammatory process. The most important pathological feature is the involvement of all layers of the bowel, not just the mucosa and the submucosa, as is characteristic of UC. Furthermore, CD is discontinuous with skip areas interspersed between one and more involved areas [10–12] (see also Chap. 10).

4.4.2 Chest Inflammation

The chest is a common site of various types of infection, acute and chronic. Such infections are frequent in the elderly and in immunosuppressed patients, including cancer patients. Common inflammatory conditions relevant to nuclear medicine include pneumonia, sarcoidosis, diffuse interstitial fibrosis, and *Pneumocystis (jirovecii) carinii* pneumonia (see also Chap. 8).

4.4.2.1 Sarcoidosis
Sarcoidosis is an inflammatory condition of uncertain etiology characterized by the presence of noncaseating granulomas involving multiple organs. Current evidence points to a genetic predisposition and exposure to as yet unknown transmissible agent(s) and/or environmental factors as etiological agents [13]. The lung is most commonly and usually the first site of involvement. The inflammatory processes extend through the lymphatics to the hilar and mediastinal nodes. The lung is involved in more than 90% of cases. Pulmonary sarcoidosis starts as diffuse interstitial alveolitis, followed by the characteristic granulomas. Granulomas are present in the alveolar septa as well as in the walls of the bronchi and pulmonary arteries and veins. The center of the granuloma contains epithelioid cells derived from mononuclear phagocytes, multinucleated giant cells, and macrophages. Lymphocytes, macrophages, monocytes, and fibroblasts are present at the periphery of the granuloma. The diagnosis is based on a compatible clinical and/or radiological picture, histopathological evidence of noncaseating granulomas in tissue biopsy specimens, and exclusion of other diseases capable of producing similar clinical or histopathological appear-

ances. Even microscopically, the noncaseating granulomas are not specific [13]. Infection by mycobacterial species other than *Mycobacterium tuberculosis* frequently leads to the production of noncaseating granulomas [14]. The disease runs a benign course with spontaneous remission of the activity though some degree of residual pulmonary function abnormality persists. Only a minority of patients develop complicated disease, which may lead to blindness, renal failure, liver failure, and heart involvement.

4.4.2.2 *Pneumocystis Carinii (Jirovecii)* Pneumonia
Pneumocystis carinii (jirovecii) pneumonia (PCP is a condition that may be endemic or epidemic). It is caused by *Pneumocystis carinii (jirovecii)*, which is a fungus. The condition is common in premature infants, debilitated children, and other immunocompromised conditions, particularly the acquired immune deficiency syndrome (AIDS). It is also seen in congenital immunodeficiency and in patients who are receiving chemotherapy and corticosteroids [15]. It is the most common infection in AIDS patients, and it remains an important cause of morbidity and mortality . Transmission is usually airborne. The pathological changes are predominantly in the lungs with an inflammatory reaction consisting of plasma cells of variable amount, monocytes, and histiocytes. The diagnosis is established through identification of the organisms in bronchial secretions obtained by bronchoalveolar lavage or bronchial washings. Gallium-67 is an important imaging modality that helps in the diagnosis and evaluation of the activity of the disease.

4.4.2.3 Idiopathic Pulmonary Fibrosis
Idiopathic pulmonary fibrosis, a sometimes fatal condition, is characterized by parenchymal inflammation and interstitial fibrosis. The pathological changes start with alveolitis followed by derangement of the alveolar-capillary units, leading to the end stage of fibrosis. There is a correlation between the inflammatory activity and the amount of gallium-67 activity in the lungs [16].

4.4.3   Renal Inflammation

Urinary tract infection (UTI) is common particularly in children. There are two main varieties of acute renal infection: cystitis (pyelitis), which is confined to the bladder or renal pelvis, and pyelonephritis, where the renal parenchyma is also involved. It is not always possible to differentiate between the two conditions on clinical grounds. The importance of the acute renal infections lies in the fact that recurrent subclinical attacks are believed to be significant in the pathogenesis of chronic pyelonephritis [17]. The number of patients with chronic kidney disease and consequent end-stage renal disease is rising worldwide (see also Chap. 7).

4.4.3.1   Acute Pyelonephritis

Many conditions and clinical situations are associated with an increased risk of pyelonephritis. Pyelonephritis is significantly more common in females than in males (more so in whites). Approximately 10–30% of women develop a symptomatic UTI at some point in their lives. Acute pyelonephritis is a bacterial infection of the kidney with acute inflammation of the pyelocaliceal lining and renal parenchyma centrifugally along medullary rays. This can occur in more than one route. Most often it occurs because of ascending infection from the lower urinary tract. Hematogenous spread to the kidney by gram positive and less likely by gram-negative organisms can also occur. Grossly, the kidney is enlarged and edematous. The cut surface may show small abscesses in the cortex, and more often there are wedge-shaped purulent areas streaking upward from the medulla, with normal areas of kidney tissue intervening in between infected zones. Frequently, the pelvis and calyces are inflamed and dilated. In severe infection, renal papillary necrosis may be present. Microscopically, there is intense inflammation, with infiltration of polymorphonuclear leukocytes throughout the interstitial tissue and abscess formation. There is destruction of the tubules, but the glomeruli and blood vessels are often unaffected.

4.4.3.2   Chronic Pyelonephritis

Chronic pyelonephritis is a chronic condition affecting the pelvis and parenchyma and resulting from recurrent or persistent renal infection. It occurs almost exclusively in patients with major anatomical anomalies, including urinary tract obstruction, calculi, renal dysplasia, or, most commonly, vesicoureteral reflux (VUR) in young children. Grossly, the kidney shows normal areas alternating with zones of scarring. Wedge-shaped scars can be seen on the subcapsular surface of the kidney. The appearance differs, depending on the presence or absence of obstruction. Chronic pyelonephritis in the presence of intra- or extrarenal obstruction shows dilatation of the pelvocalyceal system and sometimes peripelvic fibrosis. If no obstruction is present, the pelvic change is in the form of peripelvic fibrosis rather than dilatation. Microscopically, the scarred areas show changes in the interstitium and tubules. The interstitial tissue shows infiltration by predominantly lymphocytes and plasma cells. The tubules become atrophic and may collapse. The glomeruli may be normal in some cases, while in others periglomerular fibrosis is present.

4.4.4   Scrotal Inflammation

Inflammation of the epididymis (epididymis) is common, and sometimes it involves testicles (epididymo-orchitis). The condition may be infectious or noninfectious. Noninfectious may follow urinary obstruction or can be drug-induced. It can affect children and adults. Bacterial ascent through the urogenital tract is the most common etiology in acute infectious epididymitis (see Chap. 7).

4.4.5   Cellulitis

Cellulitis describes infection of the dermis and subcutaneous tissues which lead to pain, erythema, edema, and warmth. It results from disruption of the skin and invasion by microorganisms. Peripheral vascular disease and diabetes increase susceptibility to this form of infection because minor injuries to the skin in the feet or toes can serve as entry points for infection. Other patients susceptible to cellulitis include those with foreign bodies penetrating the skin, such as intravenous catheters and orthopedic hardware. There is a risk for rapid spread of infection in patients with diabetes, immunodeficiency, impaired peripheral circulation, or a history of lymphadenectomy with cellulitis [18].

4.4.6 Endocarditis

Endocarditis is the inflammation of endocardium which may be infective or noninfective. Infective endocarditis is usually caused by bacteria, commonly, streptococci or staphylococci, or fungi. It may present with fever, heart murmurs, embolic phenomena, petechiae, anemia, and endocardial vegetations. Vegetations may lead to valvular incompetence or narrowing, myocardial abscess, or mycotic aneurysm. Noninfective endocarditis on the other hand is characterized by accumulation of sterile platelet and fibrin thrombi on cardiac valves and adjacent endocardium. Noninfective endocarditis may sometimes lead to infective endocarditis. Both conditions can result in embolization and impaired cardiac function. Pathophysiologically, the condition develops in 3 stages; Bacteremia, adhesion (microorganisms adhere to the surface of abnormal or damaged endothelium), and colonization with proliferation of the microorganism leading to inflammation and formation of vegetations. The disease may lead to local and systemic sequalae. Local sequalae include myocardial abscesses, valvular regurgitation which if severe may lead to heart failure and death. Aortitis may also occur due to local spread of infection. Prosthetic valve infections are particularly associated with local consequences. Systemic complications are predominantly due to embolization from vegetations on valvular surfaces. Pulmonary infarction, pneumonia, or empyema may follow right sided lesions while left sided lesions may lead to emboli of kidneys, spleen, central nervous system, skin, and retina [19].(see Chap. 9).

4.4.7 Thyroid Gland Inflammation

Thyroiditis is a group of inflammatory thyroid diseases. It may affect the gland diffusely or focally and can be due to infection by microorganisms or noninfectious. There are many classifications and terminologies for the condition based on clinical, histopathologic, etiology, and other factors. Simply it can be classified into acute, subacute, and chronic.

Acute thyroiditis is a rare but serious form secondary to bacteria. Subacute thyroiditis is a painful, inflammatory disease of viral origin. Hashimoto's thyroiditis is chronic thyroiditis due to autoimmune pathogenesis, and patients may be euthyroid, develop hypothyroidism, or thyrotoxicosis that is usually transient. Silent and postpartum thyroiditis is also of autoimmune origin, occurring either sporadically or postpartum and clinically present with transient thyrotoxicosis. Riedel's thyroiditis is a rare chronic inflammatory disorder of uncertain etiology, characterized by dense thyroid fibrosis (see Chap. 6).

4.5 Pathophysiology of Major Skeletal Inflammations

Osteomyelitis indicates an infection involving the cortical bone as well as the marrow. Like many other pathological conditions of the bone, infections cause reactive new bone formation which—among other factors, particularly increased blood flow—is the principal reason for the accumulation of bone-seeking radiopharmaceuticals at the site of skeletal infections [20]. It is difficult to draw the line between acute and chronic osteomyelitis. Chronic osteomyelitis can occur after a duration as short as 5 days or as long as 6 weeks. Acute septic arthritis is a medical emergency, since it may result in destruction of the articular cartilage and permanent disability if treatment is delayed [21]. See Chap. 5 for more details on skeletal inflammations and their imaging.

4.6   Radiopharmaceuticals for Inflammation Imaging

Many radioisotopes have been used to detect and localize infection (see Table 4.2). Since there are limitations to the radiopharmaceuticals available for imaging infection, the search continues for better agents with ideal properties. Several mechanisms explain the uptake of the currently available radiotracers at the site of infection:

Several mechanisms explain the uptake of the currently available radiotracers at the site of infection:

1. Increased vascular permeability.
   - $^{67}Ga/^{68}Ga$-citrate
   - ^{111}In and ^{99m}Tc-human polyclonal IgG
   - ^{111}In monoclonal IgM antibody
   - ^{111}In and ^{99m}Tc-liposomes

Table 4.2 Radiopharmaceuticals for imaging inflammation/infection [22–29]

Gallium-67 citrate
Gallium-68 citrate,Gallium-68 transferrin
Labeled WBCs using ^{111}In-oxine or ^{99m}Tc-HMPAO (^{99m}Tc-hexamethylpropyleneamine oxime)
Labeled particles
Nanocolloid
Liposomes
Labeled large protein
Nonspecific immunoglobulins
Specific immunoglobulins: Polyclonal and monoclonal
Antigranulocyte monoclonal antibodies
Anti-E-selectin antibodies
Labeled receptor-specific small proteins and peptides
Chemotactic peptides
Interleukins
Labeled antibiotics: Ciprofloxacin
^{18}F-FDG
Labeled vitamin B
In-111 biotin

- ^{111}In-biotin and streptavidin
- ^{99m}Tc-nanocolloids
- ^{111}In-chloride.

2. Migration of WBCs/antibodies to the site of infection.
   - ^{111}In-and ^{99m}Tc-labeledleukocytes
   - ^{99m}Tc anti-WBC antibodies.
3. Binding to proteins at the site of infection.
   - $^{67}Ga/^{68}Ga$-citrate (lactoferrin and other iron-containing proteins).
4. Binding to WBCs at the site of infection.
   - Chemotactic peptides.
   - Interleukins.
5. Binding to bacteria.
   - ^{99m}Tc-labeled ciprofloxacin antibiotic
   - $^{67}Ga/^{68}Ga$-citrate.
6. Metabolic trapping, i.e., ^{18}F-fluorodeoxyglucose.

The multiple mechanisms of uptake of gallium by inflammatory tissue include the following:

1. Increased vascular permeability.
2. Gallium-67-binding substances at site of inflammation.
   - Transferrin (due to leakage of plasma proteins).
   - Lactoferrin (secreted with lysosomal contents of stimulated or dead neutrophils).
   - Siderophores produced by bacteria.
3. Leukocytes: direct uptake.
4. Bacteria: direct uptake.

Indium-111 leukocyte imaging accuracy is best for relatively acute infections (less than 2 weeks) but yielded a 27% false-negative rate among patients with prolonged infections [30]. On the other hand, 67 Ga imaging had its highest sensitivity in long-standing processes, with false-negative results of 19% in relatively acute infections of less than 1 week duration. Thus, 111 In- or 99 m Tc-labeled WBCs are more suitable for acute infections of short duration, while 67 Ga labeling is better for infections of longer duration. Table 4.3 lists the main advantages and

Table 4.3 Advantages and disadvantages of the main availabsputum, GI bleedingle radiopharmaceuticals for inflammation

	Gallium-67 citrate	[111]In WBC	^{99m}Tc-WBC	FDG-PET/CT
Advantages	Whole-body imaging	Whole-body imaging	Whole-body imaging\ earlier diagnosis (2–4 h). Better physical characteristics of technetium than ^{67}Ga and ^{111}In	Whole-body imaging. Early results
Disadvantages	Results after 24 h or more. Physiological liver, spleen, and bowel activity. Uptake in tumors	Tedious procedure. Results at 24 h. Physiological liver and spleen activity	Tedious procedure. Physiological bowel activity by 2 h	High radiation dose

disadvantages of the major radiopharmaceuticals used for inflammation imaging. Several monoclonal antibodies are also used to detect infections. These antibodies are mainly directed against receptors on inflammatory cells. Anti-CD15 (LeuTech) contains a murine IgM anti-CD15 monoclonal antibody. It binds to CD15 antigens expressed on the surface of human neutrophils. The basis of this is the elevated level of CD15 epitope in activated neutrophils, which should make them good targets for imaging with a monoclonal antibody. The advantages of this tracer include easy preparation since it takes about 30 min. Imaging begins immediately and diagnostic images are usually obtained within 30 min [31, 32]. Another method is the use of 99 m Tc-anti-NCA −90 Fab' fragments (nonspecific cross-reacting antigen), LeukoScan, Sulesomab. The 99 m Tc-anti-NCA −90 Fab' fragments can recognize a specific cross-reacting antigen (NCA-90) (the surface antigenic glycoprotein) on granulocytes, promyelocytes, and myelocytes [33]. LeukoScan uptake at the site of infection is explained partly by the migration of circulating antibody-labeled granulocytes to the site of infection. LeukoScan uptake is also explained by the fact that the greater proportion of the labeled antibody fragment is in a free soluble form which can easily cross capillary membranes, binding to the leukocyte once in situ. This mechanism is favored by the increased capillary permeability at the site of infection. An important advantage of LeukoScan is the 5-min preparation time. Despite the fact that LeukoScan involves

the i.v. injection of mouse proteins, no anaphylactic or other hypersensitivity reactions were observed. 99 m Tc-ciprofloxacin (Infecton) is also being used to image infection. Ciprofloxacin is a broad spectrum fluoroquinolone antibiotic. Patients receive 99 m Tc-ciprofloxacin 10 mCi, and images are obtained at 1, 3–4, and, occasionally, 24 h post injection. 99 m Tc-ciprofloxacin may be useful for distinguishing infection from inflammation. Early images of noninfectious rheumatologic inflammatory conditions were positive, but activity decreased with time [34]. 111 In- and 99 m Tc-labeled chemotactic peptide analogs have been used for detecting and localizing infections. Imaging can be performed at less than 3 h post injection, which compares favorably with the 18–24 h or more for most other agents [20]. Labeled liposomes have been used for scintigraphic imaging of infection and inflammation. The uptake of 111 In-labeled sterically stabilized liposomes (long circulating) in abscess was found to be twice as high as that of IgG, and the abscess was visualized as early as 1 h post injection [35]. 18 F-fluorodeoxyglucose (FDG) has emerged as an important diagnostic agent for infectious and noninfectious soft tissue and skeletal inflammations including inflammatory bowel disease, fevers of unknown origin, rheumatologic disorders, tuberculosis infection, fungal infection, pneumonia, abscess, postarthroplasty infections, chronic and vertebral osteomyelitis, sarcoidosis, and chemotherapy-induced pneumonitis [36–39]. Inflammatory conditions show high FDG uptake which is related to increased glucose metabolism that is produced by stimulated inflammatory cells, macrophage proliferation, and healing [40]. While uptake of FDG continues to increase at malignant sites for several hours, as can be shown by an incremental increase of the standardized uptake values (SUV), inflammatory lesions peak at approximately 60 min, and their SUV either stabilize or decline thereafter. This difference in the behavior of FDG in malignant versus inflammatory cells can be explained best by the varying levels of enzymes that degrade deoxyglucose-6- phosphate in the respective cells. Glucose-6- phosphatase dephosphorylates intracellular FDG-6-phosphate, allowing it to leave the cell. It has been shown that most tumor cells have low levels of this enzyme, while its expression is high in the mononuclear cells [41]. For this reason, imaging at two time points after administration of FDG may prove to be important in differentiating between these two common disorders.

4.7 Infection/Inflammation Imaging

Diagnosis and localization of infection by clinical and laboratory methods are often difficult. The results frequently are nonspecific, and imaging may be needed. Imaging of infection may be achieved by either nuclear medicine or other strictly morphological methods. Several nuclear medicine modalities are used to diagnose and localize soft tissue and skeletal infections. These include 111 In-labeled white blood cells, 67 Ga-citrate, IgG polyclonal antibodies labeled with 111 In or 99 m Tc, monoclonal antibodies such as antigranulocyte antibodies, 99 m Tc-HMPAO labeled white blood cells, 99 m Tc-DMSA, 99 m Tc-glucoheptonate, 99 m Tc-MDP multiphase bone scan, 111 In-labeled chemotactic peptide analogs, and 18 F-FDG. Morphological modalities including X-ray, CT, MRI, and ultrasonography are important in the diagnosis and localization of both soft tissue and skeletal inflammations. These studies are complementary to the physiological modalities of nuclear medicine.

4.7.1 Imaging of Soft Tissue Infections

The strategy for imaging soft tissue infections depends on its pathophysiological and clinical features, including whether localizing signs and symptoms are present and the location and duration of the suspected infection.

4.7.1.1 Localizing Signs Present

4.7.1.1.1 Imaging Abdominal Infections
Abdominal Abscess . Rapid and accurate diagnosis of an abdominal abscess is crucial. Delayed diagnosis is associated with higher mortality in spite of treatment. If localizing signs are suggestive of abdominal infection and morphological modalities, predominantly ultrasound and CT (Figs. 4.7 and 4.8) may be used first, according to the location of suspected infection in the abdomen. The advantages of these modalities are numerous. Most importantly they provide quick results and adequate anatomical details. These studies can be used to guide needle aspiration and abscess drainage. Ultrasound can be used portably for critically ill patients. One of the major limitations of these modalities is the inability to differentiate infected from noninfected tissue abnormalities, particularly in early stages of infection (phlegmon) before the formation of abscesses. When the results of the morphological

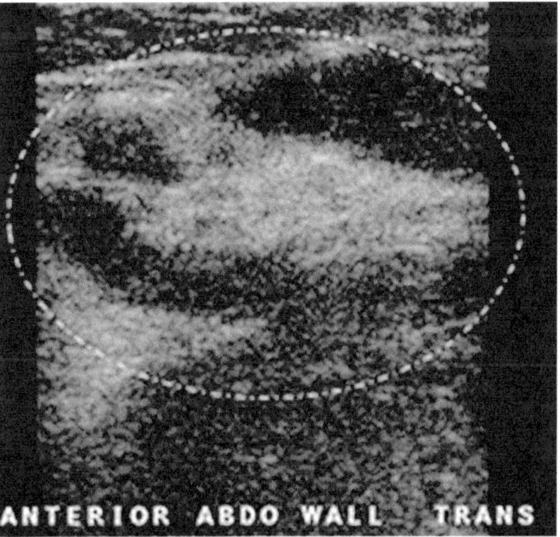

Fig. 4.7 Ultrasonography of the abdomen revealing infected hydatid liver cyst (circle)

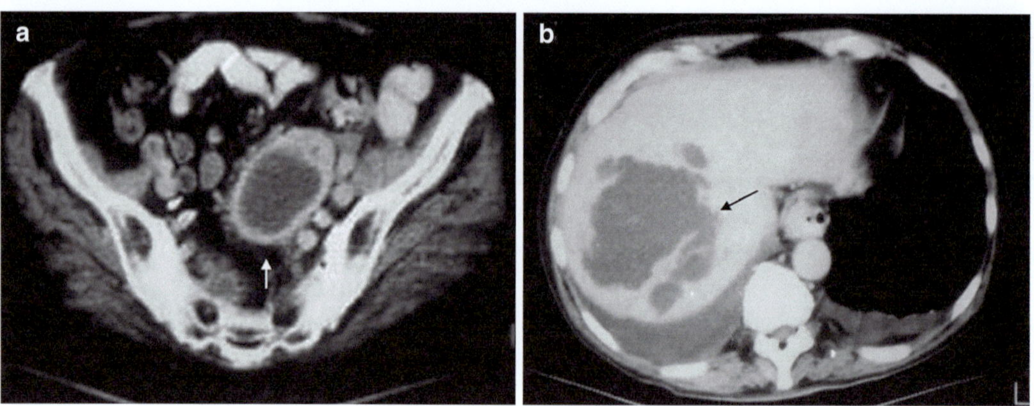

Fig. 4.8 Representative images of CT scans of the abdomen illustrating (**a**) periappendicular abscess (*arrow*) and (**b**) hepatic abscess (*arrow*)

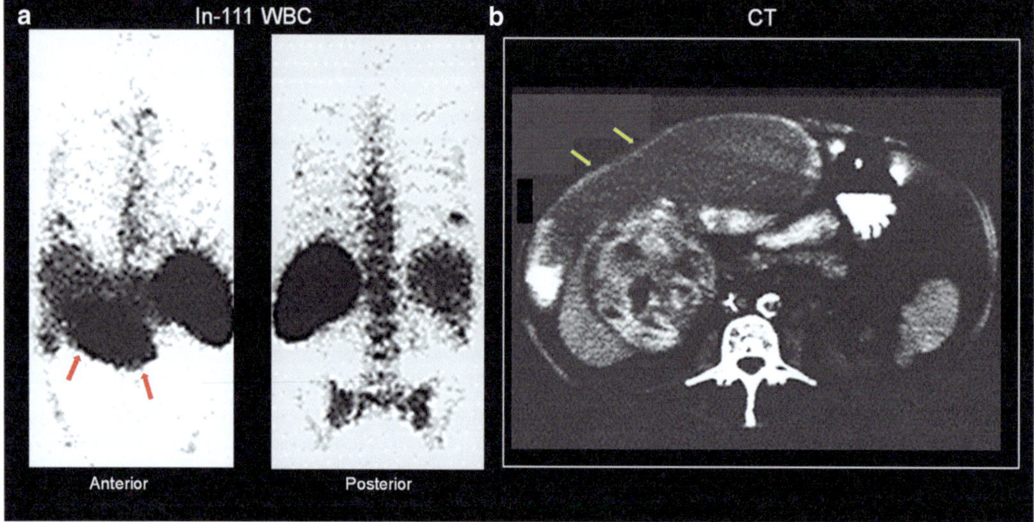

Fig. 4.9 (**a, b**) Indium-111-labeled leukocyte study (**a**) shows a large acute abdominal abscess (*arrow*) corresponding to the finding (*arrow*) on CT(**b**)

modalities are inconclusive, nuclear medicine techniques are used to detect abdominal infections. The ability to image the entire body is the major advantage of nuclear medicine modalities. Hence, radionuclide techniques are often used in cases with no localizing signs. In one study, 16% of patients suspected of having abdominal infection were shown to have extra-abdominal infections as seen on 111 In leukocyte scans [42]. Accordingly, negative morphological modalities, when used first, may be followed by whole-body nuclear imaging. Labeled WBC studies are the most specific for acute infections (Figs. 4.9 and 4.10). 67 Ga is more suitable for infection of longer duration (Fig. 4.11). 99 m Tc-HMPAO-labeled WBCs frequently used in critically ill patients after US and/or CT have yielded inconclusive results.

Inflammatory Bowel Disease (IBD). Upright chest radiography and abdominal series, barium enema and upper GI, CT scanning, MRI, or ultrasonography are used for imaging diagnosis. CT

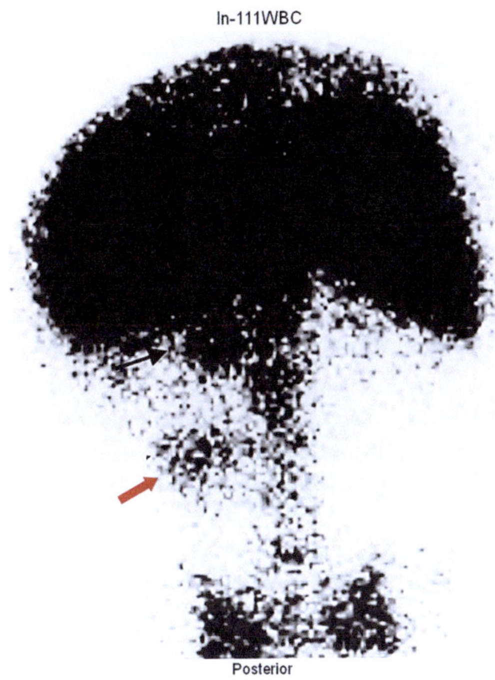

Fig. 4.10 Indium-111-labeled leukocyte scan posterior projection of the abdomen demonstrating two foci (*arrows*) of abnormal accumulation of labeled cells at the sites of the ends of a vascular graft indicating infection of the graft

scanning and ultrasonography are best for demonstrating complications such as intra-abdominal abscesses and fistulas. Evaluation of the extent of the disease and disease activity is often difficult. A wide variety of approaches depicting the different stages of the inflammatory response have been developed. Labeled WBC with 111 In or 99 m Tc is still considered the "gold standard" nuclear medicine technique for the imaging of infection and inflammation, including evaluation of IBD activity. Recently, positron emission tomography with 18 F-fluorodeoxyglucose has been shown to delineate various infectious and inflammatory disorders with high sensitivity [43, 44]. In a recent study [68], gallium, magnetic resonance imaging (MRI), and FDG-PET were compared for their ability to detect disease activity. FDG-PET showed more than twice as many lesions in the abdomen of patients with Crohn's disease as did gallium. Not all lesions shown on MRI were FDG positive, suggesting that they might represent areas of prior inflammation. FDG-PET/CT has also shown to be useful in the evaluation of its activity and response to treatment [45].

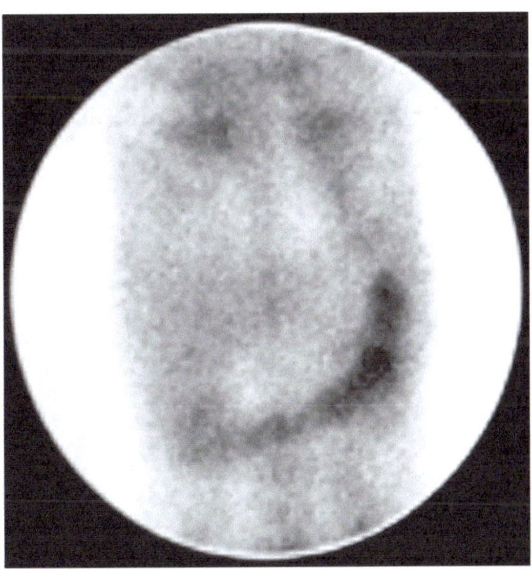

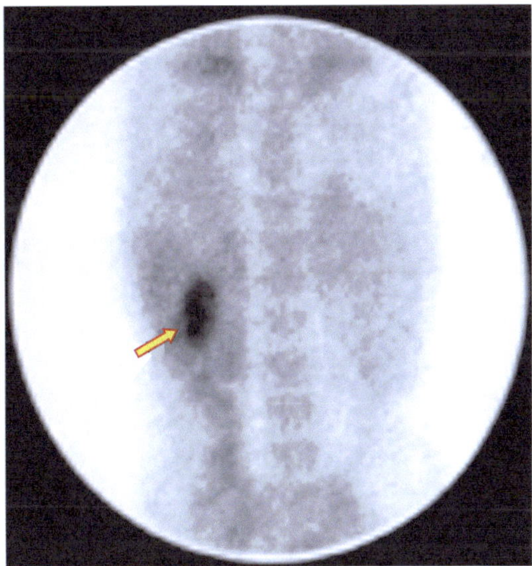

Fig. 4.11 A 72-h gallium-67 image of abdomen anterior and posterior projections for a 21-year-old female with a 6-week history of intermittent fever. No localizing signs were reported. The images demonstrate increased accumulation of gallium-67 in a perirenal abscess(*arrow*) seen in posterior view

4.7.1.1.2 Imaging Chest Infections

The role of the chest X-ray cannot be overemphasized. The chest X-ray should be used as the initial imaging modality for most chest pathologies. In many instances, however, an additional modality is needed to evaluate certain chest conditions including infections. Although CT often clearly depicts chest pathology including infections, 67 Ga still is commonly used in such cases. Siemon et al. [46] studied 67 Ga imaging in a variety of pulmonary disorders and found excellent sensitivity and specificity (Table 4.4). Gallium-67 has also been widely used in AIDS patients to detect PCP. It is highly sensitive and correlates with the response to therapy. In a study comparing 67 Ga, bronchial washing, and transbronchial biopsy in 19 patients with PCP and AIDS, 67 Ga and bronchial washing were 100% sensitive compared with 81% for transbronchial biopsy. 67 Ga is also valuable in idiopathic pulmonary fibrosis, sarcoidosis, and amiodarone toxicity. It is also useful in monitoring response to therapy of other infections including tuberculosis. In sarcoidosis, PET with 18 F-FDG allows disease activity and treatment response to be determined and is superior to 67 Ga imaging [47, 48]. 111 In-WBC imaging is less helpful, as the specificity of abnormal pulmonary uptake (either focal or diffuse) is very low. Noninfectious problems that cause abnormal uptake include congestive heart failure, atelectasis, pulmonary embolism, ARDS, and idiopathic conditions. FDG-PET has been currently used for infections including some chest infectious diseases including sarcoidosis (Fig. 4.12) and Pneumocystis jirovecii Pneumonia and interstitial lung disease (Fig. 4.13). More recently, F-18 FDG has been used for Covid-19 disease (Fig. 4.14).

Table 4.4 ^{67}Ga findings in patients with lung pathologies including infections

Pathology	Patients(n)	Ga negative(%)	Ga positive(%)
Normal	100	100	–
Active tuberculosis	197	3	97
Inactive tuberculosis	32	100	–
Pulmonary abscess	18	–	100
Asbestosis	12	–	100
Cancer	264	10	90

Data from [46]

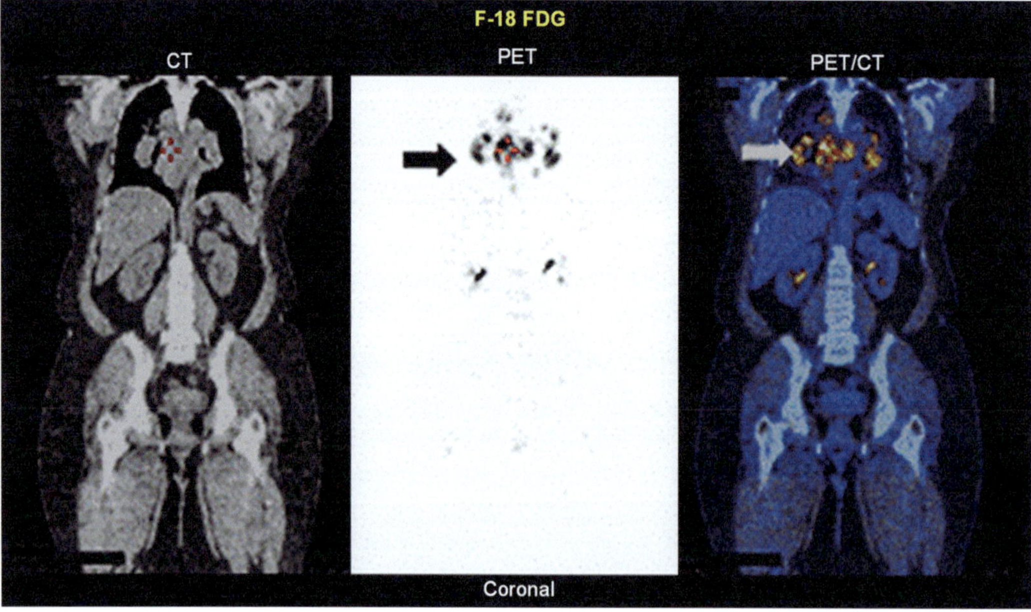

Fig. 4.12 Representative sections of F-18 FDG study in a case of pulmonary sarcoidosis illustrating uptake in bilateral hilar adenopathy (arrow)

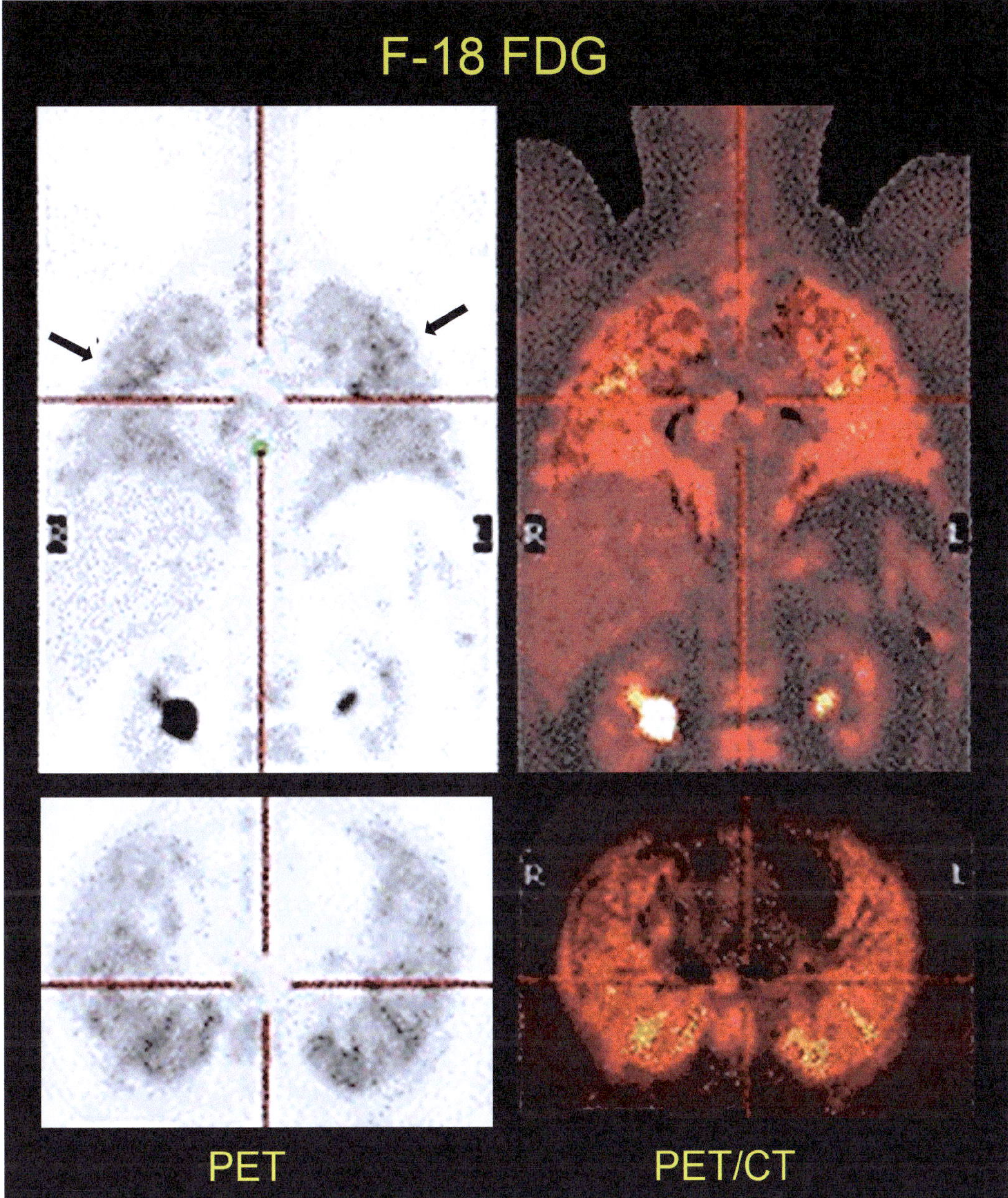

Fig. 4.13 F-18 FDG-PET/CT representative images illustrating the pattern of diffuse interstitial fibrosis with diffuse hypermetabolic activity in both lungs (arrows)

4.7.1.1.3   Imaging Renal Infections

The CT scan has good sensitivity and specificity in the diagnosis of renal infections. Ultrasound has been used frequently to evaluate the kidneys with suspected infections, even though it is not sensitive. It is used primarily to screen for obstruction or abscess when resolution of UTI is slower than expected with treatment. The sensitivity of US has been shown to be less than 60% [49, 50] and is significantly inferior to that of cortical scintigraphy (sensitivity of 86%, specificity of 81% using 99 m Tc-glucoheptonate). Positive ultrasonography can obviate the need for DMSA; however, because of a large number of false-

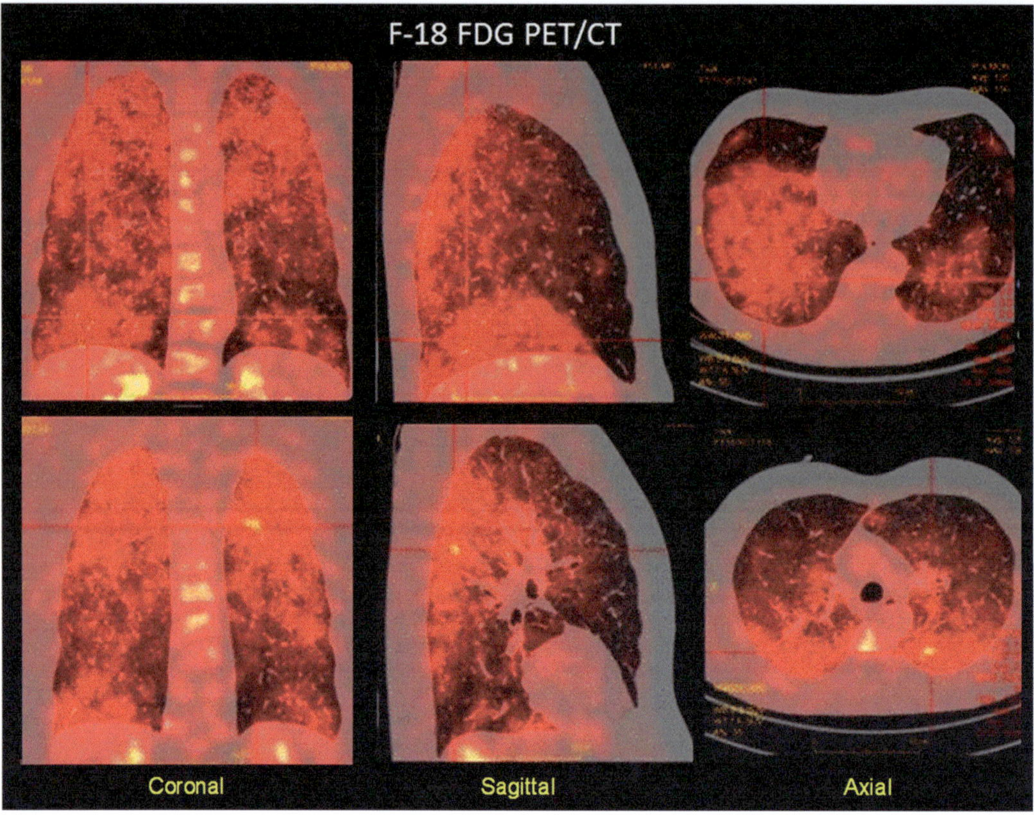

Fig. 4.14 A 70-year-old man who had interim FDG-PET/CT for his known lymphoma. No diagnosis of Covid-19 on arrival. Selected coronal sagittal and axial cuts show multiple peripheral predominantly basal infiltrates in both lungs consistent with Covid 19 which was later confirmed

negative results with reported sensitivities of 42–58% and underestimation of the pyelonephritis lesions, ultrasonography cannot replace 99 m Tc-DMSA [51, 52]. To date, 99 m Tc-DMSA is considered the most sensitive method for the detection of acute pyelonephritis in children. It also permits the photopenic area to be calculated as the inflammatory volume which correlates with the severity of infection and the possibility of scar formation even though some of the defects detected might be too small to be clinically significant. Currently US is recommended by the American Academy of Pediatrics and the National Institute for Health and Clinical Excellence (NICE) in atypical and recurrent UTI in pediatric age group [53, 54]. The pathophysiological basis of the ability of Doppler sonography in detecting acute pyelonephritis is the fact that in the acute phase of pyelonephritis, the focal decrease of renal perfusion due to edema causes vascular compression, intravascular granulocyte aggregation, or both, leading to capillary and arteriolar occlusion facilitating the detection of these hypovascular areas [55].

4.7.1.2 No Localizing Signs Present

Nuclear medicine procedures are often the imaging modalities chosen when no localizing clinical signs are present, which is common in cancer and immunosuppressed patients. The ability to screen the entire body is particularly important for such cases. The optimal choice of radiotracer again is 111-labeled white blood cells as the most specific for acute infections, but false-positive results have been reported with some tumors, swallowed infected sputum, GI bleeding, and sterile inflammation.

False-negative results have been reported in infections present for more than 2 weeks. Rarely, such false-negative results occur for infections present for only 1 week. Labeled antibodies and peptides have the potential for a specific diagnosis of infection when the localizing signs are not present. Recent studies support the use of FDG-PET in the patient with FUO and is replacing Ga-67 in cases with fever of long duration (Fig. 4.15). FDG is sensitive and its short half-life does not delay the performance of any additional radionuclide studies that might be needed. However, FDG-PET reveals infectious, noninfectious inflammatory diseases as well as malignant diseases; all are causes of fever of unknown origin.

Various chronic infectious diseases that are frequent clinical challenges are better diagnosed with the use of PET, particularly when this imaging is combined with CT. For noninfectious inflammatory diseases, FDG-PET has proved particularly helpful for the diagnosis and management of large vessels arteritis and inflammatory bowel disease [56–59]. Correlation with morphological modalities after successful radionuclide localization of infection can be of great help. For example, this correlation provides anatomical information prior to surgical interventions. Figure 4.16 illustrates suggested algorithms for the imaging diagnosis of soft tissue infections.

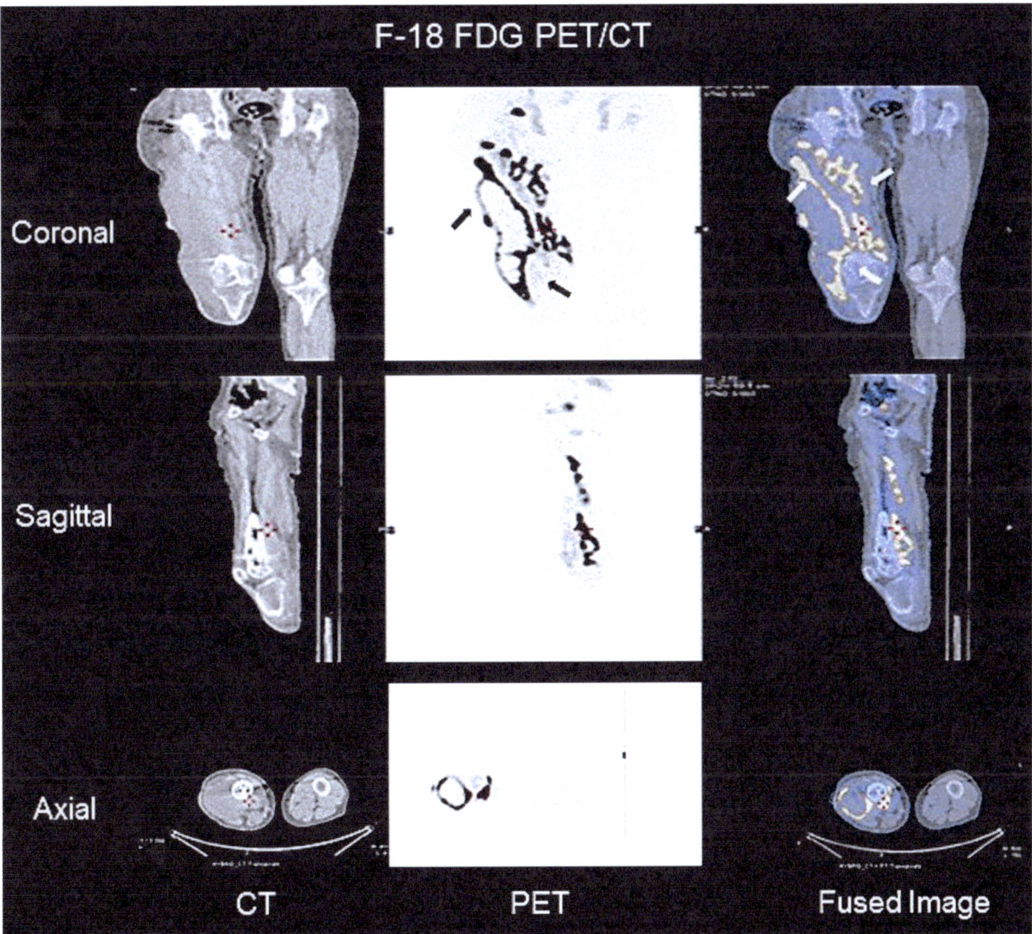

Fig. 4.15 FDG-PET study illustrating soft tissue infection with extensive uptake of the right lower extremity (arrows) of a patient with a history of traffic accident and amputation presented with fever for 3 weeks

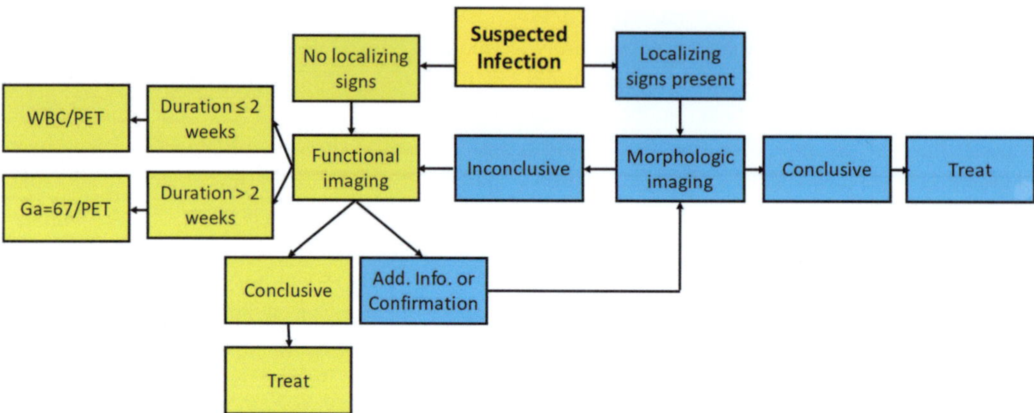

Fig. 4.16 Suggested diagnostic algorithm for soft tissue infections. Note that in case of suspected renal infection,$^{99mTc-DMSA}$scan is preferred; in infections of relatively long duration, labeled WBC may be used, but if negative, ^{67}Ga or other labeled antibodies or PET should follow before excluding chronic active infection due to possible false-negative results with labeled WBC

4.7.2 Imaging of Skeletal Infection

Several imaging techniques are being utilized for the detection of osteomyelitis including the standard radiograph, computerized tomography, magnetic resonance imaging, and several nuclear medicine modalities. The choice of modality depends on the clinical presentation, particularly its duration, the site of suspected infection, and whether the site of suspected infection has been affected by previous pathology. The pathophysiology of skeletal inflammations and relevant scintigraphic considerations are discussed in detail in Chap. 5.

References

1. Granger DN, Senchenkova E (2010) Inflammation and the microcirculation. Morgan & Claypool Life Sciences, San Rafael
2. Joost Wiersinga W, Rhodes A, Cheng AC, Peacock SJ, Prescott HC (2020) Pathophysiology, transmission, diagnosis, and treatment of coronavirus disease 2019 (COVID-19)a review. JAMA 324:782–793
3. Mc Cance KL, Huether SE (eds) (2019): Innate Immunity: Inflammation In Pathophysiology: The biologic basis for disease in adults and children, 8th edn. Elsevier, St. Louis, Missouri
4. Signore A (2013) About inflammation and infection. Signore EJNMMI Res 3:8–9
5. Nathan C (2002) Points of control in inflammation. Nature 420:846–852
6. Kumar V, Abbas A, Aster JC (2020) Robbins and Cotzan, pathologic basis of disease, 10th edn. Saunders, Philadelphia
7. Rote NSV (1998) Inflammation. In: McCance KL, Huether SE (eds) Pathophysiology, 3rd edn. Mosby, St. Louis, pp 205–236
8. Botting RM, Botting JH (2000) Pathogenesis and mechanisms of inflammation and pain: an overview. Clin Drug Investig 19(Suppl 2):1–7
9. Sirinek KR (2000) Diagnosis and treatment of intraabdominal abscesses. Surg Infect 1:31–38
10. Greth J, Torok HP, Koenig A, Folwaczny C (2004) Comparison of inflammatory bowel disease at younger and older age. Eur J Med Res 22:552–554
11. Korzenik JR (2005) Past and current theories of etiology of IBD: toothpaste, worms, and refrigerators. J Clin Gastroenterol 39:s59–s65
12. Hatoum OA, Binion DG (2005) The vasculature and inflammatory bowel disease: contribution to pathogenesis and clinical pathology. Inflammat Bowel Dis 11:304–313
13. Zumla A, James DG (1996) Granulomatous infections: etiology and classification. Clin Infect Dis 23:146–158
14. Medical Section of the American Lung Association (1997) Diagnosis and treatment of disease caused by nontuberculous mycobacteria. Am J Respir Crit Care Med 156:S1–S25
15. Wazir JF, Ansari NA (2004) *Pneumocystis carinii* infection. Update and review. Arch Pathol Lab Med 128:1023–1027
16. Beckerman C, Hoffer PB (1987) The role of gallium-67 imaging in the clinical evaluation of pulmonary disorders. In: Loken MK (ed) Pulmonary nuclear medicine. Appleton & Lange, Norwalk, p 276
17. Kasseh (1966) Pathogenesis of pyelonephritis in the kidney. In: Mostafi FK, Smith DE (eds) The kidney. Williams & Wilkins, Baltimore, pp 204–212

18. Baddour LM (2000) Cellulitis syndromes: an update. Int J Antimicrob Agents 14:113–116
19. Armstrong GP (2020. Infective endocarditis, MDS manual, 2020 update, Keynan Y, Rubinstein E (2013). Pathophysiology of infective endocarditis. Curr infect dis rep; 15:342-346]
20. Elgazzar AH, Abdel-Dayem HM (1999) Imaging skeletal infections: evolving considerations. In: Freeman LM (ed) Nuclear medicine annual. Lippincott Williams & Wilkins, Philadelphia, pp 157–191
21. Sundberg SB, Savage JP, Foster BK (1989) Technetium phosphate bone scan in the diagnosis of septic arthritis in childhood. J Pediatr Orthop 9:579–585
22. Lazzeri E, Erba P, Perri M, Doria R, Tescini C et al (2010) Clinical impact of SPECT/CT with In-111 biotin on the management of patients with suspected spine infection. ClinNucl Med 35:12–17
23. Liberatore M, Calandri E, Ciccariello G, Fioravanti M, Megna V, Rampin L, Marzola MC, Zerizer I, Al-Nahhas A, Rubello D (2010) The labeled-leukocyte scan in the study of abdominal abscesses. Mol Imaging Biol 12:563–569
24. Blazeski A, Kozloff KM, Scott PJ (2010) Besilesomab for imaging inflammation and infection in peripheral bone in adults with suspected osteomyelitis. Rep Med Imaging 3:1–11
25. Gratz S, Reize P, Pfestroff A, Höffken H (2012) Intact versus fragmented 99mTc-monoclonal antibody imaging of infection in patients with septically loosened total knee arthroplasty. J Int Med Res 40:1335–1342
26. Goldsmith SJ, Vallabhajosula S (2009) Clinically proven radiopharmaceuticals for infection imaging: mechanisms and applications. Semin Nucl Med 39:2–10
27. Sierra JM, Rodriguez-Puig D, Soriano A et al (2008) Accumulation of ^{99m}Tc-ciprofloxacin in *Staphylococcus aureus* and *Pseudomonas aeruginosa*. Antimicrob Agents Chemother 52:2691–2692
28. O'Sullivan MM, Powell N, French AP, Williams KE, Morgan JR, Williams BD (1988) Inflammatory joint disease: a comparison of liposome scanning, bone scanning and radiography. Ann Rheum Dis 47:485–491
29. Love C, Palestro CJ (2004) Radionuclide imaging of infection. J Nucl Med Tech 32:47–57
30. Sfakianakis GN, Al-SheikhW HA et al (1982) Comparison of scintigraphy with in-111 leukocytes and Ga-67 in the diagnosis of occult sepsis. J Nucl Med 23:618–626
31. Vehling D, Neurath M, Siessmeier T, Schunk K, Bartenstein P (2000) FDG-PET, antigranulocyte scintigraphy and hydro-MRI in the determination of bowel wall inflammation in Crohn's disease. In: The 47th annual meeting of the Society of Nuclear Medicine; 3–7 June 2000; St. Louis. Abstract 41
32. Kampen WU, Jaekel C, Brenner W, Czecj N, Henze E (2000) New indications for immunoscintigraphy with 99mTc-labeled anti-granulocyte antibody fragments (LeukoScan) in routine diagnostics of inflammatory diseases. In: The 47th annual meeting of the Society of Nuclear Medicine; 3–7 June 2000; St. Louis. Abstract 42
33. Becker W, Palestro CJ, Winship J, Feld T, Pinsky CM, Wolf F, Goldenberg DM (1996) Rapid imaging of infections with a monoclonal antibody fragment (Leukoscan). Clin Orthop Relat Res 329:263–272
34. Britton KE, Solanki KK, Das SS, Amaral H, Bhatnagar A, Katamihardja AHS, Malamitsi J, Moustafa H, Soroa VE, Sundram FX, Wareham DW, Padhy AK (2000) Bacterial specific imaging. [abstract]. J Nucl Med 41:11P
35. Boerman OC, Storm G, Oyen WJG, van Bloois L, van derMeer JWM (1995) Sterically stabilized liposomes labeled with in-111 to image focal infection. J Nucl Med 36:1639–1644
36. Prabhakar H, Rabinowitz C, Gibbons F, O'Donnell W, Shepard J, Aquino S (2008) Imaging features of sarcoidosis on MDCT, FDG PET, and PET/CT. AJR Am J Roentgenol 190:S1–S6
37. Love C, Marwin SE, Tomas MB, Palestro CJ (2002) Improving the specificity of 18 F-FDG imaging of painful joint prostheses. J Nucl Med 43:126P
38. Love C, Bhargava KK, Afriyie MO, Pugliese PV, Palestro CJ (2002) FDG as a screening test in patients with painful joint prostheses: a comparison with 3-phase bone scintigraphy. J Nucl Med 43:343P
39. El-Zeftawy H, LaBombardi V, Dakhel M, Heiba S, Adbel Dayem H (2002) Evaluation of 18 F-FDG PET imaging in diagnosis of disseminated *Mycobacterium avium* complex (DMAC) in AIDS patients. J Nucl Med 43:127P
40. Yamada S, Kubota K, Kubota R, Ido T, Tamahashi N (1995) High accumulation of fluorine-18-luorodeoxyglucose in turpentine-induced inflammatory tissue. J Nucl Med 36:1301–1306
41. Nelson CA, Wang JQ, Leav I, Crane PD (1996) The interaction among glucose transport, hexokinase and glucose 6-phosphate with respect to 3H-2-deoxyglucose retention in murine tumor models. Nucl Med Biol 23:533–541
42. Datz FL (1996) Abdominal abscess detection: gallium, in-111 and Tc-99 m labeled leukocytes and polyclonal and monoclonal antibodies. Semin Nucl Med 26:51–64
43. Bleeker-Rovers CP, Boerman OC, Rennen HJ, Corstens FH, Oyen WJ (2004) Radiolabeled compounds in diagnosis of infectious and inflammatory disease. Curr Pharm Des 10:2935–2950
44. Wiesner W, Steinbrich W (2003) Imaging diagnosis of inflammatory bowel disease. Ther Umsch 60:137–144
45. Spier BJ, Perlman SB, Jaskowiak CJ, Reichelderfer M (2010) PET/CT in the evaluation of inflammatory bowel disease: studies in patients before and after treatment. Mol Imaging Biol 12:85–88
46. Siemon JK, Siegfried GF, Waxman AD (1978) The use of Ga-67 in pulmonary disorders. Semin Nucl Med 3:235–249
47. Gotthardt M, Bleeker-Rovers CP, Boerman OC, Oyen WJG (2010) Imaging of inflammation by PET. Conventional scintigraphy, and other imaging techniques. J Nucl Med 51:1937–1949

48. Braun JJ, Kessler R, Constantinesco A et al (2008) 18 F-FDG PET/CT in sarcoidosis management: review and report of 20 cases. Eur J Nucl Med Mol Imaging 35:1537–1543
49. Conway JJ (1988) Role of scintigraphy in urinary tract infection. Semin Nucl Med 18:308–319
50. Mackenzie JR (1996) A review of renal scarring in children. Nucl Med Commum 17:176–190
51. Bykov S, Chervinsky L, Smolkin V, Helevi R, Garty I (2003) Power Doppler sonography versus Tc99m DMSA scintigraphy for diagnosing acute pyelonephritis in children: are these two methods comparable? Clin Nucl Med 28:198–203
52. El Hajjar M, Launay S, Hossein-Foucher C, Foulard M, Robert Y (2002) Power Doppler sonography and acute pyelonephritis in children: comparison with Tc-99 m DMSA scintigraphy. Arch Pediatr 9:21–25
53. The American Academy of Pediatrics, Subcommittee on Urinary Tract Infection, Steering Committee on Quality Improvement and Management (2011) Urinary tract infection: clinical practice guideline for the diagnosis and management of the initial UTI in febrile infants and children 2 to 24 months. Pediatrics 128(3):572–575
54. La Scola C et al (2013) Different guidelines for imaging after first UTI in febrile infants: yield, cost, and radiation. Pediatrics 131:e665–e671
55. Sakarya ME, Arslan H, Erkoc R, Bozkurt M, Atilla MK (1998) The role of power Doppler ultrasonography in the diagnosis of acute pyelonephritis. Br J Urol 81:360–363
56. Lorenzen J, Buchert R, Bohuslavizki KH (2001) Value of FDG PET in patients with fever of unknown origin. Nucl Med Commun 22:779–783
57. Buysschaert I, Vanderschueren S, Blockmans D et al (2004) Contribution of 18fluorodeoxyglucose positron emission tomography to the workup of patients with fever of unknown origin. Eur J Intern Med 15:151–156
58. Bleeker-Rovers CP, Vos FJ, Kleijn EM et al (2007) A prospective multi-center study of fever of unknown origin: the yield of a structured diagnostic protocol. Medicine (Baltimore) 86:26–38
59. Federici L, Blondet C, Imperiale A et al (2010) Value of 18F-FDG-PET/CT in patients with fever of unknown origin and unexplained prolonged inflammatory syndrome: a single Centre analysis experience. Int J Clin Pract 64(1):55–60

Musculoskeletal System 5

5.1 Anatomical and Physiological Considerations

Bones generally are classified as long bones such as femur, tibia, radius and ulna, shor bones such as bones of the writs and ankes, flat bone such as calvarium bones and irregular bones including vertebrae and some bones of the skull.

5.1.1 Bone Structure

Structure of normal adult bone can be summarized in four categories:

(a) *Gross level*

The skeleton consists of two major parts, axial skeleton and appendicular skeleton. The axial skeleton includes the skull, spine, and rib cage (ribs and sternum), while the appendicular skeleton involves the bones of the extremities, pelvic girdle, and pectoral girdle (clavicles and scapulae).

(b) *Tissue level*

Bone is divided into two types of tissues forming the skeleton: compact or cortical and cancellous, trabecular, or spongy bone. The spongy bone has a turnover rate of approximately eight times greater than the case of cortical bones and hosts hematopoietic cells and many blood cells. In mature bone, compact bone forms an outer layer (cortex), which surrounds an inner one of loose trabecular, cancellous, or spongy bone in the medulla. The architecture is arranged in the haversian system. The spongy portion contains hematopoietic cells, which produce blood cells, fat, and blood vessels. The compact bone constitutes 80% of the skeletal mass and contains 99% of the total body calcium and 90% of its phosphorus.

The appendicular skeleton is composed predominantly of cortical bone. The cortical bone is thicker in the diaphysis than in the metaphysis and epiphysis of long bones. The blood supply to the metaphysis is also different since it is rich and consists of large sinusoids, which make the flow of blood slower, a feature that predisposes to bacterial proliferation. The spine, on the other hand, is composed predominantly of cancellous bone in the body of the vertebra and compact bone in the end plates and posterior elements.

(c) *Cellular level*

Three types of cells are seen in bone: (1) osteoblasts that produce the organic bone matrix, (2) osteocyte that produces the inorganic matrix, and (3) osteoclasts which are active in bone resorption [1]. Osteoclasts are derived from the hematopoietic system in contrast to the mesenchymal origin of osteoblasts. Osteocytes are

© The Author(s), under exclusive license to Springer Nature Switzerland AG 2023

A. H. Elgazzar, *Synopsis of Pathophysiology in Nuclear Medicine*,

https://doi.org/10.1007/978-3-031-20646-7_5

derived from osteoblasts that have secreted bone around themselves [2].

(d) *Molecular level*

At the molecular level, bone matrix is composed primarily of organic matrix (approximately 35%) including collagen and glycoproteins and inorganic matrix (approximately 65%), which includes hydroxyapatite, cations (calcium, magnesium, sodium, potassium, and strontium), and anions (fluoride, phosphorus, and chloride) [3]. There is now strong evidence that the gut microbiome regulates bone homeostasis in health and disease and that prebiotic and probiotics protect against bone loss [4, 5]. Table 5.1 summarizes the major constituents of bone and their function.

Table 5.1 Bone structures and their functions

Major structural elements	Function
Bone cells	
Osteoblasts	Synthesize collagen and proteoglycans, stimulate osteoclast resorptive activity
Osteocytes	Maintain bone matrix
Osteoclasts	Resorb bone, assist with mineral homeostasis
Bone matrix	
Organic matrix	
Collagen fibers	Provide support and tensile strength
Proteoglycans	Control transport of ionized materials through matrix
Sialoprotein	Promotes calcification
Osteocalcin	Inhibits calcium/phosphate precipitation, promotes bone resorption
Laminin	Stabilizes basement membranes in bone
Osteonectin	Binds calcium to bones
Albumin	Transports essential elements to matrix
Inorganic matrix	
Calcium	Crystallizes to provide rigidity and compressive strength
Phosphate	Regulates vitamin D and thereby promotes mineralization

Modified from [1]

5.1.2 Blood Supply

Bones are richly supplied by blood and receive about 10–15% of the cardiac output [6]. The pattern of skeletal blood supply varies with the age group. In children, epiphyseal, metaphyseal, and diaphyseal vessels are present. In adults, all vessels communicate together. Nutrient and periosteal arteries feed a rich network of vessels to supply the cortex and medulla (Fig. 5.1). This vasculature takes the form of interconnecting capillaries, sinusoids, and veins. It is estimated that blood flow to cancellous bone containing marrow is 5–13 times higher than in cortical bone [7].

5.1.3 Bone Remodeling

Within all bones, a balance between osteogenesis and bone resorption continuously occurs, even in normal nonviolated bone. Remodeling occurs throughout life, with removal and replacement of bone at different rates in different parts of the skeleton. Bone remodeling is regulated by parathyroid hormone, vitamin D, and numerous other factors. It is estimated that 18% of the skeleton is replaced yearly in adults, indicating that the entire skeleton is replaced every 5 years. The process is more active in cancellous bone, with a yearly replacement rate of approximately 25% compared with 2% for compact bone [8]. Turnover varies and is affected by many factors including drugs and disease. Most bone diseases are the result of bone remodeling abnormalities [9].

5.1.4 Bone Marrow

Bone marrow is a soft tissue that is found at the inner aspect of the bones and has multiple important functions [10]. It is a hematopoietic organ involved in the production of new blood cells. Also, it has a mechanical function as it contains bone marrow mesenchymal stem cells that contribute to building the bone. In addition, bone marrow has an immune function as the hematopoietic stem cells produce multiple types of immune cells [11]. Bone marrow adipose tissue

Fig. 5.1 Same Fig. 5.1
first ed. Diagram
illustrating blood supply
to along bone

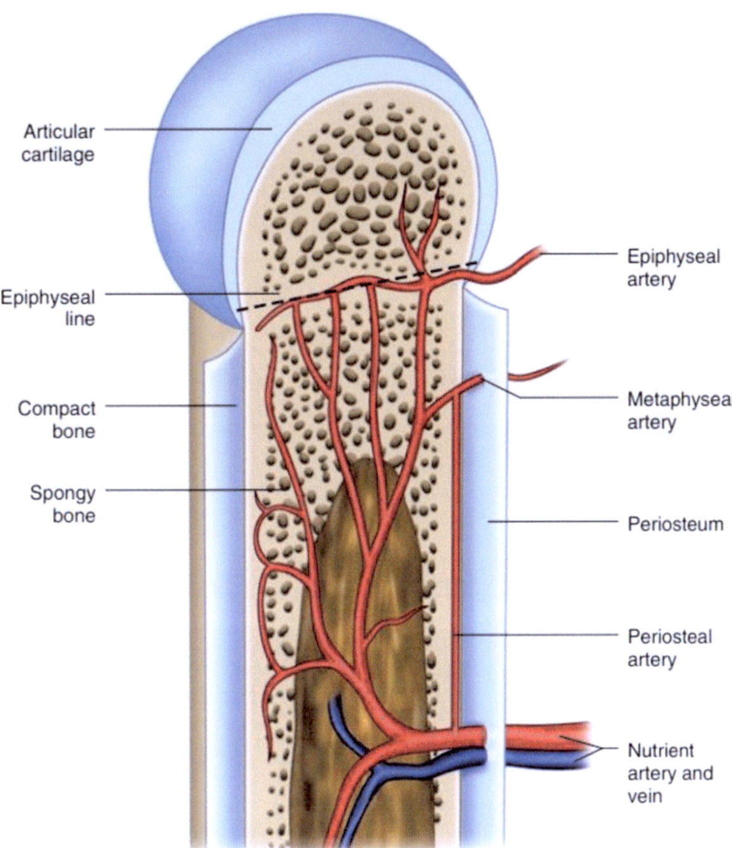

may also have a beneficial impact on skeletal health [12].

Normally, almost the entire fetal marrow space is occupied by red (hematopoietic) marrow at birth. Conversion from red to yellow, non-hematopoietically active marrow, starts in the immediate postnatal period. This process begins in the extremities and progresses in general from the peripheral to the central skeleton and from diaphyseal to metaphyseal regions in individual long bones. By approximately the age of 25 years, marrow conversion to the adult pattern is complete (Fig. 5.2). In adults, hematopoietic bone marrow usually is confined to the skull, vertebrae, ribs, sternum, pelvis, and proximal portions of the humerus and femur. Fatty marrow in other bones may contain islands of hematopoietic tissue, however, and for this reason, variations on the normal adult pattern of hematopoietic bone marrow are frequently encountered. Acquired alterations in the distribution of hema-topoietic bone marrow may be due to surgery, trauma, infection, and other destructive processes. Furthermore, with increasing demand for red cells, reconversion of yellow to red marrow may take place. This process follows the reverse order of the initial red-to-yellow marrow conversion.

5.1.5   Response of Bone to Injury

The principal response of bone to injury and disease is reactive bone formation. This reactive bone goes through stages. It is disorganized early but later may remodel to normal bone. This new disorganized bone is termed woven bone (Fig. 5.3) and is active with no lamellar arrangement.

Pathological foci containing woven bone show increased uptake of bone-imaging agents due to higher extraction efficiency.

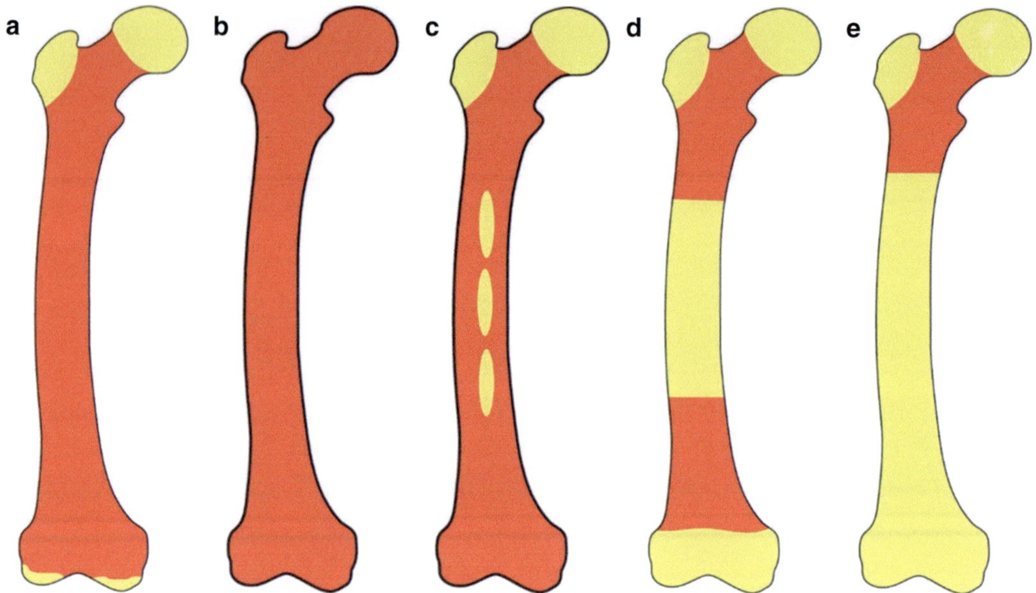

Fig. 5.2 Same Fig. 5.2 first ed. Bone marrow distribution in a long bone illustrating changes during development over the years till the adult pattern is reached by about 25 years of age: (**a**) birth; (**b**) 7-year-old; (**c**) 14-year-old; (**d**) 18-year-old; (**e**) 25-year-old

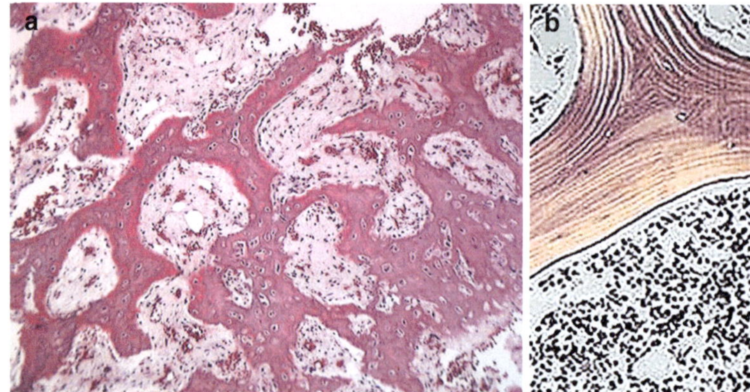
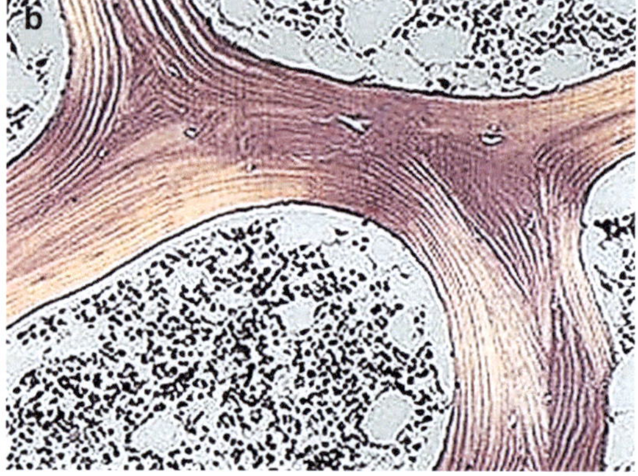

Fig. 5.3 (**a**, **b**) Photomicrographs illustrating the difference between woven and lamellar bone. The irregular and disorganized nature of woven bone (**a**) is easily seen compared to lamellar bone depicted in (**b**) The bony spicules in lamellar structure are even, with occasional lacunae containing osteocytes. Cellular marrow is seen between the spicules of bone

5.2 Bone Diseases

Bone scintigraphy shows many patterns, some specific, in a variety of benign and malignant bone diseases. Many of these patterns are better understood once the underlying pathophysiological changes of different bone diseases are appreciated.

5.2.1 Nonneoplastic Bone Diseases

5.2.1.1 Skeletal Infection/Inflammation

5.2.1.1.1 Definitions
The term osteomyelitis optimally indicates infection involving the cortical bone as well as the marrow. When infection starts in the periosteum,

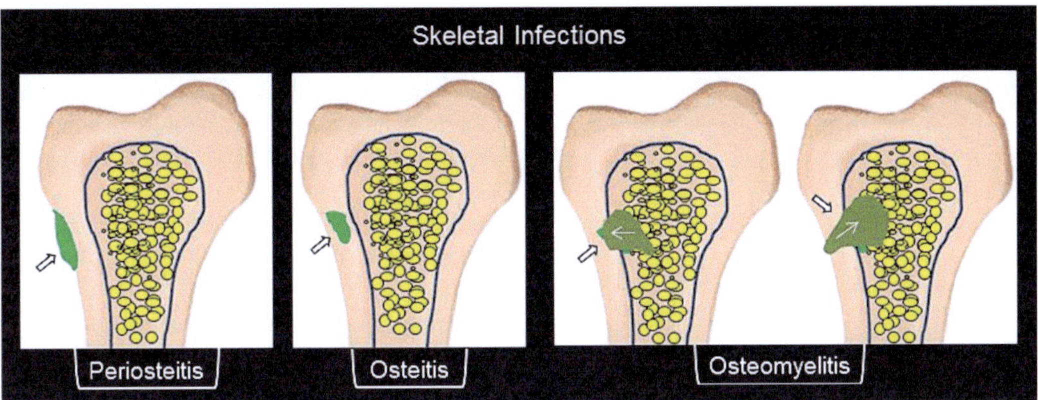

Fig. 5.4 A comparison of the extent of infection in osteomyelitis compared with the extent of infection in periostitis and in osteitis

such as in cases of direct extension bone infection, it produces periostitis. At this stage, infection may not yet involve the cortex or marrow and the condition is called infectious periostitis. When infection penetrates the cortex, the term infectious osteitis is used. When marrow is involved as well, the term osteomyelitis is applied (Fig. 5.4).

5.2.1.1.2 Classification of Osteomyelitis

The pathophysiology, imaging, and classification of osteomyelitis are challenging, varying with the age of the patient, the chronicity of infection, the route of infection, the immune and vascular status of the patient, and the affected region of the skeleton. Osteomyelitis may be classified as hematogenous and nonhematogenous [13–15]. In hematogenous osteomyelitis, the metaphyses of long bones are the most common site. Nonhematogenous osteomyelitis occurs as a result of penetrating trauma, spread of a contiguous soft-tissue infection, or inoculation (as in drug addicts). Hematogenous spread is the predominant route of infection in children aged less than 16 years and usually causes long-bone osteomyelitis [16, 17]. Hematogenous spread is less common in adults and, when it occurs, usually leads to vertebral osteomyelitis. Adult osteomyelitis is most commonly caused by contiguous spread from soft-tissue infections or direct inoculation [18]. Infantile osteomyelitis refers to that occurring prior to 1 year of age; the juvenile type occurs between 1 year and the age at closure of

the physes; adult type occurs after closure of the physes. While gram-positive bacteria such as *Staphylococcus aureus* are the most frequent cause, many different organisms have been encountered in osteomyelitis [19–22].

5.2.1.1.3 Pathophysiological Changes

Acute Hematogenous Osteomyelitis

Acute hematogenous osteomyelitis occurs most commonly in children, affecting males approximately twice as often as females. It has a predilection for the metaphyses of long bones, where blood flow is rich and relatively sluggish and bone is relatively porous in comparison to the diaphysis (Fig. 5.5). Here, the blood flows through large intramedullary venous sinusoids, a fertile site for bacterial lodgment and proliferation [14]. The process starts by implantation of organisms in the bone marrow. As infection becomes established in the marrow, it provokes acute suppurative neutrophilic infiltrates and edema with local ischemia, vasospasm, and thrombosis. Infection subsequently may spread from metaphyseal focus into the epiphysis, the joint space, the subperiosteal space, the shaft of the bone, and the surrounding soft tissues (Fig. 5.6). The disease has increased in frequency, virulence, and degree of soft-tissue involvement in recent years [23].

In children between 1 and approximately 16 years of age, the blood supply to the medullary space of bone enters through the nutrient

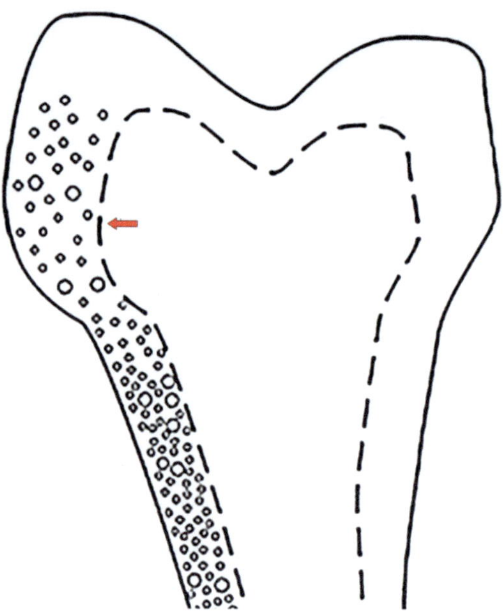

Fig. 5.5 Diagram of part of a long bone illustrating the more porous nature of the metaphysic (arrow), the most frequently affected site by hematogenous skeletal infections

artery and then passes through smaller vessels toward the growth plate. Once these vessels reach the metaphyseal side of the growth plates, they turn back upon themselves in loops to empty into large sinusoidal veins, where the blood flow is slower. The epiphyseal plate separating the epiphyseal and metaphyseal blood supplies acts as a barrier to the spread of infection (Fig. 5.7), making joint involvement less common in this age group. In this situation, infection must first break through the bone to produce joint infection (Fig. 5.7). On the other hand, in infants and adults, the terminal branches of the nutrient artery extend into the epiphysis, as there is no growth plate barrier. This vascular communication between epiphyses and metaphyses facilitates the spread of infection to adjacent joints (Fig. 5.7).

When infection lifts the periosteum, the blood supply may be impaired, causing necrosis of bone or sequestrum (Fig. 5.9). In some cases,

Fig. 5.6 Spread of hematogenous osteomyelitis

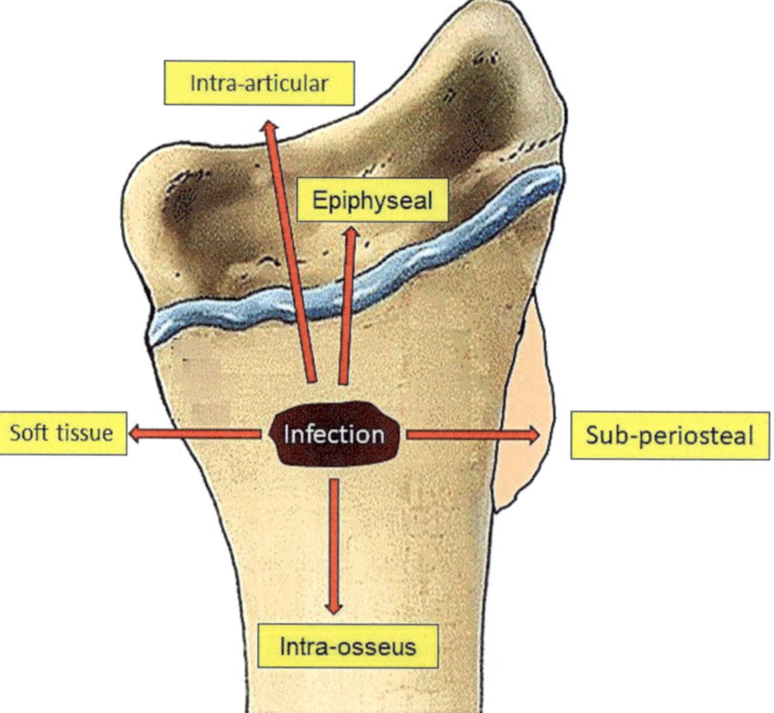

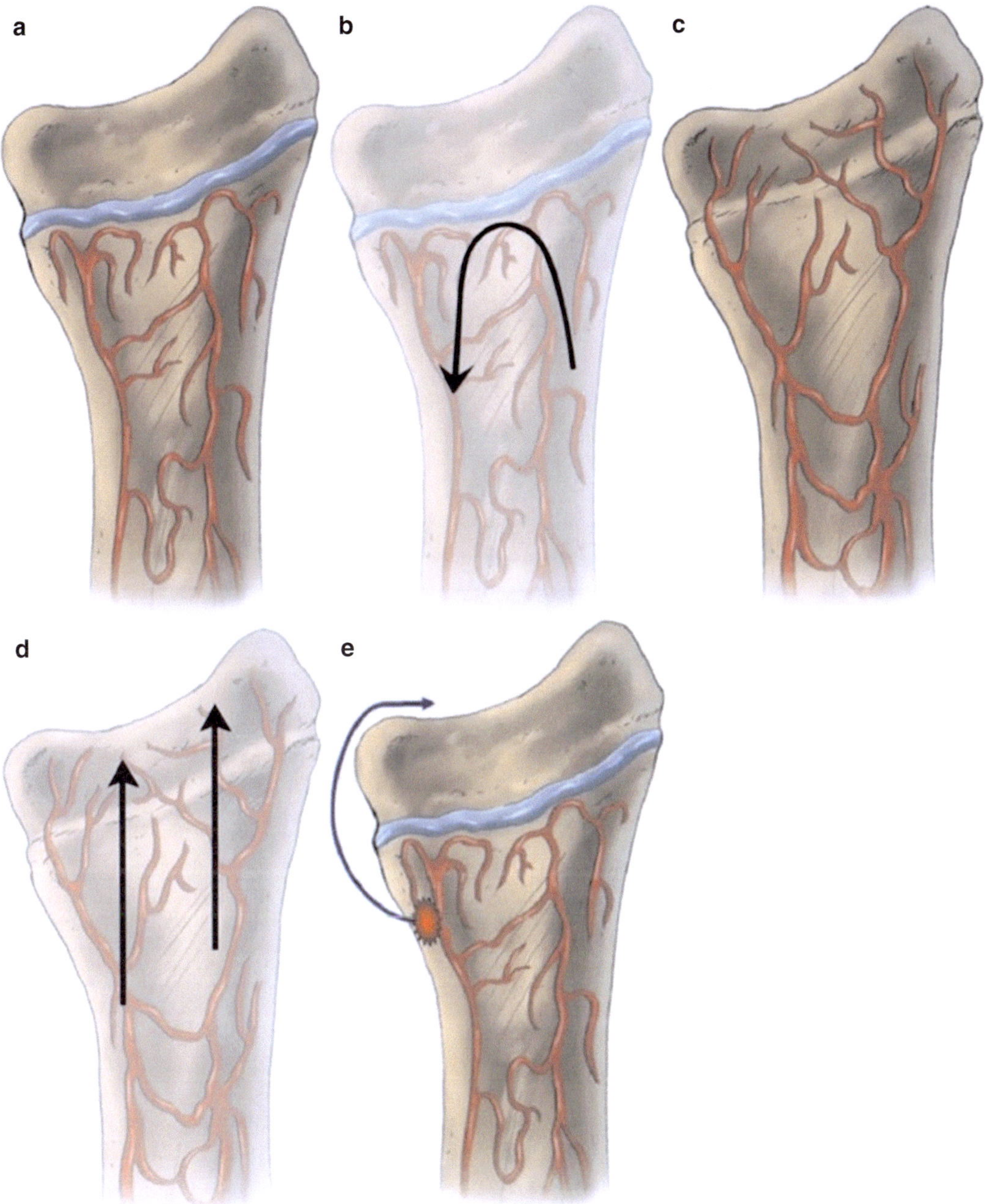

Fig. 5.7 (**a–e**) Diagram illustrating the vascular communication between the metaphysis and epiphysis of long bones. When the growth plate (**a**) is present, it acts as a barrier, and vessels turn on themselves forming loops. This acts to prevent infection that is most commonly present in the metaphysis from extending to epiphysis and adjacent joint (**b**). On the other hand, in neonates after the closure of the growth plate (**c**), infection extends more easily (**d**) to the joint since there is free vascular communication between metaphysis and epiphysis. Figure (**e**) illustrates the path of severe infection, which is able to involve the joint, when the growth plate is present, by breaking through the bone

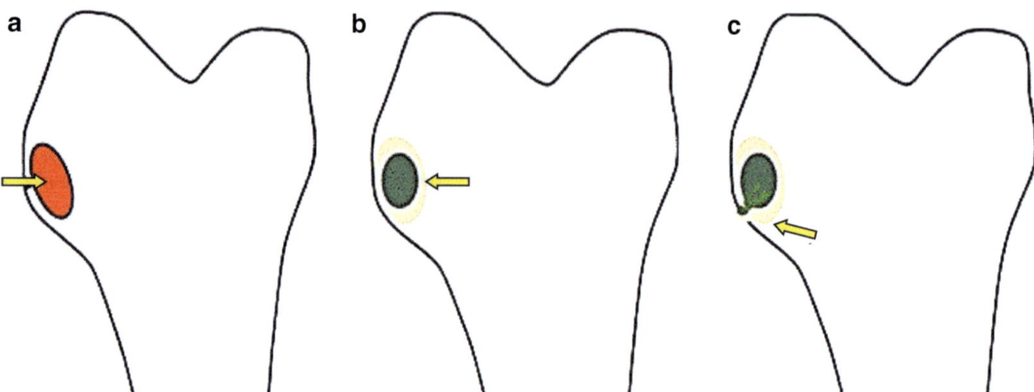

Fig. 5.8 (**a–c**) Diagrammatic representation of the sequestrum (**a**) showing the necrotic segment of bone (*arrow*) and involucrum (**b**), which has a layer of new bone formation (*arrow*) surrounding the focal infection. (**c**) illustrates cloaca with the sinus tract (arrow)

infection may stimulate osteoblastic activity, particularly from the periosteum, forming new subperiosteal bone that may envelop the infectious focus (involucrum). This osteogenesis may occasionally continue long enough to give rise to a densely sclerotic pattern of osteomyelitis that is referred to as sclerosing osteomyelitis. The infection can spread through the periosteum as the rise in intramedullary pressure may lead to rupture of the bony cortex, producing a cortical track known as a cloaca (Fig. 5.8). This causes elevation of the periosteum and disrupts the periosteal blood supply to the bone [24]. Delayed complications from acute osteomyelitis include growth arrest, fracture, soft-tissue infection, and chronic osteomyelitis [25].

Chronic Osteomyelitis

It is difficult to draw the line between acute and chronic osteomyelitis. However, it should be noted that cases of clear chronic osteomyelitis need special handling in diagnosis and management. Chronic osteomyelitis has variously been defined as symptomatic osteomyelitis with a duration ranging from 5 days to 6 weeks [26].

Since the pathology of osteomyelitis varies with age, microorganisms, prior therapy, underlying diseases, and other factors, it is somewhat inappropriate to depend only on duration of the disease to define chronicity. Chronic osteomyelitis has less marked inflammatory cell reactions and may occur without preceding acute inflam-

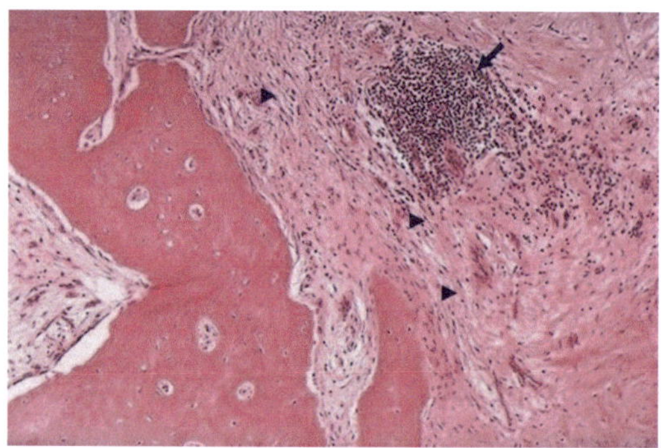

Fig. 5.9 Chronic osteomyelitis. A photomicrograph of a specimen of bone from a patient with long-standing chronic osteomyelitis. Note the presence of numerous lymphocytes (*arrow*) as well as fibrosis (*arrowheads*) within the marrow space

mation. Microscopically, chronic osteomyelitis predominantly shows lymphocytes and plasma cells rather than polymorphonuclears (Fig. 5.9). There are also fibrosis and a variable amount of necrotic tissue, and sequestra may form in some cases. The presence of necrotic tissue may also lead to draining sinuses or organization in the medullary cavity, forming a cystic cavity (Brodie's abscess) (Fig. 5.10). Because these abscesses are avascular, levels of antibiotics sufficient to eradicate the bacteria may not be achieved during treatment. Accordingly, bacteria may remain indolent for a long time (inactive disease). Reactivation of the disease may occur later, even years after the initial episode (active

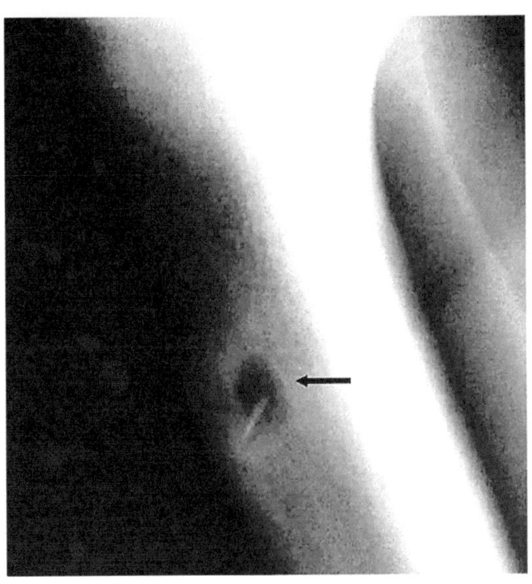

Fig. 5.10 Radiograph showing a Brodie's abscess (*arrow*)

disease). It was recently suggested that bacterial biofilm formation and bacterial invasion within the osteocyte are contributing factors to the formation of chronic and recurrent osteomyelitis [17]. It is important to evaluate patients for possible chronic disease and to either exclude or confirm the presence of chronic active infection. The continuation of intravenous antibiotic therapy and/or surgical intervention to eradicate infection will depend on that determination [27].

Vertebral Osteomyelitis (Spondylodiskitis)
Vertebral osteomyelitis is a specific form of osteomyelitis that has some unique features. It accounts for 3–5% of cases of osteomyelitis [28]. Sixty-nine percent of the patients had lumbar involvement [29] followed by the thoracic and cervical spine. Several factors predispose to vertebral osteomyelitis such as diabetes mellitus, old-age urinary tract infection, and prior back surgery.

Infection usually originates at a distant site with hematogenous extension to contiguous vertebral bodies [30] and the intervening space via the ascending and descending branches of the posterior spinal artery. Also, the venous supply of the spine allows backflow from the pelvic venous plexus due to the lack of valves [31].

The causative organism generally settles in the richly vascularized subchondral vertebral end plates with eventual progression of infection into the adjacent intervertebral disk, which is relatively avascular. In childhood, infection often starts at the disks, which are nourished by small perforating vessels. In either case, local spread of infection eventually occurs and causes end-plate destruction, disk space narrowing, and collapse. Fig. 5.11 illustrates possible ways of development of vertebral osteomyelitis. Since the disk is almost invariably involved in vertebral infections, the term spondylodiskitis is preferred [19, 20].

Diabetic Foot Osteomyelitis
Diabetic foot osteomyelitis is a unique clinical and pathological problem. It is a common complication of diabetes, particularly when angiopathy is present. It occurs in 15% of adult diabetic patients and, without prompt diagnosis and treatment, may lead to amputation. Diabetic foot infections typically begin in a wound, most often a neuropathic ulceration. Ulceration of the foot is 50 times more common in diabetics, and the incidence of amputation of the lower extremities is 25 times greater than among the general population. More than 90% of osteomyelitis of the foot of diabetic patients occurs as a result of the spread of infection from adjacent foot ulcers [22, 32].

Neuroarthropathy is characterized by destructive joint changes. A combination of factors is involved (Fig. 5.12). Loss of protective pain and proprioceptive sensation along with hyperemia secondary to loss of vasoconstrictive neural impulses is thought to result in atrophic neuropathy, occurring most frequently in the forefoot [33].

On the other hand, absence of sympathetic fibers in the presence of sensory fiber involvement tends to result in hypertrophic neuroarthropathy, which occurs most frequently in the mid- and hind foot. Since the patient continues to walk and traumatize the foot, disuse osteoporosis is usually absent. Unrelenting trauma may also result in rapidly progressive destruction, sometimes with disintegration of one or more tarsal bones within a period of only a few weeks. This is a rapidly progressive form of neuroarthropathy, which has more inflammatory reaction than oth-

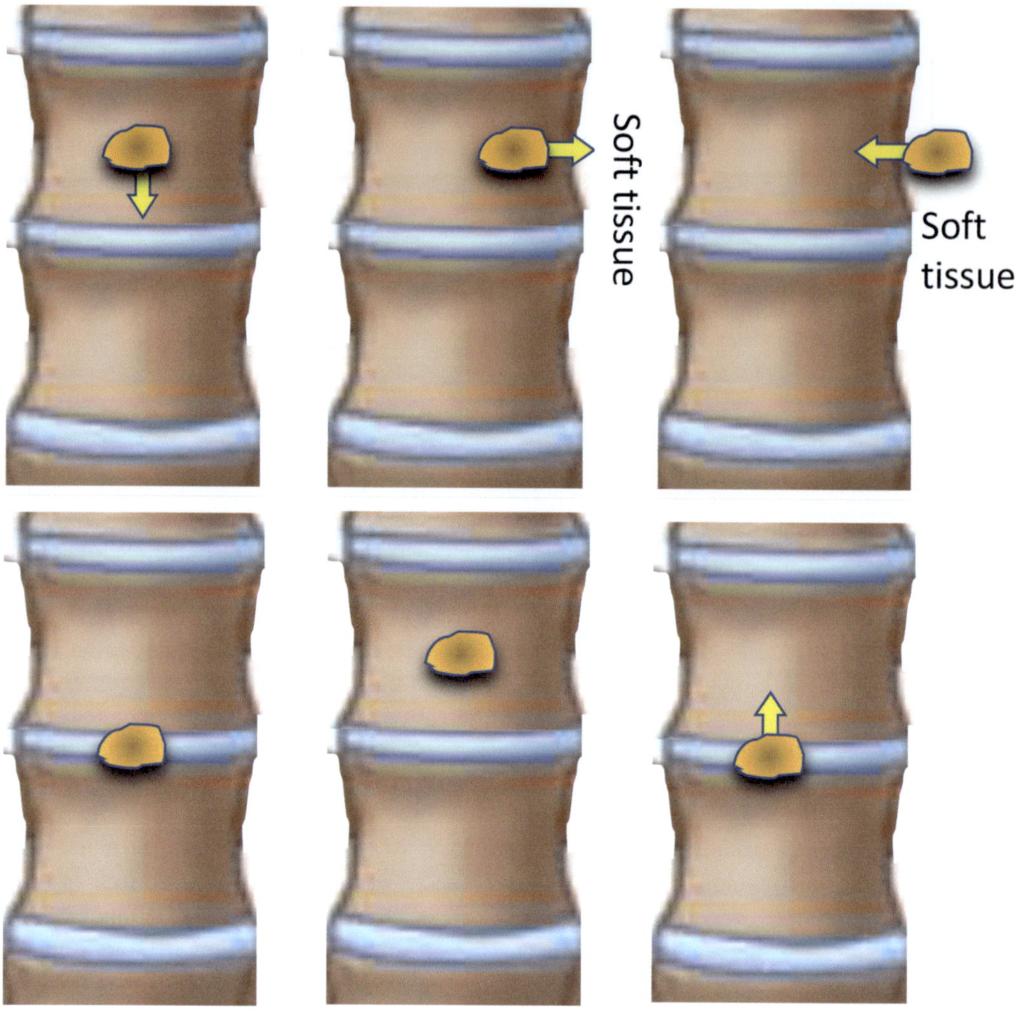

Fig. 5.11 (**a–d**) The possible ways of development and extension of infection in vertebral osteomyelitis

Fig. 5.12 Types of diabetic neuropathy (From [32], with permission)

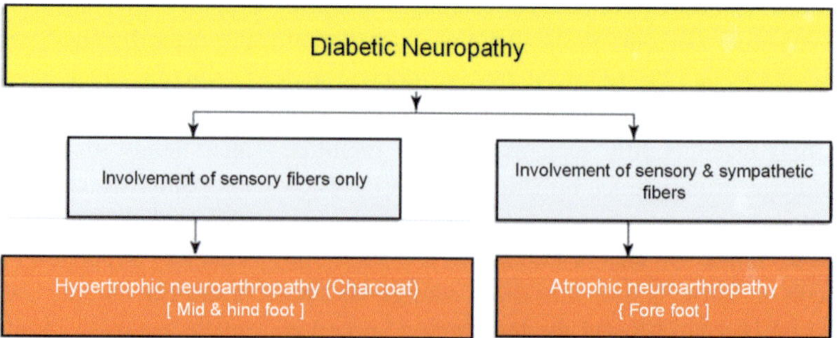

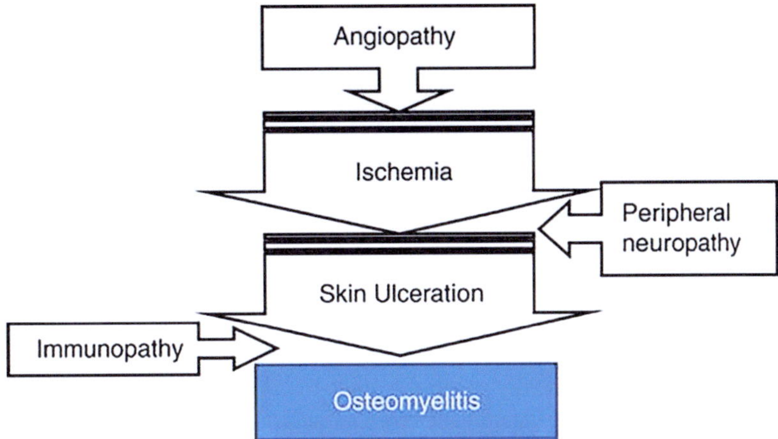

Fig. 5.13 Changes leading to skeletal infections in diabetics (Modified from [32], with permission)

erwise. A long history of diabetes mellitus with a combination of angiopathy, neuropathy, and immunopathy predisposes to pedal osteomyelitis (Fig. 5.13). Metatarsal bones and proximal phalanges are the most commonly involved sites [34, 35].

Diabetic foot osteomyelitis can affect any bone but most frequently the forefoot (90%), followed by the midfoot (5%) and the hind foot (5%) [36].

Sickle Cell Disease Osteomyelitis

In osteomyelitis associated with sickle cell disease, erythrocytes become viscous and sickle abruptly when exposed to hypoxia, since hemoglobin S is sensitive to hypoxemia. This may compromise the microvascular flow and may cause infarction, the most common skeletal complication of sickle cell disease. For symptomatic sickle cell patients, distinguishing infarction from osteomyelitis is critical. Although less common than infarctions, osteomyelitis is the second most frequent bacterial infection in children with sickle cell disease after pneumonia [37].

Osteomyelitis may occur as a primary event or may be superimposed on infarcts as the necrotic bone is a fertile site for such secondary infections. *S. aureus* and *Salmonella* are frequent causative organisms.

Periprosthetic infections: Hip and knee arthroplasties are two of the most frequent orthopedic procedures, exceeding 600,000 per year in the United States alone [38–40].

Loosening is the most common complication after hip replacements, occurring in up to 50% of femoral components and in 15% of acetabular components by 10 years after surgery.

Periprosthetic Infections

Periprosthetic infections are a clinically important complication after joint replacement. Although the incidence of infection was reported previously to be as high as 4% after the primary surgery and 32% after revision of hip arthroplasty, the currently reported incidence of infections after total hip or knee arthroplasties is only 0.5–2% and is less than 3% following revision surgery and occurs mostly within 4 months of operation [41, 42].

Infectious (Septic) Arthritis

Infectious (septic) arthritis refers to the invasion of synovial space by microbes. The synovial space contains synovial fluid, which is produced by a rich capillary network of the synovial membrane. This is a viscous fluid that serves to lubricate, nourish, and cushion the avascular joint cartilage. When the synovial space is infected, bacterial hyaluronidase decreases the viscosity of the synovial fluid. Pain is then felt with stress on the joint capsule.

Acute septic arthritis is usually caused by bacteria, while fungal and mycobacterial pathogens are seen more commonly in chronic arthritis. The lytic enzymes in the purulent articular fluid destroy the articular and epiphyseal cartilage.

Additionally, pus in the joint space increases the intracapsular pressure with epiphyseal ischemia. Concomitant osteomyelitis is not uncommon and is potentially severe [43]. A recent study reported 36% of patients with septic arthritis having concomitant bone infection, which can be called osteoarticular infection [44]. Other sequelae include dislocation, deformity, and destruction of the femoral head and neck. Hence, drainage and antibiotic therapy must be considered without delay [26, 45].

Microorganisms usually reach the joint by a hematogenous route, contagiously from an adjacent osseous infection, or through traumatic/surgical inoculation.

The joints most commonly involved in children are the hip (35%), knee (35%), and ankle (10%) [46, 47].

Chronic Nonbacterial Osteomyelitis
Chronic nonbacterial osteomyelitis is an autoinflammatory bone disorder, covering a clinical spectrum with asymptomatic inflammation of single bones at one end and chronic recurrent multifocal osteomyelitis (CRMO) at the other end. Recently, significant dysregulation of cytokine responses was demonstrated in CRMO.

Chronic nonbacterial osteomyelitis primarily affects children and adolescents but can occur in all age groups. Peak onset of the disease is between 7 years and 12 years of age with a slight female predominance. The exact molecular pathophysiology of chronic nonbacterial osteomyelitis remains largely unknown. Current knowledge indicates that bone inflammation is the net result of impaired immune responses with disbalanced cytokine expression, osteoclast differentiation and activation, osteolysis, and bone remodeling [48].

5.2.1.2 Multimodality Imaging of Skeletal Infections/ Inflammation

Several imaging modalities have been utilized for detection of osteomyelitis, including standard radiography, computerized tomography (CT), magnetic resonance imaging (MRI), and nuclear medicine techniques. The choice of modality depends on clinical presentation, duration of symptoms, site of suspected infection, previously known underlying pathology (such as fracture, infection, or tumor), and other factors [26].

5.2.1.2.1 Imaging Acute Osteomyelitis

Standard radiographs are not sensitive for early detection of osteomyelitis, as the changes are evident only after 10–21 days from the time of infection [49]. MRI has an important role in the diagnosis of osteomyelitis. In adults, MRI is reported to have a high diagnostic accuracy [95.6% sensitivity, 80.7% specificity with similar performance to PET (85% sensitivity, 92.8% specificity)]. However studies for accuracy in children are limited to draw conclusion [50]. The average overall accuracy of MRI is similar to that of multiphase bone scans. In the last decade, MRI has become an important modality for the diagnosis of acute osteomyelitis in children [23, 51], since it is sensitive for the detection of early osteomyelitis and also accurately shows the extent of disease with any associated soft-tissue extension without the risks associated with radiation exposure [52]. Accordingly, the current recommendation is to start with plain X-ray followed by MRI for the diagnosis of acute osteomyelitis [53].

Bone scintigraphy is very sensitive in the early diagnosis of osteomyelitis [27] and can show the abnormality as early as 24 h after infection [54]. Typically, there is focally increased flow, blood pool activity, and delayed uptake (Fig. 5.14). When the bone has not been previously affected by other pathological conditions (nonviolated), the bone scan has high accuracy and is a cost-effective modality for diagnosis of osteomyelitis with both sensitivity and specificity of 90–95% [27]. Osteomyelitis may present as cold lesions on bone scan and usually represent an aggressive form [55–57]. Cold foci on bone scan in cases of osteomyelitis are thought to be secondary to increased intraosseous and subperiosteal pressure. Periarticular distribution of the abnormal uptake that is largely limited to the joint capsule and has a uniform pattern indicates septic arthritis. Osteomyelitis, on the other hand, shows abnormal uptake beyond the confines of the joint

Fig. 5.14 (**a–c**) A case of osteomyelitis in a nonviolated bone as seen on 99mTc multiphase bone scan. Regionally increased flow (**a**), blood pool activity (**b**), and delayed uptake (**c**) are noted in the left distal femur

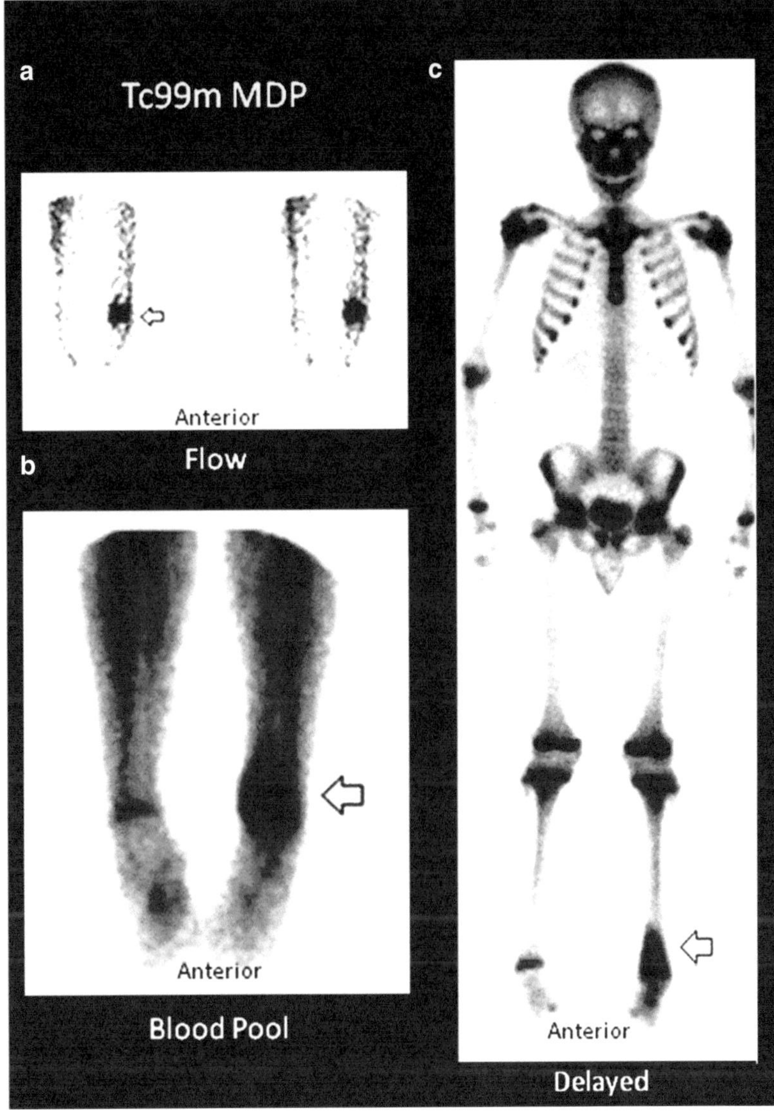

capsule or shows nonuniform uptake within the joint capsule [58, 59]. If the bone has been affected by a previous pathology (violated), particularly after orthopedic surgical procedures, the bone scan will still be highly sensitive but with poor specificity [27]. In such situations, unless the bone scan is unequivocally negative, an additional modality should be used, particularly scanning with leukocytes labeled with 111 In-oxine or 99 m hexamethylpropylene amine oxime (HMPAO). Overall, 111 In-leukocyte studies have a sensitivity of approximately 88% and a specificity of 84% for osteomyelitis [27]. This

modality is particularly useful for excluding infection in previously violated bone sites such as in postsurgical and post-traumatic condition. Combined labeled leukocytes and bone scans have a better accuracy than labeled leukocyte scans alone and can help to localize abnormal foci [60–62]. Best results for detecting osteomyelitis were observed when using combined 111 In-WBC and 99 m Tc-MDPSPECT with SPECT/CT with sensitivity in the range of 84–97% and specificity 98–100% [63].

Since labeled leukocyte scans show uptake by active bone marrow, it may be difficult to differentiate this physiological marrow uptake from abnormal uptake due to infection. Bone marrow scans using 99 m Tc-sulfur colloid or nanocolloid help in differentiation and improve the specificity [64]. SPECT/CT has proven to improve the accuracy of these imaging procedures and enhances interobserver agreement. Labeled antibodies have also been used. 111 In- or 99 m Tc-labeled human nonspecific polyclonal antibodies (IgG) and several monoclonal antibodies such as labeled antigranulocyte antibodies, anti-NCA-90 (LeukoScan), and anti-NCA-95(fanolesomab) are used to diagnose skeletal infections. Early studies suggested similar or better accuracy (90%) to WBC scan [65]. However, recent studies showed variable results and suggest that LeukoScan does not achieve the level of accuracy to replace WBC imaging for orthopedic infection.

SPECT/CT had added value in the detection of osteomyelitis. In a study on 85 children suspected of having osteomyelitis, bone scan with SPECT/CT was significantly superior to planar scan and changed the diagnosis and treatment planning in 14/85 (16.5%) patients. It increases the accuracy of diagnosis in the evaluation of osteomyelitis compared to planar three-phase bone scintigraphy/SPECT. Planar bone scan/SPECT predicted the correct diagnosis in 82% of patients with proven osteomyelitis, while SPECT/CT predicted the correct diagnosis in 98% of patients. Additionally, SPECT/CT was statistically more successful in the detection of chronic osteomyelitis and useful in differentiating chronic from acute osteomyelitis (kappa value of 0.541 for planar scan/SPECT and 0.944 for SPECT/CT) [25].

5.2.1.2.2   Imaging Other Forms of Osteomyelitis

Diabetic Foot Osteomyelitis
Despite its limitation, plain X-ray has been and still the first imaging modality to consider in patients with a suspicion of diabetic foot osteomyelitis. Bone scanning is very sensitive but not specific for detecting infection in diabetics. ^{67}Ga is not helpful in resolving the question of osteo-

myelitis in the diabetic foot, since it is also usually positive in noninfected neuroarthropathy. Indium-111 leukocyte imaging is both sensitive and specific for diabetic foot infections. Combined bone/labeled leukocyte imaging improves the accuracy of diagnosis of foot osteomyelitis and its differentiation from soft-tissue infection. False-positive results however can still occur in some cases of noninfected neuroarthropathy. SPECT/CT (Fig. 5.15) imaging for diabetic foot osteomyelitis with ^{99m}Tc-MDP and In-111-labeled leucocyte scans is more accurate in diagnosing and localizing infection compared with conventional planar imaging.

Additionally, it provided clear guidance and promoted many limb salvage procedures. Its use was associated also with considerably reduced length of hospitalization [66, 67]. Combined ^{111}In-labeled leukocyte and ^{99mTc}-sulfur colloid marrow scans further improve the specificity, differentiating marrow uptake of labeled leukocytes from uptake by actual bone infection. Simultaneous SPECT/CT of ^{99m}Tc-sulfur colloid (SC) and ^{111}In white blood cells (WBC) provides essentially perfect spatial registration of the tracers within anatomical sites of interest [68]. PET/CT also provides faster results (typically within 2 h). However, the reported results are not consistent although a recent systemic review and meta-analysis compared MRI, labeled leucocyte scintigraphy, and FDG-PET/CT for the detection of diabetic foot osteomyelitis to a reference standard of bone biopsy. Despite the comparable sensitivity of all the different imaging modalities, ranging from 89 to 93%, the specificity of 99mTc-HMPAO-labeled leucocyte scintigraphy and FDG-PET/CT (92%) was higher than MRI (75%) [66]. SPECT/CT with In-111-labeled leukocyte combined with bone or bone marrow scan is currently the best imaging modality for diagnosing diabetic foot osteomyelitis [67].

Vertebra; Osteomyelitis
Gadolinium-enhanced magnetic resonance imaging (MRI) is the imaging technique of choice to evaluate spinal infection [69]. It has excellent sensitivity and specificity (96% and 94%, respectively) [70, 71]. If MRI is not conclusive or there

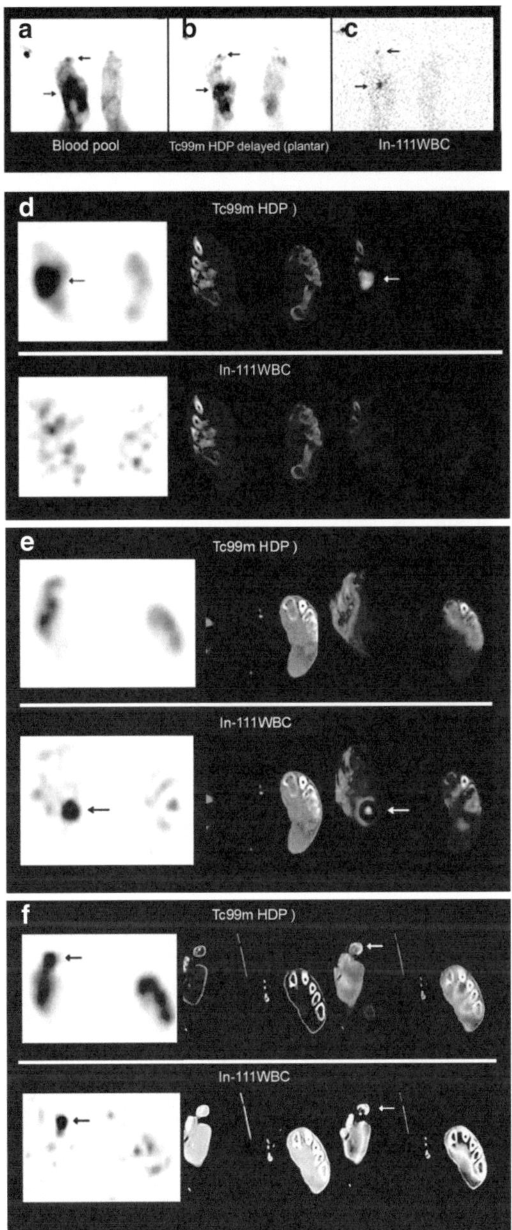

Fig. 5.15 A 59-year-old male diabetic patient S/P right great toe amputation presented with discharging ulcers on the right foot plantar surface referred to rule out osteomyelitis. Planar images (**a**) demonstrate foci of increased blood pool activity involving the probable distal third toe and mid right foot. The delayed bone scan plantar image (**b**) demonstrates foci of increased radiotracer uptake in the same regions. On the planar 111In-WBC plantar image (**c**) there are two foci of abnormal uptake also probably in the same areas (*arrows*). In the selected dual-isotope SPECT/CT transaxial slices, there is increased 99mTc-HDP uptake in the right intermediate and lateral cuneiforms and inter-cuneiform joint without corresponding abnormality on the simultaneously obtained 111In-WBC images (*arrows*). These findings are consistent with arthritic changes. (**d**) In the adjacent dual-isotope SPECT/CT transaxial slices, there is increased 111In-WBC uptake in a region of plantar ulcer without corresponding abnormal uptake on 99mTc-HDP bone scan consistent with soft-tissue infection (*arrows*). (**e**) In another dual-isotope SPECT/CT transaxial slices (**f**) there is focal increased uptake in the right third distal phalanx on both bone scan and In-WBC scan images consistent with a small focus of osteomyelitis (*arrows*). Based on these images, the patient was effectively treated with soft-tissue debridement of the large plantar ulcer and distal right third toe partial amputation as well as antibiotics and was saved from a major foot amputation (Courtesy of Dr. S. Heiba with thanks)

is a contraindication for its use, F-18-PET/CT is the functional modality of choice with Ga-67 SPECT as an alternative [72–76].

A recent prospective study on 32 patients using ^{18}F-FDG-PET/CT and MRI reported 100% sensitivity for both modalities and a specificity of 90.9% for ^{18}F-FDG-PET/CT and 91.7% for MRI. MRI detected more epidural/spinal abscesses [77].

Chronic Active Osteomyelitis

The radiological diagnosis of chronic active osteomyelitis is neither sensitive nor specific, while bone scintigraphy is very sensitive but not specific. ^{67}Ga citrate imaging is more specific than bone scanning for chronic osteomyelitis. False positives still occur in conditions such as healing fractures, tumors, and noninfected prostheses. Combined ^{99m}Tc-MDP and ^{67}Ga scans can be helpful in making the diagnosis of active disease. As Tumeh et al. [78] suggested, when ^{67}Ga uptake exceeds ^{99m}Tc-MDP uptake in intensity or differs in spatial distribution, active osteomyelitis usually is present.

F-18-FDG-PET has been found valuable to assess the activity of chronic osteomyelitis by confirming the presence of metabolically active infection and guide appropriate treatment [79, 80]. A meta-analysis study showed that FDG-PET not only is the most sensitive (96%) imaging modality for detecting chronic osteomyelitis but also has a greater specificity (91%) than radiolabeled WBC scintigraphy, bone scintigraphy, or MR [81]. From several studies reported, the overall sensitivity is 95–100% and specificity is 86–100% for FDG-PET [79–84].

Periprosthetic and Post-traumatic Infection

Making the distinction between mechanical failure of a prosthesis and infection is not easy. Combined ^{111}In-WBC and ^{99m}Tc-sulfur colloid SPECT/CT is an adequate method to diagnose prosthetic bone and joint infections [85]. With a sensitivity of 100%, specificity of 91%, and accuracy of 95%, it seems to be significantly better than FDG-PET. ^{99m}Tc-WBC is a very sensitive tool (95%) for imaging of infection in patients with metallic implants. Specificity is also high (93–100%) with SPECT/CT, but it seems dramatically lower (53%) in case of ^{99m}Tc-WBC SPECT alone. The improvement of specificity by addition of CT to SPECT is of substantial importance, as has been shown in multiple studies [86, 87]. FDG-PET has been shown to be useful in detecting infections and differentiating it from loosening in patients with hip and knee prostheses [88, 89]. The same concept is applied for detecting infection after trauma utilizing combined ^{111}In-WBC and ^{99m}Tc-sulfur colloid SPECT/CT.

Osteomyelitis in Patients with Sickle Cell Disease

Differentiating bone infarct from osteomyelitis clinically is difficult. Initial radiographs either are normal or show nonspecific changes. On bone scintigraphy, the findings vary. If bone scintigraphy is performed a week after the onset of symptoms, healing of the infarct may cause increased uptake rather than the typical pattern of cold defect. To add more difficulty, osteomyelitis may also cause cold defects rather than increased uptake [59, 90, 91]. Addition of ^{67}Ga or 99mTc-sulfur colloid imaging to bone scans enhances the specificity and can resolve the majority of diagnostic problems related to osteomyelitis in patients with sickle cell disease [91].

Infectious (Septic) Arthritis

Ultrasonography and also MRI are mainly used for identifying the condition [92]. Bone scan is not routinely used, and the condition can be seen when bone scan is performed for suspected osteomyelitis. However, it has been reported that identifying joint involvement and distinguishing bone from joint infection can be achieved in up to 90% of cases using bone scintigraphy [93, 94].

Figure 5.16 presents an updated algorithm for the diagnosis of skeletal infection, and Table 5.2 summarizes the findings correlated to the pathophysiologic changes of skeletal infections.

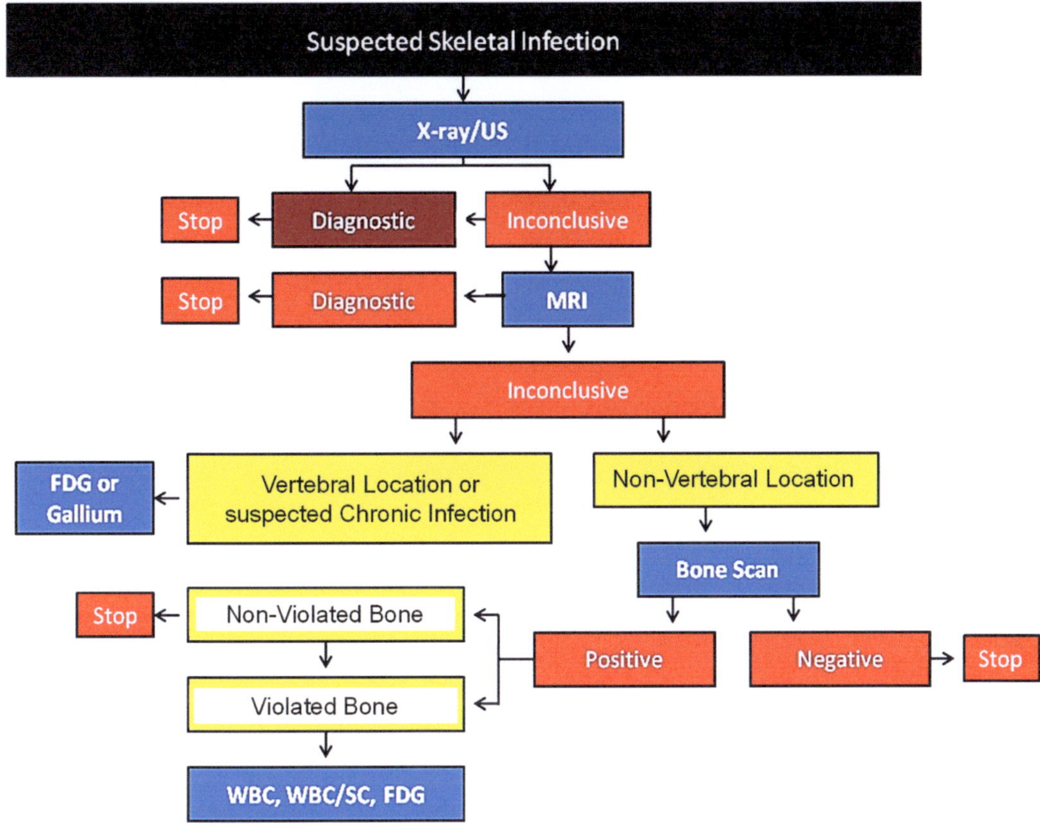

Fig. 5.16 Algorithm for the diagnosis of skeletal infection utilizing multiple modalities based on the location and understanding pathophysiology of the suspected infection

Table 5.2 Correlation of imaging findings and pathophysiological features of infection

Pathological change at the site of infection	Imaging pattern
Vasodilation of blood vessels	Increased flow and blood pool activity on bone scan, increased ^{67}Ga- and ^{99m}Tc-nanocolloid accumulation
Increased permeability and chemotaxis	Increased accumulation of ^{111}In- or ^{99m}Tc-labeled WBC
Increased secretion of iron-containing globulin by injured and stimulated WBC	Increased accumulation of ^{67}Ga
Formation of woven bone	Increased uptake of ^{99m}Tc-MDP on delayed images with persistent accumulation beyond 3–4 h
Increased expression of glucose transporters	Increased accumulation of 18F-FDG on activated inflammatory cells

5.2.2   Avascular Necrosis (Osteonecrosis)

Avascular necrosis of bone results from imbalances between oxygen demand and supply to osseous tissues. There are many causes for osteonecrosis (Table 5.3).

In some cases, the underlying cause cannot be determined, and in this situation the term primary, idiopathic, or spontaneous osteonecrosis is used.

Following the interruption of blood flow, the blood-forming and mesenchymal cells of the marrow as well as the primitive osteoblasts are affected first and die within 6–12 h after the interruption of the blood supply. Bone cells including osteocytes and mature osteoblasts die 12–48 h later, followed by the fat cells, which are most

Table 5.3 Causes of osteonecrosis

Trauma (e.g., fracture or dislocation)
Hemoglobinopathies (e.g., sickle cell anemia)
Exogenous or endogenous hypercortisolism (e.g., corticosteroid medication, Cushing's syndrome)
Renal transplantation
Alcoholism
Pancreatitis
Dysbaric (e.g., caisson disease)
Small-vessel disease (e.g., collagen vascular disorders)
Gaucher's disease
Hyperuricemia
Irradiation
Synovitis with elevation of intra-articular pressure (infection, hemophilia)
Idiopathic (spontaneous osteonecrosis)

Table 5.5 Osteochondrosis

Involved bone	Disease
Capital femoral epiphysis	Legg-Calvé-Perthes disease
Metatarsal head	Freiberg's disease
Carpal lunate	Kienböck's disease
Tarsal navicular	Köhler's disease
Capitellum of humerus	Panner's disease
Phalanges of the hand	Thiemann's disease
Tibial tuberosity	Osgood-Schlatter disease
Proximal tibial epiphysis	Blount disease
Vertebral body	Scheuermann's disease
Patella	Sinding-Larsen-Johansson
Calcaneus	Sever's disease
Ischiopubic synchondrosis	Van Neck's disease

Table 5.4 Cell death after blood supply interruption

Cell	Time of death after interruption of blood supply
Blood-forming cells	6–12 h
Mesenchymal cells	6–12 h
Primitive osteoblasts	6–12 h
Bone cells including osteocytes and mature osteoblasts	12–48 h
Fat cells	2–5 days

resistant to ischemia and die 2–5 days after the interruption of blood flow (Table 5.4). This sequence of events may explain why the bone marrow scintigraphic changes of decreased uptake appear earlier than the bone scan abnormalities. The bone marrow is affected earlier than the bone cells, which are relatively more resistant to ischemia [95, 96].

The reparative process is initiated and carried out by neovascularization through the collateral circulation, advancing from the periphery of the area of necrosis, or by recanalization of occluded vessels. This granulation tissue provides all the elements necessary for the formation of bone matrix and new bone deposition by young osteoblasts. This repair process may be altered. Often, bone collapse results from structural weakening and external stress. Bone collapse and cartilage damage can result in significant deformity [95, 96].

When osteonecrosis occurs in growing skeleton, it is included in the group of disorders collectively called osteochondrosis. Osteochondrosis involves the epiphyses or apophyses of the growing bones. The process is due to osteonecrosis in some cases and trauma or stress in others (Table 5.5) [97]. In addition to avascular necrosis, osteochondrosis often demonstrates similar pathological features such as transchondral fractures, reactive synovitis, and cyst formation. Some common forms of osteonecrosis are described below.

Modified from [98].

Generally, the common sites affected by osteonecrosis include the femoral head, humeral head, knee, femoral and tibial metadiaphysis, scaphoid, lunate, and talus [99].

Although MRI has been considered the gold standard diagnostic modality for osteonecrosis, the disease can be diagnosed even at a very early stage using nuclear medicine imaging techniques. Available literature suggests that SPECT/CT bone scan and ^{18}F-sodium fluoride PET/CT have similar or better results in comparison to MRI in the evaluation of osteonecrosis of the femoral head. They also provide both morphological and functional information about the diseased part and, therefore, can indicate whether the disease is active or healed [100].

5.2.2.1 Post-Traumatic Osteonecrosis

Following a fracture, bone death of variable extent on either side of the fracture line is relatively common. Necrosis of a relatively large segment of bone following fracture or dislocation, however, is generally restricted to sites that possess a vulnerable blood supply with few arterial anastomoses. Examples include the femoral head, the body of the talus-scaphoid bone, and the humeral head [101].

Other locations include the carpal hamate and lunate and the tarsal navicular bone. These bones are characterized by an intra-articular location and limited attachment of soft tissue, in addition to the peculiarities of their blood supply [95].

5.2.2.2 Legg-Calvé-Perthes Disease

This condition represents osteonecrosis of the femoral head in pediatric populations, especially boys 4–7 years old. The blood supply to the adult femoral heads is via the circumflex femoral branches of the profunda femoris artery. This adult pattern of femoral head vascularity usually becomes established after closure of the growth plate at approximately 18 years of age. In infancy and childhood, variable vascular patterns can be noted. The changing pattern of femoral head vascular supply with age may explain the prevalence of Legg-Calvé-Perthes disease in children between the ages of 4 and 7 years and the high frequency of necrosis following femoral neck injury in this age group. Fractures of the femoral neck, more often intracapsular than extracapsular fractures, are the most common cause. Others include dislocation of the hip and slipped capital femoral epiphysis.

MRI is a very useful modality in the diagnosis and predicting the course of the disease particularly later in the fragmentation stage [102, 103].

Bone scintigraphy is also useful although it is currently infrequently used. For bone scintigraphy, pinhole imaging must be used routinely in this young-age-group patients with suspected Legg-Calvé-Perthes disease rather than parallel hole. Additionally, since the anterolateral aspect of the femoral head (the principal weight-bearing region) is typically involved, but no region of the head is necessarily spared and involvement is usually not uniform, pinhole imaging using frog leg and straight anterior position is recommended for better resolving of the abnormalities in this condition. Pinhole imaging is preferred to SPECT

in the diagnosis of this condition in children as it provides magnification while preserving the resolution of images.

Bone scintigraphy is sensitive as well as specific for the diagnosis of this condition showing typically a cold area with or without a rim of increased uptake. It has the advantage of detecting early necrosis of the femoral head after surgical treatment of slipped capital femoral epiphysis [104].

5.2.2.3 Dysbaric Osteonecrosis

This type of osteonecrosis occurs in patients subjected to a high-pressure environment, such as deep-sea divers. The exact cause of ischemia is debated. Immobilization of gas bubbles blocking the vascular channels is considered to be the major factor by many investigators. The presence of intravascular gas bubbles is seen even after ultrasound, and other techniques [105] have documented asymptomatic decompression. Shoulders, hips, knees, and ankles are commonly involved in this type.

5.2.2.4 Sickle Cell Disease Necrosis

Sickle Cell Disease Necrosis. Sickle cell disease is a relatively common hereditary hematological disorder. The disease is caused by the replacement of glutamic acid of B-chains with valine. The disease has numerous consequences; one of the most common is injury to bone. Osteonecrosis and osteomyelitis are the most common bony complications [106].

The bone manifestations occur similarly in other hemoglobinopathies and affect most commonly femora, tibiae, and humeri [107, 108].

Since sickle cell osteonecrosis most commonly involves the femoral and humeral heads although it can affect any bone of the skeleton, it is possible that the increased length of the nutrient arteries supplying the marrow in the long bones makes them more susceptible to occlusion. Necrosis of the femoral head is one of the significant skeletal disorders in sickle cell disease patients. Neonates who have sickle cell disease do not often develop osteonecrosis because of the high fetal hemoglobin level. Although the pathogenesis of the vascular occlusion leading to an infarct is not entirely clear, vaso-occlusion of the marrow is considered to be one of the main culprits in sickle cell crisis. Since hemoglobin S is sensitive to hypoxemia, erythrocytes become viscous and sickle abruptly when exposed to hypoxia. Although the exact pathophysiology of this condition in sickle cell disease patients is not entirely clear, it is proposed to be due to red cell sickling and repetitive vaso-occlusion leading to tissue hypoxia, inflammation, and subsequent bone necrosis (infarct), the most common skeletal complication of sickle cell disease and which subsequently results in collapse. Signs of acute infarction can include warmth, tenderness, erythema, and swelling over the site of vaso-occlusion [107]. However, these clinical signs are nonspecific and may also occur in acute osteomyelitis, which may occur as a primary event or may be superimposed on infarcts as necrotic bone is a fertile site for such secondary infections [107, 108].

Thus, recognition of bone marrow infarction often relies on the use of imaging modalities. MRI is useful for determining the anatomic site and the extent of acute infarcts. and contributes to differentiating acute infarcts from acute osteomyelitis [109, 110].

However, it has not been found to have the specificity or sensitivity of radionuclide studies by some researchers [108].

The scintigraphic diagnosis may be straightforward using bone scan, which shows photon-deficient areas in early stages. SPECT and pinhole are very valuable particularly in resolving a photon-deficient area in the middle of the increased uptake at the reparative process. In this stage, it can be difficult to differentiate osteonecrosis from osteomyelitis, and adding ^{67}Ga or bone marrow scanning may be essential. Acute chest syndrome in sickle cell patients is characterized by chest pain that can mimic several pulmonary disorders including pulmonary embolism and pneumonia [111]. This condition is believed to be a sequel of osteonecrosis of the ribs and is usually associated with pulmonary infiltrates on chest X-ray. Whole-body imaging cannot be overemphasized and should include ribs in addition to the area of interest if different.

5.2.2.5 Idiopathic (Primary or Spontaneous) Osteonecrosis

This is a unique entity with cases presenting with no clear underlying disorders. The femoral head is the most common site involved in osteonecrosis in general [100]. It is usually bilateral and can lead to secondary osteoarthritis. It may also affect the femoral condyles, tibial plateau, wrists, and humoral heads.

5.2.2.6 Spontaneous Osteonecrosis of the Femoral Head

Although no specific cause is recognized for this condition, the most popular hypothesis is an abnormality of fat metabolism, leading to marrow fatty infiltration or vascular embolization [112].

Legg-Calvé-Perthes disease represents a juvenile form of idiopathic osteonecrosis of the femoral head [113].

Primary osteonecrosis of the femoral head affects adult men more frequently than women and is usually seen between the fourth and seventh decades of life. Unilateral and bilateral involvement may be detected. The reported incidence of bilateral disease has varied from 35 to 70%, influenced predominantly by the method of examination and the length of follow-up. Despite the high frequency of bilateral involvement, it usually first manifests as a unilateral symptomatic condition that can be related to osseous collapse in the more severely affected sites. The pathological findings are virtually identical to those in other varieties of osteonecrosis. To demonstrate photopenia in the femoral head, SPECT (85%) is more sensitive than planar imaging (55%) [98].

5.2.2.7 Spontaneous Osteonecrosis of the Knee

5.2.2.7.1 Spontaneous Osteonecrosis of the Knee *(SONK)*

Although osteonecrosis around the knee is observed in association with steroid therapy, sickle cell anemia, other hemoglobinopathies, and renal transplantation, it may also occur in a spontaneous or idiopathic fashion. This entity occurs most characteristically in the medial femoral condyle. It can also affect the medial portion of the tibial plateau, the lateral femoral condyle, or the lateral portion of the tibial plateau alone or in combination with the medial femoral condyle. It characteristically affects older women and is characterized by abrupt onset of knee pain. Signs of localized tenderness, stiffness, effusion, and restricted motion may also be present. Unilateral involvement predominates over bilateral involvement. Initially, radiographs are normal. Weeks or months pass before changes in the weight-bearing articular surface of the medial femoral condyle can be seen. The pathogenesis of this condition is not clear. Vascular insufficiency associated with age is a proposed etiology. Traumatic microfractures in the subchondral bone with secondary disruption of the local blood supply have also been suggested. A predominant role of meniscus injury in the pathogenesis of spontaneous osteonecrosis has also been proposed. X-rays are usually normal at the time of presentation and may even remain so for the entire course of the disease. Bone scintigraphy is a more sensitive modality and is usually helpful in early detection. Scintigraphy may reflect the likely pathogenesis of microfractures with vascular disruption. In the first 6 months, there is increased flow, blood pool activity, and uptake on delayed images. From 6 months to approximately 2 years, blood flow decreases as well as the blood pool activity, while delayed uptake may persist. After 2 years, the bone scan tends to return to normal except in patients who develop joint collapse and secondary osteoarthritis [114].

Osteochondritis dissecans (which affects young patients and does not classically involve the weight-bearing surface of the femoral condyle) should not be confused with spontaneous osteonecrosis. Also, osteoarthritis, commonly affecting the knee, is usually limited to the subchondral bone, whereas osteonecrosis tends to involve the adjacent shaft.

5.2.3 Complex Regional Pain Syndrome-1 (CRPS-1)

Complex regional pain syndrome-1 is a clinical syndrome which has been defined according to the criteria of the International Association for the Study of Pain (IASP) as a clinical syndrome characterized by pain, allodynia, hyperalgesia, edema, abnormal vasomotor and sudomotor activity, movement disorder, joint stiffness, regional osteopenia, and dystrophic soft-tissue changes [115].

The pathophysiology of CRPS-1 (RSD) is not well understood. It is believed that an imbalance between the sympathetic and neuroceptive sensory systems occurs after an event, usually traumatic. Normally, afferent C and A delta fibers carry information from skin neuroceptors to neurons in the dorsal horn of the spinal cord. From this region, information is transferred to higher central nervous system levels and also directed through sympathetic neurons and their efferent fibers. These sympathetic fibers control the tone of distal arterioles and capillaries. It is postulated that trauma, which could be trivial, causes an alteration or imbalance of these nociceptive-sympathetic contact sites, resulting in vasomotor disturbances, pain, and dystrophic changes which form the features of this condition. It is now believed that the pathophysiology of this syndrome is, at least in part, a disease of both the central and peripheral nervous systems [116].

Synovial histopathological changes have been found in patients with CRPS-1. The most common changes are proliferation of synovial cells, subsynovial fibrosis, and vascular proliferation.

Vascular changes can be demonstrated on bone scintigraphy blood pool images, which show increased periarticular activity. A unifying pathophysiological mechanism in CRPS-1 can be proposed, related to an initial triggering injury causing an imbalance between the nociceptors and the autonomic nervous system (sympathetic and parasympathetic) to the affected area. As a result, vasomotor disturbances take place with vasodilatation as a prominent feature, leading to increased blood flow to the synovial and osseous tissues. The synovium reacts with cell proliferation and eventually secondary fibrosis. There is a lack of inflammatory cellular infiltration. The adjacent bone undergoes increased turnover locally, with some resorption. This explains the presence of radiographic and bone scintigraphic changes typical of CRPS-1, as well as changes at the level of the synovium. The clinical course of the condition, which may be underrecognized and could vary with the location, consists of three stages: acute, dystrophic, and atrophic [117].

The first stage is characterized clinically by pain, stiffness, tenderness, and swelling of the involved joint. In stage 2, there is still pain, tenderness, and wasting of subcutaneous tissues and muscles. Thickened fascia and loss of color with cold skin are also seen. Stage 3 may last for months or becomes chronic. This stage is characterized by pronounced wasting of the muscles and subcutaneous tissue. The skin is atrophic, and smooth-appearing contractures are frequent.

Three-phase bone scintigraphy is the most sensitive modality for the diagnosis of the condition [118]. The scintigraphic pattern depends on the duration or stage of the disease [119].

In the first or acute stage (20 weeks), all three phases of bone scan typically show increased activity (Fig. 5.17). After 20 and up to 60 weeks during the dystrophic phase, the first two phases are normalized, while the delayed-phase images show increased periarticular uptake. After 60 weeks (atrophic phase), the flow and blood pool images show decreased perfusion, with normal uptake on delayed images. In children with CRPS-1, decreased perfusion and uptake are the most common manifestations (Table 5.6). A unilateral decrease in the metaphyseal band of activity may be the most striking feature.

Radiopharmaceuticals other than ^{99m}Tc-MDP have also been reported to have potential use in the diagnosis. These include Tc-99 m-labeled human serum albumin [120] combined with N-13 ammonia and 6-[F-18] fluorodopamine [121], F-18 FDG, Tc-99 m sestamibi [122], In-111 octreotides, and I-123 MIBG [123].

N-13-ammonia radioactivity has been reported to be less on the affected side than in the unaffected side, while the F-18 FDG activity is symmetrical. Accordingly, FDG activity is high in the affected side [124]. I-123 MIBG on the other hand was found to be decreased in the affected side reflecting the impaired sympathetic dysfunction with congruent reduction in perfusion [125].

Recently, F-18 FDG-PET/MRI was found to have improved sensitivity over conventional MRI in the detection of musculoskeletal changes, specially in early stages before the onset of irreversible muscle or skin atrophy [126].

5.2.4 Fibrous Dysplasia

Fibrous dysplasia is a benign, developmental, noninheritable condition. It is relatively common, although the etiology is not known. The condition may involve a single bone (monostotic) or multiple bones (polyostotic) and typically results in enlargement and deformity of the involved bone. Pathologically, it is characterized by slow, progressive replacement of the medullary cavity of bone by fibrocollagenous tissue containing poorly formed and randomly arranged trabeculae of woven bone, islands of cartilage, and cystic formations of varying size. The cytoplasm of osteogenic cells within the bone spicules and of the stellate and spindle-shaped cells in the stroma stains histochemically for alkaline phosphatase. A study using C-11 methionine PET in two cases of fibrous dysplasia indicated the presence of viable tumorlike cells [127].

Elevated serum alkaline phosphatase levels have been observed in about one-third of patients, usually with the polyostotic form. Alkaline phosphatase is not a sensitive indicator of the disease but correlates with its extent and severity. This finding indicates the presence of active osteoblasts with increased blood flow and blood pool activity and increased uptake of bone-imaging agents [119].

The lesions are monostotic in 70–80% of patients and polyostotic in up to 30% of cases [47]. Multiphase bone scan shows intense uptake

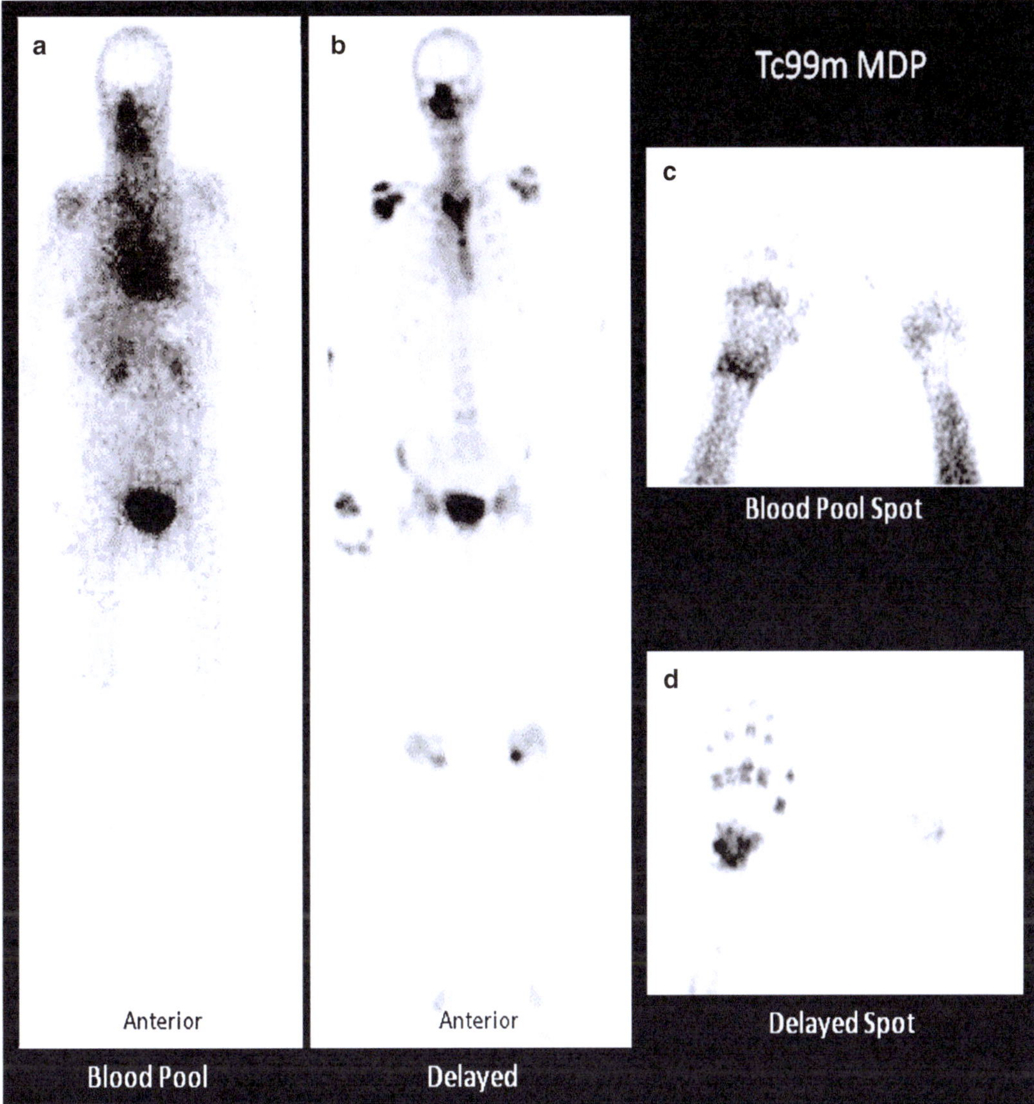

Fig. 5.17 (**a–d**) 99 m Tc-MDP whole-body and spot images of a 40-year-old male with CRPS-1 (RSD) involving the right upper extremity. Whole-body blood pool image (**a**) shows increased activity in the right shoulder wrist and hand. Delayed whole-body and spot images (**b**, **d**) show periarticular increased uptake in the right shoulder, elbow, wrist, and hand. Blood pool spot image (**c**) and delayed spot image (**d**) of the hands clearly demonstrate the blood pool and delayed increased activity around the joints

(Fig. 5.18), reflecting hyperemia as well as osteoid matrix, which is almost always asymmetrical. However, not every case has intense uptake since rarely it shows barely increased uptake probably due to concurrent bone infarct. F-18 NaF has also been found to be useful in the evaluation of the disease activity and correlates quantitatively with the clinical outcomes [128]. The condition may be associated with an endocrine abnormality (McCune-Albright syndrome), which includes precocious puberty and abnormal skin pigmentation in the form of café au lait spots [129].

5.2.5 Trauma

Trauma to the musculoskeletal system may affect bone, cartilage, muscles, and joints. To each of

Table 5.6 Scintigraphic patterns of CRPS-1

Pattern on bone scans	Flow on angiogram	Blood pool	Uptake in delayed images
Typical	Increased	Increased	Increased
Atypical			
In children and adolescents	Decreased	Decreased	Increased
Paralysis, immobilization	Decreased	Decreased	Increased
Subacute	Normal	Normal	Increased
Late phase of CRPS-1	Normal, decreased	Normal, decreased	Variable
Persistent use of painful limb	Decreased	Decreased	Decreased

Modified from [27] with permission

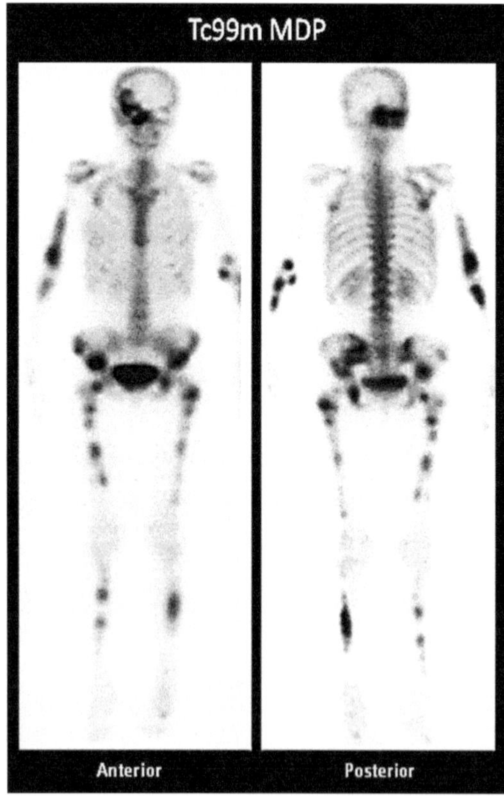

Fig. 5.18 Nineteen-year-old girl with known polyostotic fibrous dysplasia. Tc-99 m MDP anterior and posterior whole-body images demonstrating increased osteoblastic activity in multiple bones including facial bones and skull, bilateral forearm bones, humeri, femora, tibiae, right scapula, and both sides of the pelvis

these structures, trauma may cause immediate damage and late changes.

5.2.5.1 Fractures

A fracture is defined as a break in the continuity of a bone. Fractures can be classified according to several features. Based on the extent of the break, fractures are classified as complete or incomplete. A complete fracture breaks the bone all the way through, while with incomplete fracture, the bone is broken but stays as one piece. Fractures are also classified as open (previously called compound) if the skin is broken and closed (previously called simple) when the skin at the site of fracture is not broken [119].

At sites of preexisting abnormalities that weaken the bone, a minimal force that usually would not cause the fracture of a normal bone may produce a pathological fracture. A transchondral fracture (osteochondritis dissecans) represents fragmentation and separation of portions of cartilage or cartilage and bone. This type is most prevalent in adolescents and occurs typically in the head of the femur, ankle, kneecap, elbow, and wrist [119].

The role of scintigraphy in fracture diagnosis is limited to those cases of radiologically occult fractures, fractures of the small bones of the hands and feet, and fractures of abused children. SPECT/CT has an additional benefit in localizing the findings particularly.

5.2.5.1.1 Stress Fractures

Stress fractures are due to repeated stress, each episode of which is less forceful than required to fracture the bony cortex. The stress fracture is not as thought due to repeated traumatic microfractures.

It is a focal area of increased bone turnover secondary to the repeated stress. The process starts with resorption cavities before being coupled by an osteoblastic response to replace the absorbed bone. The process of rarefaction is faster than the osteoblastic process and will progress if the individual continues stressful activity and trauma. Complete fracture through the zone of rarefaction may occur. If this occurs in normal bones, the resulting fractures are called fatigue fractures, while if they occur on abnormal bones, as in osteoporosis, they are termed insufficiency fractures. Bone scintigraphy is much more sensitive than standard radiographs in detecting stress fractures. If scintigraphy is performed in the acute phase of less than 4 weeks, the flow and blood pool images show increased activity. Later, only delayed uptake will be seen. The delayed uptake is typically focal or fusiform, involving less than one-fifth of the bone (Fig. 5.19). The pattern of uptake of stress fractures is different from the pattern of a shin splint, which is another consequence of stress also known as medial tibial stress syndrome and occurs in the same patient population as fatigue fractures. The pain usually occurs on the anterior part of the tibia due to repetitive activity-related trauma to the tissues surrounding tibia. Pain from shin splints can be generalized across the lower two-thirds of the tibia; in contrast, pain from a stress fracture is localized [130]. Shin splints typically show normal flow and blood pool images, with an elongated linear pattern of increased uptake on delayed images (Fig. 5.20). They are most commonly found in the tibiae and may coexist with fatigue fractures in the same patient. The scintigraphic pattern seen with shin splints is due to subperiosteal bone formation [131].

5.2.5.1.2 Spondylolysis

Spondylolysis is a condition in which there is a loss of continuity of bone of the neural arch of the vertebra due to trauma or more likely due to stress. The gap or loss of continuity most commonly occurs at the junction of the lamina when the vertebra is viewed from above or between the superior and inferior articular processes (pars interarticularis or facet joints) when viewed from the side (Fig. 5.21). This condition most frequently affects the fourth and fifth lumbar vertebra, may or may not be symptomatic, and usually does not result in any neurological deficit but is a common cause of low back pain, particularly in children and young adults [132]. The diagnosis is principally radiological (CT, MRI), and scintigraphy is reserved for detection of radiologically occult stress changes and for assessing metabolic activity of the condition. Typically, a focal area of increased uptake is seen in the region of the pars interarticularis (Fig. 5.22). SPECT is much more sensitive than planar imaging in detecting the abnormality. SPECT/CT is preferred to SPECT

Fig. 5.19 (**a**) Representative images of a ^{99m}Tc-MDP bone scan for a 23-year-old man with an 8-week history of right-shin pain. There is fusiform focus of prominent increased uptake in the shaft of the right fibula illustrating the pattern of fatigue fracture. (**b**) Another example of stress fracture in the foot with focally increased flow and blood pool with corresponding focus of increased uptake on delayed images

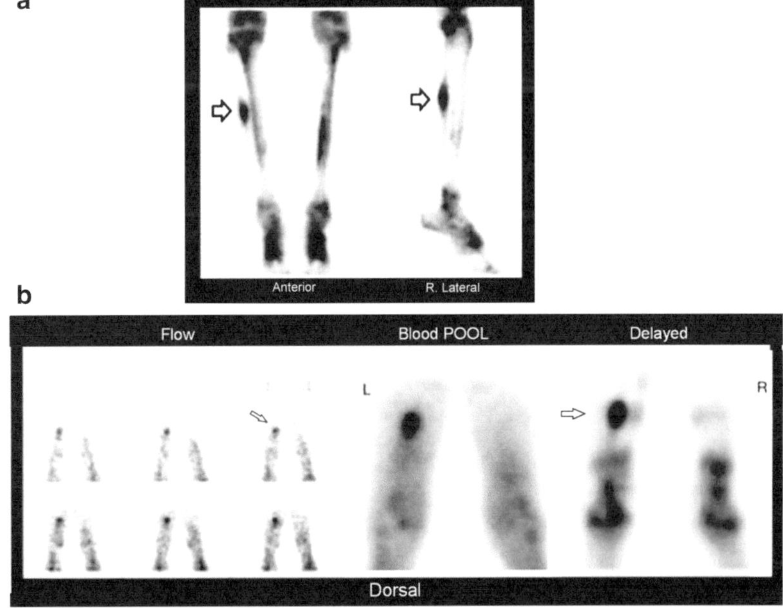

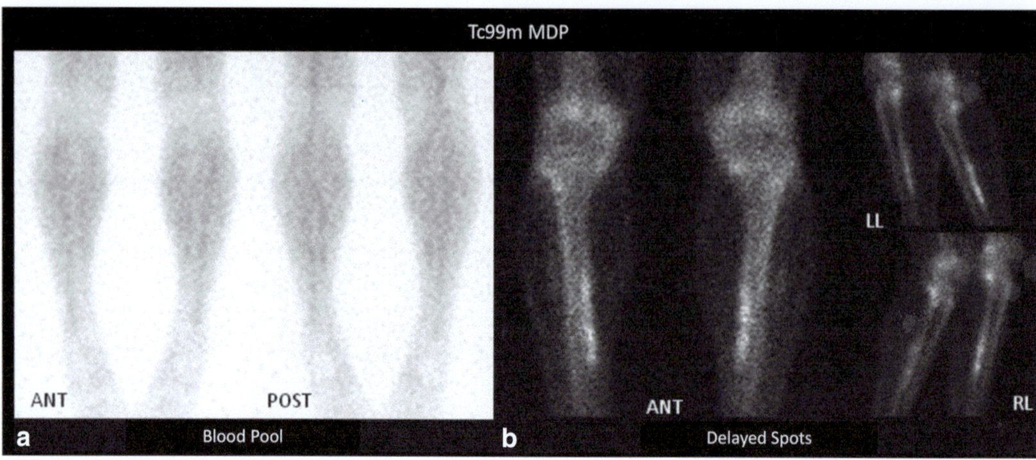

Fig. 5.20 Tc99m MDP whole-body and spot images for a 33-year-old military man with a history of lower back pain and bilateral leg pain more over the medial aspects for 1-year duration. Blood pool images (**a**) are unremark- able. Delayed spot images of the legs (**b**) demonstrate increased linear uptake over the tibial bone bilaterally postero-medially indicating bilateral medial tibial stress syndrome (shin splint)

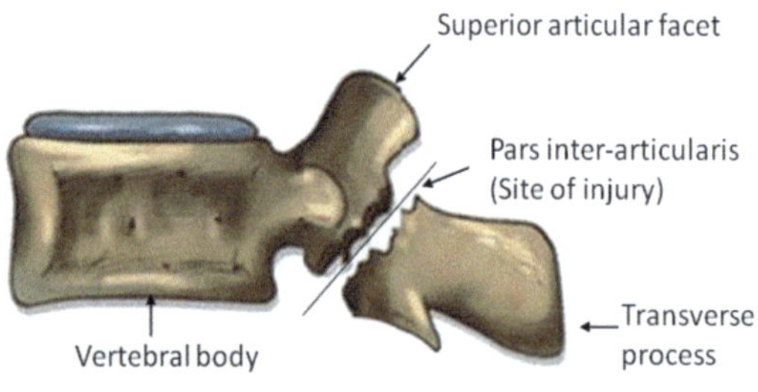

Fig. 5.21 A diagram illustrating the site of injury causing spondylolysis as seen from lateral view of the vertebra

only [133]. Spondylolisthesis is the forward or occasionally backward movement of one vertebra over another (Fig. 5.23a–c) as a result of fracture of the neural arch. It is again most commonly seen in the fifth lumbar vertebra (Fig 5.24), in which there is a forward shift of L5 on the sacrum [132]. It is less commonly seen at L4. In addition to parallel-hole high-resolution acquisition, pinhole and/or SPECT is needed, along with correlation with plain radiographs of the lumbar spine.

5.2.5.2 Fracture Healing

Fracture union is simply defined as sufficient growth of the bone across the fracture line. Several factors affect the fracture healing, and if disturbances happen, delayed, non-, or malunion could result. *Delayed union* indicates that union does not occur at the expected time, which is difficult to be determined and varies with the site of fracture although overall it is usually 3–4 months after the fracture. *Nonunion* indicates failure of the bone ends to grow together. Instead of a new bone, dense fibrous material fills the gap between the broken ends and uncommonly by fibrocartilaginous tissue. Occasionally, the gap between the bone ends contains a space filled with fluid. In this case, the term false joint or *pseudoarthrosis* is applied, and persistent uptake of ^{99m}Tc-diphosphonate continues to be seen after the usual period of healing or postoperative changes. *Malunion* describes healing of a bone in a non-anatomical orientation.

5.2.6 Growth Plate Injury

The physis, or growth plate, is recognized as the site of endochondral ossification and is responsible for a bone's growth in length. Although the band of increased uptake seen on scintigraphic bone images is referred to as the growth plate, it actually does not correspond to the lucent band present on a bone radiograph that is also referred to as the growth plate. The radionuclide growth

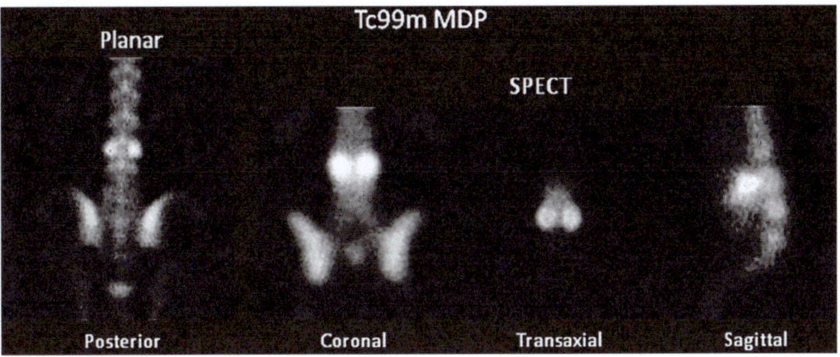

Fig. 5.22 Tc-99 m MDP spot planar image of the pelvis and lumbar spine and selective coronal, transaxial, and sagittal SPECT slices of the lumbar spine demonstrating increased uptake in both sides of the L3 vertebra corresponding to the area of pars interarticularis

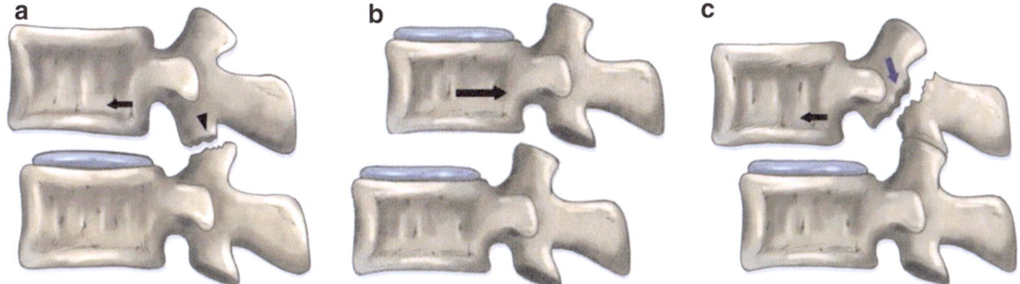

Fig. 5.23 Spondylolisthesis without spondylolysis (a). Apophyseal joint osteoarthritis allows the inferior articular processes to move anteriorly, producing forward subluxation of the superior vertebra on the inferior vertebra. (b) Spondylolisthesis without spondylolysis but with backward subluxation of the superior vertebra. (c) Spondylolisthesis with spondylolysis. The bilateral defects through the pars interarticularis allow anterior displacement of vertebral body on its neighbor, but the alignment of the apophyseal joints is normal (Adapted from Resnick [101]) (Fig. 5.24)

plate corresponds to the dense band of bone in the metaphysis adjacent to the radiographic growth plate and is described in radiographic anatomy as the zone of provisional calcification.

On scintigraphy, a key to the comparison of growth plate uptake is having both plates symmetrically positioned on the same large view. Two- or three-phase imaging is recommended in growth plate evaluation. Both flow and blood pool images show information on plate activity.

They often show differences in plate function more clearly than the delayed images [134]. The normal physis scintigraphic appearance of the growth plate changes with age. In the infant and young child, the physis has a thicker, oval-shaped appearance. With maturation, it becomes linear, and in adolescence, the closing physis shows progressively decreasing activity.

Physiological status of the growth plate is difficult to evaluate using morphological imaging.

Segmental closure can be better identified using pinhole view and quantitation [135]. SPECT imaging was found useful to detect and locate decreased metabolism associated with post-traumatic closure of the physeal plate which predicts growth arrest and deformities. Pinhole magnification imaging is superior to SPECT and is the preferred method of imaging. Injury to the physis or growth plate in children may lead to growth arrest and/or angular deformities in the limbs.

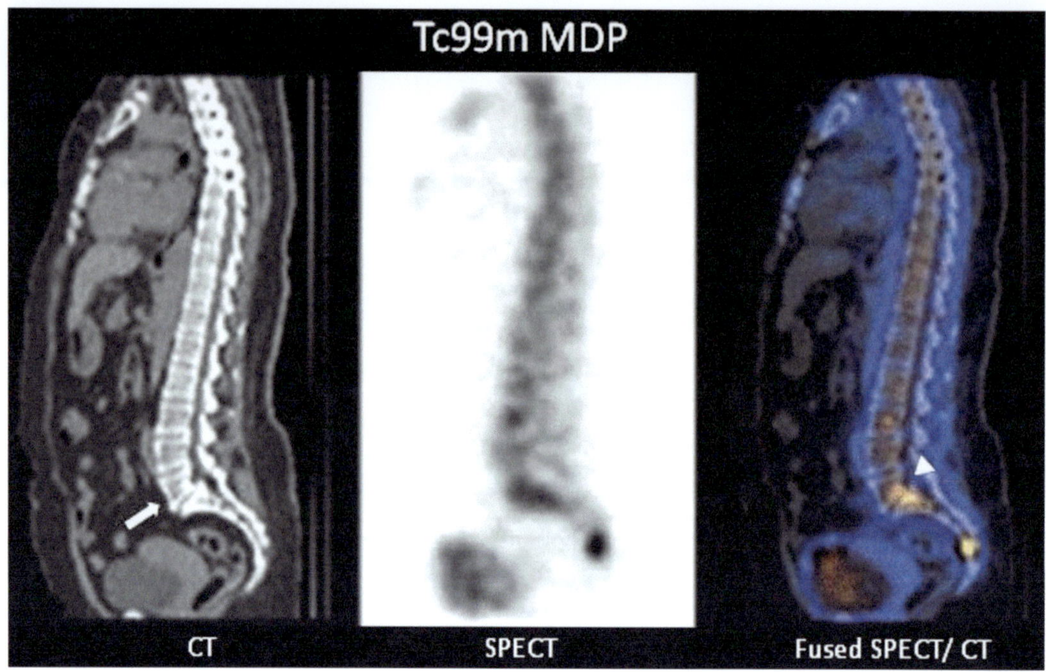

Fig. 5.24 Selected SPECT/CT sagittal cuts in a case with known spondylolisthesis with forward shift of L5 on S1 vertebra (arrow) and uptake seen clearly at the site (arrowhead)

5.2.7 Metabolic Bone Diseases

The osseous bone response to injury, regardless of the type, is characterized by increased remodeling and new bone formation in an attempt to repair the damage or to contain the noxious insult.

This process is evidenced by focal increased uptake of bone-seeking agents. In contrast, in metabolic bone disease, a general imbalance of the processes of bone formation and resorption is present. The net effect resulting from these two processes determines the scintigraphic patterns observed in metabolic bone disease. Metabolic bone disease, however, is usually linked to alterations of calcium metabolism by one or more number of physiological factors [136]. Increased rates of bone turnover are present in most metabolic bone disorders (Table 5.6) often associated with decreasing calcium content of the affected bone. This explains why most metabolic disorders result in generalized increased radiopharmaceutical uptake on bone scintigraphs, reflecting

this increased bone turnover. The regulation of calcium and bone metabolism is multifactorial and complex. Parathyroid hormone (PTH) plays an important role in these mechanisms by acting on two major mechanisms. The two main actions are (1) to increase resorption of calcium and magnesium and (2) to decrease phosphate reabsorption. The effect of PTH on bone is also modulated by vitamin D and is mainly to promote the efflux of calcium from bone, acting through osteoclasts. In some disorders, however, abnormal bone formation has a more localized character as in the case of hypertrophic osteoarthropathy, the pathogenesis of which is still poorly understood, although neurovascular abnormalities may be present.

5.2.7.1 Paget's Disease (Osteitis Deformans)

The etiology of Paget's disease is not known; viral infection has been suggested, although direct recovery of a virus has not been made. The skeletal distribution of Paget's disease suggests that the disease predominates in bones containing red marrow and may be dependent on the blood supply. Normal hematopoietic bone marrow may be replaced by loose fibrous connective tissue. With time, the increased osteoblastic and osteoclastic activity ceases, marrow abnormalities return to normal, and the affected bones become sclerotic. The chronic acceleration of remodeling may lead to enlargement and softening of the bones affected. Paget's disease begins with active and excessive resorption (resorption or lytic phase), which may progress rapidly and results in softening of the bone. Pathological fractures frequently occur, particularly of the femur and tibia. In this phase, the bone trabeculae are slender and very vascular. Giant osteoclasts are present and have been shown to take up 57Ga. This is followed by a mixed phase characterized by accelerated formation as well as resorption of bone. If bone formation predominates, this can be called the osteoblastic phase and the term mixed can be reserved for those with approximately equal resorption and formation. The final phase (the sclerotic or burned-out phase) is characterized predominantly by new bone formation, more disorganized structure, thick trabeculae, and less prominent vascular sinusoids [137].

The morphology of the resorptive phase of Paget's disease is characterized by the presence of increased numbers of large multinucleated osteoclasts that may assume bizarre shapes and contain as many as 100 nuclei; normal osteoclasts have five to ten nuclei. In the mixed phase, a profusion of osteoblasts and osteoclasts, evidence of high bone turnover, coexists in a matrix of highly vascularized fibrous tissue. The late sclerotic phase is characterized by a disordered mosaic pattern of thickened lamellae containing irregular patterns of cement lines where waves of bone formation have succeeded in areas of previous bone resorption. Although Paget's disease is diagnosed economically with standard radiographs, other modalities are needed, particularly scintigraphy, given the limitations of the standard radiographs. MRI can add diagnostic value in the diagnosis of Paget's disease, by demonstrating marrow changes when present, and can contribute to a noninvasive diagnosis of Paget's disease in atypical presentations.

On multiphase bone scan, dynamic flow and early static images show varying degrees of hyperemia at the sites of involvement depending on the stage of the disease; the earlier the phase, the more the hyperemia. On delayed static images, Paget's disease appearance depends on the stage of the disease. During the active lytic phase, involvement of Paget's disease is characteristically seen as intense increased uptake, which is uniformly distributed throughout the region affected (Fig. 5.25). An exception to this characteristic pattern of the early phase is the skull pagetic lesion, which shows intense uptake at the periphery of the lesion while the center is cold which is referred to as osteoporosis circumscripta.

With time, the disease activity gradually decreases toward the sclerotic phase, and uptake of the bone-imaging agents decreases as well. The sclerotic phase may show practically no abnormal uptake of the radiopharmaceuticals, and hence, the disease can be detected by X-ray and missed by bone scanning. This is in contrast to the early lytic phase when bone scan is much more sensitive than radiographs. The bone scan will identify approximately 15–30% of lesions not visualized on X-rays [138]. Conversely, in about 5% of cases, the radiograph may demonstrate diffuse pagetic involvement, for example, of the pelvis, whereas the bone scan reveals little uptake of the isotope [139]. The disease is often nonuniform within the skeleton. Individual involved bones can simultaneously present more than one stage of the disease process, reflecting variations of the duration of the disease at different sites. Paget's disease may show absent and expanded bone marrow uptake or a mixture of both. This can be explained by the presence of areas of advanced, sclerotic disease with active bone marrow and areas of earlier active disease with replaced bone marrow. Since 111In-WBCs are taken up by hematopoietic bone marrow, uptake is therefore seen in areas of Paget's disease with active marrow. This can mimic the uptake in infection, particularly when it is focal.

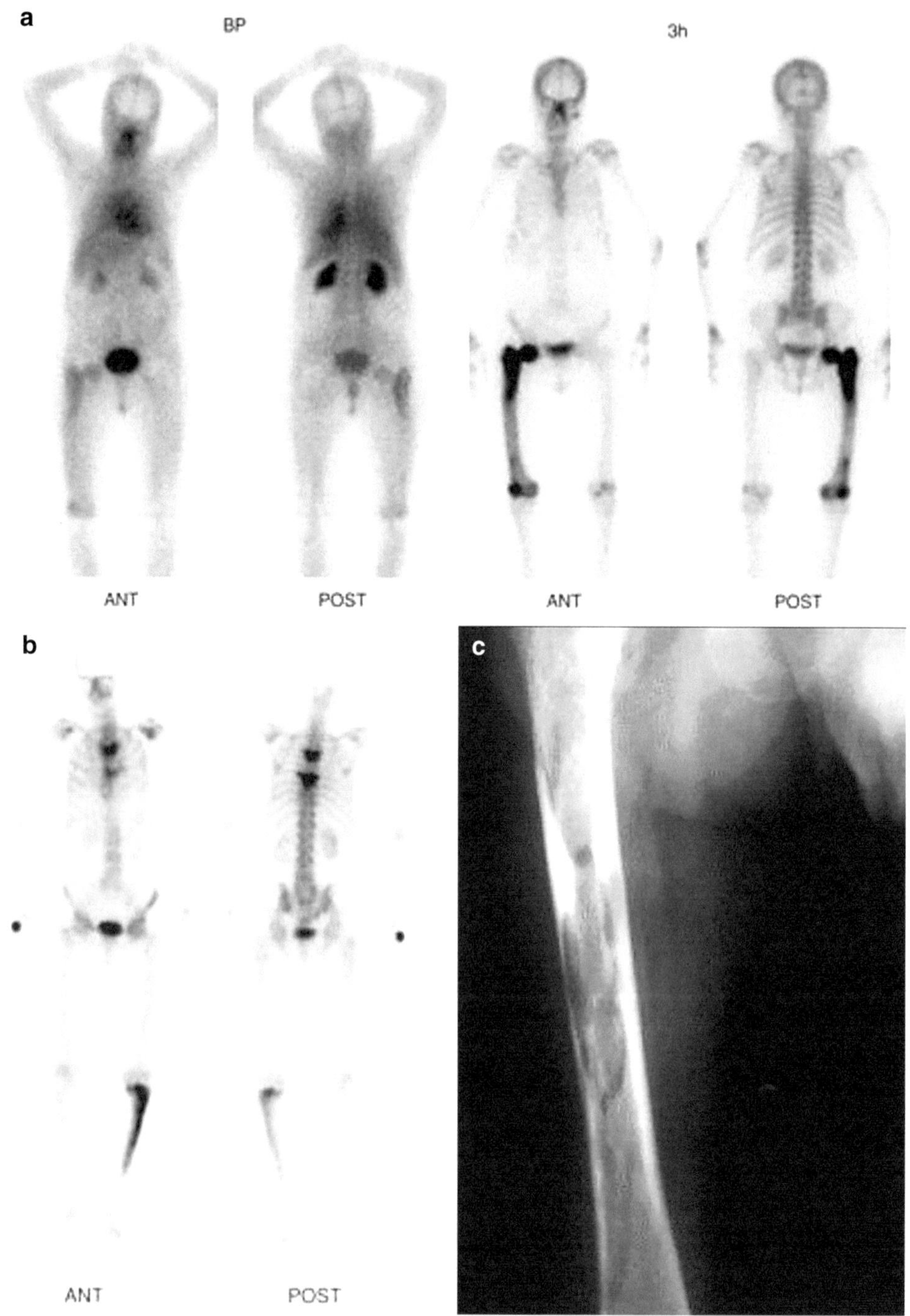

Fig. 5.25 76 y/o female with lytic lesion in the right tibia. Monostotic Paget's disease. There is diffusely increased blood pool activity in the right tibia more obvious proximally with corresponding increased delayed uptake. (**a**) the increased uptake involves the entire tibia but with grades of uptake from mild to intense represent-ing uptake patterns in early active phase and delayed phases. (**b**) demonstrates an example of polyostotic type of the disease affecting more than one location (thoracic spine and left tibia). (**c**) Radiograph of a femur affected with Paget's disease demonstrating the typical osteolytic pattern (flame shaped) of the disease

5.2.7.2 Osteoporosis

Bone mass gradually increases during childhood and increases rapidly once the skeleton approaches maturity, and longitudinal skeletal growth slows till it reaches the peak bone mass in the second decade although this is somewhat controversial [140]. At maturity, black men have denser skeleton than white men and black women, whereas white women have the least dense bones. Generally, men have an average 20% greater peak bone mass than women [138]. After reaching its peak, bone mass begins to decrease at a rate of 0.25–1% per year. Osteoporosis is the most common metabolic disorder of the skeletal system. It affects approximately 20 million older Americans, 90% of whom are postmenopausal [141]. Osteoporosis is "a condition in which bone tissue is reduced in amount increasing the likelihood of a fracture. In other words, the bone is qualitatively normal but quantitatively abnormal. The basic mechanism behind this condition is decreased bone formation (osteoid formation), even though calcium deposition may be normal. The disease develops when the process of bone resorption and formation (remodeling cycle) is disrupted, leading to an imbalance.

The complete remodeling cycle that consists of activation of basic multicellular units, bone resorption, and bone formation normally takes about 4 months in adults. In patients with osteoporosis, this remodeling cycle may require up to 2 years. This can be attributed to an increase in the number of activated basic multicellular units, leading to resorption at more sites, increased rate of resorption, increased frequency of activation of basic multicellular units, and delay in bone formation.

Osteoporosis also occurs when the numbers of osteoblasts and osteoclasts in bone are inadequate.

There are numerous causes of osteoporosis, many of which are metabolic in nature (Table 5.7). The types of osteoporosis not considered metabolic in nature include juvenile osteoporosis, which affects younger individuals and is idiopathic rather than metabolic. The disease may be generalized, involving the major portions of the

Table 5.7 High turnover disorders

Generalized disorders
Primary hyperparathyroidism
Renal osteodystrophy(certain forms)
Type 1 (postmenopausal) osteoporosis
Localized disorders
Focal osteoporotic syndromes
Disuse atrophy
CRPS-1 (RSD)
Transient osteoporosis
Paget's disease
Stress fractures

axial skeleton, or regional, in one segment of the appendicular skeleton. Both compact and spongy bones are lost, but loss of spongy bone exceeds that of compact bone.

Bone densitometers measure the radiation absorption by the skeleton to determine bone mass of the peripheral, axial, and total skeleton. Although osteoporosis sometimes is obvious on plain radiographs, quantification of bone density from plain radiographs is difficult and inaccurate. Dual-energy X-ray absorptiometry (DXA) however is the most widely used technique and is considered the gold standard method for the measurement of bone mineral density (BMD). It has the advantages of good precision, short scan times, and stable calibration.

5.2.7.3 Osteomalacia and Rickets

Osteomalacia is due to abnormal mineralization of bone, predominantly as a result of vitamin D deficiency, with a decrease in bone density secondary to lack of both calcium and phosphorus.

Note that in osteomalacia the amount of osteoid (bone formation) is normal, while osteoid is decreased in osteoporosis. In other words, there is inadequate and delayed mineralization of osteoid in spongy and compact bones, which have a normal remodeling cycle as opposed to delayed cycles in osteoporosis. Simply, in osteomalacia, the osteoid tissue is normal in amount but soft since it lacks calcium, while in osteoporosis there is a lack of osteoid tissue as a whole.

If osteomalacia occurs in growing bones prior to closure of the growth plate, it is called infantile osteomalacia or rickets. Growing bones fail to mineralize and become soft, with resultant deformities. Growth plates and metaphysis are disorganized in patients with rickets, with a decrease in the length and width of the growth plates.

5.2.7.4 Bone Changes of Hyperparathyroidism

Overactivity of the parathyroid gland(s) results in excess secretion of parathyroid hormone, which promotes bone resorption and consequently leads to hypercalcemia and hypophosphatemia. Primary, secondary, and tertiary hyperparathyroidism all share elevated serum calcium and parathyroid hormone. Primary hyperparathyroidism is caused by benign adenoma in approximately 80% of cases. Hyperplasia is generally the cause in the remainder of cases, and carcinoma is a very rare cause. Secondary hyperparathyroidism is due to compensatory hyperplasia in response to hypocalcemia. For example, this may occur in long-standing renal failure. Reduced renal production of 1,25-dihydroxyvitamin D3 (active metabolite of vitamin D) leads to decreased intestinal absorption of calcium, resulting in hypocalcemia. Failure of the tubules to excrete phosphate results in hyperphosphatemia. Hypocalcemia is compensated for by parathyroid hyperplasia and excess production of parathyroid hormone [141]. Tertiary hyperparathyroidism describes a condition of persistent parathyroid hormone overproduction (even after a low calcium level has been corrected) as a result of autonomous hyperplastic parathyroid tissue. In all forms of hyperparathyroidism, there is increased bone resorption associated with increased osteoblastic activity, leading to increased uptake of bone-seeking radiopharmaceuticals. This is least prominent in primary compared with other forms of hyperparathyroidism. After parathyroidectomy for primary or secondary hyperparathyroidism, hypocalcemia is generally transient, and normal parathyroid tissue recovers function quickly (usually within 1 week) even after long-term suppression. Severe and prolonged hypocalcemia may occur in some cases despite normal or even elevated levels of parathyroid hormone leading to hungry bone syndrome [142].

5.2.7.4.1 Renal Osteodystrophy

Renal osteodystrophy is a metabolic condition of the bone associated with chronic renal failure. The major skeletal changes of the disease include osteitis fibrosa, osteitis fibrosa cystica, rickets, osteomalacia, osteosclerosis, and extraosseous calcification including tumoral calcinosis. Osteitis fibrosa is characterized by extensive medullary fibrosis and increased osteoclastic resorption linked to PTH hypersecretion. When cystic lesions are present, it forms cystitis fibrosa cystica. Osteomalacia is mainly due to vitamin D insufficiency, hypocalcemia, acidosis, aluminum toxicity, and, exceptionally, hypophosphatemia. It should be mentioned that aluminum overload directly inhibits the osteoblast [143–145]. Currently, the disease is believed to occur in three major types: high turnover disease (most common), low turnover disease, and mixed disease [146]. The low turnover type may present with osteomalacia and osteoporosis, which can also occur in the high turnover disease. The mixed form shows both osteomalacia and osteitis fibrosa. Differentiation of different forms is usually based on clinical data, laboratory findings, and standard radiographs although it can be difficult. Scintigraphically, diffusely increased uptake with increased skeletal-to-renal uptake ratio occurs in high turnover form. This uptake may be homogenous or heterogeneous with focal findings depending on the predominant pathophysiological process. One or more of the typical finding of metabolic bone disease on bone scan may be seen (Table 5.8). Low turnover form shows typically decreased uptake unless complicated by a focal pathology. A mixture of those findings is seen in mixed form.

5.2.7.5 Hypertrophic Osteoarthropathy

Hypertrophic osteoarthropathy is a rheumatic disorder characterized by bone pain, joint pain, and nearly always clubbing of fingers and/or toes. Two types of hypertrophic osteoarthropathy are recognized: primary and secondary. The primary type (also called pachydermoperiostosis) is less common and occurs in adolescence, with

Table 5.8 Etiology and classification of osteoporosis

Primary
1. Involutional
Type I: Postmenopausal
Type II: Age related (senile)
2. Idiopathic
Juvenile
Adult
Secondary
1. Prolonged immobilization
2. Steroid therapy
3. Diabetes mellitus
4. Prolonged heparin administration
5. Sickle cell disease
6. Cushing's syndrome
7. Rheumatoid arthritis
8. Scurvy
9. Multiple myeloma
10. Osteogenesis imperfecta (brittle bone disease)
11. Disuse or immobilization of a limb (regional osteoporosis)

Table 5.9 Main types of joint disease with major examples

A. Inflammatory joint disease
1. Infectious
Infectious arthritis
2. Noninfectious
Rheumatoid arthritis
Crystal deposition arthropathies (gouty arthritis, CPPD)
Sacroiliitis
Neuropathic joint disease
Spondyloarthropathies
Ankylosing spondylitis
Psoriatic arthritis
Reactive arthritis (formerly Reiter's disease)
Inflammatory bowel disease-associated arthritis
B. Noninflammatory joint disease
1. Primary osteoarthritis
2. Secondary osteoarthritis

spontaneous arrest of the process in young adulthood. A variant has been reported in a family [147]. The secondary form follows a variety of pathological conditions, predominantly intrathoracic. Lung cancer and other intrathoracic malignancies, benign lung pathologies, and cyanotic heart disease are common causes. Abdominal malignancies, hepatic and biliary cirrhosis, and inflammatory bowel disease are less common causes [148]. Nasopharyngeal carcinoma has also been reported as a cause [81]. Pathologically, the condition is a form of periostitis and may be painful. Additionally, clubbing of fingers and toes, sweating, and thickening of skin may also be seen. In the tubular bones, there is periosteal new bone formation. This pathological feature explains the typical scintigraphic pattern of diffusely increased uptake along the cortical margins of long bones, giving the appearance of "parallel tracks." The scintigraphic abnormalities are usually confined to diaphyseal regions, although they may also occur in the epiphyseal bone. The changes are usually bilateral but can be unilateral in approximately 15% of cases [148]. The tibiae and fibulae are affected most commonly, followed by the distal femur, radius, ulna, hands, feet, and distal humerus. Scapula, patella,

maxilla, mandible, and clavicle are less frequently affected and rarely the ribs and pelvis. The condition has no prognostic significance as there was no significant difference in survival between lung cancer patients with and others without hypertrophic osteoarthropathy. The changes disappear following successful treatment of the lung cancer or other inciting pathology.

5.2.8 Arthropathy

No unified classification for the many types of joint diseases is available. Arthropathies are grouped into two main categories: inflammatory and noninflammatory [149] (Table 5.9). Table 5.10 summarizes the typical features of common arthropathies on bone scintigraphy.

5.2.8.1 Soft-Tissue Calcification

Pathological calcification is classified mainly into three types:

5.2.8.1.1 Dystrophic Calcification

Dystrophic calcification is the calcification of dying or dead tissue. The mechanism appears to be increased calcium-binding capacity of the exposed denatured proteins of the injured cells,

Table 5.10 Typical scintigraphic findings of major joint diseases

Disease	Scintigraphic findings
Rheumatoid arthritis	Symmetric uptake involving small and large joints
Gouty arthritis	Uptake of metatarsophalangeal joint of the great toe and large joints, commonly symmetric
Ankylosing spondylitis	Symmetric intense tracer uptake in both sacroiliac joints and spine
Osteoarthritis	Uptake of large joints, symmetric in primary type
Reactive arthritis	Asymmetric uptake of large and small joints and spine
Psoriatic arthritis	Asymmetric uptake of large and small joints typically of upper extremity including fingers and spine
Infectious arthritis	Uptake involving a large joint
Enteropathic arthritis	Uptake of large joints (asymmetric), sacroiliac joints (symmetric), and spine

which preferentially bind with phosphate ions which in turn react with calcium and form calcium deposits. Examples include calcification in infarcted myocardial muscle, in atheromas, in amyloid tissue, and in the centers of tumors.

5.2.8.1.2 Metastatic Calcification

Metastatic calcification describes the calcification of viable, undamaged, normal tissue as a result of hypercalcemia associated with increased calcium phosphate product, locally or systemically. This can be due to metabolic abnormalities as with renal failure, hypervitaminosis D, and hyperparathyroidism or due to increased bone demineralization from bone tumors or disseminated metastases.

5.2.8.1.3 Heterotopic Bone Formation

(Heterotopic ossification) Heterotopic bone formation, or increased ectopic osteoblastic activity, is defined as the presence of bone in soft tissue where it does not normally exist. In the vast majority of cases, the condition is acquired. Rarely, it can be congenital [150]. The pathogenesis of heterotopic bone formation is still debated. However, it is believed to be secondary to the transformation of pluripotent mesenchymal cells,

present in the connective tissue septa within the muscle, into the osteogenic cell line. The acquired form of heterotopic bone formation often occurs after trauma. Other associated conditions include burns, sickle cell disease, hemophilia, tetanus, poliomyelitis, multiple sclerosis, toxic epidermal necrolysis, and cancer. It also occurs infrequently in the absence of a precipitating event or condition. Heterotopic bone formation includes the specific entity myositis ossificans: a post-traumatic skeletal muscle ossification usually occurring next to long bones. In many clinical practices, myositis ossificans is usually seen among patients who have sustained trauma such as operative procedures (e.g., total hip arthroplasty), fractures, dislocations, and direct trauma to muscle groups (mainly quadriceps femoris and brachialis muscles). Additional reported sites include abdominal incisions, wounds, and gastrointestinal tract. Anatomically, HBF is always extra-articular, but it may be attached to the joint capsule without disrupting it. Occasionally, HBF may be attached to the cortex of adjacent bone with or without cortical disruption. Tumoral calcinosis describes heterotopic bone formation that has large amounts of bone formation resembling tumor masses. The incidence of heterotopic bone formation varies greatly in different patient populations. It has been reported to be between 20 and 25% among spinal cord injury patients, while 10–20% of closed head injury patients develop heterotopic bone formation [151, 152]. The onset of heterotopic bone formation has been reported to range from 4 to 12 weeks after injury, most commonly at 2 months, but it has also been reported to occur as early as 20 days post-injury. The most commonly involved areas, in decreasing order, are the hips, knees, shoulders, and elbows. Rarely, it can occur in the foot. The course of acquired heterotopic bone formation is relatively benign in 80% or more of cases. The remaining patients often develop significant loss of motion, and ankylosis occurs in up to 10%. Clinical, laboratory, radiographic, and scintigraphic criteria have been used to follow the course of heterotopic bone formation and to assist in treatment. The most sensitive imaging modality for early detection of heterotopic bone

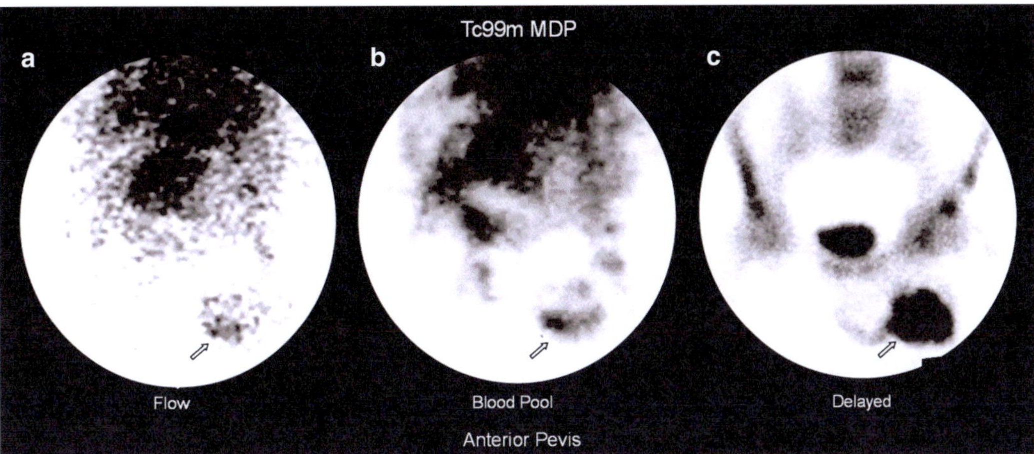

Fig. 5.26 (**a–c**) Multiphase bone scan showing increased flow (**a**), blood pool (**b**), and delayed (**c**) soft-tissue uptake in the left thigh (*arrows*) and illustrating the finding of immature heterotopic bone formation

formation is multiphase bone scintigraphy. Blood flow and pool images have detected incipient heterotopic bone formation as early as 2.5 weeks after injury, with delayed scintigraphs becoming positive about 1 week later. These scintigraphic findings precede positive radiographs by 1–4 weeks [153]. The condition is classified as immature when flow and blood pool activity are increased (Fig. 5.26). When flow and blood pool patterns normalize or stabilize after showing decreasing activity, the condition is considered to be mature. As heterotopic bone progresses from immature to mature, the three-phase bone scan typically shows progressive reduction in the activity of all three phases. The majority of bone scans return to baseline within 12 months, although many patients reach the mature phase much earlier or much later. Since surgical intervention during the immature phase often leads to recurrence, serial bone scans are useful in monitoring the activity of the disease, so as to determine the appropriate time for surgical removal of heterotopic bone with minimal risk of recurrence. SPECT/CT is helpful since it clarifies the location of abnormal uptake and helps in alleviating the confusion with bone infections [154]. The congenital forms include the rare form of heterotopic ossification called myositis ossificans progressiva, or fibrodysplasia ossificans progressiva [88, 89], and the very rare progressive osseous heteroplasia (progressive and potentially debilitating disorder). Myositis ossificans progressiva is an autosomal dominant congenital disease often associated with other skeletal abnormalities including malformation of the great toes and shortening of digits, as well as other clinical features such as deafness and baldness.

5.3 Neoplastic Bone Disease

5.3.1 Primary Bone Tumors

Various primary tumors originate from the bone. Based on the cell of origin, primary tumors can be classified as osteogenic, chondrogenic, collagenic, or myelogenic.

5.3.1.1 Osteogenic Tumors

Osteogenic tumors originate from bone cell precursors, the osteoblasts, and are characterized by formation of bone or osteoid tissue. These tumors include osteoid osteomas, osteosarcomas, and osteoblastomas.

5.3.1.1.1 Osteoid Osteoma

The benign tumor osteoid osteoma is the most common in children, particularly boys. Typically, it presents in the lower extremities, the pelvis, or less commonly the spine. Patients frequently report nocturnal pain, which is relieved by aspirin. It is characterized by its small nidus size of less than 2 cm, self-limited growth, and tendency to cause extensive reactive changes in the surrounding bone tissue. The lesion classically presents with severe pain at night that is dramatically relieved by non-steroidal anti-inflammatory drugs (NSAIDs). The tumor has been shown to express very high levels of prostaglandins, particularly PGE2 and PGI2. High local levels of these prostaglandins are presumed to be the cause of the intense pain seen in patients with this lesion. Studies have shown strong immunoreactivity to cyclooxygenase-2 (COX-2) in the nidus of the tumor but not in the surrounding reactive bone. COX-2 is one of the mediators of increased production of prostaglandins by osteoid osteomas and may be the cause of the secondary changes depicted by MRI [155]. The usual sites of involvement include bones of the lower extremities, pelvis, and spine.

5.3.1.1.2 Osteoblastoma

Osteoblastoma is a tumor related to osteoid osteoma and has almost identical histological appearance, but the nidus is larger in size measuring more than 2 cm. It is commonly seen in the spine and can occur in any other location. For the appendicular skeleton, the lower extremity is the most common location for osteoblastoma where 35% of the lesions occur.

5.3.1.1.3 Osteogenic Sarcoma

Osteogenic sarcoma is an osteogenic tumor with sarcomatous tissue. It is the most common malignant bone-forming tumor and has the appearance of callus containing compact or cancellous bone, produced by anaplastic cells and sometimes chondroid and fibrinoid tissue. The male-to-female ratio is 3/2. Sixty percent of cases occur before the age of 20. A secondary peak incidence is found between 50 and 60 years of age, mainly in patients with a history of prior radiation therapy years earlier. The vast majority of the tumors involve the metaphyses of long bones particularly in the distal femur, with 50% around the knee region.

5.3.1.2 Chondrogenic Tumors

All tumors that produce cartilage, primitive cartilage, or cartilage-like substance are called chon-drogenic. The most common malignant chondrogenic tumor is chondrosarcoma. Two types of this malignant tumor are recognized: (a) primary chondrosarcoma, occurring mainly in patients aged 50–70 years, and (b) secondary chondrosarcoma, which is derived from the benign chondrogenic tumor enchondroma and occurs more frequently in patients aged 20–30 years. Chondrosarcoma is more common in men than in women, often arising in the metaphysis or diaphysis of long bones, particularly the femur and the pelvis. The neoplasm consists of hyaline cartilage with bands of anaplastic cells and fibrous tissue. The tumor may infiltrate the joint spaces located near the end of the long bone. Chondroma is the benign chondrogenic tumor which is an uncommon benign tumor that characteristically forms mature cartilage. The tumor is encapsulated with a lobular growing pattern. It is formed of chondrocytes (cartilaginous cells) that resemble normal cells and produce cartilaginous matrix. It is found mostly in the small bones of the hand and/or feet, although it can also occur in long, tubular bones, primarily the humerus, femur, and ribs. Occasionally, focal areas of myxoid degeneration may result in a mistaken diagnosis of chondrosarcoma. Chondromas are classified according to their location in enchondroma within the medullary cavity of bone, periosteal chondroma found on the surface of the bone, and soft-tissue chondroma found in the soft tissue. The primary significance of enchondroma is related to its complications, most notably pathological fracture, and a small incidence of malignant transformation. Enchondromas are usually solitary but may be multiple. Multiple enchondromas occur in three distinct disorders: Ollier disease is a non-hereditary disorder characterized by multiple enchondromas with a predilection for unilateral distribution. Maffucci syndrome is another non-hereditary disorder which is less common than Ollier disease. This syndrome features multiple hemangiomas in addition to enchondromas. The third form is metachondromatosis, which consists of multiple enchondromas and osteochondromas, and it is the only one of the three disorders that is hereditary as autosomal dominant [156].

5.3.1.3 Collagenic Tumors

Collagenic tumors are primary bone tumors that produce fibrous connective tissue. A fibrosarcoma is a malignant collagen-forming tumor that occurs most frequently in patients between 30 and 50 years of age but also is encountered in younger and older age groups. It is slightly more common among women. A secondary form may occur following Paget's disease, radiation therapy, and long-standing osteomyelitis. The tumor is most frequently located in the metaphysis of the femur or tibia. It begins in the marrow cavity and infiltrates the trabeculae. Histological examination typically reveals collagen, malignant fibroblasts, and occasionally giant cells.

5.3.1.4 Myelogenic Tumors

Myelogenic tumors originate from various cells in the bone marrow.

5.3.1.4.1 Myeloma

A myeloma originates from the plasma cells of the reticuloendothelial element of the bone marrow and may be solitary (85%) or multifocal (multiple myeloma). It is a highly malignant tumor that occurs more commonly in patients above 40 years of age and more frequently in men and blacks. It affects mainly the spine, pelvis, ribs, skull, and proximal bones of the extremities. Pain progresses over time during the course of the disease, and pathological fractures may take place. Patients may develop renal failure, anemia, and thrombocytopenia, and their urine shows Bence Jones protein. The tumor has a poor prognosis, and radiation and chemotherapy have limited success.

5.3.1.4.2 Ewing's Sarcoma

Ewing's sarcoma is a malignant tumor originating from the bone marrow that is most frequently encountered between the ages of 5 and 15 years, and it is rare after the age of 30. It is more common in males and in whites. It is characterized by chromosomal translocation between chromosomes 11 and 22. Typically, it occurs in the diaphysis of long bones such as the femur and tibia and in flat bones such as the pelvis; however, any bone may be involved. After arising from the marrow, Ewing's sarcoma breaks through the bone cortex to form a soft-tissue mass which does not contain osteoid. The tumor metastasizes early to the lung, other bones, lymph nodes, bone marrow, liver, spleen, and central nervous system. Often, the prognosis is poor, particularly if the tumor involves the pelvis rather than the long bones. Morphological imaging modalities play a major role in evaluating the local extent of the primary tumors of bone. MRI has become the examination of choice for local staging. Bone scintigraphy, on the other hand, has a limited role in local staging but is still the modality of choice for detecting distant metastases. Positron-emission tomography (PET) is used on an individual basis, particularly to evaluate the response to therapy. Thallium-201 also plays a role in evaluating the response to therapy and in differentiating benign from malignant lesions [157].

5.3.1.4.3 Giant Cell Tumor

Giant cell tumor is difficult to classify although many practitioners include it with myelogenic tumors since it is believed to originate from the fibrous tissue of the bone marrow. While giant cell tumor may occur in persons between 10 and 70 years of age, it is more commonly encountered in those between 20 and 40 years old, with women afflicted more often than men from the metaphyseal-epiphyseal region of long bones. The tumor occurs mainly around the knee (50%), in the radius, and in the humerus. It has a high recurrence rate, often extending locally into adjacent soft tissues; distant metastases, however, occur more rarely. It consists particularly of osteoclast-like giant cells and anaplastic stromal cells, with a minor component of osteoid and collagen.

5.3.1.4.4 Bone Hemangiomas

Bone hemangiomas are benign, malformed vascular lesions, overall constituting less than 1% of all primary bone neoplasms. They occur most frequently in the vertebral column (30–50%) and skull (20%) but can occur anywhere in the body, and thus any bone can be affected including the long bones, short tubular bones, and ribs. It is multiple in approximately one-third of cases particularly within the vertebral column. Osseous hemangioma generally occurs more commonly in females than males, with a ratio of 3:2. Bone hemangiomas are usually asymptomatic lesions discovered incidentally on imaging or postmortem examination and mostly encountered in the middle age. Vertebral hemangiomas are the most common benign tumor of the spinal column, and they occur most frequently in the lower thoracic and upper lumbar spine. Long-bone hemangiomas are uncommon and are found mainly in the tibia, femur, or humerus. They have a predilection for the metaphyseal or diaphyseal regions but can involve the epiphyses and even extend across the joint space. Skull hemangiomas affect most commonly the frontal bone. Gross pathology usually reveals well-demarcated, unencapsulated lesions with cystic red cavities. Microscopic examination shows hamartomatous proliferations of vascular tissue within endothelial lined spaces. There are four histological variants of hemangioma, classified according to the predominant type of vascular channel: cavernous, capillary, arteriovenous, and venous. These types can coexist. Bone hemangiomas are predominantly of the cavernous and capillary varieties. Cavernous hemangiomas most frequently occur in the skull, whereas capillary hemangiomas predominate in the vertebral column; overall, the former type is most common in bone [158].

5.3.1.5 Imaging of Primary Bone Tumors

Morphological imaging modalities play a major role in evaluating the local extent of the primary tumors of bone. MRI has become the examination of choice for local staging. Functional nuclear medicine imaging plays a minor role in evaluating the local extent of the primary bone tumors. However, utilization of several radiotracers including ^{99m}Tc-MDP, thallium-201, Tc99m MIBI, ^{67}Ga, F-18-sodium fluoride, and F18 FDG helps in making diagnosis, grading, and evaluating the response to chemotherapy.

Bone scintigraphy is still very useful for detecting distant metastases. Combining MRI with FDG-PET (PET/MR) adds the benefit of providing physiological information that can guide and assess treatment [159]. The effective radiation dose of whole-body FDG-PET/MR is more than 50% lower than for FDG-PET/CT [160], which makes PET/MR especially attractive for imaging particularly in pediatric and young age group [161].

5.3.1.5.1 Imaging of Major Specific Tumors

Osteoid Osteoma

Characteristically, the tumors are intracortical and diaphyseal in location, although they occasionally involve the metaphysis. On standard radiographs, the characteristic appearance is a small, less than 1.5–2 cm, cortically based radiolucency (nidus) surrounded by marked sclerosis and cortical thickening, combined with the classic clinical history of pain, worse at night, that is relieved by aspirin. On CT, an area of increased bone density surrounding a lucent nidus is typical of this tumor. Scintigraphically, there is a focal area of increased flow, increased blood pool activity, and increased delayed uptake. A specific scintigraphic pattern of a double density may be seen as more intense uptake corresponding to the nidus and a peripheral less intense activity (Fig. 5.27). Symptoms of osteoid osteoma are cured by removing the nidus. The nidus of the tumor must also be removed during surgery to avoid regrowth. SPECT may help to localize an osteoid osteoma before surgery, and a gamma probe is a useful operating room tool for localizing this tumor [162]. Osteoblastoma: This tumor is related to osteoid osteoma and affects most commonly spine and lower extremities. Scintigraphically, osteoblastoma shows intense uptake similar to osteoid osteoma. Radiographically, a pattern of lysis with or without a rim of surrounding sclerosis is characteristic. Extensive surrounding sclerosis is usually absent; however, surrounding inflammatory changes are often identified on MRI. Osteochondroma: This tumor could appear as sessile/pedunculated (exostosis) or sessile. The lesions, particularly the pedunculated, have a central core of cancellous bone surrounded by a shell of cortical bone and covered by a cap of hyaline cartilage. It can be familial and multiple forming the entity of hereditary multiple exostosis that is discovered in childhood. Standard radiographs and CT scan usually are enough to detect the lesions; however, bone scan is particularly useful to detect multiplicity and follow up patients with hereditary disease since there is a risk of malignant transformation in up to 30% of cases [162]. Scintigraphically, a variable degree

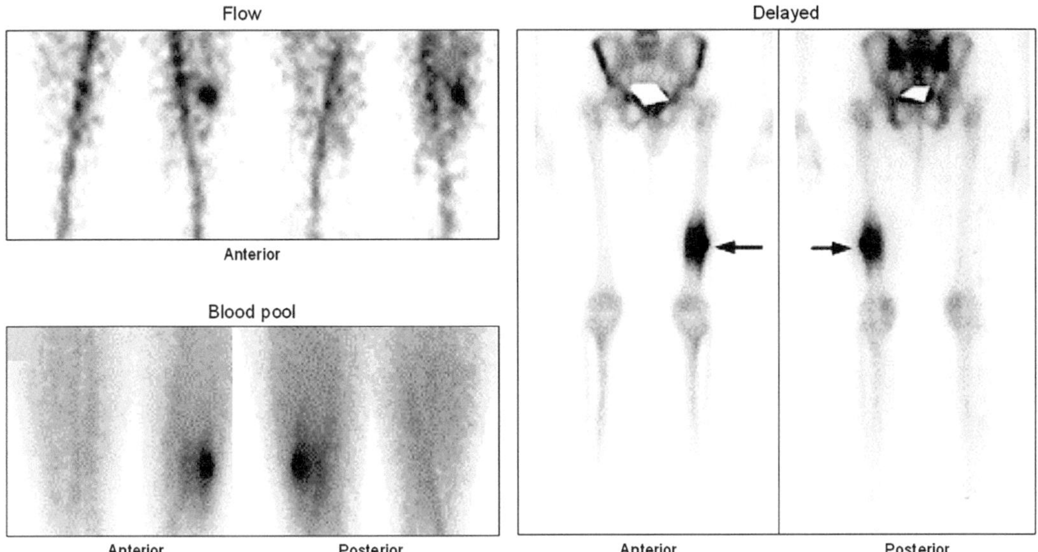

Fig. 5.27 (a–c) Flow (a), blood pool (b), and delayed (c) images of a patient with osteoid osteoma of the left femur showing intense flow and blood pool activity and on delayed images the specific pattern of double intensity (*arrow*)

of uptake is seen which may reflect the lesion's activity; however, active peripheral lesions particularly if small may not show enough uptake to be detected on bone scans [162].

Hemangioma

Multiphase 99 m Tc-MDP bone scintigraphy may reveal increased tracer uptake in all phases (perfusion, blood pool, and delayed), with uptake, most marked in the delayed static images. SPECT may be helpful in vertebral hemangiomas [163].

Osteogenic Sarcoma

Scintigraphically, osteogenic sarcoma presents as an area of intense uptake (Fig. 5.28). Rarely, the tumor may present as a cold lesion. CT and particularly MRI are superior to bone scan in evaluating the extent of the tumor. Bone metastases are extremely rare at presentation. And the initial bone scan yield is small, but it is a justified procedure on presentation because the results may profoundly alter the treatment of the patient and is indicated in all patients routinely during follow-up even if they are asymptomatic.

More recently, 18F-FDG-PET/CT demonstrated superior sensitivity over BS for detecting osseous metastases, supporting the use of 18F-FDG-PET/CT for staging of osteosarcoma

[164]. A meta-analysis study compared PET and PET/CT to bone scan in the diagnosis. Recurrence and evaluation of response to therapy found that FDG has a pooled sensitivity of 91% and a specificity of 93% for detecting recurrence of osteosarcoma. The study demonstrated that ^{18}F-FDG-PET and PET/CT are very accurate for the diagnosis, staging, and recurrence monitoring and the follow-up of the response of tumor to the therapy (Fig. 5.29) of osteosarcoma [165].

Myeloma

Traditional staging of myeloma depends partially on the extent of the disease evaluated by full skeletal survey. The tumor presents on radiographs as osteolytic areas due to demineralization of bone by the tumor. 99 m Tc-MDP, 99 m Tc-MIBI, and thallium-201 have all been used to image multiple myeloma [166]. Imaging plays an important role in the management of patients with multiple myeloma. Standard radiograph has traditionally been the standard imaging modality; however, it has low sensitivity in detecting osteolytic lesions and inability to evaluate response to therapy. Accordingly, other modalities are being used including whole-body low-dose CT, whole-body MRI, and ^{18}F-FDG PET/CT. In large studies, whole-body low-dose CT (WBLDCT) was found to be superior to whole-

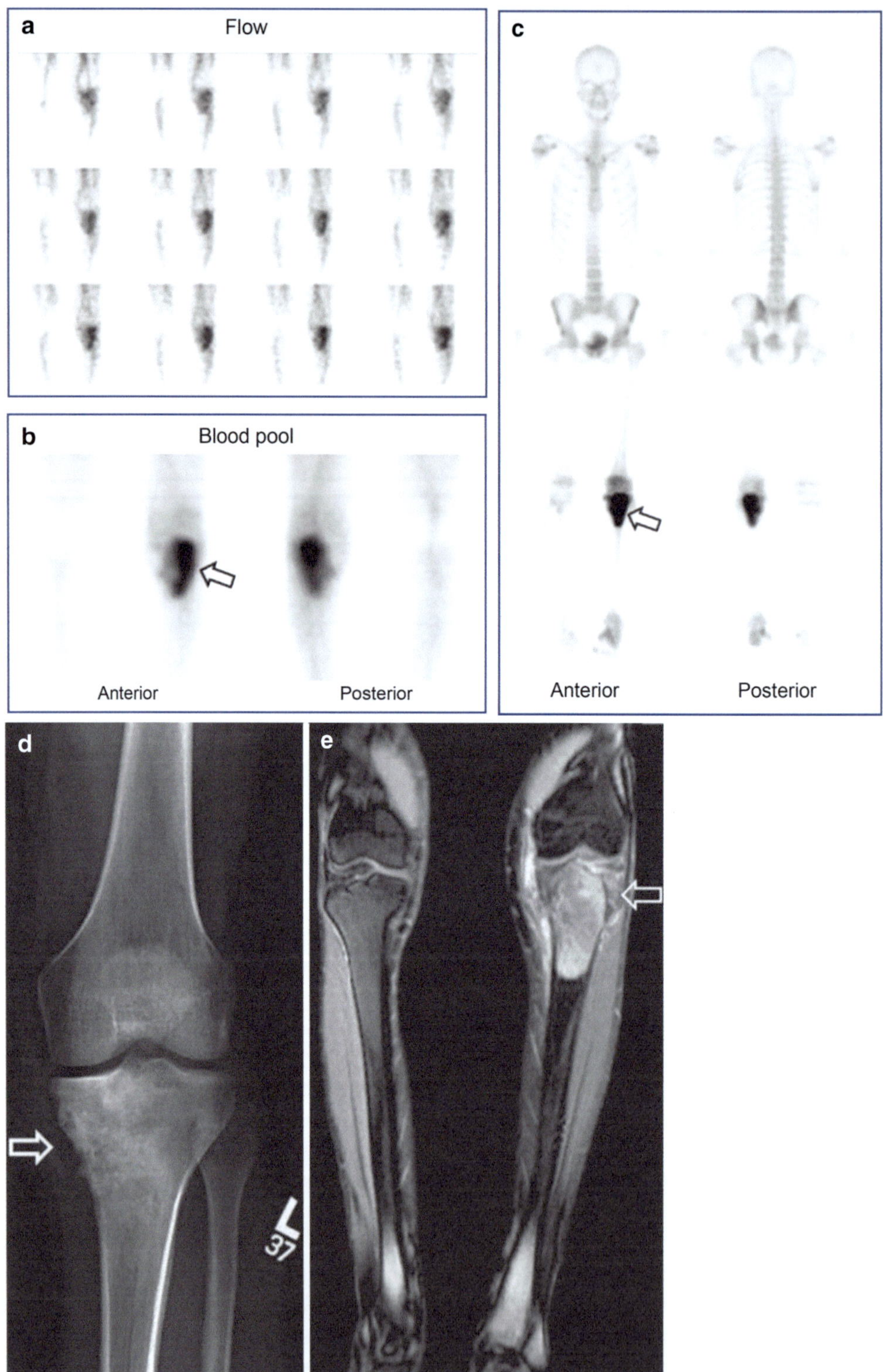

Fig. 5.28 A 14-year-old male with pain and swelling of the left upper leg proven later to be osteogenic sarcoma. Bone scan showing hypervascularity (**a**, **b**) and intense delayed uptake (**c**) corresponding to the X-ray (**d**) and MRI (**e**) findings. Note the mildly diffuse increased uptake in the bones of the left lower extremity due to disuse. No distant metastases. Note the outlines of the tumor on MRI images, which is superior to bone scan in regional staging of the tumor

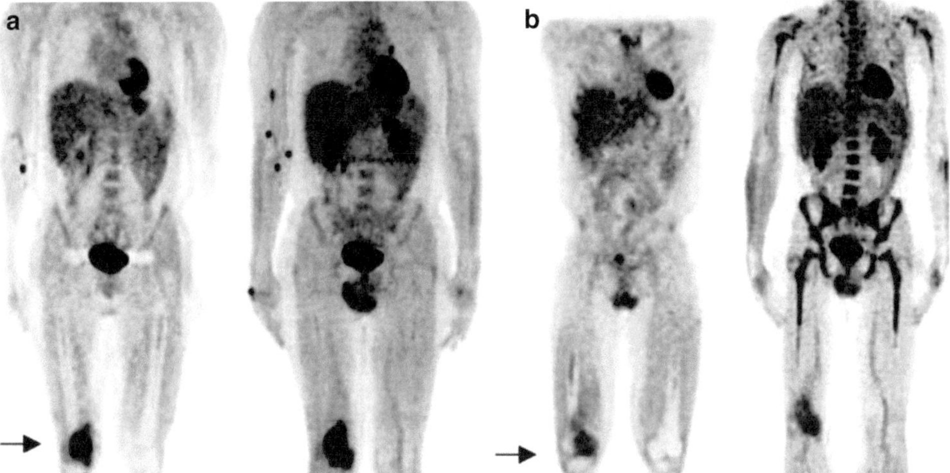

Fig. 5.29 (**a, b**) ^{18}F-FDG-PET study of a patient with osteogenic sarcoma of the distal right femur showing increased uptake and SUV of 9.6. (**b**) Follow-up study obtained after chemotherapy shows a significant decrease of the initial uptake with a drop of SUV to 4.2, indicating a good response

body X-ray in detecting osteolytic lesions due to higher sensitivity and accuracy and in particular in the spine and pelvis [167, 168].

The European Myeloma Network and the European Society for Medical Oncology guidelines have recommended WBLDCT as the imaging modality of choice for the initial assessment of multiple myeloma-related lytic bone lesions. Magnetic resonance imaging is the gold standard imaging modality for detection of bone marrow involvement, while FDG-PET/CT provides valuable prognostic data and is the preferred modality for response to therapy assessment [169]. Bone scan is viewed to be in general unreliable for staging, although a study reviewing the literature comparing the usefulness of conventional skeletal radiography and bone scans in diagnosing the osteolytic lesions of myeloma shows that bone scintigraphy, considered by many to have no role in the detection of osteolytic lesions of myeloma, is in fact more sensitive than radiography in detecting lesions in the ribs, scapula, and spine. Although cold areas are commonly seen on bone scans, increased uptake is a common scintigraphic pattern. This should not contradict the fact that myeloma is the most common tumor to cause cold lesions on bone scan. Ga-68-PSMA PET/CT was reported recently to show intense uptake in a case of multiple myeloma, which may also suggest the possibility of theranostics with 177Lu-PSMA. Tumor neoangiogenesis is the mechanism attributed to increased 68Ga-PSMA uptake in such nonprostatic malignancies [170].

5.3.2 Metastatic Bone Disease

Metastasis means "the transfer of disease from one organ or part to another not directly connected with it." In general, several events are required for the metastatic spread of tumors (Fig. 5.30). The sequence of these events is as follows: 1. Neoplastic cells separate from primary tumors. 2. They gain access to an efficient lymphatic channel or blood capillary. 3. They survive the transport. 4. They attach to the endothelium of a distant capillary bed. 5. They exit the vessel. 6. They develop a supporting blood supply for the cells at the new site. The pathophysiology of skeletal metastases includes two major events, transport of viable tumor cells to bone and interaction of these cells with osseous tissue.

5.3.2.1 Methods of Tumor Cell Transport

In addition to direct extension, tumor cells are transported to produce metastases by the following methods:

5.3.2.1.1 Lymphatic Spread

Lymphatic spread is relatively unimportant for the transport of tumor cells to distant bones.

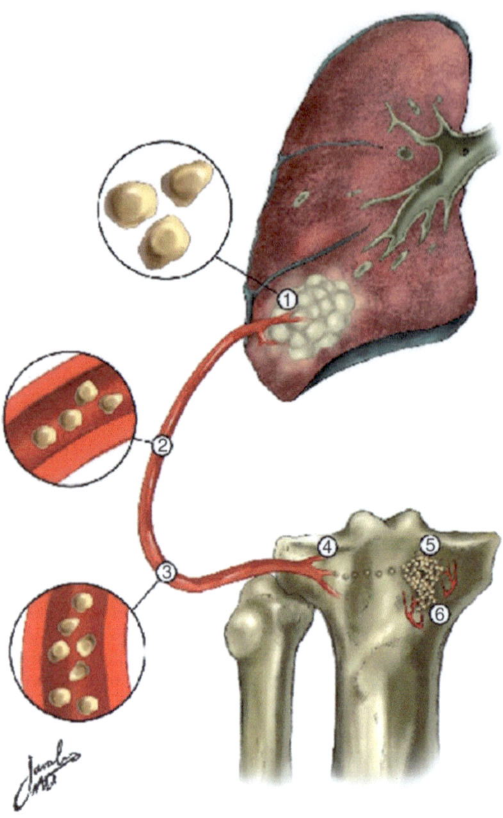

Fig. 5.30 Sequential events generally required for metastatic spread of tumors

5.3.2.1.2 Hematogenous Spread

Hematogenous spread is a major way of transporting malignant cells to the skeleton; it may happen through the arterial system or through the venous system, particularly the vertebral plexus of the veins of Batson [171]. This vertebral plexus consists of an intercommunicating system of thin-walled veins with low intraluminal pressure. The plexus has extensive communication with veins in the spinal canal and with the caval, portal, intercostal, pulmonary, and renal systems.

Intraspinal Spread

Intraspinal dissemination allows secondary deposits in the spinal canal to develop in patients with intracranial tumors.

5.3.2.2 Bone Response to Metastases

Hematogenous metastasis in human beings generally begins in the medullary cavity and then involves the cortex. Accordingly, intramedullary injection of tumor cell suspension is used experimentally. There are two types of osseous response to metastasis: 1. Bone resorption: There is increased bone resorption secondary to malignant disease. Osteoclasts, tumor cells, tumor cell extracts, monocytes, and macrophages may all be involved in the process. 2. Bone formation: This response to tumor occurs in two ways: (a) Stromal bone formation is the earlier and quantitatively less important mechanism of bone formation associated with metastasis. (b) Reactive bone formation occurs in response to bone destruction. Immature woven bone is deposited and subsequently converted to lamellar bone [166]. Bone scan is viewed to be in general unreliable for staging, although a recent study reviewing the literature comparing the usefulness of conventional skeletal radiography and bone scans in diagnosing the osteolytic lesions of myeloma shows that bone scintigraphy, considered by many to have no role in the detection of osteolytic lesions of myeloma, is in fact more sensitive than radiography in detecting lesions in the ribs, scapula, and spine. Although cold areas are commonly seen on bone scans, increased uptake is the most common scintigraphic pattern [172]. This should not contradict the fact that myeloma is the most common tumor to cause cold lesions on bone scan.

5.3.2.3 Distribution of Bone Metastases

The distribution of skeletal metastases varies with the type of primary malignant tumor and age. However, metastases typically involve the axial skeleton, which is the region rich in red bone marrow. Factors favoring the predominant involvement of the red marrow include a large capillary network, a sluggish blood flow, and suitability of this tissue for the growth of tumor emboli. It is estimated that blood flow is 5–13 times higher to cancellous bone containing marrow than to cortical bone. In decreasing order, the usual locations of bone metastases are the vertebral column, pelvic bones, ribs, sternum, femoral and humeral shaft, and skull. Less common sites of skeletal metastases include the mandible, patella, and bones of the extremities distal to the elbows and knees. The involvement of the spine as the most common site by metastasis can be explained by Batson's venous plexus that provides direct com-

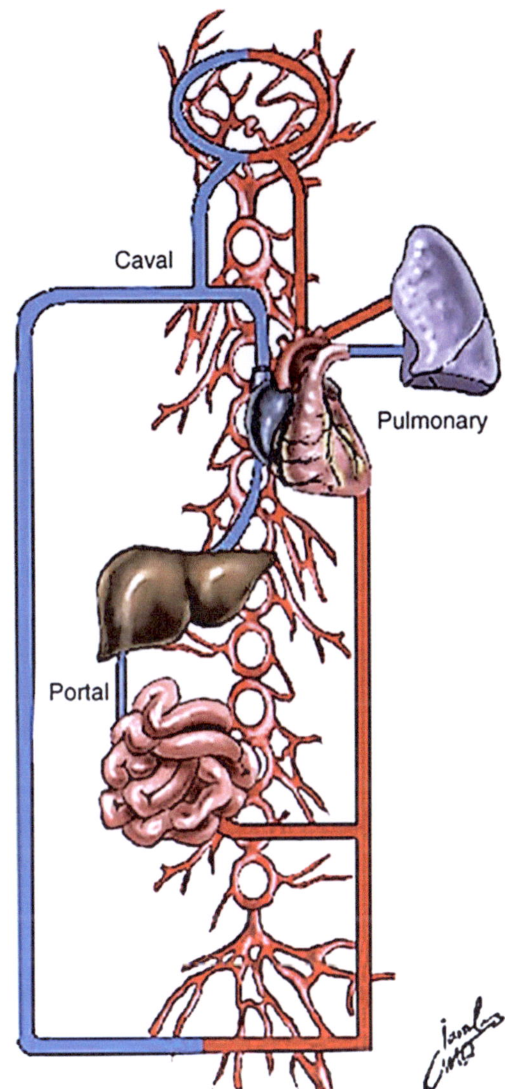

Fig. 5.31 Batson's plexus

munication between the spine and numerous other locations in the body (Fig. 5.31) and large amount of bone mass. Within the spine, the thoracic and cervical areas involving the lumbar region are the most commonly affected. Within the vertebra, metastases are more common in the vertebral body than in the posterior elements. Possible explanations for the low frequency of metastases in the distal portion of the extremities are (1) the blood supply, which is essentially limited to the arterial route, and (2) the relative absence of red marrow, which is a suitable soil for the growth of metastatic tumor cells.

5.3.2.4 Classification of Bone Metastases

Bone metastases can be classified on the basis of several factors, including number of lesions, location, calcium content (as seen on radiographs), and patterns of bone response. The skeleton might at times respond to the various metastatic foci of a tumor in a uniform manner. However, this is not constant. Sometimes, bone metastases show, for example, purely osteoblastic or mixed osteoblastic/osteolytic lesions in certain sites and purely osteolytic lesions in others [173]. Based on the pattern of bone response, metastases can be classified as follows:

- Purely osteolytic: typically arising from carcinomas of the thyroid, kidney, adrenal, uterus, and gastrointestinal tract.
- Purely osteoblastic: arising from carcinoma of the prostate and less often from bronchial carcinoid, carcinoma of the nasopharynx and stomach, neuroblastomas, and medulloblastomas.
- Mixed osteolytic/osteoblastic: arising from carcinomas of the breast, lung, cervix, ovary, and testis.

5.3.2.5 Sources of Bone Metastases

Since the vast majority of metastatic bone lesions appear in the middle and older age groups, certain tumors are known to be common sources of bone metastases. The following primary tumors are the most common to metastasize to bone: prostate, breast, kidney, lung, and thyroid. Bladder and uterine carcinomas are less common sources. In children, skeletal metastases come from neuroblastoma, Ewing's sarcoma, and osteosarcoma. In men, carcinoma of the prostate accounts for 50% of bone metastases, while in women, breast cancer accounts for 70% of such metastases. Following is a brief presentation of the relevant pathological considerations concerning the major sources of skeletal metastases.

5.3.2.5.1 Breast Cancer

Breast cancer is a common source of skeletal metastases. The average incidence of metastases is low at less than 5% in clinical stages 1 and 2, although it ranges from 0 to 40%. In clinical stage 3, the incidence of bone metastases is

20–45%. A recent study reported 22% incidence in patients during a mean of 8.4 years [174]. The tumor usually produces osteolytic or mixed osteolytic/osteoblastic lesions. Rarely, breast cancer gives rise to only osteoblastic lesions. The bone metastases develop most rapidly during the first 2 years. Pain is not a good predictor of bone metastases, since such metastases are found in asymptomatic breast cancer patients and in only 50% of patients with constant pain. Bone scan is recommended as the first imaging modality in asymptomatic patients with X-ray added for assessing abnormal uptake. MRI-PET/CT are used when abnormalities on bone scan cannot be classified on X-ray.

5.3.2.5.2 Prostate Cancer

Prostate cancer is also a common source of bone metastases that are characteristically osteoblastic. Metastases to bone are found in 8–35% of patients at the time of diagnosis. Bone scintigraphy has a crucial role in detecting metastases since it is more sensitive than other imaging and laboratory modalities. Pain has a low predictive value in their detection.

5.3.2.5.3 Lung Cancer

Lung cancer produces skeletal metastases in three ways: (a) via lymphatic spread to mediastinal nodes with direct extension to bone; (b) via lymphatic spread to para-aortic nodes, followed by direct extension to bone; and (c) via invasion of pulmonary veins, followed by transport of tumor through the arterial circulation to any part of the skeleton, including the appendicular. The lesions are predominantly osteolytic and mixed, although only osteoblastic lesions can occur in a minority of cases, particularly those with small cell and adenocarcinoma. Among the four major types of lung cancer, small cell is the most aggressive, followed by large cell and adenocarcinoma, and squamous cell is the least aggressive [175].

5.3.2.5.4 Renal Cell Carcinoma

Renal cell carcinoma produces skeletal metastases rather commonly. Although symptoms related to metastases might be the presenting feature, these symptoms are inconsistent and pain is not a

reliable predictor. The tumor produces skeletal metastases through (a) lymphatic channels to para-aortic, hilar, paratracheal, and/or mediastinal nodes with invasion of bone later and (b) invasion of renal veins which lead to the inferior vena cava, right atrium, and then pulmonary vessels, to be disseminated to bones. The metastatic lesions are predominantly osteolytic and in some cases expansile [176].

5.3.2.6 Sequelae of Skeletal Metastases

Bone metastases may result in local or generalized changes.

Local consequences include the following:

1. Bone Destruction

Both direct and indirect mechanisms of bone destruction are involved in the bone loss associated with tumor invasion of bone [177].

Direct stimulation of bone loss: Tumors cause increased osteoclastic activity and consequently bone destruction through secretion of tumor-derived substances that directly stimulate osteoclasts. These substances include parathyroid hormone-related protein, transforming growth factor alpha, transforming growth factor beta, and prostaglandins.

Indirect stimulation of bone loss by tumors occurs, on the other hand, by substances secreted by the tumor that stimulate first the immune cells (T cells) or activated bone cells, which in turn release osteoclast-stimulating cytokines such as tumor necrosis factor (TNF) and interleukin-1 (IL-1), which increase the osteoclastic activity and cause bone destruction (Fig. 5.32).

2. Pathological Fractures: Metastases cause weakening of the involved bones and may lead to fractures in the vertebrae (compression fractures) or long bones, most commonly affecting the proximal portion of the femur.

3. Periosteal New Bone Formation: In general, periosteal reaction due to metastases is minimal if present compared with significant new bone formation in association with primary bone tumors.

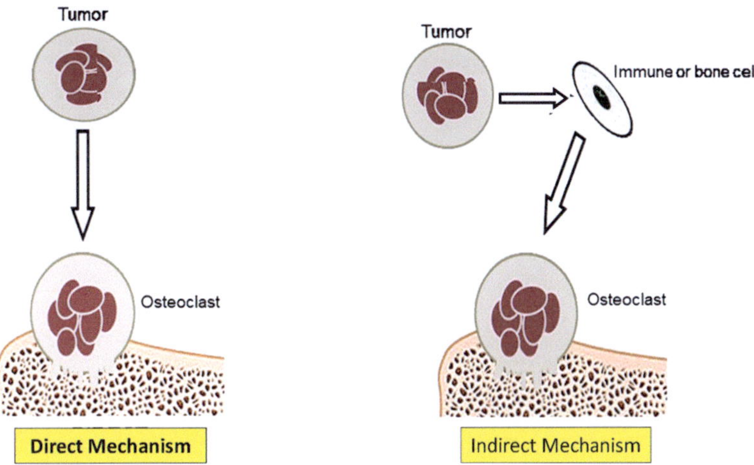

Fig. 5.32 Direct and indirect mechanisms of bone destruction associated with tumor invasion of bone

4. Soft-Tissue Extension: Soft-tissue masses may infrequently present regionally in association with metastases. This occurs particularly with rib lesions in association with myeloma and in the pelvis in association with colon cancer.
5. Bone Expansion: This occurs with both osteolytic and osteoblastic lesions. Carcinomas of the prostate, kidney, and thyroid and hepatocellular carcinoma are particularly known to cause expansile metastatic lesions.

Generalized or metabolic consequences include the following:

1. Hypercalcemia: This can be associated with metastases due to destruction of bone but also with primary tumors not associated with skeletal metastases. Hypercalcemia occurs in up to 20% of cancer patients.
2. Hypocalcemia: An unidentified humoral substance capable of stimulating osteoclasts in some cancer patients with skeletal metastases is proposed to be the underlying mechanism behind the presence of hypocalcemia in up to 15% of cancer patients.
3. Osteomalacia: In some patients with skeletal metastases, depressed levels of 1,25-hydroxyvitamin D3, hypocalcemia, and hypophosphatemia are recognized and associated with generalized weakness and pain of bones and muscles (oncogenic osteomalacia).

5.3.2.7 Imaging of Metastatic Bone Disease

In general, four main modalities are routinely utilized clinically to assess bone, the third most common site of metastatic diseases, for existence of metastatic lesions. These modalities include standard radiography, CT scan, bone scintigraphy, and MRI [178].

5.3.2.7.1 Appearance of Bone Metastases on Bone Scan

Bone scan is the most widely used modality and is the most practical and cost-effective screening technique for assessing the entire skeleton. In addition, bone scan is very sensitive in detecting the disease. However, there is a variable false-negative rate in assessing lesions in certain locations particularly in the spine and in those confined to bone marrow [109]. On bone scans, metastases have different patterns:

Typical pattern: The most common and typical pattern of bone metastases is that of multiple, randomly distributed foci of increased uptake (Fig. 5.33), usually in the axial skeleton, following the distribution of certain bone marrow including the shoulder girdle, with relatively less extensive involvement of the ribs. Multiple fractures and multifocal infection may simulate this pattern.

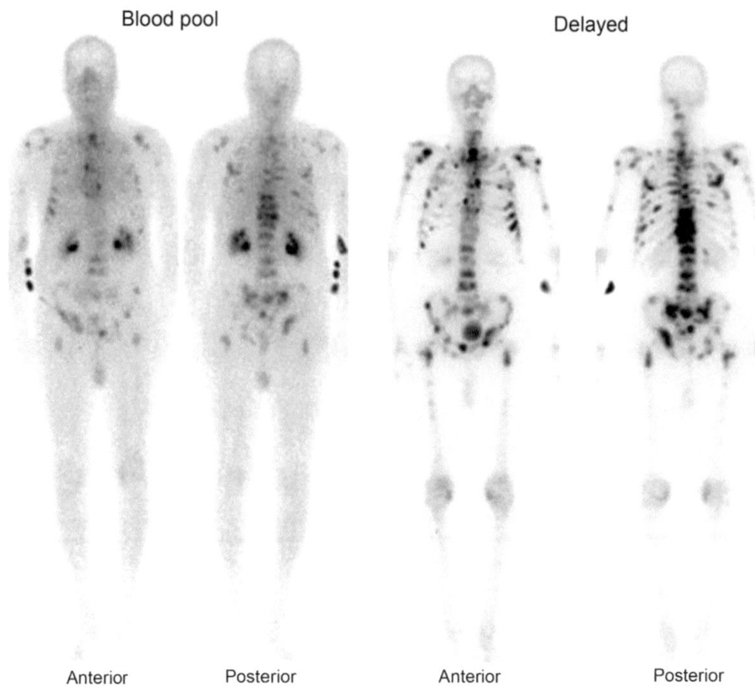

Fig. 5.33 Whole-body blood pool and delayed scans of a 77-year-old male with advanced carcinoma of the prostate. PSA 99 ng/µl. Patient was referred to rule out metastases. The scan shows the typical pattern of metastatic bone diseases of randomly distributed foci of increased uptake

Atypical patterns include the following:

1. Solitary Lesions: These occur in the axial and in the appendicular skeleton in a variable percentage of patients. The incidence of malignancy in solitary lesions varies with the location. The incidence is highest in the vertebrae. These lesions are commonly asymptomatic and are not suspected clinically. Less than half of these lesions are evident on X-rays. These facts further emphasize the importance of obtaining a bone scan of the entire skeleton routinely in patients with cancer.

2. Cold Lesions: Aggressive tumors may cause cold lesions at the time of presentation. This is seen frequently in multiple myeloma and renal cell carcinoma, although the most common pattern of multiple myeloma on bone scan is hot spots [179].

3. Equilibrium Pattern: Hot lesions may have a relatively normal appearance with time, reflecting a point of equilibrium between osteoblastic activity and bone destruction by the tumor. It appears that skeletal lesions may evolve through increased uptake, the equilibrium phase, and then decreased uptake. The second phase can result in minimal abnormalities of focal, nonuniform, minimally increased uptake, or even near-normal patterns that can be missed on scan. This phenomenon has been observed and studied particularly in rib lesions [180].

4. Diffuse Pattern: With advanced metastatic disease, the entire axial skeleton may be involved by a load of tumor cells causing increased extraction of radiopharmaceutical. This pattern may be interpreted as normal depending on the display intensity and should also be differentiated from other causes of diffusely increased uptake in the skeleton (superscan) such as hyperparathyroidism and other metabolic bone diseases and Paget's disease. A superscan secondary to metastases shows increased uptake that is usually confined to the axial skeleton, while in case of metabolic disorders, it also involves the skull, mandible, sternum, and metaphyses of long bones. Preferential increase of uptake at the osteochondral junctions and joint renal activity are additional features of metabolic disease on assorted superscans.

5. Flare Pattern: Therapy producing healing at the tumor site results in several pathological changes as seen on scintigraphy. As the term healing implies, inflammatory changes with increasing blood flow occur early after ther-

apy. Since the tumors are in bones, reactive bone formation increases with successful therapy. Following radiation therapy, there is increased activity on blood pool images and delayed images may be seen early on due to inflammatory reaction. Later, these changes disappear and decreased uptake is typically seen. It should be noted that the effects of therapeutic radiation depend on the time after treatment and the dose. Follow-up scans are more frequently obtained after chemotherapy than after radiation therapy, and the changes that are seen continue for longer periods. Early increased activity on blood pool and delayed images is noted, followed by decreasing activity that can be normalized. Increasing activity may be significant and continue for several months even with successful therapy. This phenomenon may include the appearance of small, new lesions due to healing at the sites of preexisting small or cold lesions that were not resolved on earlier scans.

6. Symmetrical Pattern: Occasionally, symmetrical uptake due to metastases is seen in certain tumors as neuroblastoma and in case of bone marrow involvement in leukemia. This pattern is particularly seen in distal femoral and proximal tibial metaphyses.

Table 5.11 summarizes the important correlation between common pathological changes of bone and scintigraphic findings.

Table 5.11 Scintigraphic pathologic correlation

Pathological etiology	Scintigraphic pattern on bone scan
Osteoblastic response	Increased uptake
Increased vascularity	Increased flow and blood pool activity
Angiogenesis	Increased blood pool activity
Bone destruction (infarction, rapidly growing aggressive metastasis)	Cold areas
Large destructive lesion with a rim of new bone formation	Doughnut pattern
Paget's disease, some primary or metastatic tumors	Bone expansion
Arthritis, complex regional pain syndrome-1	Periarticular increased uptake
Equilibrium of bone destruction and bone formation	Near-normal appearance

Imaging Metastases with Other Modalities

MRI has been found to detect more vertebral metastases than bone scan. F18-sodium fluoride and FDG-PET are increasingly evaluated for detection of bone metastases (Fig. 5.34) and have been shown to be more sensitive than bone scan [181–184].

F-18-sodium fluoride (NaF) PET/CT is used for bone imaging with some established indications. The uptake mechanism of 18F-fluoride resembles that of 99mTc-methylene diphosphonate (MDP), with better pharmacokinetic characteristics including faster blood clearance and twofold higher uptake in bone resulting in a better target-to-background ratio and excellent image quality with higher spatial resolution superior to standard bone scanning. After diffusing into the extracellular fluid of bone, the fluoride ion is exchanged for a hydroxyl group in the bone crystal and forms fluoroapatite, which then deposits on the bone surface. 18F-fluoride is very sensitive for the detection of both lytic and sclerotic bone lesions; however, benign bone lesions (degenerative change, fractures, Paget's disease, enchondroma, and osteoma) will also demonstrate increased tracer uptake of 18F-sodium fluoride. The use of low-dose CT in conjunction with 18F-fluoride PET improves sensitivity and specificity and improves the ability to distinguish benign from malignant lesions [116, 185, 186]. There is no definite evidence yet that 18F-fluoride PET is overall more sensitive in detecting bone metastases to justify replacing conventional bone scan although in certain tumors it is more sensitive.

F-18-FDG-PET/CT was found to have a very high PPV of 98% in the evaluation of bone malignancy when the two portions of the examination are in agreement and when bone window of CT is used. It can also help better differentiate whether FDG-avid lesions are truly located within bone versus adjacent soft tissue [187, 188].

Compared to ⁹⁹ᵐTc-MDP and 18F-fluoride, 18F-FDG-PET is found to be more sensitive for the detection of bone metastases secondary to lung cancer. For metastases of breast cancer, 18F-FDG appears to be more sensitive for lytic lesions, but less sensitive for sclerotic ones. Conversely, 18F-FDG-PET is also less sensitive in the detection of bone metastases from prostate cancer. Accordingly, posttreatment studies which

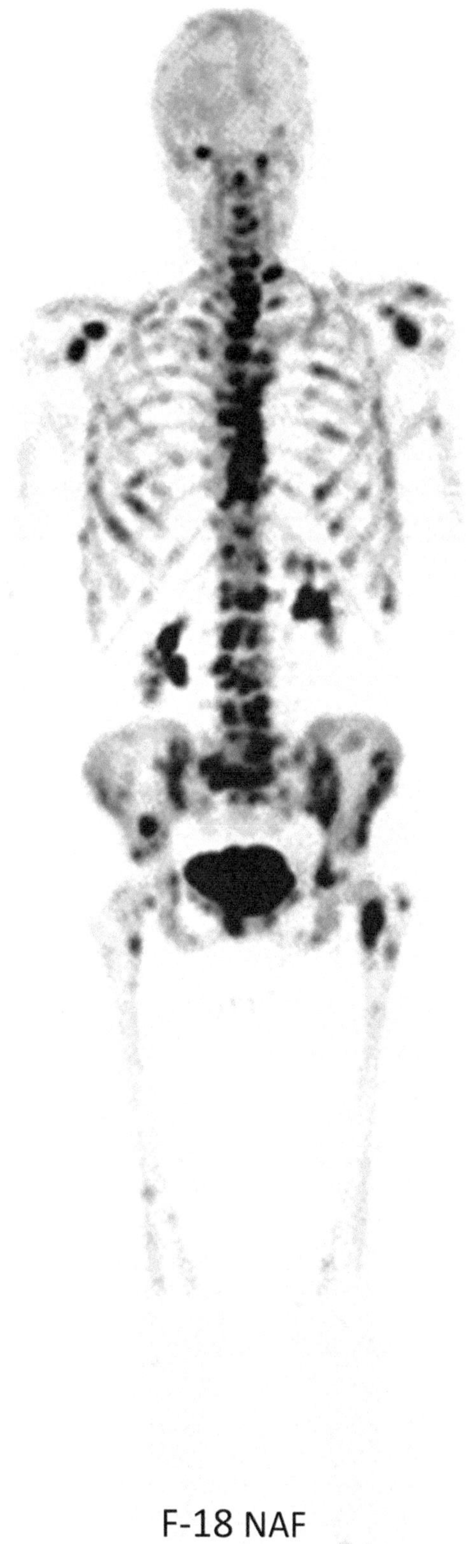

Fig. 5.34 F-18-sodium fluoride bone PET study in a patient with lung cancer illustrating multiple metastases with excellent resolution

often result in sclerotic lesions are negative with 18F-FDG imaging because they have healed and no longer have viable tumor [189].

Combined sodium fluoride and FDG-PET has also been used and has added benefit. In a comparative study, the diagnostic accuracy of whole-body MR imaging, bone scintigraphy, and FDG-PET for the detection of bone metastases in children was determined. Twenty-one patients exhibited 51 bone metastases. Sensitivities for the detection of bone metastases were 90, 82, and 71% for FDG-PET, whole-body MR imaging, and bone scintigraphy, respectively. False-negative lesions were different for the three imaging modalities, mainly depending on lesion location. Most false-positive lesions were seen with FDG-PET [190]. Another study of 55 patients with malignant lymphoma also showed that FDG-PET is more sensitive but, in contrast, more specific than bone scintigraphy [191]. It is important to remember that PET provides direct visualization of metastases, while bone scan visualizes the reactive bone in response to the presence of metastases. FDG-PET can help differentiate flare from progression and evaluate the tumor status when bone scan is stable (Fig. 5.35) [191].

^{18}F-fluoride however also shows increased uptake in benign bone lesions including degenerative change, fractures, Paget's disease, enchondroma, and osteoma. The use of low-dose CT in conjunction with 18F-fluoride PET improves sensitivity and specificity and improves the ability to distinguish benign from malignant lesions [116, 185, 186].

PET/CT studies are valuable in the evaluation of metastatic bone disease and in following patients with bone-dominant metastases. However, there is no definite evidence yet that 18F-fluoride PET is more sensitive in detecting bone metastases to justify replacing conventional bone scan.

PET imaging with 18F-fluoro-2-deoxyglucose (18F-FDG) has also been used to identify bone metastases. 18F-FDG is directly taken by tumor cells and consequently detects cortical and marrow involvement. This indicates that this radiotracer will be best for lytic lesions. Since 18F-FDG-PET has low uptake in normal red marrow, it allows for early detection of malignant bone marrow involvement preceding detection of bone metastases by bone scan using diphosphonates. 18F-FDG-PET

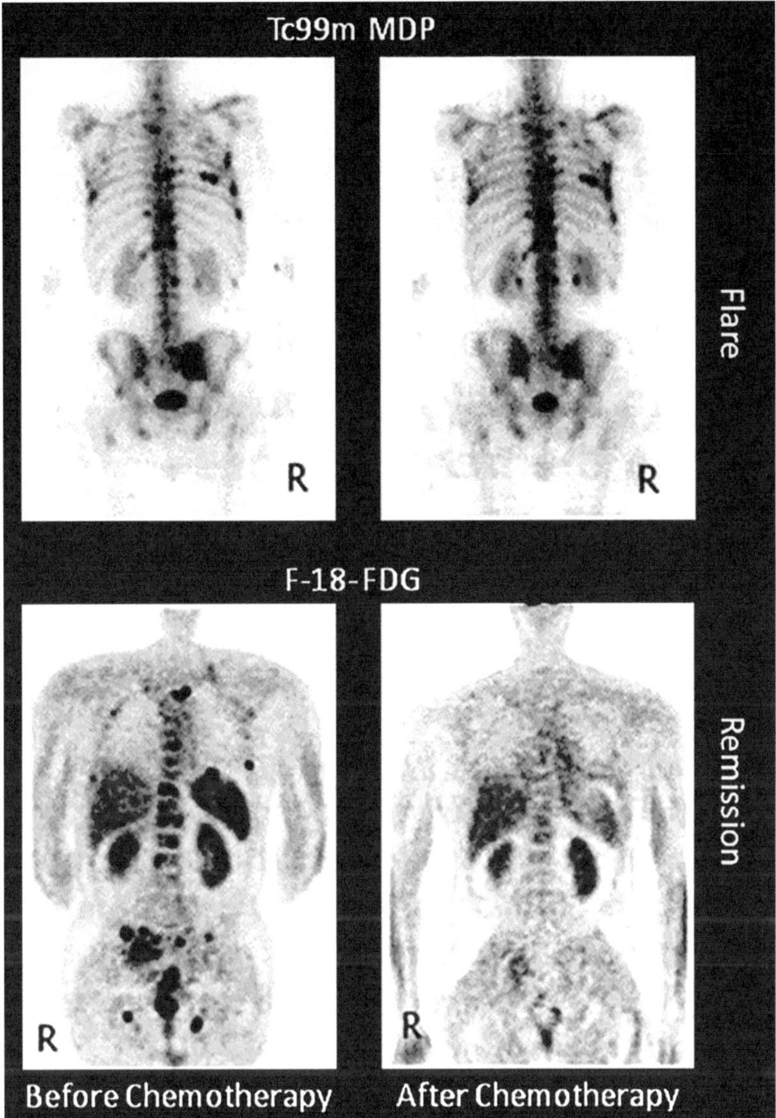

Fig. 5.35 A 55-year-old man recently diagnosed with non-small right lung cell cancer. BS (*top left*) and PET (*bottom left*) in the staging showed multiple bone metastases, with a different distribution, probably due to the lytic/blastic behavior. The patient was treated with chemotherapy. Eight months after treatment, BS remained similar (*top right*). PET scan showed resolution of previous lesions (*bottom right*). On the basis of the PET findings, BS results should be interpreted as representing a persistent bone reaction, not active metastatic disease (Figure printed with permission from [191])

can detect all three types of skeletal metastases including lytic, blastic, and mixed, but preferably 18F-FDG-PET is more sensitive for detection of lytic rather than osteoblastic metastases which are usually less aggressive lesions [192–194].

Cook et al. found that 18F-FDG-PET has slightly decreased sensitivity for predominantly osteoblastic lesions but has higher overall sensitivity due to more frequent occurrence of osteolytic bone metastases [195].

Compared to ^{99m}Tc-MDP and 18F-fluoride, 18F-FDG-PET is found to be more sensitive for the detection of bone metastases secondary to lung cancer. For metastases of breast cancer, 18F-FDG appears to be more sensitive for lytic lesions, but less sensitive for sclerotic ones. Conversely, 18F-FDG-PET is also less sensitive in the detection of bone metastases from prostate cancer. Accordingly, posttreatment studies which often result in sclerotic lesions are negative with 18F-FDG imaging because they have healed and no longer have viable tumor [189].

FDG-PET/CT was found to have a very high PPV of 98% in the evaluation of bone malignancy when the two portions of the examination are in agreement and when bone window of CT is used. It can also help better differentiate whether FDG-avid lesions are

Table 5.12 Role of PET in primary and metastatic bone tumors

Detection of metastatic bone disease
Evaluation of response to therapy of primary or metastatic bone disease
Detection of recurrence of primary bone malignancies
Early differentiation of progression and flare of metastatic bone disease seen on bone scan
Evaluation of solitary bone lesion

truly located within bone versus adjacent soft tissue [187, 188].

Most recently, fluorocholine (18F) (FCH) PET/CT seems to be promising in the detection of bone metastases in patients with prostate cancer. Several clinical studies have found increased sensitivity of combined NaF/FDG-PET/CT for detection of osseous lesions when compared with separate NaF PET/CT and FDG-PET/CT [196–200].

Several tumor-targeted radiotracers have been introduced for molecular imaging of bone metastases, particularly 68Ga PSMA, which is very useful in the detection and follow-up of prostatic cancer metastases [201] Table 5.12 summerizes the role of PET in primary and metastatic bone malignacies.

References

1. Mourad LA (1998) Structure and function of the musculoskeletal. In: McCane KL, Huether SE (eds) pathophysiology, 3rd edn. Mosby, Philadelphia, pp1405–1434
2. Föger-Samwald U, Dovjak P, Azizi-Semrad U, Kerschan-Schindl K, Pietschmann P (2020) Osteoporosis: Pathophysiology and therapeutic options. EXCLI journal 19:1017–1037. https://doi.org/10.17179/excli2020-2591
3. Clarke BL, Khosla S (2010) Physiology of bone loss. Radiol Clin North Am 48:483–495
4. Pacifici R (2018) Bone Remodeling and the Microbiome. Cold Spring Harb Perspect Med. 2(8):a031203. https://doi.org/10.1101/cshperspect.a031203
5. McCabe L, Britton RA, Parameswaran N (2015) Prebiotic and Probiotic Regulation of Bone Health: Role of the Intestine and its Microbiome. Curr Osteoporos Rep. 13(6):363–371
6. Watson EC, Ralf H (2018) Adams. Biology of Bone: The Vasculature of the Skeletal System. Cold Spring Harb Perspect Med 8:a031559
7. Tondevold E, Eliasen P (1982) Blood flow rates in canine cortical and cancellous bone measured with tc 99 m, labeled human albumin microspheres. Acta Orthop Scand 53:7–11
8. McCarthy EF (1997) Histopathologic correlates of positive bonescan. Semin Nucl Med 27:309–320
9. Ralston SH (2017) Bone structure and metabolism. Medicine 45(9):560–564
10. Andrea Benova A, Tencerova M. (2020) Obesity-Induced Changes in Bone Marrow Homeostasis. Front Endocrinol, 12 May 2020 .
11. Tencerova M, Kassem M (2016) The bone marrow-derived stromal cells: commitment and regulation of adipogenesis. Front Endocrinol 7:127
12. Muruganandan S, Govindarajan R, Sinal CJ (2018) Bone Marrow Adipose Tissue and Skeletal Health. Curr Osteoporos Rep 16:434–442
13. Haas DW, McAndrew M (1996) Bacterial osteomyelitis in adults: evolving considerations in diagnosis and treatment. Am J Med 101:550–561
14. Cierny G, Mader JT, Pennick H (1985) A clinical staging system of adult osteomyelitis. Contemp Orthop 10:17–37
15. Mandell JC, Khurana B, Smith JT et al (2018) Osteomyelitis of the lower extremity: pathophysiology, imaging, and classification with an emphasis on diabetic foot infection. Emerg Radiol. 25:175–188
16. Jaramillo D (2011) Infection: musculoskeletal. Pediatr Radiol 41(Suppl 1):S127–S134
17. Hofstee et al (2020) Current concepts of osteomyelitis from pathologic mechanisms to advanced research methods. Am J Pathol 190:1151–1163
18. Calhoun JH, Manring MM (2005) Adult osteomyelitis. Infect Dis Clin North Am. 19:765–786
19. Torda AJ, Gottlieb T, Bradbury R (1995) Pyogenic vertebral osteomyelitis: analysis of 20 cases and review. Clin Infect Dis 20:320–328
20. Song KS, Ogden JA, Ganey T, Guidera KT (1997) Contiguous discitis and osteomyelitis in children. J Pediatr Orthop 17:470–477
21. Babinchak TJ, Riley DK, Rotheram EB (1997) Pyogenic vertebral osteomyelitis of the posterior elements. Clin Infect Dis 25:221–224
22. Lipsky BA, Berendt AR, Cornia PB, Pile JC, Peters EJ, Armstrong DG et al (2012) 2012 Infectious Diseases Society of America clinical practice guideline for the diagnosis and treatment of diabetic foot infections. Clinical infectious diseases 54(12):e132–e173
23. Jaramillo D, Dormans JP, Delgado J, Laor T, St Geme JW III (2017) Hematogenous osteomyelitis in infants and children: imaging of a changing disease. Radiology 283:629–643
24. Lee YJ, Sadigh S, Mankad K, Kapse N, Rajeswaran G (2016) The imaging of osteomyelitis. Quantitative imaging in medicine and surgery 6(2):184–198

25. Arıcan P, Okudan B, Şefizade R, Naldöken S (2019) Diagnostic Value of Bone SPECT/CT in Patients with Suspected Osteomyelitis. Molecular imaging and radionuclide therapy 28:89–95

26. Elgazzar AH, Abdel-Dayem HM (1999) Imaging skeletal infections: evolving considerations. In: Feeman LM (ed) Nuclear medicine annual. Lippincott/Williams and Wilkins, Philadelphia, pp 157–191

27. Elgazzar AH, Abdel-Dayem HM, Clark J, Maxon HR (1995) Multimodality imaging of osteomyelitis. Eur J Nucl Med 22:1043–1063

28. Issa K, Diebo BG, Faloon M, Naziri Q, Pourtaheri S, Paulino CB, Emami A (2018) The Epidemiology of Vertebral Osteomyelitis in the United States From 1998 to 2013. Clin Spine Surg. 31:E102–E108

29. Mete B, Kurt C, Yilmaz MH, Ertan G, Ozaras R, Mert A, Tabak F, Ozturk R (2012) Vertebral osteomyelitis: eight years' experience of 100 cases. Rheumatol Int 32:3591–3597

30. Zimmerli W (2010) Clinical practice. Vertebral osteomyelitis. N Engl J Med 18(362):1022–1029

31. Batson OV (1967) The vertebral system of veins as a means for cancer dissemination. Progress in Clinical. Cancer 3:1–18

32. Bamberger DM, Daus GP, Gerding DN (1987) Osteomyelitis in the feet of diabetic patients: long term results, prognostic factors, and the role of antimicrobial and surgical therapy. Am J Med 83:653–660

33. Schwartz GS, Berenyi MR, Siegel MW (1969) Atrophic arthropathy and diabetic neuritis. Am J Roentgenol Radium Ther Nucl Med 106:523–529

34. Horwitz SH (1993) Diabetic neuropathy. Clin Orthop 296:78–85

35. Gold RH, Tang DTF, Crim JR, Seeger LL (1995) Imaging the diabetic foot. Skeletal Radiol 24:563–571

36. Malhotra R, Chan CS, Nather A (2014) Osteomyelitis in the diabetic foot. Diabetic Foot & Ankle 5:24–45

37. Mandell GA (1996) Imaging in the diagnosis of musculoskeletal infections in children. Curr Probl Pediatr 26:218–237

38. Rand JA (1995) Preoperative planning for total knee arthroplasty. In: Dennis DA, Paprosky WG, Rosenberg AG (eds) Callaghan JJ. Orthopedic knowledge update. Hip and knee reconstruction. American Academy of Orthopedic Surgeons, Rosemont

39. American Academy of Orthopaedic Surgeons (1995) Proceedings of the American Academy of Orthopaedic Surgeons. AAOS, Rosemont, pp 255–263

40. Griffiths HJ (1995) Orthopedic complications. Radiol Clin North Am 33:401–410

41. Harris WH, Sledge CB (1990) Total hip and total knee replacement (part I). N Engl J Med 323:725–731

42. Johnson JA, Christie MJ, Sandler MP, Parks PF Jr, Horma L, Kayle JJ (1988) Detection of occult infection following total joint arthroplasty using sequential technetium-99 m HDP bone scintigraphy and Indium-111 WBC imaging. J Nucl Med 29:1347–1353

43. Calvo C, Núñez E, Camacho M, Clemente D, Fernández-Cooke E et al (2001) Epidemiology and Management of Acute, Uncomplicated Septic Arthritis and Osteomyelitis. The Pediatric Infectious Disease Journal 35:1288–1293

44. Manz, N., Krieg, A.H., Heininger, U. Ritz N (2018) al. Evaluation of the current use of imaging modalities and pathogen detection in children with acute osteomyelitis and septic arthritis. Eur J Pediatr 177, 1071–1080

45. Barton LL, Dunkle LM, Habib FH (1987) Septic arthritis in childhood: a 13-year review. Am J Dis Child 141:898–900

46. Mathews CJ, Weston VC, Jones A, Field M, Coakley G (2012) Bacterial septic arthritis in adults. Lancet. 375(9717):846–855

47. Silberstein EB, Elgazzar AH, Fernandez-Uloa M, Nishiyama H (1996) Skeletal scintigraphy in non-neoplastic osseous disorders. In: Henkin RE, Bles MA, Dillehay GL, Halama JR, Karesh SM, Wagner PH, Zimmer AM (eds) Textbook of nuclear medicine. Mosby, New York, pp 1141–1197

48. Hofmann SR, Schnabel A, Rösen-Wolff A, Morbach H, Girschick HH, Hedrich CM (2016) Chronic Nonbacterial Osteomyelitis: Pathophysiological Concepts and Current Treatment Strategies. The Journal of Rheumatology 43:1956–1964. https://doi.org/10.3899/jrheum.160256

49. Waldvogel FA, Medoff G, Swartz MN (1970) Osteomyelitis: a review of clinical features, therapeutic considerations and unusual aspects, part I. N Engl J Med 282:198–205

50. Llewellyn A, Jones-Diette J, Kraft J, Holton C, Harden M, Simmonds M (2019) Imaging tests for the detection of osteomyelitis: a systematic review. Health Technol Assess 23:1–128

51. Manz N, Krieg AH, Heininger U, Ritz N et al (2018) Evaluation of the current use of imaging modalities and pathogen detection in children with acute osteomyelitis and septic arthritis. Eur J Pediatr 177:1071–1080

52. Kan JH, Hilmes MA, Martus JE, Yu C, Hernanz-Schulman M (2008) Value of MRI after recent diagnostic or surgical intervention in children with suspected osteomyelitis. AJR Am J Roentgenol 191:1595–1600

53. Liu C, Bayer A, Cosgrove SE, Daum RS, Fridkin SK et al (2011) Clinical practice guidelines by the infectious diseases society of America for the treatment of methicillin-resistant Staphylococcus aureus infections in adults and children: executive summary. Clin Infect Dis. 52:285–292

54. ConnollyLP CSA, Drubach LA, Jaramillo D, Treves ST (2002) Acute hematogenous osteomyelitis of children: assessment of skeletal scintigraphy based diagnosis in the Era of MRI. J Nucl Med 43:1310–1315

55. Tuson GE, Hoffman EB, Mann MD (1994) Isotope bone scanning for acute osteomyelitis and septic arthritis in children. J Bone Joint Surg (Br) 75B:305–310

56. Handmaker H, Giammona ST (1984) Improved early diagnosis of acute inflammatory skeletal-articular diseases in children: a two radiopharmaceutical approach. Pediatrics 73:551–559

57. Pennington WT, Mott MP, Thometz JG, Sty JR, Metz D (1999) Photopenic bone scan osteomyelitis: a clinical perspective. J Pediatr Orthop 19:595–598

58. Sundberg SB, Savage JP, Foster BK (1989) Technetium phosphate bone scan in the diagnosis of septic arthritis in childhood. J Pediatr Orthop 9:579–585

59. Gilday DL, Paul DJ, Paterson J (1975) Diagnosis of osteomyelitis in children by combined blood pool and bone imaging. Radiology 117:331–335

60. Johnson JE, Kennedy EJ, Shereff MJ, Patel NC, Collier BD (1995) Prospective study of bone, In-111 labeled white blood cell and gallium scanning for the evaluation of osteomyelitis in the diabetic foot. Foot Ankle Int 17:10–15

61. Grerand S, Dolan M, Laing P, Bird M, Smith ML, Klenerman L (1995) Diagnosis of osteomyelitis in neuropathic foot ulcers. J Bone Joint Surg (Br) 78B:51–55

62. Ezuddin S, Yuille D, Spiegelhoff D (1992) The role of dual bone and WBC scan imaging in the evaluation of osteomyelitis and cellulitis using both planar and SPECT imaging. J Nucl Med 33:839

63. Vander-Bruggen W, Bleeker-Rovers CP, Boerman OC, Gotthardt M, WJG O (2010) PET and SPECT in osteomyelitis and prosthetic bone and joint infections: a systematic review. Semin Nucl Med 40:3–15

64. Seabold JE, Nepola JV, Marsh JL et al (1991) Postoperative bone marrow alterations: potential pitfalls in the diagnosis of osteomyelitis with In-111-labeled leukocyte scintigraphy. Radiology 180:741–747

65. Hakki S, Harwood SJ, Morrissey MA et al (1997) Comparative study of monoclonal antibody scan in diagnosing orthopedic infection. Clin Orthop 335:275–285

66. Lauri C, Tamminga M, Glaudemans AWJM et al (2017) Detection of osteomyelitis in the diabetic foot by imaging techniques: a systematic review and meta-analysis comparing MRI, white blood cell Scintigraphy, and FDG-PET. Diabetes Care 40:1111–1120

67. Filippi L, Uccioli L, Giurato L, Schillaci O (2009) Diabetic foot infection: usefulness of SPECT/CT for 99mTc-HMPAO-labeled leukocyte imaging. J Nucl Med 50(7):1042–1046

68. Heiba S, Kolker D, Ong L, Sharma S, Travis A, Teodorescu V, Ellozy S, Kostakoglu L, Savitch I, Machac J (2013) Dual-isotope SPECT/CT impact on hospitalized patients with suspected diabetic foot infection: saving limbs, lives, and resources. Nucl Med Commun 34:877–884

69. Modic M, Palestro CJ, Love C, Miller TT (2006) Infection and musculoskeletal conditions: imaging of musculoskeletal infections. Best Pract Res Clin Rheumatol. 20:1197–1218

70. Duarte RM, Vaccaro AR (2013) Spinal infection: state of the art and management algorithm. Eur Spine J 22:2787–2799

71. Cassar-Pullicino VN (2004) MR imaging of spinal infection. Semin Musculoskelet Radiol 8:215–229

72. Palestro CJ (2016) Radionuclide imaging of musculoskeletal infection: a review. J Nucl Med 57:1406–1412

73. Seifen T, Rettenbacher L, Thaler C, Holzmannhofer J, Mc Coy M, Pirich C (2012) Prolonged back pain attributed to suspected spondylodiscitis: the value of 18F-FDG PET/CT imaging in the diagnostic work-up of patients. Nuklearmedizin 51:194–200

74. Fuster D, Tomás X, Mayoral M et al (2015) Prospective comparison of whole-body 18F-FDG PET/CT and MRI of the spine in the diagnosis of haematogenous spondylodiscitis. Eur J Nucl Med Mol Imaging 42:264–271

75. Ioannou S, Chatziioannou S, Pneumaticos SG, Zormpala A, Sipsas NV (2013) Fluorine-18 fluoro2-deoxy-D-glucose positron emission tomography/computed tomography scan contributes to the diagnosis and management of brucellar spondylodiskitis. BMC Infect Dis 13:73

76. Riccio SA, Chu AKM, Rabin HR, Kloiber R (2015) Fluorodeoxyglucose positron emission tomography/computed tomography interpretation criteria for assessment of antibiotic treatment response in pyogenic spine infection. Can Assoc Radiol J 66:145–152

77. Kouijzer IJ, Scheper H, De Rooy JW, Bloem JL, Janssen MJ, van Den Hoven L et al (2018) The diagnostic value of 18 F–FDG-PET/CT and MRI in suspected vertebral osteomyelitis–a prospective study. Eur J Nucl Med Mol Imaging 45(5):798–805

78. Tumeh SS, Aliabadi P, Weissman BN, McNeil BJ (1986) Chronic osteomyelitis: bone and gallium scan patterns associated with active disease. Radiology 158:685–688

79. Demirev A, Weijers R, Geurts J, Mottaghy F, Walenkamp G, Brans B (2014) Comparison of [18 F] FDG PET/CT and MRI in the diagnosis of active osteomyelitis. Skeletal radiology 43(5):665–672

80. Lankinen P, Seppänen M, Mattila K, Kallajoki M, Knuuti J, Aro HT (2017) Intensity of 18F-FDG PET uptake in culture-negative and culture-positive cases of chronic osteomyelitis. Contrast Media Mol Imaging 2017:9754293

81. Basu S, Chryssikos T, Houseni M, Malay DS, Shah JH, Zhuang M et al (2007) Potential role of FDG PET in the setting of diabetic neuro-osteoarthropathy: can it differentiate uncomplicated Charcot's neuro-arthropathy from osteomyelitis and soft-tissue infection? Nucl Med Commun 28:465–472

82. Guhlmann A, Brecht-Krauss D, Sugar G, Glatting G, Kotzerke J, Kinzi L, Reske SN (1998) Chronic osteomyelitis: detection with FDG PET and cor-

relation with histopathologic findings. Radiology 206:749–753

83. Zhuang HM, Duarte PS, Poudehnad M et al (2000) The exclusion chronic osteomyelitis with F-18 fluorodeoxyglucose positron tomography imaging. Clin Nucl Med 25:281–284

84. De Winter F, Dierckx R, De Bondt P et al (2000) FDG PET as a single technique is more accurate than the combination bone scan/white blood cell scan in chronic orthopedic infection (COI). J Nucl Med 41:59 (Abstract)

85. Palestro CJ (2015) Radionuclide imaging of osteomyelitis. Semin Nucl Med 45:32–46

86. van der Bruggen W, Bleeker-Rovers CP, Boerman OC, Gotthardt M, Oyen WJ (2010) PET and SPECT in osteomyelitis and prosthetic bone and joint infections: a systematic review. Semin Nucl Med 40:3–15

87. Mariani G, Bruselli L, Kuwert T, Kim EE, Flotats A, Israel O, Dondi M, Watanabe N (2010) A review on the clinical uses of SPECT/CT. Eur J Nucl Med Mol Imaging 37:1959–1985

88. Zhuang H, Durate PS, Pourdehnad M et al (2001) The promising role of F-18-FDG PET in detecting infected lower limb prosthesis implants. J Nucl Med 42:44–48

89. Chacko TK, Zhuang H, Stevenson K, Moussavian B, Alavi A (2002) The influence of the location of fluodeoxyglucose uptake in periprosthetic infection in painful; hip prosthesis. Nucl Med Commun 23:851–855

90. Greyson ND, Tepperman PS (1984) Three-phase bone studies in hemiplegia with refl ex sympathetic dystrophy and the effect of disuse. J Nucl Med 25:423–429

91. Amunden TR, Siegel MJ, Siegel BA (1984) Osteomyelitis and infarction in sickle cell hemoglobinopathies: differentiation by combined technetium and gallium scintigraphy. Radiology 153:807–812

92. Porrino J, Richardson ML, Flaherty E, Albahhar M, Ha AS, Mulcahy H, Chew FS (2019) Septic Arthritis and Joint Aspiration: The Radiologist's Role in Image-Guided Aspiration for Suspected Septic Arthritis. Semin Roentgenol 54:177–189

93. Jaramillo D, Treves ST, Kasser JR, Harper M, Sundel R, Laor T (1995) Osteomyelitis and septic arthritis in children. Appropriate use of imaging to guide treatment. AJR Am J Roentgenol 165:399–403

94. Sundberg SB, Savage JP, Foster BK (1989) Technetium phosphate bone scan in the diagnosis of septic arthritis in childhood. J PediatrOrthop 9:579–585

95. Mc Affe JG, Roba RC, Majid M (1995) The musculoskeletal system. In: Wagner HN (ed) Principles of nuclear medicine, 2nd edn. Saunders, Philadelphia, pp 986–1020

96. Graham J, Wood SK (1976) Aseptic necrosis of bone following trauma. In: Davidson JK (ed) Aseptic necrosis of bone. Excerpta Medica, Amsterdam, p 101

97. Achar S, Yamanaka J (2019) Apophysitis and osteochondrosis: Common causes of pain in growing bones. American family physician 99:610–618

98. Collier BD, Carrera GF, Johnson RP, Isitman AT, Hellman RS, Knobel J et al (1985) Detection of femoral head avascular necrosis in adults by SPECT. J Nucl Med 26:979–987

99. Murphey MD, Foreman KL, Klassen-Fischer MK, Fox MG, Chung EM, Kransdorf MJ (2014) From the radiologic pathology archives imaging of osteonecrosis: radiologic-pathologic correlation. Radiographics 34:1003–1028

100. Agrawal K, Tripathy SK, Sen RK, Santhosh S, Bhattacharya A (2017) Nuclear medicine imaging in osteonecrosis of hip: Old and current concepts. World journal of orthopedics 8:747–753

101. Resnick D (1989) Bone and joint imaging. Saunders, Philadelphia, pp 979–999

102. Laine JC, Martin BD, Novotny SA, Kelly DM (2018) Role of advanced imaging in the diagnosis and management of active Legg-Calve-Perthes disease. JAAOS-Journal of the American Academy of Orthopaedic Surgeons 26(15):526–536

103. de Sanctis N, Rondinella F (2000) Prognostic evaluation of Legg-Calvé-Perthes disease by MRI. Part II: pathomorphogenesis and new classification. J PediatrOrthop 20:463–470

104. Fragniere B, Chotel F, VargasBarreto B, Berard J (2001) The value of early postoperative bone scan in slipped capital femoral epiphysis. J PediatrOrthop B 10:51–55

105. Resnick D, Niwayama G (1998) Osteonecrosis: diagnostic techniques and complications. In: Resnick D, Niwayama G (eds) Diagnosis of bone and joint disorders second editions. Saunders, Philadelphia, p 3268

106. Smith JA (1996) Bone disorders in sickle cell disease. Hematol Oncol Clin North Am 10:1345–1346

107. Keeley K, Buchanan GR (1982) Acute infarction of long bones in children with sickle cell anemia. J Pediatr 101:170–175

108. Skaggs DL, Kim SK, Green NW, Harris D, Miler JH (2001) Differentiation between bone infarct and acute osteomyelitis in children with sickle-cell disease with use of sequential radionuclide bone-marrow and bone scans. J Bone Joint Surg Am 83:1810–1813

109. Jain R, Sawhney S, Rizvi SG (2008) Acute bone crises in sickle cell disease: the T1 fat-saturated sequence in differentiation of acute bone infarcts from acute osteomyelitis. Clin Radiol. 63:59–70

110. Bouden AK, Kaïs C, Abdallah NB, HoudaKraiem N, Jamoussi MM (2005) MRI contribution in diagnosis of acute bone infarcts in children with sickle cell disease. Tunis Med. 83:344–348

111. Sisayan R, Elgazzar AH, Webner P, Religioso DG (1996) Impact of bone scintigraphy on clinical management of a sickle cell patient with recent chest pain. Clin Nucl Med 21:523–526

112. Kim HK (2012) Pathophysiology and new strategies for the treatment of Legg-Calvé-Perthes disease. J Bone Joint Surg Am 94:659–669

113. Kawai K, Maruno H, Watanabe Y, Hirohata K (1980) Fat necrosis of osteocytes as a causative factor in idiopathic osteonecrosis inheritable hyperlipemic rabbits. Clin OrthopRelat Res 153:273

114. Greyson ND, Lotem MM, Gross AE (1982) Radionuclide evaluation of spontaneous femoral osteonecrosis. Radiology 142:729–735

115. Janig W, Baron R (2003) Complex regional pain syndrome: mystery explained? Lancet Neurol 2:687–697

116. Sheth S, Colletti PM (2012) Atlas of sodium fluoride PET bone scans: atlas of NaF PET bone scans. ClinNucl Med 37:e110–e115

117. Shehab D, Al-Jarralah K, Al-Awadhi A et al (1999) Reflex sympathetic dystrophy: an under-recognized entity in Kuwait. APLAR J Rheumatol 3:343–347

118. Cappello ZJ, Kasdan ML, Louis DS (2012) Meta-analysis of imaging techniques for the diagnosis of complex regional pain syndrome type I. J Hand Surg 37:288–296

119. Mourad A (1998) Alterations of musculoskeletal function. In: McCance KL, Huether SE (eds) Pathophysiology, 3rd edn. Mosby, Philadelphia, pp 1435–1485

120. Blockx P, Driessens M (1991) The use of Tc-99-m-HSA dynamic vascular examination in the staging and therapy monitoring of reflex sympathetic dystrophy. Nucl Med Commun 12:725–731

121. Goldstein DS, Tack C, Li TS (2000) Sympathetic innervation and function in reflex sympathetic dystrophy. Ann Neurol 48:49–59

122. Sankaya A, Sankaya I, Pekindil G, Firat MF, Pekindil Y (2001) Technetium-99m sestamibi limb scintigraphy in post-traumatic reflex sympathetic dystrophy: preliminary results. Eur J Nucl Med 28:1517–1522

123. Haensch C, Jorg J, Lerch H (2002) I-123 metaiodobenzyl-guanidine uptake of the forearm shows dysfunction of sympathetic mediated neuro-vascular transmission in complex regional pain syndrome 1 (CRPS 1). J Neurol 249:1742–1743

124. Yoon D, Xu Y, Cipriano PW, Alam IS, Mari Aparici CA, Tawfik VL et al (2021) Neurovascular, muscle, and skin changes on [18F] FDG PET/MRI in complex regional pain syndrome of the foot: A Prospective Clinical Study. Pain Med 23:339–346. https://doi.org/10.1093/pm/pnab315

125. Bernateck M, Rolke R, Birklein F et al (2007) Successful intravenous regional block with low-dose tumor necrosis factor α antibbody Infliximab for treatment of complex regional pain syndrome. Anesthesia Analgesia 105:1148–1151

126. Yoon D, Xu Y, Cipriano V, Tawfik V, Curtin C, Carroll I, Biswal S (2019) Musculoskeletal changes on [18F]FDG PET/MRI from complex regional pain syndrome in foot. J Nucl Med 60(supplement 1):94. (abstract)

127. Tsuyuguchi N, Ohata K, Morino M, Takami T, Goto T, Nishio A, Hara M, Sunada I (2002) Magnetic resonance imaging and [11c] methyl-L-methionine positron emission tomography of fibrous dysplasia-two case reports. Neurol Med Chir 42:341–345

128. Papadakis GZ, Manikis GC, Karantanas AH, Florenzano P, Bagci U et al (2019) 18F-NaF PET/CT imaging in fibrous dysplasia of bone. J Bone Min Res 34:1619–1631

129. Kairemo KJ, Verho S, Dunkel L (1999) Imaging of McCune Albright syndrome using bone single photon emission computed tomography. Eur J Pediatr 158:123–126

130. Amin I, Moroz A (2017) Medial Tibial Stress Syndrome (Shin Splints). In: Musculoskeletal Sports and Spine Disorders. Springer, Cham, pp 281–282

131. Holder LE, Michael RH (1984) The specific scintigraphic pattern of shin splints in the lower leg: concise communication. J Nucl Med 25:865–869

132. Chung CC, Shimer AL (2021) Lumbosacral Spondylolysis and Spondylolisthesis. Clinics in Sports Medicine 40(3):471–490

133. Gaddikeri S, Matesan M, Alvarez J, Hippe DS, Vesselle HJ (2018) MDP-SPECT Versus Hybrid MDP-SPECT/CT in the Evaluation of Suspected Pars Interarticularis Fracture in Young Athletes. Journal of Neuroimaging 28(6):635–639

134. Mandell GA (1998) Nuclear Medicine in pediatric orthopedics. Semin Nucl Med 28:95–115

135. Harcke HT, Mandell GA (1993) Scintigraphic evaluation of the growth plate. Semin Nucl Med 23:255–273

136. Fragniere B, Chotel F, Vargas BB, Berard J (2001) The value of early postoperative bone scan in slipped capital femoral epiphysis. J Pediatr Orthop B 10:51–55

137. King MA, Maxon HR (1984) Paget's Disease: the role of nuclear medicine in diagnosis and treatment. In: Silberstein EB (ed) Bone scintigraphy. Futura publishing Company, Mount Kisco, New York, pp 333–345

138. Christiansen C, RIIS BJ (1989) Optimizing bone mass in the permenopause. In: Kleerehoper M, Krane SM (eds) Clinical disorder of bone and mineral metabolism. Mary AnLiebert, Inc, New York, p 189

139. Renier JC, Audran M (1997) Polyostotic Paget's disease. A search for lesions of different durations and for new lesions. Rev RhumEngl Ed 54:233–242

140. Gillespy T, Gillespy MP (1991) Osteoporosis. RadiolClin North Am 29:77–84

141. Cooper C, Aihie-Sayer A (1994) Osteoporosis: recent advances in pathogenesis and treatment. Q J Med 87:203–209

142. Brasier AR, Nussbaum SR (1988) Hungry bone syndrome: clinical and biochemical predictors of its occurrence after parathyroid surgery. Am J Med 84:654

143. Dabbagh S (1998) Renal osteodystrophy. Curr Opin Pediatr 10:190–195

144. Cicconetti A, Maffeini C, Piro FR (1999) Differential diagnosis in a case of brown tumor caused by primary hyperparathyroid ism. Minerva Stomatol 48:553–558

145. Rt L, Hensinger RN (1997) Slipped capital femoral epiphysis associated with renal failure osteodystrophy. J Pediatr Orthop 17:205–211

146. Yalcinkaya F, Ince E, Tumer N, Ensari A, Ozkaya N (2000) Spectrum of renal osteodystrophy in children on continuous ambulatory peritoneal dialysis. Pediatr Int 42:53–57

147. Seggewiss R, Hess T, Fiehn C (2003) A family with a variant form of primary hypertrophic osteoarthropathy restricted to the lower extremities. Joint Bone Spine 70:230–233

148. Ali A, Tetalman MR, Fordham EW et al (1980) Distribution of hypertrophic pulmonary osteoarthropathy. AJR Am J Roentgenol 134:771–780

149. McCarthy D (ed) (1984) Arthritis and allied conditions. Lea and Fabiger, Philadelphia

150. Elgazzar AH, Martich V, Gelfand MJ (1995) Advanced fi brodysplasia ossifi cans progressiva. Clin Nucl Med 20:519–521

151. Orzel JA, Redd TG (1985) Heterotopic bone formation: clinical, laboratory and imaging correlation. J Nucl Med 26:125–132

152. Choi YH, Kim KE, Lim SH, Lim JY (2012) Early presentation of heterotopic ossification mimicking pyomyositis – two case reports. Ann Rehabil Med 36:713–718

153. Shehab D, Elgazzar A, Collier BD (2002) Heterotopic ossifi cation. J Nucl Med 43:346–353

154. Ghanem M, Elgazzar AH (2012) The added value of SPECT/CT., Hassan F, Enayat M, Mohammed F, Vijayanathan S, Gnanasegaran G (2012) Heterotrophic ossification in a patient suspected of having osteomyelitis: additional value of SPECT/CT. Clin Nucl Med 37:170–171

155. Kawaguchi Y, Hasegawa T, Oka S, Sato C, Arima N, Norimatsu H (2001) Mechanism of intramedullary high intensity area on T2-weighted magnetic resonance imaging in osteoid osteoma: a possible role of COX-2 expression. Pathol Int 51:933–937

156. Flemming DJ, Murphey MD (2000) Enchondroma and chondrosarcoma. Semin Musculoskelet Radiol 4(1):59–71

157. Elgazzar AH, Malki AA, Abdel-Dayem HM, Sahweil A, Razzak S, Jahan S, Elsayed M, Omar YT (1989) Role of thallium 201 in the diagnosis of solitary bone lesions. Nucl Med Commun 10:477–485

158. Resnik D, Kyriakos M, Greenway GD (2002) Tumors and tumor-like lesions of bone. Diagnosis of bone and joint disorders, 4th edn. Saunders, Philadelphia, pp 3979–3985

159. Gupta A (2018) Ewing Sarcoma. In: PET/MR Imaging. Springer, Cham, pp 9–11

160. Weber W (2020) Clinical PET/MR. In: Molecular Imaging in Oncology. Springer, Cham, pp 747–764

161. Gholamrezanezhad A, Guermazi A, Salavati A, Alavi A (2018) Evolving Role of PET-Computed Tomography and PET-MR imaging in assessment of musculoskeletal disorders and its potential revolutionary impact on day-to-day practice of related disciplines. PET clinics 13(4):xiii-xiv

162. Yildiz C, Erler K, Atesalp AS, Basbozkurt M (2003) Benign bone tumors in children. Curr Opin Pediatr. 15:58–67

163. Moser RP Jr, Masewell JF (1987) An approach to primary bone tumors. Radiol Clin North Am 25:1049–1093

164. Hurley C, McCarville MB, Shulkin BL, Mao S, Wu J, Navid F et al (2016) Comparison of ^{18}F-FDG-PET-CT and bone scintigraphy for evaluation of osseous metastases in newly diagnosed and recurrent osteosarcoma. Pediatr Blood Cancer 63:1381–1386

165. Liu F, Zhang Q, Zhou D et al (2019) Effectiveness of ^{18}F-FDG PET/CT in the diagnosis and staging of osteosarcoma: a meta-analysis of 26 studies. BMC Cancer 19:323. https://doi.org/10.1186/s12885-019-5488-5

166. Murthy NJ, Rao H, Friedman AS (2000) Positive findings on bone scan in multiple myeloma. South Med J 93:1028–1029

167. Hillengass J, Moulopoulos LA, Delorme S, Koutoulidis V, Mosebach J, Hielscher T, Terpos E (2017) Whole-body computed tomography versus conventional skeletal survey in patients with multiple myeloma: a study of the International Myeloma Working Group. Blood cancer journal 7(8):e599–e599

168. Gleeson TG, Moriarty J, Shortt CP et al (2009) Accuracy of whole-body low-dose multidetector CT (WBLDCT) versus skeletal survey in the detection of myelomatous lesions, and correlation of disease distribution with whole-body MRI (WBMRI). Skeletal Radiol 38:225–236

169. Zamagn E, Tacchetti P, Cavo M (2019) Imaging in multiple myeloma: How? When? Blood 133:644–651

170. Sasikumar A, Joy A, Pilla MRA, Nanabala R, Thomas B (2016) G-68a-PSMA PET/CT Imaging in Multiple Myeloma. Clin Nucl Med 42:e126–e127

171. Batson OV (1940) The function of the vertebral veins and their role in the spread of metastases. Ann Surg 112:138

172. Alexandrakis MG, Kyriakou DS, Passam F, Koukouraki S, Karkavitsas N (2001) Value of Tc-99 m sestamibi scintigraphy in the detection of bone lesions in multiple myeloma: comparison with Tc-99 m methylene diphosphonate. Ann Hematol 80:349–353

173. Mihailović J, Freeman LM (2012) Bone: from planar imaging to SPECT & PET/CT. Arch Oncol 20:117–120

174. Harries M, Putushothatham A (2014) Incidence of bone metastases and survival after a diagnosis of

bone metastases in breast cancer patients. Cancer Epidemiology 38":427–434

175. Resnick D, Niwayama G (1998) Skeletal metastases. In: Resnick D, Niwayama G (eds) Diagnosis of bone and joint disorders, 2nd edn. Saunders, Philadelphia, pp 3945–4010

176. Shutte H (1979) The influence of bone pain on the results of bone scans. Cancer 34:2039–2043

177. Ripamonti C, Fulfaro F, Ticozzi C, Casuccio A, De Conno F (1998) Role of pamidronate disodium in the treatment of metastatic bone disease. Tumori. 84:442–455

178. Rybak LD, Rosenthal DI (2001) Radiological imaging for the diagnosis of bone metastases. Q J Nucl Med 45:53–54

179. Goris ML, Basso LV, Etcublanaas E (1980) Photopenic lesions in bone scintigraphy. ClinNuclMed 5:299–301

180. Sy WM, Westring DW, Weinberger G (1975) Coldlesions on bone imaging. J Nucl Med 15:1013–1015

181. Daldrup-Link HE, Franzius C, Link TM, Laukamp D, Sciuk J, Jurgens H, Schober O, Rummeny EJ (2001) Whole-body MR imaging for detection of bone metastases in children and young adults: comparison with skeletal scintigraphy and FDG PET. AJR Am J Roentgenol 177:229–236

182. Kao CH, Hsieh JF, Tsai SC, Ho YJ, Yen RF (2000) Comparison and discrepancy of 18F-2-deoxyglucose positron emission tomography and Tc-99m MDP bone scan to detect bone metastases. Anticancer Res 20:2189–2192

183. Moog F, Kotzerke J, Reske SN (1999) FDG PET can replace bone scintigraphy in primary staging of malignant lymphoma. J Nucl Med 40:1407–1413

184. Schirrmeister H, Guhlmann A, Elsner K, Kotzerke J, Glatting G, Rentschler M, Neumaier B, Trager H, Nussle K, Reske SN (1999) Sensitivity in detecting osseous lesions depends on anatomic localization: planar bone scintigraphy versus F18 PET. J Nucl Med 40:1623–1629

185. Segall G, Delbeke D, Stabin MG, Even-Sapir E, Fair J, Sajdak R, Smith GT (2010) SNM practice guideline for sodium 18F-fluoride PET/CT bone scans. J Nucl Med 51:1813–1820

186. Yen RF, Chen CY, Cheng MF, Wu YW, Shiau YC, Wu K, Hong RL, Yu CJ, Wang KL, Yang RS (2010) The diagnostic and prognostic effectiveness of F-18 sodium fluoride PET-CT in detecting bone metastases for hepatocellular carcinoma patients. Nucl Med Commun 31:537–545

187. Taira AV, Herfkens RJ, Gambhir SS, Quon A (2007) Detection of bone metastases: assessment of integrated FDG PET/CT imaging. Radiology 243(1):204–211

188. Costelloe CM, Chuang HH, Chasen BA, Pan T, Fox PS, Bassett RL, Madewell JE (2013) Bone windows for distinguishing malignant from benign primary bone tumors on FDG PET/CT. J Cancer 4:524–530

189. Gnanasegaran G, Cook G, Fogelman I (2007) Musculoskeletal system. In: Biersac HJ, Freeman LM (eds) Clinical nuclear medicine. Springer, Berlin, pp 241–262

190. Daldrup-Link HE, Franzius C, Link TM, LaukampD SJ, Jurgens H, Schober O, Rummeny EJ (2001) Whole-body MR imaging for detection ofbone metastases in children and young adults: comparison with skeletal scintigraphy and FDG PET.AJR. Am J Roentgenol 177:229–236

191. Garcia JR, Simo M, Soler M, Perez G, Lopez S, Lomena F (2005) Relative roles of bone scintigraphy and positron emission tomography in assessing the treatment response of bone metastases. Eur J Nucl Med Mol Imaging 32:1243–1244

192. Blake GM, Park-Holohan SJ, Cook GJ et al (2001) Quantitative studies of bone with the use of 18F-fluoride and 99mTc-methylene diphosphonate. SeminNucl Med 31:28–49

193. Cook GJ, Fogelman I (2001) The role of positron emission tomography in skeletal disease. SeminNucl Med 31:50–61

194. Even-Sapir E (2005) Imaging of malignant bone involvement by morphologic, scintigraphic, and hybrid modalities. J Nucl Med 46:1356–1367

195. Cook GJ, Houston S, Rubens R et al (1998) Detection of bone metastases in breast cancer by 18-FDG PET: differing metabolic activity in osteoblastic and osteolytic lesions. J ClinOncol 16:3375–3379

196. Kruger S et al (2009) Detection of bone metastases in patients with lung cancer: 99mTc-MDP planar bone scintigraphy, 18F-fluoride PET or 18F-FDG PET/CT. Eur J Nucl Med Mol Imaging 36:1807

197. Iagaru A et al (2012) Prospective evaluation of (99m) Tc MDP scintigraphy, (18)F NaF PET/CT, and (18) F FDG PET/CT for detection of skeletal metastases. Mol Imaging Biol 14:252

198. Jadvar H et al (2012) Prospective evaluation of 18F-NaF and 18F-FDG PET/CT in detection of occult metastatic disease in biochemical recurrence of prostate cancer. ClinNucl Med 37:637

199. Lin FI et al (2012) Prospective comparison of combined 18F-FDG and 18F-NaF PET/CT vs. 18F-FDG PET/CT imaging for detection of malignancy. Eur J Nucl Med Mol Imaging 39:262

200. Iagaru A, Mittra E, Mosci C, Dick DW, Sathekge M, Prakash V, Gambhir SS (2013) Combined 18F-fluoride and 18F-FDG PET/CT scanning for evaluation of malignancy: results of an international multicenter trial. Journal of nuclear medicine 54(2):176–183

201. Karamzade-Ziarati N, Manafi-Farid R, Ataeinia B, Langsteger W, Pirich C, Mottaghy FM, Beheshti M (2019) Molecular imaging of bone metastases using tumor-targeted tracers. Q J Nucl Med Mol Imaging. 63:136–149

6.1 The Thyroid Gland

6.1.1 Anatomical and Physiological Considerations

6.1.1.1 Anatomy

The thyroid gland develops from the foramen cecum of the tongue, to which it is connected by the thyroglossal duct. It descends during fetal life to reach the anterior neck by about the seventh week. Absent or aberrant descent results in ectopic locations, including the sublingual region and superior mediastinum.

The normal adult thyroid gland weighs 14–19 g and is barely palpable. It is generally smaller in women than in men and is barely palpable [1, 2]. The thyroid is located in the mid to lower anterior neck, with the isthmus in front of the trachea, usually just below the cricoid cartilage, and the lobes on the sides of the trachea (Fig. 6.1a). Ectopic thyroid gland can occur in multiple locations particularly sublingual (Fig. 6.1b). In older individuals with shorter necks, the thyroid may lie at or just above the suprasternal notch, and it may often be partly substernal. The thyroid gland moves cephalad during swallowing, a characteristic that aids in palpation and in distinction of thyroid from non-thyroid neck masses.

6.1.1.2 Physiology

The thyroid gland regulates a spectrum of physiological activities such as growth, metabolism, homeostasis, and cell proliferation and differentiation through the secretion of thyroid hormones. The thyroid follicle consists of a colloid center, which acts as a storage site for thyroid hormone, surrounded by epithelial cells (Fig. 6.2). The thyroid epithelial cell has a transport mechanism, also referred to as trapping, that enables thyroid concentration of iodide [3].The sodium dependent iodide transport activity of the thyroid gland is mainly attributed to the functional expression of the Na+/I- Symporter (NIS) localized at the basolateral membrane of thyroid epithelial cells. Symporter activity is influenced primarily by pituitary thyroid stimulating hormone (TSH), which increases the transport of iodide. The trapped iodide subsequently undergoes organification and incorporation into thyroid hormones.

Synthesis of hormone takes place in thyroglobulin, a glycoprotein, which is produced in the thyroid cell and extruded into the colloid. Iodine combines with tyrosine in thyroglobulin to form monoiodotyrosine (MIT) and diiodotyrosine (DIT). Subsequently, the iodotyrosines are coupled, with the formation of thyroxine (T_4) and triiodothyronine (T3). The coupling reaction also is mediated by peroxidase.

A. H. Elgazzar, *Synopsis of Pathophysiology in Nuclear Medicine*,
https://doi.org/10.1007/978-3-031-20646-7_6

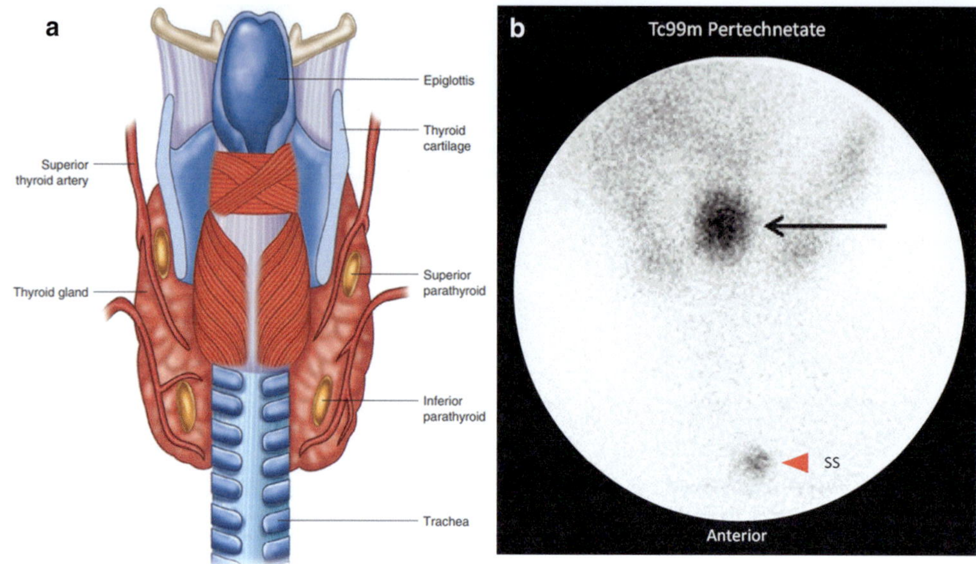

Fig. 6.1 Diagram (**a**) showing typical locations of the thyroid and parathyroid glands (**b**) is a tc99m thyroid scan image illustrating an ectopic location of functioning thyroid tissue in the sublingual location (arrow)

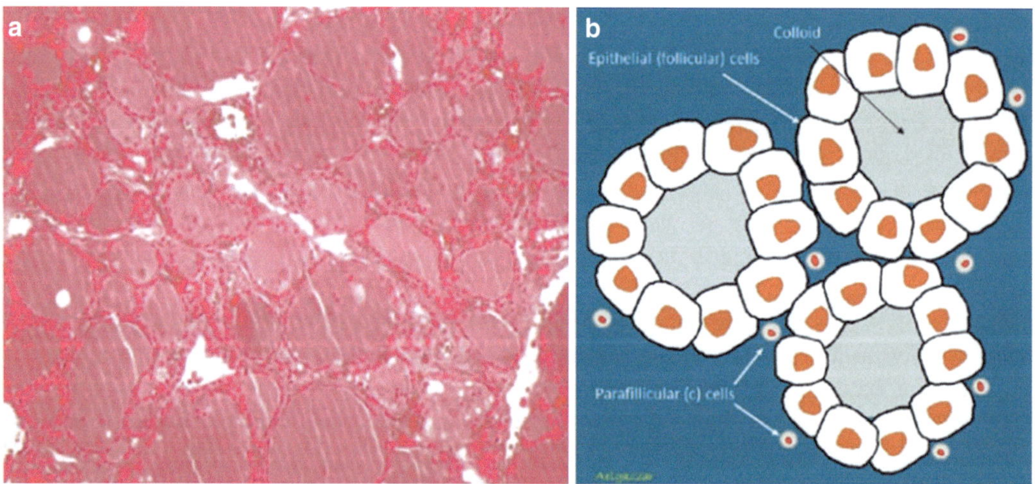

Fig. 6.2 Thyroid follicle. (**a**) Low-power field images of thyroid gland tissue showing the follicles lined by follicular cells and filled with colloid. (**b**) Diagram illustrating thyroid follicles and cells

Release of thyroid hormones occurs in response to TSH where a small amount of colloid is engulfed by the epithelial cell and proteolyzed, with release of T_3 and T_4, which diffuse into the circulation. Thyroglobulin not undergoing proteolysis also enters the circulation in small quantities. The serum thyroglobulin has been used as a tumor marker in differentiated thyroid cancer. Thyroglobulin decreases and eventually becomes undetectable following thyroidectomy and ^{131}I ablation, and its subsequent rise indicates a recurrence. TSH stimulation, by promoting colloid endocytosis, increases the amount of thyroglobulin released. Consequently, the serum thyroglobulin is a more reliable tumor marker at high TSH levels [4, 5].

Most of the circulating thyroid hormones are bound to plasma proteins, the free fraction comprising about 0.05% of T_4 and 0.2% of T_3. Only the free hormone has metabolic effects, and it is a more accurate measure of thyroid function than the total hormone, which varies with plasma proteins levels. T_3 is considered the active hormone. About 20%–30% of the circulating T_3 is secreted by the thyroid gland and the remainder is produced by monodeiodination of T_4 in extrathyroid tissues, notably the liver, kidney, brain, and pituitary [5]. Decrease in the peripheral conversion of T_4 to T_3 is a basis for the use of some antithyroid drugs. Most antithyroid drugs generally block one or more steps in the synthesis and metabolism of thyroid hormone.

6.1.1.3 Role of Iodine Metabolism in Thyroid Physiology

Iodine is needed for the production of thyroid hormones. Since the body does not make iodine, it is an essential part of diet. The mean daily turnover of iodine by the thyroid is approximately 60–95 µg in adults in iodine-sufficient areas. The body of a healthy adult contains 15–20 mg of iodine, 70–80% of which is in the thyroid. Iodine is a trace element that is ingested in several chemical forms. Most forms of iodine are reduced to iodide in the gut. Iodide is nearly completely absorbed in the stomach and duodenum [6]. In the basolateral membrane of the thyroid cell, the sodium/iodine symporter transfers iodide into the thyroid across a concentration gradient 20–50 times that of plasma by active transport [6]. Under normal circumstances, plasma iodine has a half-life of approximately 10 h, but this is shortened if the thyroid is overactive, as in iodine deficiency or hyperthyroidism.

Degradation of T4 and T3 in the peripheral tissues releases iodine that re-enters the plasma iodine pool. Most ingested iodine is eventually excreted in the urine. Only a small amount appears in the feces.

6.1.1.3.1 Effect of Iodine Insufficiency
Iodine is an integral part of the thyroid hormones thyroxine (T4) and triiodothyronine (T3). Severe iodine deficiency results in depleted iodine stores and a failure to sustain normal thyroid hormone levels. Reduced synthesis of thyroid hormone is compensated, at least in part, by increased TSH secretion, resulting eventually in goiter formation.

Because an adequate supply of thyroid hormone is needed for fetal neurological development, maternal and fetal hypothyroidism resulting from iodine deficiency is associated with varying degrees of neuropsychological deficits including cretinism .

6.1.1.3.2 Effect of Excessive Iodine
When intrathyroid iodine concentrations are significantly increased, the rate of thyroid hormone synthesis is decreased, with a reduction in iodothyronine synthesis and decrease in the DIT/MIT ratio. This response is referred to as the Wolff-Chaikoff effect.

Continued exposure to large amounts of iodine would eventually lead to hypothyroidism, with compensatory increase in TSH and development of goiter. While this does occur occasionally, adaptation or escape from the effects of chronic iodide excess is more likely. The inhibitory effect of iodides on thyroid function is utilized clinically for prompt control of severe hyperthyroidism and thyroid storm. In Graves' disease, large doses of iodide decrease not only hormone synthesis but also hormone release [7, 8]. Since escape from the inhibitory effect is likely, iodide therapy is only a short-term measure for lowering thyroid hormone levels rapidly.

Iodine excess may lead to hyperthyroidism or hypothyroidism [6, 9]. Iodine-induced hyperthyroidism, referred to as Jod-Basedow, characteristically occurs in persons with hyperplastic thyroid glands. Hyperthyroidism occurring after iodine supplementation in endemic goiter areas is a classical example. Iodine-containing medical products, including amiodarone, radiographic dyes, and kelp, also have the potential to cause Jod-Basedow [10, 11]. Amiodarone, a cardiac antiarrhythmic drug, is a benzofuranic product with a very high iodine content, is associated with either hypo- or hyperthyroidism development.

Figure 6.3 summarizes the mechanism of hormonal interactions related to thyroid gland.

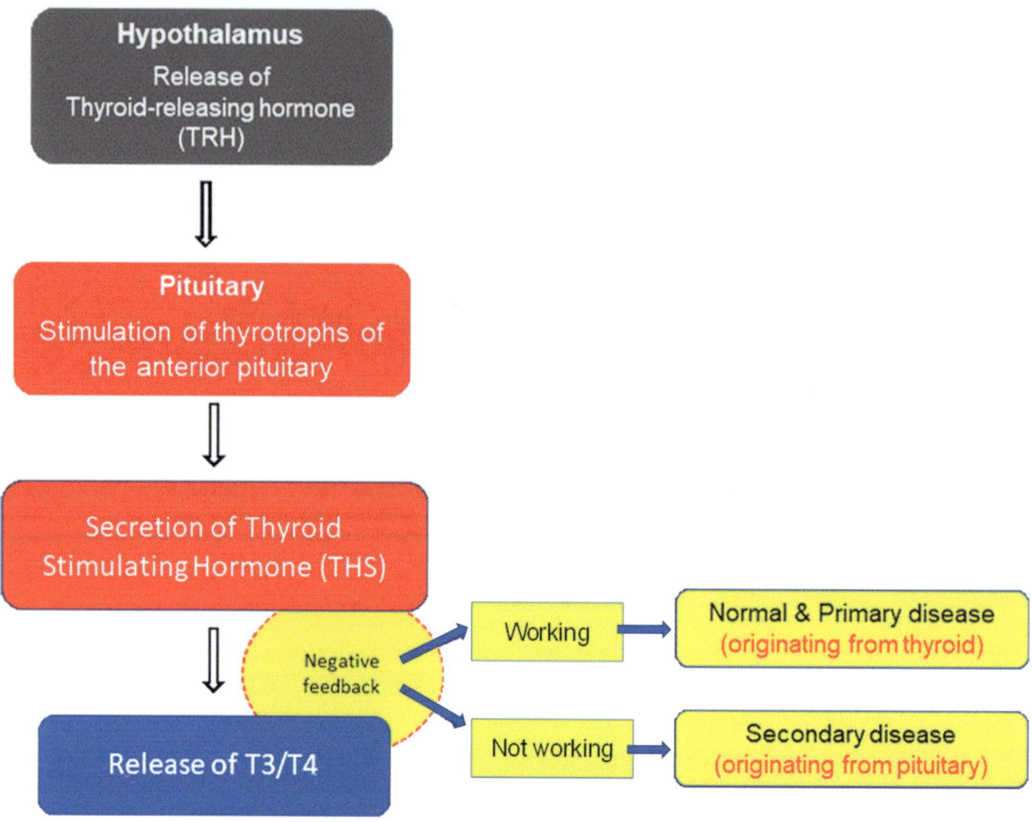

Fig. 6.3 Simple illustration of different hormones related to thyroid function and pathology

6.1.2 Radiopharmaceuticals for Thyroid Imaging

6.1.2.1 Technetium-99 M-Pertechnetate

Technetium-99 m-pertechnetate is widely used for imaging the thyroid gland. It is trapped by the thyroid, but unlike iodine, it does not undergo organification and remains in the gland for a relatively short duration. Therefore, imaging is done about 20–30 min after intravenous administration of the radiotracer. Approximately 5–10 mCi (185–370 MBq) are used. The thyroid-to-background activity ratio is not as high as that with radioiodine, so that ^{99m}Tc-pertechnetate is unsuitable for imaging to search for metastatic thyroid carcinoma, which usually functions poorly compared with normal thyroid tissue.

Imaging of ectopic mediastinal thyroid tissue also may be suboptimal due to high blood and soft tissue background activity.

6.1.2.2 Iodine-123

Iodine-123 (^{123}I) has ideal characteristics for imaging the thyroid gland, with a short physical half-life of 13 h, absence of beta emissions, and high uptake in thyroid tissue relative to background [12]. However, it is less readily available and more expensive than ^{99m}Tc-pertechnetate. ^{123}I undergoes organic binding in the thyroid gland, and imaging is usually done 4–24 h after oral administration of 200–400 μCi (7.4–14.8 MBq) of radiotracer. Because of its superior biodistribution characteristics, ^{123}I is preferred over ^{99m}Tc-pertechnetate for imaging of poorly functioning and ectopic thyroid glands. [123]I also may be used for whole-body imaging in differentiated thyroid cancer. Approximately 2–4 mCi (74–148 MBq) of the radiotracer are used for this purpose.

6.1.2.3 Iodine-131
Iodine-131 (^{131}I) may be used for the measurement of thyroid uptake, which requires only very small amounts of radiotracer. It is no longer used for routine imaging of the thyroid gland but continues to be valuable for the detection of metastases and recurrences in differentiated thyroid cancer [4, 13, 14]. Following appropriate patient preparation to increase TSH levels, 2–4 mCi (74–148 MBq) of ^{131}I are administered orally and imaging is performed 48–96 h later. Radioiodine imaging has diagnostic as well as prognostic value. Iodine-avid tumors tend to be well-differentiated histological features and a favorable prognosis, whereas tumors that do not accumulate iodine are likely to be less differentiated and more aggressive [4, 15, 16].

Iodine-131 delivers a high radiation absorbed dose to the thyroid, with relative sparing of non-thyroid tissues. It is therefore ideal for the treatment of thyroid disease and used extensively in the management of Graves' disease, toxic nodular goiter, and differentiated thyroid cancer.

6.1.2.4 Fluorine-18 Fluorodeoxyglucose (^{18}F-FDG)
Positron emission tomography (PET) with ^{18}F-FDG is used in evaluating a variety of neoplasms including differentiated thyroid cancer. In differentiated thyroid cancer, FDG may be used to identify metastases not visualized at radioiodine imaging and to assess prognosis. Lesions that accumulate FDG tend to follow a more aggressive course than lesions that are not FDG-avid [17]. Whole-body FDG-PET, therefore, is useful in evaluating high-risk thyroid cancer. Patient preparation is similar to that for radioiodine scintigraphy, since the uptake and diagnostic sensitivity of FDG are increased by TSH stimulation [18].

Focal uptake of FDG within the thyroid gland, an occasional finding at evaluation of non-thyroid cancers, may be related to a benign or malignant pathology [16]. In patients with thyroid nodules with indeterminate FNA, FDG-PET/CT has a moderate ability to correctly discriminate malignant from benign lesions [19]. It may be a reliable option to reduce unnecessary diagnostic surgeries particularly if it is negative at the site of a solitary nodule. On the other hand, diffusely increased FDG uptake in the thyroid gland was found to be associated with chronic thyroiditis and thyroid dysfunction [20].

6.1.3 Major Thyroid Disorders

The most relevant thyroid conditions that commonly need imaging for diagnosis and management include nodular disease, inflammatory conditions, autoimmune disorders, and thyroid cancer.

6.1.3.1 Pathophysiology

6.1.3.1.1 Nodular Thyroid Disease
Thyroid nodules are common. The prevalence ranges from 4% to 10% in general adult and 0.2–1.5% in children [21] and is greater in countries affected by iodine deficiency. The incidence of thyroid nodules inapparently normal thyroid glands is greater than 50% in autopsy series. Studies using high frequency ultrasound in detecting nodules showed a varying prevalence of up to 68% [22, 23], higher in females compared to males and increasing with age [23].

Most thyroid nodules are benign, particularly when multiple. Malignancy in clinical thyroid nodules is reported to occur in 5–20% of nodules and is higher in males [24]. Mortality due to thyroid cancer is generally very low.

Types of Thyroid Nodules
Thyroid nodules represent wide spectrum of thyroid diseases. In a normal sized gland or a diffuse goiter, thyroid nodules may be solitary or multiple. In multinodular goiters, a nodule may become clinically dominant in terms of growth,

dimensions, and functional characteristics. A clinicopathological classification of thyroid nodules subdivides nodules into nonneoplastic nodules, true neoplastic nodules (benign or malignant), and micronodules.

Nonneoplastic Nodules (Pseudo-Nodules)

These nodules may be seen in patients with thyroid hyperplasia and inflammatory or autoimmune thyroid diseases:

(a) Glandular hyperplasia arising spontaneously or following previous partial thyroidectomy.
(b) Rare forms of thyroid hemiagenesis which may present as hyperplasia of the existing thyroid tissue, mimicking a thyroid nodule.
(c) Hashimoto's thyroiditis associated nodules, indicative of lymphocyte infiltration.
(d) Nodules found during the initial phase of subacute thyroiditis, resulting from the inflammatory process.

Neoplastic Nodules

Based on scintigraphy, thyroid nodules are classified into functioning (hot) nodules which are able to concentrate radioactive iodine or technetium-99 m pertechnetate and non-functioning (cold) which show radiotracer uptake less than that in normal thyroid tissue. Hot nodules represent from 3% to 20% of thyroid nodules, according to the geographical origin of the patients as their incidence is higher in countries where iodine deficiency is still present. They are 3–4 times more frequent in females and tend to occur in those older than 40 years. In the great majority of cases, hot nodules are benign. Cold nodules account for more than 80% of all thyroid nodules. Three types of nodules are distinguished by ultrasonography: cystic, solid, and mixed (containing solid and cystic components). Cystic nodules (10–20% of all nodules) are almost always benign. Thyroid cancer is found in approximately 10% of cold nodules (solitary and multiple) that are solid or mixed at ultrasonography. More than 75% of malignant nodules are differentiated thyroid cancer of the follicular epithelium (papillary and follicular) with excellent prognosis. The other types of cancer are rare and include anaplastic or undifferentiated carcinoma (2–14% of all thyroid carcinomas),

medullary thyroid carcinoma representing 5–10% of thyroid carcinomas and originating from the calcitonin-producing parafollicular C cells of the thyroid [25–27]. Lymphoma and metastases to thyroid are other uncommon malignancies.

Micronodules

Micronodules describe nodules of 1 cm or less in diameter. These nodules are discovered increasingly by the commonly used ultrasonography. In the absence of other suspicious clinical criteria, they only require to be followed by repeated thyroid ultrasonography.

6.1.3.1.2 Thyroiditis

Thyroiditis, a group of inflammatory thyroid diseases affecting the gland diffusely or focally and can be infectious, due to microorganisms, or non-infectious. Based on clinical, histopathologic, etiological, and other factors, many classifications and terminologies for the conditions have been proposed. Simply it can be classified into acute, subacute, and chronic [27]. Figure 6.4. shows that classification which is modified to be more inclusive.

Acute Thyroiditis

Acute thyroiditis also called acute suppurative thyroiditis is a rare but serious form secondary to bacteria. Acute thyroiditis requires immediate parenteral antibiotic therapy before abscess formation begins.

Subacute Thyroiditis

Subacute thyroiditis or destructive thyroiditis is characterized by cell membrane breakdown and consequently release of excessive amounts of thyroid hormone into the circulation. The usual causes are autoimmune thyroid disease, viral infection, and amiodarone treatment. Less commonly, thyroiditis may be related to treatment with certain drugs such as interferon alpha, interleukin-2, lymphokine-activated killer (LAK) cells, and lithium. These therapeutic agents probably exacerbate existing autoimmune thyroid disease [27–29].Bacterial thyroiditis is currently rarely seen.

Thyroiditis is typically painful and usually resolves spontaneously. Hyperthyroidism in the

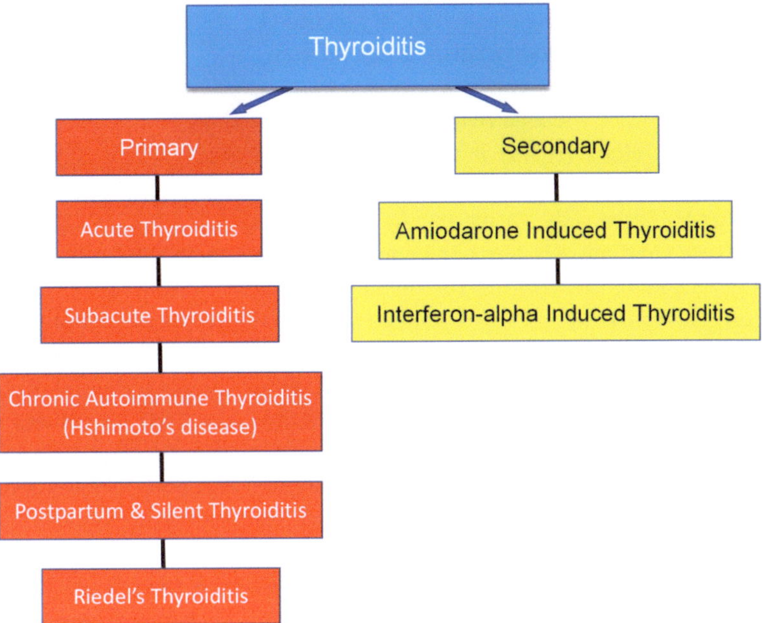

Fig. 6.4 Classification of thyroiditis

active phase is followed by transient hypothyroidism before restoration of the euthyroid state, usually in 6–12 months. Treatment usually consists of β-adrenergic blockers in the hyperthyroid phase and analgesics for pain. Protracted thyroiditis may require glucocorticoids.

Viral subacute thyroiditis, also known as de Quervain's thyroiditis, usually occurs after an upper respiratory tract infection. The disorder tends to be seasonal and may occur in clusters, occasionally causing mini epidemics. It usually presents as a painful and tender goiter, associated with general malaise and possibly fever. Inflammation frequently begins in one lobe of the thyroid and gradually spreads to involve the entire gland. Permanent hypothyroidism is uncommon.

Postpartum Thyroiditis

Postpartum thyroiditis, also known as painless or subacute lymphocytic thyroiditis, is the principal thyroid disorder in postpartum women. It may be considered an accelerated form of autoimmune thyroid disease, attributed to suppression of immune-related disorders during pregnancy with a rebound after childbirth [30, 31].

For the same reason, Graves' disease also may occur in the postpartum period, though less frequently, and a strong association with insulin-dependent diabetes mellitus, an autoimmune condition, has been noted.

Postpartum thyroiditis, like other forms of destructive thyroiditis, is a self-limited, but tends to reoccur in subsequent pregnancies. Permanent hypothyroidism occurs in 20%–25% of patients over a period of 5 years. Elevated thyroid peroxidase (anti-microsomal) antibodies during pregnancy are associated with a sharp increase in postpartum thyroiditis.

Amiodarone-Induced Thyroiditis

Amiodarone is an iodine-rich benzofuran derivative used to treat and prevent cardiac arrhythmias. It may precipitate a number of thyroid conditions including thyroiditis, which appears to be related to a cytotoxic effect [10, 11]. Thyroid hormone synthesis may increase or decrease. Other actions of amiodarone include blocking peripheral conversion of T4 to T3, binding of T3 to its receptors, and thyroid release of T3 and T4. These effects may permit the use of amiodarone in very selected cases of hyperthyroidism [32].

Since amiodarone and its metabolite desethylamiodarone have long half-lives of up to 100 days, the thyroid-related effects can be protracted and occasionally may begin after stopping the drug. Amiodarone-induced thyroiditis generally requires treatment with a glucocorticoid. Permanent hypothyroidism is uncommon.

Interferon-Alpha Induced Thyroiditis

Interferon alpha (IFNα) is an important drug therapy for several malignant and nonmalignant diseases, especially hepatitis C. Interferon induced thyroiditis is a major clinical problem for patients receiving interferon therapy. Studies have shown that up to 15% of patients with hepatitis C receiving IFNα develop clinical thyroid disease, and up to 40% were reported to develop thyroid antibodies. Interferon-alpha induced thyroiditis can be classified as autoimmune type and non-autoimmune type. Autoimmune interferon-alpha induced thyroiditis may be manifested by the development of thyroid antibodies with or without clinical disease, Clinical disease includes both autoimmune hypothyroidism (Hashimoto's thyroiditis) and autoimmune thyrotoxicosis (Graves' disease). Non-autoimmune thyroiditis can manifest as subacute (destructive thyroiditis) or as hypothyroidism with negative thyroid antibodies [33, 34].

Autoimmune Thyroiditis (Hashimoto's Disease). See Following Section

6.1.3.1.3 Autoimmune Thyroid Disease

Autoimmune thyroid disease is often observed together with other autoimmune diseases. The coexistence of two or more autoimmune diseases in the same individual is referred to as polyautoimmunity. The occurrence of polyautoimmunity has led to a hypothesis that the affected patients suffer from a generalized dysregulation of their immune system [35].

Autoimmune thyroid disease comprises two major entities, Hashimoto's disease (chronic autoimmune thyroiditis and variants) and Graves' disease. Variants of Hashimoto's disease include subacute thyroiditis, which occurs typically in the postpartum period, and atrophic thyroiditis. The predisposing factors of the disease are listed in Table 6.1 [36–39].

Hashimoto's Disease

Elevation of thyroid peroxidase antibodies is characteristic of Hashimoto's disease.

Table 6.1 Predisposing factors for autoimmune thyroid disease

Genetic predisposition
Immune system dysregulation
Iodine excess
Cigarette smoking
Female gender
Psychological stress
Infection

Antithyroglobulin antibodies may also be elevated. Hormone synthesis is impaired with immune thyroid disease compensatory increase in TSH secretion, which stimulates thyroid function and growth. Eventually, many patients become hypothyroid. Both overt and subclinical hypothyroidism related to autoimmune disease are widely prevalent in iodine-sufficient regions [40].

Exacerbation of Hashimoto's disease, frequently occurring in the postpartum period, is a cause of subacute thyroiditis.

Graves' Disease

Graves' disease is associated with high levels of thyrotropin receptor autoantibodies(TRAB) that stimulate thyroid growth, and thyroid hormone synthesis and release [39, 41]. Most organ systems are affected by Graves' disease, the cardiovascular manifestations being the most apparent. Increased heart rate and contractility increase the cardiac output. These effects are related to a direct inotropic effect of T3, decreased systemic vascular resistance, increased preload related to a higher blood volume, and heightened sensitivity to sympathetic stimulation. Blood volume is increased by activation of the renin–angiotensin–aldosterone system caused by the reduction in systemic vascular resistance, and by increased erythropoietin activity. Overt cardiac failure may result from severe and prolonged hyperthyroidism, but is rarely seen today. Atrial fibrillation is not an uncommon complication, occurring in up to 15% of patients with hyperthyroidism [42, 43].

Autoimmune Interferon Induced Thyroiditis

The entire spectrum of autoimmune thyroid diseases (AITD) has been described in patients receiving IFNα: Graves' disease (GD), Hashimoto's thyroiditis (HT), and the presence of thyroid antibodies (TAb's) without clinical disease [33, 34].

6.1.3.1.4 Thyroid Cancer

In most areas of the world, the incidence of thyroid cancer of follicular origin is increasing. Currently, the incidence is approximately 4/100,000 in males and and 13.5/100,000 in females. Mortality is stable, at approximately 0.5/100,000 [44]. Based on the histologic classification nuclear medicine has a very important role in the management of thyroid cancer. Table 6.2 Summarizes the classification of thyroid cancer. (See Chap. 10).

Table 6.2 Types of Thyroid Cancer and main features

Type	Main features
Papillary carcinoma	Most common thyroid malignancy (85%). Derived from the follicular epithelium Has papillary growth pattern with psammoma bodies Has characteristic nuclear changes
Follicular variant papillary carcinoma	Follicular architecture with the characteristic papillary thyroid nuclear pattern
Papillary microcarcinoma	Added relatively recently Of less than 10 mm in size
Follicular carcinoma	Represents 10–20% of thyroid cancers Derived from follicular epithelium with evidence of capsular and/or vascular invasion but without nuclear changes characteristic of papillary thyroid cancer Have a slightly poorer prognosis than papillary cancer. Metastatic spread is hematogenous most commonly to the lung and bone
Oncocytic or Hurthle cell carcinoma	Hurthle cell can occur in any thyroid tumor More commonly associated with follicular carcinomas Prognosis is worse for comparative stage mainly due to poor radioiodine uptake
Poorly differentiated thyroid cancer	Formed of poorly differentiated cells Has a poor prognosis
Anaplastic carcinoma	Formed of undifferentiated (anaplastic) cells Aggressive and has generally short clinical course and poor prognosis

6.1.3.2 Thyroid Scintigraphy

6.1.3.2.1 Nodular Disease

When thyroid nodule is discovered, the main problem is distinguishing between a benign and a malignant lesion. This problem has largely been solved by fine-needle biopsy which makes that distinction when performed by experienced cytologists. Nevertheless, nodules labeled as indeterminate by cytology remains a challenge [45]. Neck ultrasound plays a pivotal role in the diagnosis, and several ultrasound stratification systems have been proposed in order to predict malignancy and help clinicians in therapeutic and follow-up decision. Despite new technologies in thyroid imaging, diagnostic surgery in 50–70% of patients with indeterminate cytology is still performed.

The role of thyroid scintigraphy is reserved to the assessment of the functional activity of the nodules and when functional autonomy is suspected (Figs. 6.5, 6.6, and 6.7). Thyroid scintigraphy is performed then when serum TSH is suppressed or low in a patient with a single nodule and in all patients with multinodular goiter, regardless of the TSH result. Iodine-123 and ^{99m}Tc-pertechnetate are routinely used for imaging thyroid nodular disease.

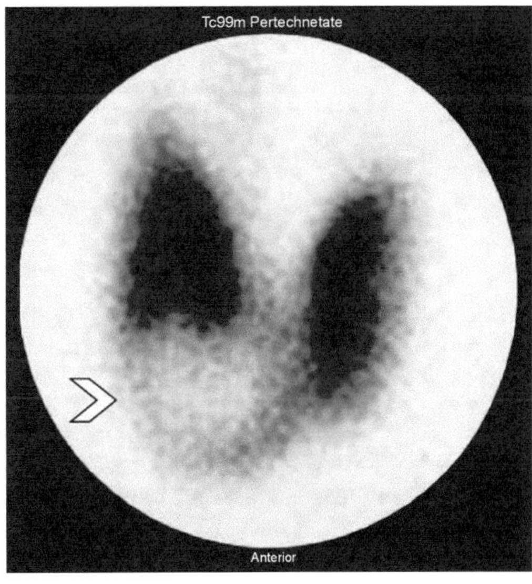

Fig. 6.5 Solitary nodule.^{88m}Tc-pertechnetate thyroid scan anterior pinhole images showing a large solitary cold nodule (*arrow*)

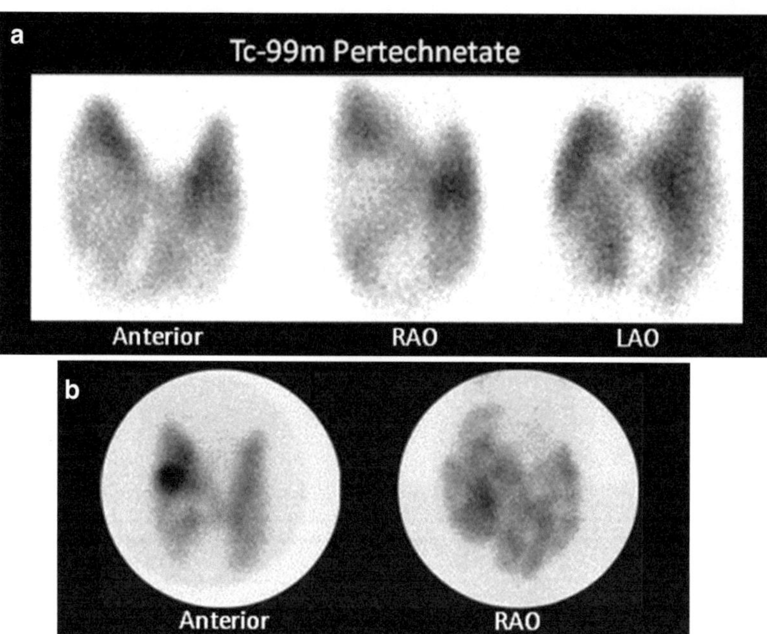

Fig. 6.6 Two examples of multinodular goiter as it appears on scintigraphy. (**a**) Shows multiple cold nodules, while (**b**) represents a mixture of cold and hot nodules

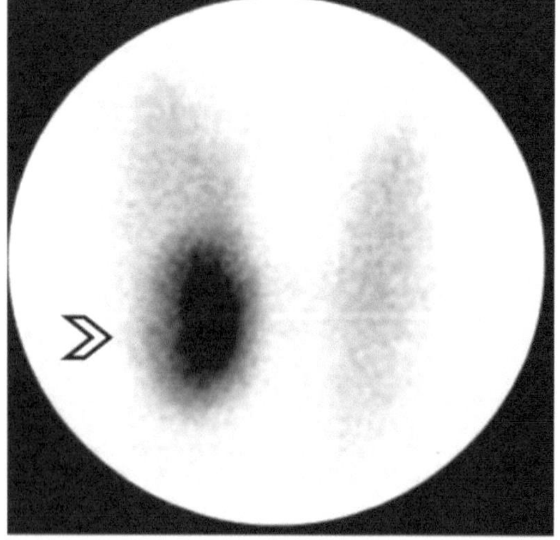

Fig. 6.7 A study showing a toxic nodule in the right lower lobe (*arrow*) with suppression of the remainder of the gland

The acquisition of multiple projections is important as more than 30% of nodules can be missed with anterior views and only seen on the oblique views [55] ^{18}F-FDG PET has low specificity (63%) in the diagnosis of thyroid nodules but can help to select patients who need surgery when cytology is inconclusive in view of its high (100%) negative predictive value for thyroid cancer [45].

Whole-body ^{131}I and FDG-PET have a role in the investigations and follow-up of thyroid cancer (see Chap. 10). On FDG-PET scans, a normal thyroid gland demonstrates absent or low-grade FDG uptake. FDG-PET may incidentally identify thyroid uptake. In general, a diffuse uptake by the thyroid gland is considered to be benign and very likely secondary to thyroiditis and/or hypothyroidism, while a focal uptake of the thyroid on FDG-PET is defined as an incidentaloma, which is more clinically significant due to its high risk of malignancy ranging from 25% to 50% [46, 47].

6.1.3.2.2 Thyroiditis

Poor radioiodine/^{99m}Tc-pertechnetate uptake in the thyroid gland is the hallmark of subacute thyroiditis of any etiology (Fig. 6.8). Decreased tracer uptake is related to TSH suppression by excessive thyroid hormone released from damaged follicles and to decreased hormone synthesis in the damaged gland. The thyroid uptake and scan normalize with resolution of thyroiditis.

Scintigraphy is frequently used in some thyrotoxic patients to differentiate autoimmune thyroiditis, with low uptake, from Graves' disease, with high uptake [41].

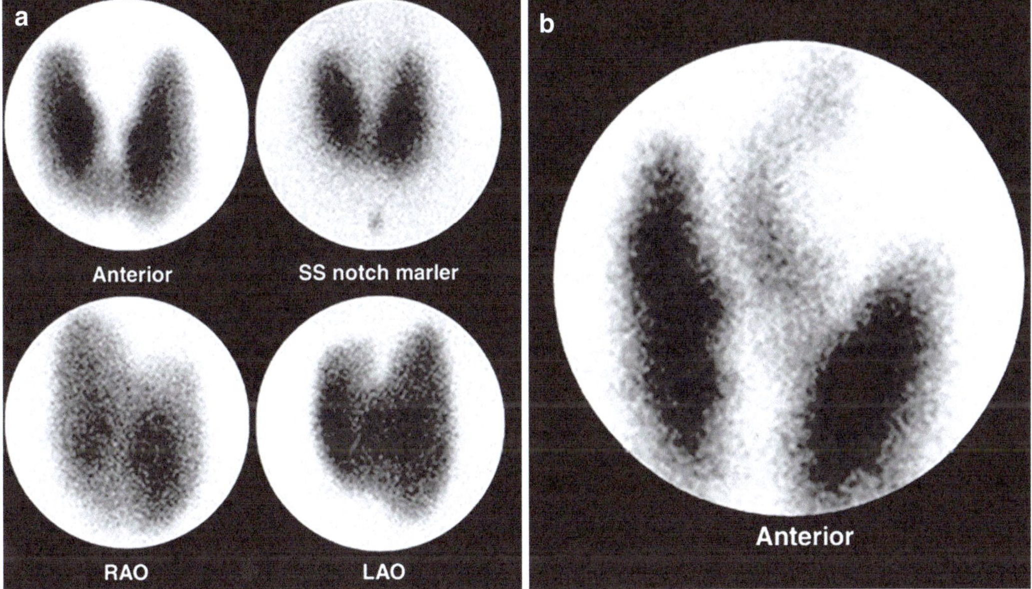

Fig. 6.8 Thyroiditis (**a**, **b**). (**a**) ^{99m}Tc-pertechnetate thyroid scan in an 8-year-old girl with a recent history of upper respiratory infection. The scan shows poor uptake by the thyroid gland with poor delineation of its outlines. The thyroid uptake was 0%. SS notch: suprasternal notch. (**b**) Microscopic illustration of thyroiditis with a focus of inflammatory cells (*arrow*) surrounded by thyroid follicles (Courtesy of Professor Magda El-Monayeri with thanks)

Fig. 6.9 (**a**) Graves' disease. ^{99m}Tc-thyroid scan illustrating the pattern of Graves' disease. There is uniform increased radionuclide distribution with low background activity. (**b**) Anterior view of tc99m pertechnetate illustrating Grave's disease with visualized pyramidal lobe and decreased background uptake

A thyroid uptake/scan may be worthwhile in amiodarone-related hyperthyroidism, which may be due to Jod-Basedow or thyroiditis. A low thyroid uptake is frequently found in patients treated with amiodarone and is nondiagnostic, while a normal or high uptake suggests that Jod-Basedow is likely. The thyroid uptake measurement also helps determine the feasibility of ^{131}I treatment in refractory cases.

Scintigraphy is nonspecific in Hashimoto's disease. The thyroid gland is usually symmetrically enlarged with uniform tracer distribution, and the 24-h radioactive iodine uptake is normal. In subacute thyroiditis resulting from exacerbation of Hashimoto's disease, tracer uptake is typically absent or very low.

6.1.3.2.3 Graves' Disease

Graves' disease typically shows uniformly increased tracer uptake in a diffusely enlarged thyroid gland (Fig. 6.9a), frequently with visualization of a pyramidal lobe and decreased background activity of various degrees based on the severity of the condition (Fig. 6.9b). However, atypical appearances, particularly in Graves' disease superimposed on nodular goiter, are occasionally encountered. If needed, TRAB measurement may assist in confirming the diagnosis. The 24-h radioactive iodine uptake is elevated and, typically, much higher than in toxic nodular goiter [42, 48].

6.2 Parathyroid Gland

6.2.1 Anatomic and Physiologic Considerations

Normal parathyroid glands are derived from the pharyngeal pouches, the upper glands from the endoderm of the fourth pouch, and the lower glands from the third pouch. The parathyroid glands are typically located on the thyroid gland (Fig. 6.1).Occasionally one or more glands may be embedded in the thyroid. The normal position of the superior parathyroids is at the cricothyroid junction, above the anatomical demarcation of the inferior thyroid artery and the recurrent laryngeal nerve [44]. The inferior parathyroids are more widely distributed mostly anterolateral or posterolateral to the lower thyroid gland [45]. The accessory glands that can be variously located in humans, from the cricoid cartilage down into the mediastinum [46, 49], are derived from the numerous dorsal and ventral wings of the pouches. Normally, human beings have four glands, but more or fewer than this number are found in some individuals [47]. Among healthy adults, 80–97% have four parathyroids; approximately 5% have fewer than four glands, and 3–13% have supernumerary glands [45].

The normal glands usually measure 4–6 mm in length, 2–4 mm in width, and 0.5–2 mm in thickness. The glands are usually ovoid or bean shaped but may be elongated, flattened into a leaf-like structure, or multilobulated [41]. The weight of the glands is usually 30 mg each, with the largest normal gland not exceeding 70 mg. The total weight of the glands is less than 210 mg, and the total parenchymal cell weight is less than 145 mg [50]. In normal glands, parenchymal

Table 6.3 Cells of the parathyroid glands and their functions

Cell type	Major ultrastructural feature	Function
Chief cell	Slightly eosinophilic cytoplasm, few mitochondria	The active endocrine cell, producing the parathyroid hormone
Oxyphil cell	Rich eosinophilic cytoplasm, tightly packed mitochondria	May be able to produce parathyroid hormone
Transitional oxyphil cell	Less eosinophilic cytoplasm	Variant of oxyphil cell
Clear cell	Foamy and water-clear cytoplasm	Unknown, fundamentally inactive

cells are predominantly chief cells which contain cytoplasmic fat droplets. Oxyphilic and transitional oxyphilic cells are sparsely present in children and young adults and increase to 4–5% of the parenchymal cells in old age. These cells tend to form nodules if they increase in number and have a very small amount of fat or no fat at all in their cytoplasm. Ultrastructurally, oxyphil cells are characterized by the presence of closely packed mitochondria, while chief cells contain moderate to high mitochondrial content. Water-clear cells are vacuolated with distended organelles. Each of the three cell types may contain varying amounts of lipid droplets and residual bodies. Table 6.3 summarizes the types of parathyroid cells and their function.

Parathyroid hormone has four principle actions: (a) to increase calcium absorption from the gastrointestinal tract; (b) to stimulate osteoclastic activity, resulting in resorption of calcium and phosphate from bone; (c) to inhibit phosphate reabsorption by the proximal renal tubules; and (d) to enhance renal tubular calcium reabsorption. Parathyroid hormone secretion is controlled mainly by the extracellular calcium concentration. The parathyroid cell surface is thought to be equipped with a cation-sensitive receptor mechanism through which ambient calcium regulates the cytosolic calcium ($Ca^{2+}i$) concentration and parathyroid hormone secretion.

Activation of this receptor causes also activation of protein kinase C [41]. 1,25-dihydroxy cholecalciferol reduces the secretion of parathyroid hormone independent of any changes in calcium concentration. Parathyroid hormone is metabolized in Kupffer's cells of the liver.

In patients with hyperparathyroidism, pathological parathyroid cells show defective sensing of ambient calcium. The cellular basis of this abnormality is unknown, although increased protein kinase C activity within abnormal parathyroid cells may be the mechanism. Pathological parathyroid glands also have an increased parenchymal cell content, although the extent of hypercalcemia appears more closely related to the defective secretory regulation than to increased parenchymal cell mass [42].

6.2.2 Hyperparathyroidism

Hyperparathyroidism has been diagnosed with increasing frequency in recent years due to awareness of the disease and to the laboratory advancement that allowed for routine chemistry screening. The condition is characterized by excess secretion of parathyroid hormone. The resulting biochemical changes, including increased levels of serum calcium and increased urinary excretion of calcium, may result in calcium wastage, nephrocalcinosis, urolithiasis, bone disease, and neuropsychiatric disturbances. Hyperparathyroidism may occur as a primary, secondary, or tertiary disease. It can also occur as eutopic and ectopic disease. In addition, it may have a familial origin, as in multiple endocrine neoplasia (MEN).

6.2.2.1 Primary Hyperparathyroidism
Primary hyperparathyroidism occurs due to neoplastic or hyperplastic parathyroid glands or when nonparathyroid tumors such as bronchogenic or renal cell carcinomas secrete ectopically parathyroid hormone or a biologically similar product. The incidence in the United States has been estimated at approximately 27.7 cases per 100,000 population per year [48]. The condition is more prevalent in females than males by a ratio

of 3 to 1. More than 80% of patients with primary hyperparathyroidism have a solitary adenoma. Hyperplasia—predominantly of chief cells—occurs in less than 20% of patients. Parathyroid carcinoma is the cause in less than 1% of patients, and very rarely the condition is due to ectopic secretion of parathyroid hormone [51, 52].

Primary hyperparathyroidism occurs as part of MEN. MEN is a hereditary syndrome that involves hyperfunctioning of two or more endocrine organs. Primary hyperparathyroidism, pancreatic endocrine tumors, and anterior pituitary gland neoplasms characterize type 1 MEN. MEN2A is defined by medullary thyroid carcinoma, pheochromocytoma (about 50%), and hyperparathyroidism caused by parathyroid gland hyperplasia (about 20%). MEN2B is defined by medullary thyroid tumor and pheochromocytoma. Both MEN1 and MEN2 are inherited autosomal dominant cancer syndromes. The gene responsible for MEN1 is a tumor suppressor gene located on chromosome 11.

Primary hyperparathyroidism is also associated with thyroid pathology in 15–70% of patients [53, 54]. This includes thyroid carcinoma which has been reported in the range of 1.7–6.2% of patients with primary hyperparathyroidism [53–55].

6.2.2.2 Secondary Hyperparathyroidism
Secondary hyperparathyroidism occurs when there is a condition causing chronic hypocalcemia such as chronic renal failure, malabsorption syndromes, dietary rickets, and ingestion of drugs such as phenytoin, phenobarbital, and laxatives, which decrease intestinal absorption of calcium. Secondary hyperparathyroidism is simply a compensatory hyperplasia in response to hypocalcemia. In this condition, reduced renal production of 1,25-dihydroxy vitamin D_3 (active metabolite of vitamin D) leads to decreased intestinal absorption of calcium, resulting in hypocalcemia. Tubular failure to excrete phosphate results in hyperphosphatemia. Hypocalcemia along with hyperphosphatemia is compensated by hyperplasia of the parathyroids to overproduce PTH.

6.2.2.3 Tertiary Hyperparathyroidism

Tertiary hyperparathyroidism describes the condition of patients who develop hypercalcemia following long-standing secondary hyperparathyroidism due to the development of autonomous parathyroid hyperplasia, which may not regress after correction of the underlying condition, as with renal transplantation.

6.2.2.4 Eutopic Parathyroid Disease

Parathyroid disease with typical location of glands (eutopic) represents 80–90% of all cases. There is a relatively fixed location for the superior parathyroids and are found close to the dorsal aspect of the upper thyroid [44, 45]. On the other hand, inferior parathyroids have a more widespread distribution, which is closely related to the migration of the thymus. Inferior parathyroids are mostly located inferior, posterior, or lateral to the lower thyroid [44]. They may be very close to the thyroid and may be covered by or attached to the thyroid capsule and are sometimes adjacent to or surrounded by remnant thymic tissue. Interestingly, the parathyroid glands demonstrate a remarkably constant symmetry, which is helpful in the surgical exploration of eutopic disease [45].

6.2.2.5 Ectopic Parathyroid Disease

Superior parathyroid adenoma may have an abnormal supero-posterior mediastinal position, such as a retropharyngeal, retroesophageal, or paraesophageal site or the tracheoesophageal groove. The frequency of ectopia (up to 39%) is similar for the right and left superior parathyroids [56]. Intrathyroid superior parathyroid adenomas are rare.

The more common ectopic inferior parathyroids are a well-established entity responsible for 10–13% of all cases of hyperparathyroidism [56]. Ectopic tissue can occur from the angle of the mandible to the mediastinum according to the developmental and migratory aberrations. These sites include the mediastinum, thymus, aortopulmonary window, carotid bifurcation, and rarely thyroid, carotid sheath, vagus nerve, retroesophageal region, thyrothymic ligament, and pericardium [56, 57].

6.2.3   Parathyroid Adenoma

Parathyroid adenoma is a benign tumor that is usually solitary, although multiple adenomas are found in a low percentage. The tumor in general is more common in women and varies in weight from less than 100 mg to more than 100 g. The most commonly found adenomas, however, weigh 300 mg to 1 g. The size was found to correlate to the degree of hypercalcemia.

Microscopically, the vast majority of typical adenomas are formed predominantly of chief cells, although a mixture of oxyphil cells and transitional oxyphil cells is also common. Adenomas formed of water-clear cells are very rare. A rim of parathyroid tissue is usually present outside the capsule of the adenoma and can serve to distinguish it from parathyroid carcinoma. The chief cells in adenomas are usually enlarged, and their nuclei are larger and more variable in size than in normal chief cells. Nuclear pleomorphism may be prominent; this is not considered a sign of malignancy but a criterion for discriminating adenoma from hyperplasia, which lacks this feature. The following variants (Table 6.4) of parathyroid adenoma may be recognized.

6.2.3.1 Solitary Adenoma

Solitary adenoma is found in 80–85% of patients with primary hyperparathyroidism [67]. There is no significant predominance in location among the four parathyroids with each responsible for approximately 25% of all solitary adenomas [56]. The remaining tumor-free parathyroid glands associated with single adenomas usually have lower weight and parenchymal cell mass than the average normal glands and show signs of secretory in activity on electron microscopy [41].

6.2.3.2 Double or Multiple Adenomas

Double or multiple adenomas occur in up to 12% of cases of primary hyperparathyroidism [50, 58]. These patients have more prominent symptoms and usually have higher parathyroid hormone and alkaline phosphatase levels than those with a solitary parathyroid adenoma or hyperplasia. Preoperative detection of double or multiple adenomas with any imaging modality is not reliable [60].

Table 6.4 Variants of parathyroid adenoma [50, 58–66]

Type	Major features	Imaging
Solitary adenoma	Found in 80–85% of patients with primary hyperparathyroidism	^{99m}Tc-MIBI with high sensitivity
	Composed of chief cells or mixture of chief, oxyphil, or transitional oxyphil cells	
Double/multiple	Occurs in up to 12% of cases of primary hyperparathyroidism	Detection with any imaging modality is not reliable
	Bilateral in 55–88% of cases	^{99m}Tc-MIBI has a sensitivity of less than 37%
	More prominent symptoms and higher parathyroid hormone and alkaline phosphatase levels than with a solitary adenoma or hyperplasia	
Cystic adenoma	Central necrosis or cystic degeneration of adenomas	May not be visualized on ^{99m}Tc-MIBI studies
	Accounts for less than 9% of all parathyroid adenomas	
	Frequently associated with hyperparathyroidism	
Lipoadenoma	Composed of hyperfunctioning parathyroid tissue and fatty stroma	Target-to-background ratio may be low due to the high adipose content
Oncocytic adenoma	Rare subtype formed of 80–100% oxyphil cells	^{99m}Tc-MIBI with high sensitivity

6.2.3.3 Cystic Adenoma

Cystic adenomas are thought to represent central necrosis or cystic degeneration of adenomas [63]. Contrary to the asymptomatic true parathyroid cysts which are due to embryologic vestiges of the third and fourth pharyngeal pouches or enlargement of microcysts within the parathyroid as a manifestation of colloid retention [64], cystic adenomas are frequently associated with hyperparathyroidism.

6.2.3.4 Lipoadenoma

Parathyroid lipoadenoma, composed of hyperfunctioning parathyroid tissue and fatty stroma, is a rare entity that occurs in patients beyond the fourth decade of life.

6.2.3.5 Oncocytic Adenoma

A rare subtype has been reported to be associated with hyperparathyroidism. It is found in the sixth or seventh decades and like the typical adenomas is more common in women [66].

6.2.4   Parathyroid Hyperplasia

Parathyroid hyperplasia affects the glands to varying degrees, and commonly one or two glands are of normal size even though microscopic signs of endocrine hyperfunction are present, at least focally, in all glands. Chief cell

Table 6.5 Classification of parathyroid hyperplasia

Type	Major pathological features
Primary hyperplasia	Uniform chief cells with some oxyphil and transitional oxyphil cells
Secondary hyperplasia	
Diffuse (classic) type	Cords, sheets, or follicular arrangement of cells replacing the stromal fat cells. Oxyphil cells are more frequent in this type. This type is in distinguishable from the primary type
Adenomatous-nodular type	Cells are grouped in large islands or nodules. Necrosis is seen more frequently than in diffuse type

hyperplasia is the most common and is composed of chief cells or a mixture of chief cells and to a lesser extent oxyphil cells. The cells are arranged diffusely, in nodules, or in a mixture of both patterns. Water-clear cell hyperplasia is rare and is characterized by substantial enlargement of most parathyroid glands. The large water-clear cells are usually arranged in a diffuse pattern [68].

In primary hyperparathyroidism, hyperplasia affects the glands asymmetrically. In secondary hyperparathyroidism, the hyperplastic glands are more uniformly enlarged than with primary chief cell hyperplasia, with two histological types (Table 6.5). In the tertiary form, the glands are more often markedly and asymmetrically enlarged.

Pathologically, it is difficult to differentiate primary chief cell hyperplasia of only one gland from adenoma. Both contain large numbers of active chief cells with cells characterized by aggregated arrays of rough endoplasmic reticulum and a large, complex Golgi apparatus with numerous vacuoles and vesicles. Secretory granules are frequently present in these cells. These changes indicate that most of these cells are in thermoreactive phases of parathyroid hormone synthesis and secretion [69]. Molecular biology techniques used on pathological parathyroid tissue have shown that cell proliferation is monoclonal in many sporadic adenomas and in the largest glands of multiple endocrine neoplasia type I. This monoclonality has not been found in the smaller parathyroid glands of multiple endocrine neoplasia or in sporadic hyperplasia. Additionally, rearrangement of parathyroid hormone gene in chromosome 11 was observed in sporadic adenomas.

6.2.5 Parathyroid Carcinoma

Parathyroid carcinoma is a rare cause of hyperparathyroidism which can arise in any parathyroid gland, including ectopic and mediastinal, although the usual site of involvement is the normally located parathyroids. The tumor is found predominantly in patients between the ages of 30 and 60 years, with no sex preference and is usually functioning. The tumors tend to be larger than adenomas and appear as lobulated, firm, and encapsulated masses that often adhere to the surrounding soft tissue structures. The involved glands usually weigh more than 1 g, and the diagnosis is restricted histologically to the lesions displaying infiltrative growth into vessel or capsule, since pleomorphism can be seen in many adenomas.

6.2.6 Hyperfunctioning Parathyroid Transplant

Autotransplantation of parathyroid tissue is performed in cases of recurrent, persistent type1

MEN and symptomatic secondary hyperparathyroidism in association with total parathyroidectomy. After total parathyroidectomy, the most normal glands, usually one or two, are used for the graft. They are diced into small fragments with each fragment placed in an individual bed beneath a muscle health and between muscle fibers [70]. A graft site in the forearm is preferred for accessibility. The graft may be functional in 8–9 days after surgery [50]. After autotransplantation, recurrent hyperparathyroidism occurs in approximately 14% of cases [71]. A hyperfunctioning graft in the forearm is easily demonstrated with Doppler US or ^{99m}Tc-sestamibi scintigraphy [71].

6.2.7 Consequences of Hyperparathyroidism

Excess secretion of parathyroid hormone promotes bone resorption and consequently leads to hypercalcemia and hypophosphatemia. The clinical presentation and complications of hyperparathyroidism depend on the rapidity of development and the degree of hypercalcemia. They can be grouped into genitourinary, gastrointestinal and musculoskeletal, neuropsychiatric, and others (Table 6.6).

The five disease-specific symptoms are muscle weakness, polydipsia, dry skin and itching, memory loss, and anxiety. Overall the symptoms, particularly the disease-specific ones, show significant decline after successful parathyroidectomy [72].

6.2.8 Preoperative Parathyroid Localization

Surgery is the major and only current curative modality in treating primary hyperparathyroidism. Identifying the glands can be difficult, however, particularly with removal of multiple glands and with reoperation [73]. Although the success rate is high in experienced hands, up to 25% of the initial explorations fail because the abnormal glands cannot be located. Prolonged exploration

Table 6.6 Consequences of hyperparathyroidism

Types of abnormality	Presentation
Genitourinary	Nephrolithiasis
	Nephrocalcinosis
	Renal insufficiency
	Polyuria
	Nocturia
	Decreased urine concentrating ability
Gastrointestinal	Nausea
	Vomiting
	Constipation
	Increased thirst
	Loss of appetite
	Abdominal pain
	Peptic ulcers
	Heartburn(hypercalcemia causes increased gastric acidity)
	Pancreatitis
Musculoskeletal	Myopathy
	Muscle weakness
	Osteoporosis
	Osteomalacia
	Bone and joint pains
	Renal osteodystrophy
	Pseudogout
Neuropsychiatric	Memory loss
	Anxiety
	Sleepiness
	Confusion
	Lassitude, coma
	Depression
	Impaired thinking
	Psychosis
Others	Fatigue
	Hypertension
	Pruritis
	Metastatic calcification including cardiocalcinosis
	Band keratopathy (present in the medial and lateral aspects of the cornea)

was also found to result in a high incidence of recurrent laryngeal nerve damage [73]. Surgical re-exploration with violated anatomy is even more difficult and hazardous and can often be unrewarding.

Preoperative localization of parathyroid lesions is thus desirable to reduce the incidence of missed lesions and to help avoid prolonged neck exploration. Since surgeons' experience with neck exploration is decreasing due to the reduced incidence of thyroid surgery with the expanding use of iodine-131 for therapy of hyperthyroidism, preoperative localization of parathyroid lesions is even more important than before.

In recent years, minimal access parathyroid surgery (small incisions with gamma probe or endoscopic assistance) is increasingly becoming the operation of choice for single parathyroid adenomas [74]. Compared with bilateral neck exploration, it has a shorter hospital stay, less morbidity, and better cosmetic result [74]. The development of this minimally invasive surgical techniques has placed an even greater emphasis on preoperative localization [75].

The forms that preoperative localization can take include computed tomography (CT), ultrasound, magnetic resonance imaging (MRI), arteriography, selective venous sampling, ^{99m}Tc-sestamibi (MIBI) scintigraphy, ^{18}F-fluorodeoxyglucose positron emission tomography (FDG-PET), and ^{11}C-methionine PET. The morphological imaging modalities, such as CT, ultrasound, and MRI, have the disadvantage that they cannot distinguish functional parathyroid tissue from other types of tissue. However, they provide excellent image resolution and contrast. Overall their accuracy is inadequate and varies.

6.2.9   Scintigraphic Localization

Scintigraphy using ^{99m}Tc-sestamibi (MIBI) is currently the preferred nuclear medicine method for parathyroid imaging. It is the most sensitive and cost-effective modality for preoperative localization of hyperfunctioning parathyroid tissue. Due to a wide variation in scintigraphic techniques [76], the reported sensitivities of MIBI scan range from 80 to 100%. The mechanism of uptake of this radiopharmaceutical by abnormal parathyroid cells is not fully understood although the mitochondria have been implicated in its uptake [77]. P-glycoprotein, a membrane transport protein encoded for by the multidrug resistance (MDR) gene, may also be additionally responsible for uptake, since it transports other products with structural similarity to MIBI [78]. The uptake and retention of MIBI by the abnormal neoplastic and hyperplastic lesions are probably due to the alterations in the biology of the abnormal parathyroid cells, as noted earlier, and mitochondria are probably the site of retention. The size and the cellularity of the abnormal gland are also factors in the visualization and correlate with its MIBI uptake (Fig. 6.10) [79, 80]. Additionally, the ectopic disease (Fig. 6.11) may affect the degree of visualization and SPECT with or without CT is better to be used.

Our group found that the amount of mitochondria (Fig. 6.11) in adenoma oxyphil cells correlates with the degree of uptake [81].

The protocol for MIBI parathyroid scintigraphy varies regarding timing of acquisition, SPECT and SPECT/CT. However the study principle is to acquire early and delayed (Figs. 6.12 and 6.13). ^{123}I or pertechnetate thyroid imaging for comparison or subtraction is only occasionally needed on an individual basis (e.g., presence of thyroid nodule).

SPECT/CT has proven to be most accurate in localizing parathyroid glands (Fig. 6.14) and is currently the recommended procedure. It has proven to be a useful tool for preoperative assessment, not only for ectopic glands but also for patients with previous neck surgery. It also increases reporting confidence for physicians [82, 83]. It has been reported to be 94% accurate in detecting parathyroid adenoma and 92% in accurate localization [84].

PET has been also investigated for localizing parathyroid glands. Initial studies using FDG showed conflicting results in imaging the parathyroid glands in primary hyperparathyroid-

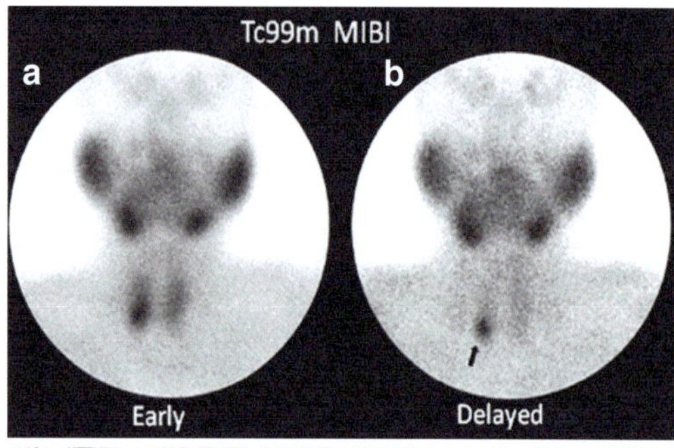

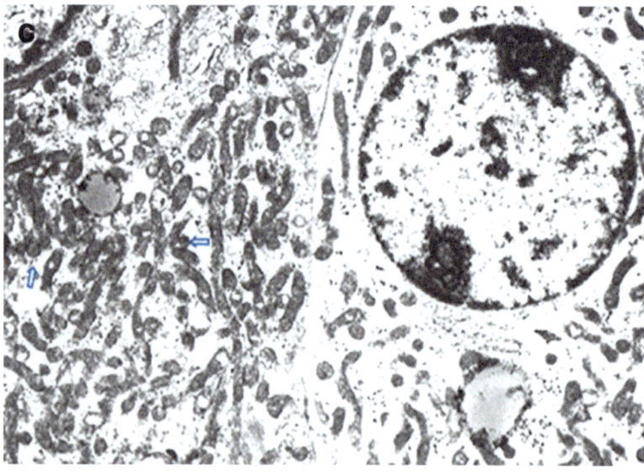

Fig. 6.10 Tc99m-sestamibi study for a patient with biochemically proven hyperparathyroidism. Early images (**a**) show a focus of increased uptake in the region of the right lower pole of the thyroid gland which, in the delayed image (**b**), retains the activity(arrow) with clearance of thyroid uptake consistent with adenoma. Surgery was performed, and the lesion was pathologically proven to be adenoma. Sample was sent for electron microscopic study. Electron microscopic photograph (**c**) of this parathyroid adenoma illustrates cells packed with mitochondria (arrows)

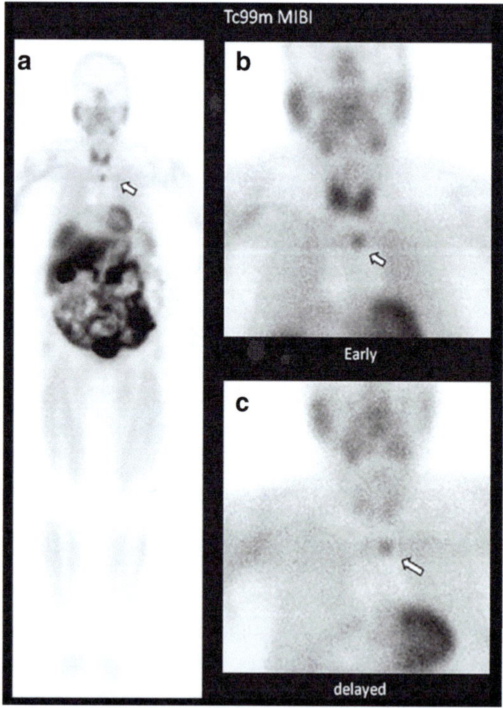

Fig. 6.11 Ectopic parathyroid adenoma (*arrow*) seen on Tc99m MIBI study. Early whole body (**a**) and spot image (**b**) with retained activity on delayed spot image (**c**)

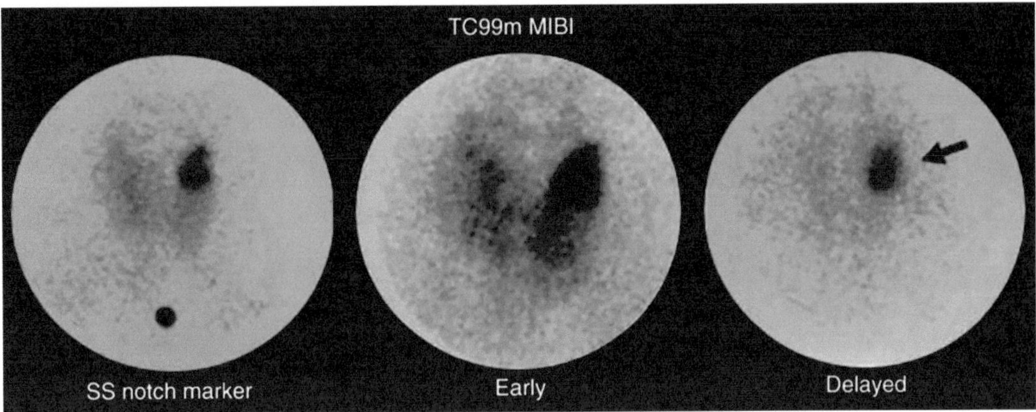

Fig. 6.12 ^{99m}Tc-sestamibi study acquired 15–90 min post injection using pinhole collimator. The delayed image shows differential clearance of activity from the thyroid gland with retained and intense uptake by a large parathyroid adenoma (*arrow*)

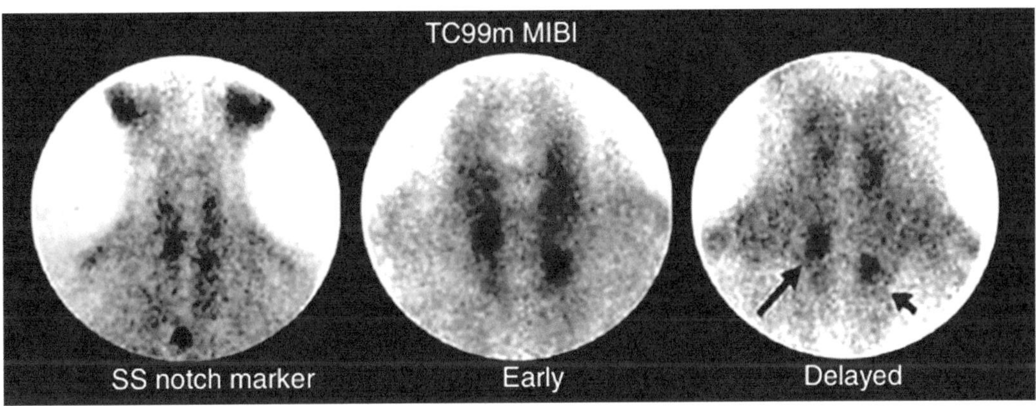

Fig. 6.13 Hyperplastic parathyroid glands (*arrows*) with persistent uptake on delayed ^{99m}Tc-sestamibi image

ism. ^{11}C-methionine PET was suggested to be more promising than FDG in parathyroid localization [85]. In a large recent study of 171 patients ^{18}F-fluorocholine (FCH) PET/CT, correct detection was calculated at 96% and 90%, on a per patient-based and per lesion-based analysis, respectively [86].

6.2.10 Atypical Washout of Radiotracer

As outlined the diagnosis of parathyroid tumor with ^{99m}Tc-sestamibi scintigraphy is based on the differential washout rate between the thyroid and diseased parathyroids. A typical radiotracer clearance whether fast parathyroid or delayed thyroid gland washout will limit the efficacy of detection of parathyroid disease with dual-phase ^{99m}Tc-sestamibi scintigraphy as well as using the intraoperative probe.

Early parathyroid washout is frequently seen in parathyroid hyperplasia; the detection rate for this entity is approximately half of that for parathyroid adenoma [71]. Scintigraphy performs worse in cases of multisite hyperplasia, in which only the most prominent radiotracer-avid gland is visualized. In addition, rapid washout from a parathyroid adenoma has been attributed, without unanimous confirmation, to the histological composition of the adenoma [71]. Modifying the imaging protocol with additional interval scanning between the

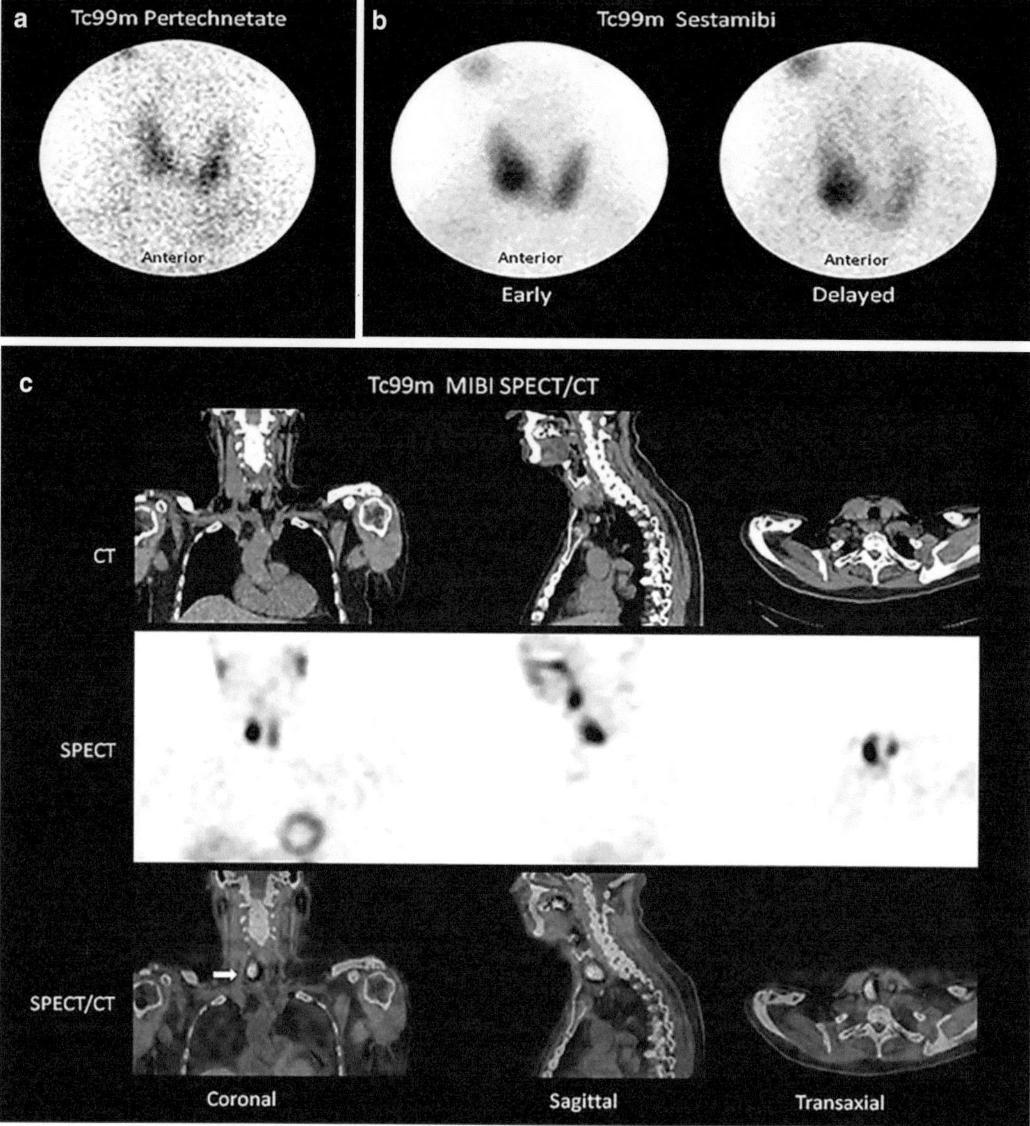

Fig. 6.14 A 70 -year-old male with osteoporosis who is on rheumatoid arthritis treatment. He has hypercalcemia and high parathyroid hormone (PTH) levels. Tc-99 m pertechnetate thyroid scan (**a**) and Tc-99msestamibi planar (**b**) with SPECT/CT (**c**) were performed. The thyroid scan (**a**) is grossly normal with no focal abnormalities. There is a focus of increased uptake on early sestamibi image (**b**) in the region of the right lower pole of the thyroid which does not show significant washout of activity and becomes more prominent on delayed image. There is normal washout of activity from the thyroid gland. Based on planar images, scintigraphic findings are consistent with parathyroid adenoma at the region of the right lower pole. Selected SPECT/CT images (**c**) demonstrate that this focal activity is located posterior to the lower pole of the right lobe (arrow). Note that SPECT/CT better located the lesion as compared to planar imaging

standard 15-min and 2–4-h acquisitions may be helpful in demonstrating rapid washout.

Delayed radiotracer washout from the thyroid parenchyma makes dual-phase scintigraphic assessment difficult. It was observed that the delay varies, and significant washout may not occur even several hours after injection of the radiotracer. This retention of ^{99m}Tc-sestamibi occurs

Table 6.7 Causes of false-positive ^{99m}Tc-sestamibi parathyroid studies

Lymph nodes
Supraclavicular
Axillary
Hyperplastic thymus[a]
Sarcoidosis[b]
Carcinoid tumor
Malignant tumors

[a]Confused with an intrathymic or mediastinal parathyroid adenoma

[b]Thorax

in thyroid diseases such as multinodular goiter, Hashimoto's thyroiditis, thyroid adenoma, and thyroid carcinoma owing to the hypermetabolic characteristics of these diseases [61]. Extended delayed-phase imaging of ^{99m}Tc-sestamibi along with in-depth clinical examination may be useful in the diagnosis of concomitant thyroid and parathyroid disease [73].

As rapid washout and small size of parathyroid glands would cause false-negative localization studies, several pathologies can also cause false-positive studies (Table 6.7).

6.2.11 Intraoperative Probe Localization

Localization using intraoperative gamma probe has recently gained popularity. The patient is injected 2 h before surgery, and the probe is used to detect the higher level of activity after exploration by the surgeon. On the day of surgery, the patients receive the same dose of MIBI as for imaging and is taken to the operating room. Prior to skin incision, counts over 4 quadrants in the neck as well as over the mediastinum are obtained using a gamma probe [74].

6.3 Adrenal Gland

6.3.1 Anatomical and Physiological Considerations

The adult adrenal glands weigh 8–10 g and lie above and slightly medial to the upper pole of both kidneys. The outer cortex comprises 90% of the adrenal weight, the inner medulla about 10%. The cortex is rich with vessels and receives its main blood supply from branches of the inferior phrenic artery, renal arteries, and the aorta. These small arteries for man arterial plexus beneath the capsule and then enter a sinusoid system that penetrates the cortex and medulla, draining into a single central vein in each gland [75].

Histologically, the adult adrenal cortex is composed of three zones: an outer zona glomerulosa which produces aldosterone, a zona fasciculata, and an inner zona reticularis. The zona fasciculata is the thickest layer and produces cortisol and androgens; its cells are large and contain more lipid and thus are termed clear cells. The zona reticularis produces weak androgens. The zona fasciculata and reticularis are regulated by adrenocorticotropic hormone(ACTH).

Cholesterol within the adrenal cortex is the starting point for synthesis of multiple adrenal hormones. Therefore, a radioactive cholesterol is useful in evaluating the functional status of adrenocortical lesions. The adrenal medulla is composed histologically of chromaffin cells, which are large ovoid columnar cells arranged in clumps or cords around blood vessels and surrounded by capillaries and sinusoids. They have large nuclei and a well-developed Golgi apparatus; they have a large number of granules containing catecholamines. The adrenal medulla also contains some sympathetic ganglia. The cells of adrenal medulla are innervated by preganglionic sympathetic fibers. Most of the blood supply to the hormonally active cells of the medulla is derived from a portal vascular system arising from the capillaries in the cortex. There is also a network of lymphatics that drain into a plexus around the central vein [76]. The adrenals provide adjustment of heart performance and vascular tone. Epinephrine is found essentially only in the adrenal medulla, and constituting greater than 80% of its output. Norepinephrine is synthesized by adrenergic neurons and cells of the adrenal medulla; therefore, a radioactive norepinephrine analog is used to evaluate adrenomedullary lesions.

6.3.2   Adrenal Cortex

6.3.2.1 Pathophysiology

6.3.2.1.1   Primary Aldosteronism (Conn's Syndrome)

In primary aldosteronism (Conn's syndrome), there is increased production of aldosterone by abnormal zona glomerulosa (adenoma or hyperplasia) leading to hypertension through the increased reabsorption of sodium and water from the distal tubules. A benign adenoma accounts for 75% of cases of this syndrome; it is usually small, ranging from 0.5 to 1.5 cm in diameter. It is more common in women than in men (3:1) and usually occurs between the ages of 30 and 50 years. Bilateral, or rarely unilateral, micro-or macro nodular adrenal hyperplasia accounts for most of the remaining cases. Two types of familial hyper aldosteronism have recently been identified: Type I is glucocorticoid suppressible and associated with bilateral hyperplasia, and type II is associated with adrenocortical adenoma. Adrenal carcinoma is a very rare cause of this syndrome. The patients typically come to medical attention because of clinical signs of hypokalemia or detection of previously unsuspected hypertension during the course of a routine physical examination. The diagnosis is principally a biochemical one (low plasma renin activity and a high level of aldosterone); imaging is required to localize the lesion and identify its multiplicity. The diagnostic information provided by CT or MRI in localizing adenomas is both accurate and practical, and they are the initial approach of choice. Some smaller adenomas which are not clearly visualized by CT can be depicted by scintigraphy.

6.3.2.1.2   Cushing's Syndrome

The most common pathological cause of this syndrome is the stimulation of the zona fasciculata by excess ACTH from the pituitary gland (Cushing's disease) or, less commonly, the ectopic production of ACTH (as in small cell lung cancer and neural crest tumors) or corticotropin-releasing factor (CRF) (as in bronchial carcinoid and prostate cancer). Stimulating this zona may lead to bilateral adreno cortical hyperplasia, which is nodular in 25% and diffuse in 75% of cases. Cushing's syndrome may also be due to autonomous adrenal cortisol production (30–40% of cases) due to adrenal adenoma or hyperfunctioning adrenal carcinoma. ACTH-induced Cushing's disease is more common in adults (25–45 years) and is at least three times more common in women than in men. Cushing's disease resulting from ectopic ACTH secretion is more common in older adults, particularly men. Adrenal tumors rather than pituitary tumors are more common in children, especially girls. Twenty percent of nonfunctional adrenocortical carcinomas tend to be highly malignant, with weights exceeding 1 kg.

6.3.2.1.3   Hyperandrogenism

Hyperandrogenism can be the result of hypersecretion of androgens (causing virilization) or estrogens (causing feminization) from the zona reticularis of the adrenal cortex by primary adrenocortical hyperplasia and rarely by adrenal tumors, though the most common cause of this syndrome is polycystic ovary disease (POD). In POD, the chronic anovulation associated with increased circulating LH levels results in increased ovarian stromal stimulation, which leads to increased ovarian androgen production. A testosterone-secreting adrenal adenoma may contain the crystalloids characteristic of Leydig's cells [77].

6.3.2.2 Scintigraphy for Adrenal Cortex

6.3.2.2.1   Radiolabeled Cholesterol Analogs

NP(^{131}I-7-iodomethyl-19-norcholesterol)-59(NP-59) is the classic nuclear medicine study used to evaluate some disease processes related to the adrenal cortex. Its main uses are documented cases of adrenal excess secretion and negative or equivocal CT or MRI findings. This radio pharmaceutical is a cholesterol analog that is bound to and transported by low-density lipoproteins (LDL) to specific LDL receptors on adrenocortical cells; therefore, endogenous hypercholesterolemia may limit the number of receptors available for radio cholesterol localization through competitive inhibition. Once liberated from LDL, NP-59 is esterified but is not further converted to steroid hormones [78]. This scan should be done only on patients with clinically hyperfunctioning adrenal cortex verified by lab results, CT, or MRI.

The normal distribution is seen in the liver, gallbladder, and colon. In 90% of cases, the right adrenal gland is more cephalad and deeper than the left adrenal gland. In two thirds of normal subjects, the activity in the right adrenal appears greater than that in the left in the posterior projection; this is because the right adrenal occupies a more posterior location than the left adrenal. In some instances, the gallbladder can be confused with the right adrenal. In the lateral view, the gallbladder is located anteriorly. In difficult cases, cholecystokinin can clear the gallbladder activity. Interfering colonic activity can be reduced by cathartics. Although count rates are low, single-photon emission computed tomography (SPECT) can be performed and may separate adrenals from gut and liver activity.

In primary aldosteronism, early unilateral increased uptake indicates adrenal adenoma, whereas bilateral increased uptake suggests bilateral adrenal hyperplasia. Pituitary ACTH-producing adenoma or ectopic ACTH secretion can result in bilateral adrenal hyperplasia manifested by bilateral symmetric increased uptake, with ectopic causes producing more uptake of NP-59; this pattern may be asymmetric in the macronodular form of hyperplasia. Adrenal adenoma causes unilateral increased uptake, whereas adrenocortical carcinoma gives rise to bilateral nonvisualization. In hyperandrogenism, early bilateral uptake is compatible with hyperplasia, and early (<5 days) unilateral uptake or markedly asymmetric visualization is indicative of adrenal adenoma.

6.3.2.2.2 Positron Emission Tomography Imaging

Since adrenal adenomas are relatively common (2–9%) in the general population, incidental detection of adrenal lesions poses a diagnostic challenge, particularly in patients with a previous clinical history of malignancy [87, 88].

CT is used as the first-line diagnostic modality for screening and determining the nature of the adrenal lesions, and MRI is often performed to further characterize indeterminate masses seen on CT. ^{18}F-FDG-PET can help in differentiating malignant from benign adrenal lesions in patients with proven malignancy or in patients with incidentally detected adrenal tumors on CT or MRI studies [88–90]. However, some adenomas show increased FDG tracer uptake similar to cancer and some do not. It has been suggested that the functional state of an adenoma is a factor determining the intensity of uptake, with $^{18F\text{-}FDG}$ uptake being increased in functioning adrenal masses [91]. SUV value can help differentiate adrenal cortical adenomas from adrenal cortical carcinomas [90].

6.3.3 Adrenal Medulla

6.3.3.1 Pathophysiology

Neuroendocrine tumors are a heterogeneous group of usually slow-growing tumors that arise from neuroendocrine cells from various organs, including adrenal in addition to lung, thymus, thyroid, stomach, duodenum, small bowel, large bowel, appendix, pancreas, and skin (see Chap. 12).

6.3.3.1.1 Pheochromocytoma

Pheochromocytoma is a rare tumor arising from chromaffin cells of the adrenal medulla. Most pheochromocytomas produce excessive amounts of norepinephrine, attributable to autonomous functioning of the tumor, although large tumors may secrete both norepinephrine and epinephrine [92] and in some cases also dopamine. The release of catecholamine into the circulation causes hypertension, tremor, tachycardia, and other signs. Other catecholamine-producing tumors (e.g., chemodectoma and ganglioneuroma) may also cause a syndrome similar to that seen with pheochromocytoma. Furthermore, they may also produce some active peptides such as somatostatin, ACTH, and calcitonin.

Pheochromocytomas vary in size from less than 1 g to several kilograms; in general, they are small, most weighing under 100 g. They are vascular tumors, tend to be capsulated, and commonly contain cystic or hemorrhagic areas. The cells tend to be large and contain typical catecholamine storage granules. Multinucleated cells, pleomorphic nuclei, mitosis, and extension into capsule and vessels are sometimes seen but do not indicate that the tumor is malignant. The chromogranin existing within secretory granules in the tumor tends to form *Zellballen* (cell balls); these structures are surrounded by sustentacular cells. Five to ten percent of cases are malignant, and malignancy is determined by the only biological behavior of the tumor. It is estimated that 0.1% of hypertensive patients have pheochromocytoma. More than 90% of patients with pheochromocytoma exhibit hypertension, which is sustained in two thirds of patients. These tumors are observed more frequently in women than in men and at all ages, including infancy; they are most common in the fifth and sixth decades [92].

Although most patients with functioning tumors have symptoms (sweating, palpitation, headache, dyspnea, and anxiety), most of the time, these vary in intensity, and in about half of the patients, they are paroxysmal.

6.3.3.1.2 Neuroblastoma

Neuroblastoma is a malignant tumor of the sympathetic nervous system, accounting for up to 10% of childhood cancers and 15% of cancer deaths among children. Seventy-five percent of neuroblastoma patients are younger than 4 years. The tumor is usually more than 5 cm in the largest diameter and tends to extend across the midline; it has the potential to mature into pheochromocytoma or ganglioneuroma. Metastases are the first manifestation in up to 60% of cases. The electron microscopic appearance of NB cells is distinctive. The malignant neuroblasts exhibit peripheral dendritic processes containing longitudinally oriented microtubules, neurosecretory granules, and filaments in the cytoplasm. Neuroblastomas readily infiltrate the surrounding structures and metastasize to the regional lymph nodes, liver, lungs, and bones; metastases to the orbit may result in proptosis [93]. Areas of necrosis, hemorrhage, calcifica-

tion, and cystic changes are frequently present. Around one third of cases are found in the adrenal gland, another third in other abdominal sites, and 20% in the posterior mediastinum. More than 90% of these tumors produce catecholamine in excess, but they rarely cause typical clinical syndromes. Severe diarrhea may be caused by secretion of vasoactive intestinal peptides by the neuroblastoma.

6.3.3.1.3 Ganglioneuroma

Ganglioneuroma is a benign tumor found in older children and young adults, with no sex predilection. Forty percent of the patients are over 20 years of age. Up to 30% of these tumors occur in the adrenal medulla and 43% in the posterior mediastinum. Histologically, the tumor consists of mature ganglion cells and is well encapsulated; it is frequently calcified and rarely hormone active.

6.3.3.2 Scintigraphy for Adrenal Medulla

6.3.3.2.1 Metaiodobenzylguanidine

Metaiodobenzylguanidine (MIBG) is a guanethidine analog chemically similar to noradrenaline. Following i.v. injection, MIBG is rapidly cleared from the vascular compartment; however, a small amount remains in the thrombocytes. It localizes in storage granules of adrenergic tissue (referred to as synaptosomes) by means of energy- and Na-dependent mechanisms (type 1), and it is not metabolized to any appreciable extent. Neural crest tumors have these synaptosomes in abundance.

The normal distribution of ^{123}I-MIBG is to the salivary gland, liver, urinary bladder, gastrointestinal tract, lung, myocardium, normal adrenal gland, thyroid, spleen, and uterus [94–97]; in small children, uptake may also be seen in the nape of the neck, which is currently believed to be related to accumulation in brown adipose tissue [98].

Eighty-five percent of the injected dose is excreted unchanged by the kidneys. Imaging is performed at 24 and 48 h after injection of ^{131}I-MIBG and at 6 and 24 h after injection of

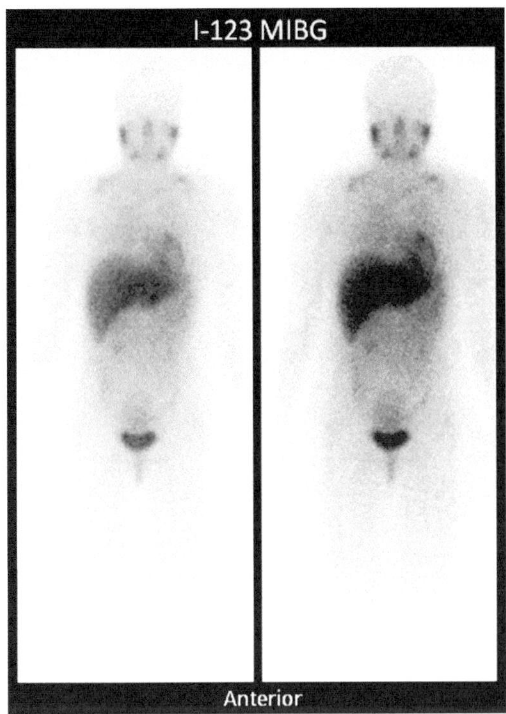

Fig. 6.15 A 32-year-old male with suspected pheochromocytoma. Anterior ^{123}I-MIBG whole-body image with different intensity is shown. There is increased uptake at the supraclavicular region bilaterally. This pattern is due to uptake by brown fat. The remainder of the study shows also physiological distribution of the radiotracer with no abnormalities

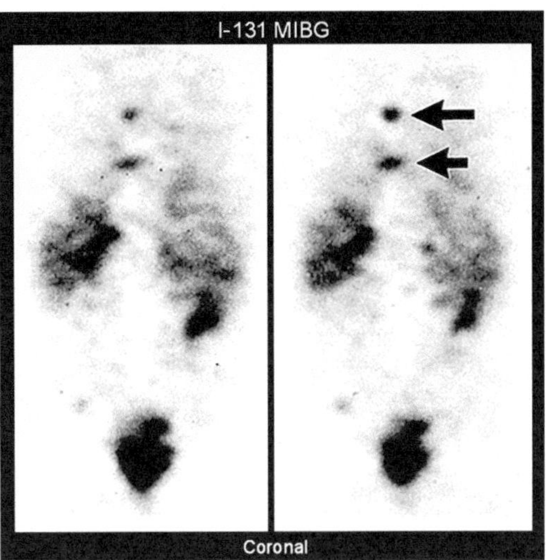

Fig. 6.16 Representative coronal images from a SPECT ^{131}I-MIBG study for a patient with neuroblastoma, showing metastases to the spine (*arrows*)

^{123}I-MIBG (Fig. 6.15). When SPECT is used (Figs. 6.16 and 6.17), increased certainty is achieved in interpreting the studies [95]. It is worthy of mention that ^{123}I is better than ^{131}I, especially in the pediatric population, because of the lower radiation exposure to the adrenals in addition to the superior image quality of the former. The sensitivity of ^{131}I-MIBG in pheochromocytoma is 80–90% and specificity is more than 90%; positive MIBG uptake in benign solitary pheochromocytoma occurs in about 90% of patients [99]; tumors as small as 1–2 cm in diameter were detected especially with ^{123}I [100] (Fig. 6.18).

MIBG is localized in other neuroendocrine tumors to a lesser degree, including carcinoid, medullary thyroid carcinoma, and paraganglioma. Indium-111 octreotide (a somatostatin analog) is less accurate in the detection of pheochromocytoma, probably due to normal physiological uptake in the liver, spleen, and kidneys and blocking of somatostatin receptors by endogenous somatostatin.

Radiolabeled MIBG imaging is now a well-established examination in the diagnostic evaluation of neuroblastoma. ^{123}I is preferred especially in pediatric patients (dose 3–5 mCi) due to its favorable dosimetry and superior image quality; scintigraphy can be performed as early as 4 h after injection. Elevated catecholamine levels are not necessary for the detection of NB by MIBG. The sensitivity of MIBG in NB is 91%. Somatostatin analog scintigraphy has been reported to visualize MIBG-negative tumor sites in patients with NB. MIBG is essential as a prelude to ^{131}I-MIBG therapy. In the follow-up of the patients with high-risk neuroblastoma, MIBG Imaging using SPECT/CT has been found to significantly improve planar method interpretation and provides positive positive impact on patient management [101]. Recently the use of low-dose ^{124}I-MIBG PET/CT for monitoring neuroblastoma in children and evaluate tumor burden

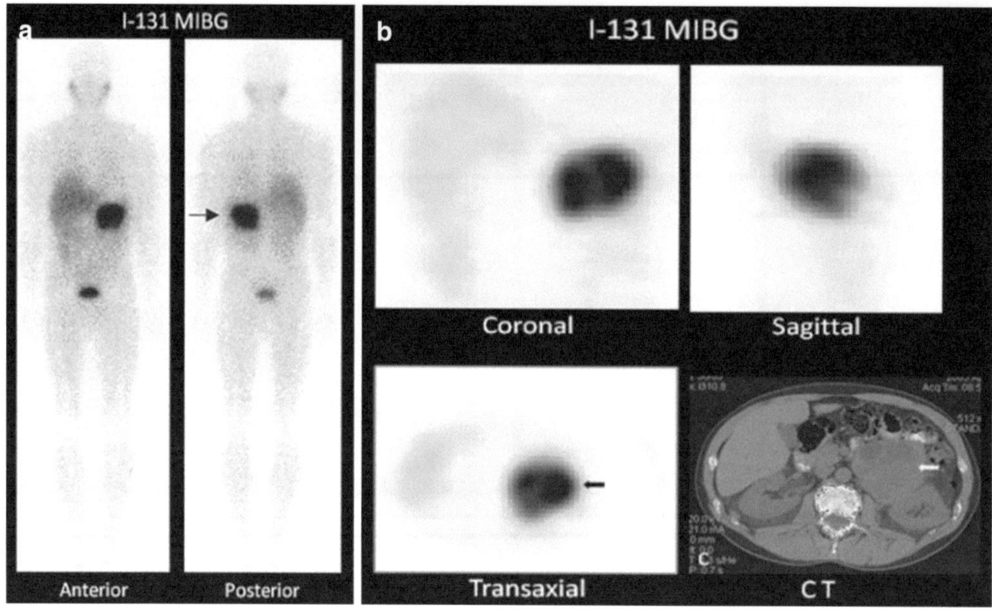

Fig. 6.17 A planar (**a**) and SPECT (**b**) ^{131}I-MIBG study and a CT section of a patient with a large pheochromocytoma (*arrows*)

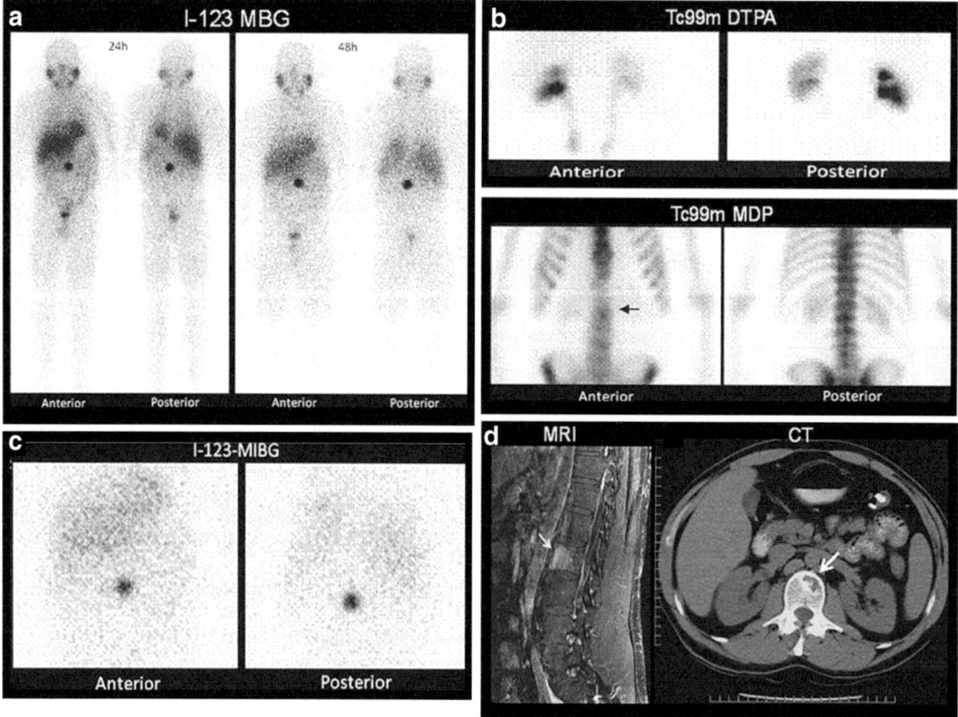

Fig. 6.18 123 I -MIBG whole body (**a**) of a patient with known pheochromocytoma who was referred for back pain. The study shows a focal area of increased uptake in the midline of the abdomen. Forty-eight hours spot image (**b**) was acquired, and 99mTc-DTPA study (**c**) was also obtained for comparison and lesion appeared away from the kidneys. The study was correlated with 99mTc-MDP spot images of the thoracolumbar spine (**d**) which showed questionable focal abnormality in the midlumbar spine corresponding to the location of I-123 abnormal uptake. MRI (**e**) and CT (**f**) scans were obtained and show a lesion in L-3 representing metastatic pheochromocytoma

showed better tumor detection capability compared to ^{123}I-MIBG planar imaging and SPECT/CT [102]. Other PET agents are also being used since approximately 10% of the neuroblastomas are non MIBG avid [103].

6.3.3.2.2 Indium-111 Octreotide

In healthy human beings, somatostatin, a natural neuropeptide, is produced in various tissues, including the nervous system, endocrine pancreas, and gastrointestinal tract. Somatostatin inhibits the secretion of several hormones, most importantly GH and TSH.

Neuroendocrine (including adrenal medulla) and non-neuroendocrine organs have surface receptors that bind to somatostatin. Octreotide, a somatostatin analog with a half-life of 120 min, is used to evaluate the tumors that contain these receptors, in which case it binds to somatostatin receptor subtypes 2 and 5. Among these tumors are pheochromocytoma, neuroblastoma, paraganglioma, and others including pancreatic tumors and carcinoid.

Octreotide is usually tagged with [111]In (Fig. 6.19), although ^{123}I has also been used in the past. It is recommended that octreotide therapy be withheld for at least 72 h prior to the injection of the radiopharmaceutical. Following i.v. injection of a standard dose of 6 mCi, static images are obtained at 4 and 24 h. SPECT images through the region of interest are then obtained at 4 h and at 24 h and later if needed (Figs. 6.20 and 6.21). This radiopharmaceutical is excreted via glomerular filtration. In a normal patient, octreotide activity is identified in the thyroid, kidneys, liver, spleen, pituitary, gallbladder, and, to a lesser extent, the bowel on delayed images. The kidney and spleen receive the highest absorbed dose. A focal area of intense early radiotracer uptake is considered to be pathological, indicating primary neoplasm or metastasis. A false-negative scan is seen in cases where the tumor is small, has few somatostatin receptors, or both. ^{111}In-octreotide scanning is highly sensitive for detecting tumors greater than 1.5 cm. Since the expression of somatostatin receptors in neuroblastomas is variable with less receptors in more advanced disease, an accurate sensitivity of ^{111}In-octreotide is not readily definable. In children, several studies

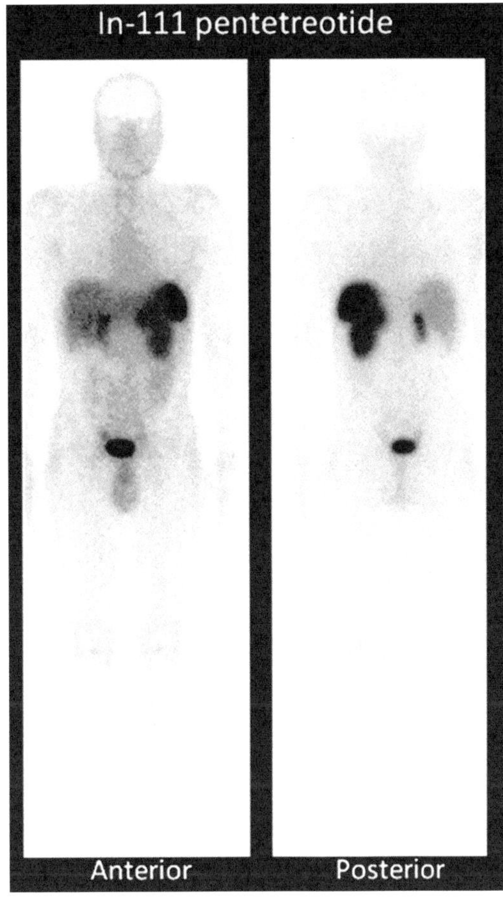

Fig. 6.19 Normal distribution of In-111 pentetreotide includes intense uptake in the spleen as well as uptake in the liver and activity in the kidneys and urinary bladder. Bowel activity is seen usually at 24 h. The pituitary and the thyroid glands may be faintly visualized. Biliary excretion of the tracer occurs with occasional visualization of the gallbladder. Note that the right kidney is smaller than the left in this case

have compared ^{111}In-octreotide with MIBG scintigraphy for imaging neuroblastoma; the sensitivity of the former ranged from 55 to 70% and that of the latter 83–94% [104–108]. Several studies reported MIBG-negative tumor sites detected by ^{111}In-pentetreotide in patients with neuroblastomas [104–108].

[111]In-octreotide is currently the agent of choice for nuclear medicine imaging of head and neck paraganglioma, though it is insensitive for lesions less than 1 cm. The recent introduction of SPECT/CT has greatly improved the sensitivity of ^{111}In-octreotide scintigraphy [109].

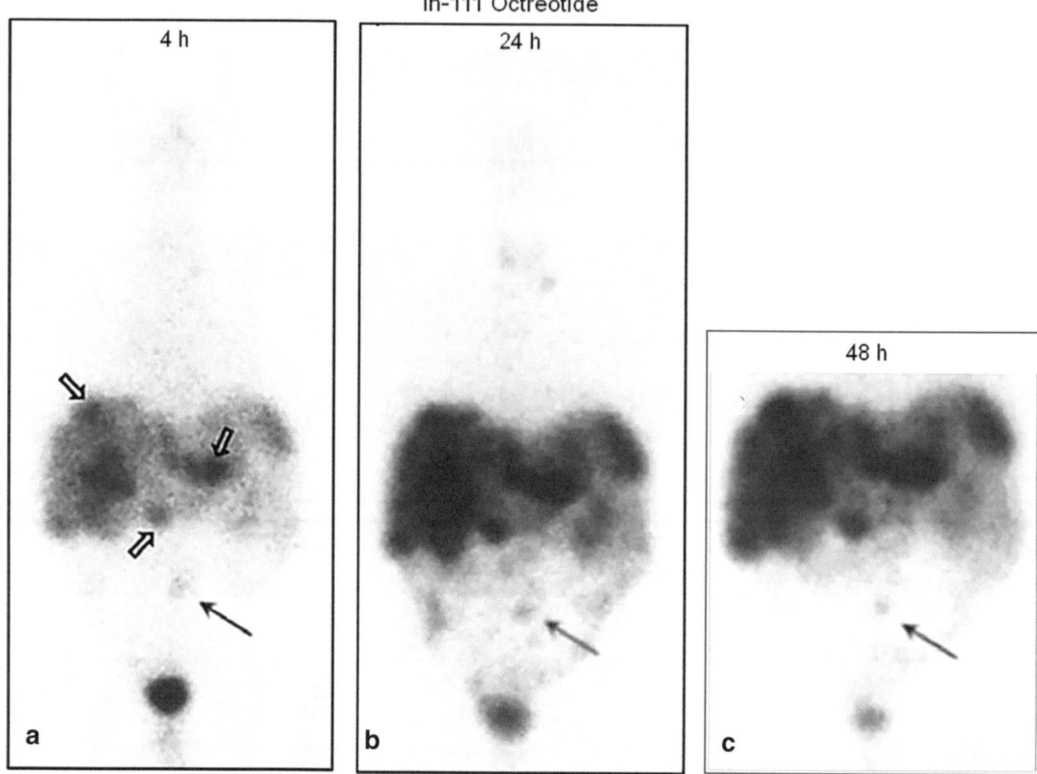

Fig. 6.20 ^{111}In-octreotide imaging study obtained at 4 (**a**), 24 (**b**), and 48 (**c**) h after i.v. injection of 6 mCi of the radiopharmaceutical. The images illustrate—in addition to the foci of metastatic carcinoid to the liver—the physiological uptake in the liver, spleen, kidneys, bowel, and urinary bladder. Note that delayed imaging (C) and/or SPECT may be needed to differentiate physiological activity such as in the bowel from true disease (*arrow*) such as in this case

It was suggested that ^{111}In-DTPA-D-Phe-1-- octreotide might be useful for radiation therapy of patients with surgically incurable tumors having high somatostatin receptor densities such as carcinoid [110].

6.3.3.2.3 Positron Emission Tomography Imaging

PET has been used to evaluate adrenal masses. The higher spatial resolution of PET scanners (Figs. 6.22, 6.23 and 6.24) enables the detection of small tumors not seen with ^{123}I-MIBG. Malignant adrenal tumors can be detected with FDG-PET, but its use in these cases is limited due to the low specificity. FDG-PET/ CT can help detect certain malignant lesions particularly the minority which are not detected by MIBG. ^{11}C-hydroxyephedrine, the first available positron-emitting tracer of the sympathetic nervous system, was found useful in the detection of pheochromocytomas, with a high level of accuracy [111]. Its uptake reflects catecholamine transport and storage and neuronal reuptake. In detecting metastatic pheochromocytomas, (^{18}F) dopamine was found to be a superior to ^{131}I-MIBG [112–114]. PET imaging is used for the detection, localization, staging, and follow-up of neuroendocrine tumors. It can also be used to determine SSTR status of the tumor and for selecting patients with metastatic disease for SSTR radionuclide therapy with Lutetium-177 (Lu-177)- or Yttrium-90 (Y-90)-labeled soma-

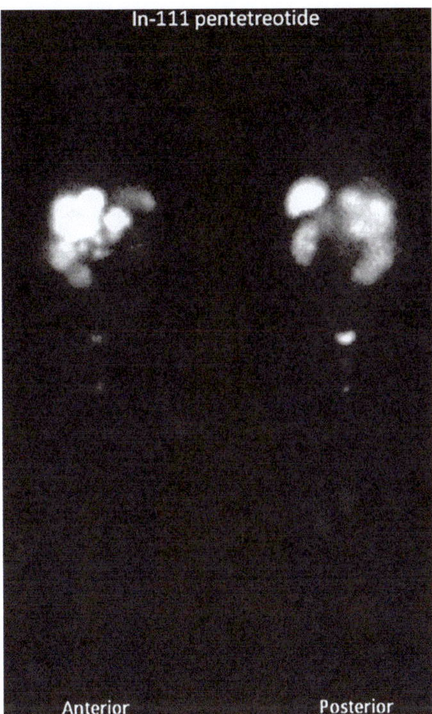

Fig. 6.21 Fifty-three-year-old female presented with carcinoid symptoms for 6 months. She was found to have metastatic disease to the liver and pancreas. In-111 pentetreotide anterior and posterior whole-body planar images at 24 h. Images reveal multiple foci of increased activity in the liver and abdomen consistent with SSTR-positive metastatic disease. SPECT/CT would better locate the abdominal disease

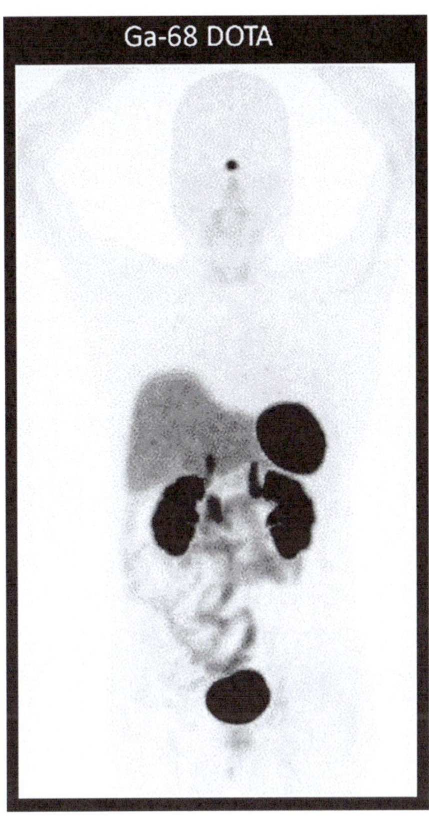

Fig. 6.23 Normal distribution of Ga-68 DOTA peptides includes intense uptake in the spleen with uptake in the pituitary gland, liver, adrenals, and pancreatic head and activity in the kidneys, bowel, and bladder. Salivary and thyroid glands show mild uptake. The prostate gland and breast glandular tissue may show diffuse low uptake. Physiological uptake in the pancreatic head may mimic focal tumor. Uptake in adrenals may be prominent

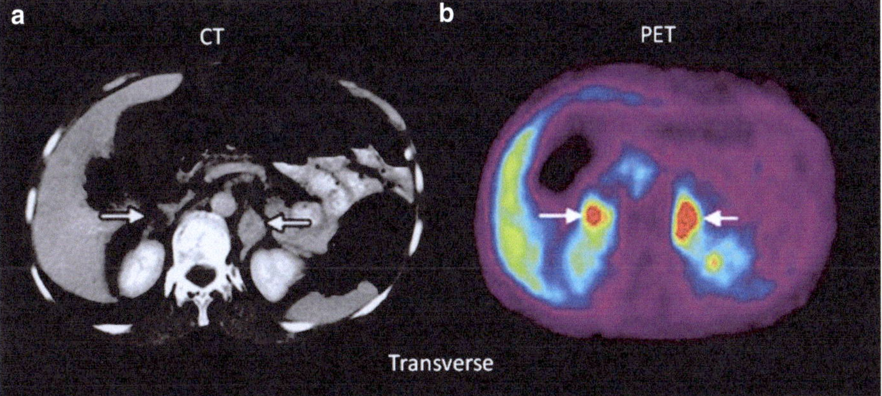

Fig. 6.22 (**a**, **b**) Transverse images obtained in a patient with multiple endocrine neoplasia type 2 and an increase in urinary catecholamine levels. A CT image shows bilateral adrenal tumors (*arrows*) and a 2-cm-diameter tumor on the right side and a 4-cm-diameter tumor on the left side adrenal lesions (*arrows*). HED PET image (**b**) shows intense uptake in both. Surgery revealed bilateral pheochromocytomas (From Anderson et al. [115] with permission)

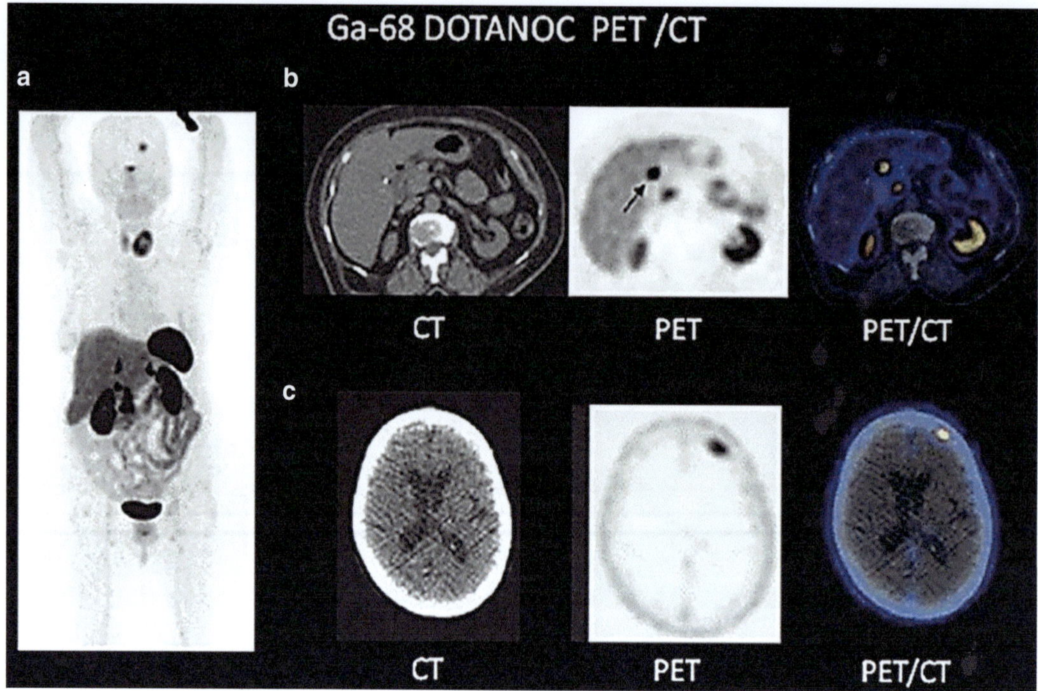

Fig. 6.24 Scintigraphic studies for a 74-year-old woman with duodenal 1 cm polyp, grade 1 carcinoid tumor, for staging. Ga-68 DOTANOC PET/CT whole-body MIP (**a**) and selected transaxial CT, PET, and PET/CT fusion images of the abdomen (**b**) and head (**c**) are shown. There is a focal uptake in the duodenal carcinoid (arrow) which is higher than liver activity. Incidentally, focal uptake is also seen in the left frontal region due to benign meningi-oma and markedly and heterogeneously increased uptake in the enlarged left thyroid lobe which can be due to medullary thyroid carcinoma, well-differentiated thyroid carcinoma, or carcinoid metastases. Physiological uptake is seen in the pituitary gland, right thyroid lobe, liver, spleen, both adrenal glands, pancreatic head, and bowel with excreted activity in the kidneys and bladder

tostatin analogs. 68-Ga-DOTATATE and 64-Cu-DOTATATE are radiolabeled somatostatin analogs for the diagnosis and pretreatment evaluation of neuroendocrine tumors with PET.

PET imaging with Ga-68 DOTA peptides is more accurate and detects more lesions than Octreoscan in carcinoid tumors and other neuroendocrine tumors [112]. Figures 6.23 and 6.22 illustrate normal and abnormal Ga-68 DOTA TATE studies.

6.3.4 Incidental Adrenal Mass

Incidental detection of adrenal lesions is a diagnostic challenge in adrenal adenomas which are relatively common (2–9%) in the general population. This is particularly important in patients with a previous clinical history of malignancy. Incidental adrenal lesions are detected in about 2–5% of contrast-enhanced abdominal CT examinations making the diagnosis of adrenal incidentaloma a common clinical problem [116]. In these cases, the patients should be screened for pheochromocytoma clinically and biochemically. Adrenal incidentalomas are uncommon in patients younger than 30 years but increase in frequency with age; they occur equally in males and females. Adrenocortical adenoma accounts for 36–94% of incidentalomas detected in patients without a history of malignancy [116]. Only about 10% of incidental adrenal masses are functional [116]. Accordingly, NP-59 would not been appropriate radiotracer for adrenal incidentaloma because 90% of adrenal masses cannot incorporate NP-59 in their cells. Metomidate is an inhibitor of 11ß-hydroxylase, a key enzyme in the biosynthesis of cortisol and aldosterone by the adrenal cortex. ^{11}C-metomidate is a promising PET tracer to identify incidentalomas of adrenocortical origin [117]. Khan et al. reported on the value of ^{11}C-metomidate in evaluation of adrenocortical cancer [118].

FDG-PET can help detect certain malignancy in adrenal incidentalomas particularly when they occur in patients with known extra-adrenal malignancies. The prevalence of adrenal metastases discovered by FDG-PET has been reported to be as high as 9.9% in several studies. The upstaging resulting from FDG-PET can play an important role in modifying the plans of therapeutic strategies. In some patients, the adrenal metastasis can be the first manifestation of a cancer [119].

References

1. Nurunnabi ASM, Alim A, Sabiha M, Manowara B, Monira K, Shamim A (2010) Weight of the human thyroid gland a Postmortem study. Bangladesh J Med Sci 9(1):44–48.
2. Ellis H (2007) Anatomy of the thyroid and parathyroid glands. Surgery (Oxford) 25:467–468
3. Alotaibi H, Tuzlakoğlu-Öztürk M, Tazebay UH (2017) The thyroid Na+/I- symporter: molecular characterization and genomic regulation. Mol Imaging Radionucl Ther 26(Suppl 1):92–101
4. Sarkar SD (1996) Thyroid pathophysiology. In: Sandler MP, Coleman RE, Th. Wackers FJ (eds) Diagnostic nuclear medicine. Williams and Wilkins, Baltimore, pp 899–909
5. Cooper DS (2005) Antithyroid drugs. N Engl J Med 352:905–917
6. Bidart JM, Mian C, Lazar V, Russo D, Filetti S, Caillou B et al (2000) Expression of pendrin and the Pendred syndrome (PDS) gene in human thyroid tissues. J Clin Endocrinol Metab 2000(85):2028–2033
7. Koukkou EG, Roupas ND, Markou KB (2017) Effect of excess iodine intake on thyroid on human health. Minerva Med 108:136–146
8. Malozowski S, Chiesa A (2010) Propylthiouracil-induced hepatotoxicity and death. Hopefully, never more. J Clin Endocrinol Metab 95:3161–3163.
9. Mitchell AM, Manley SW, Morris JC, Powell KA, Bergert ER, Mortimer RH (2001) Sodium iodide symporter (NIS) gene expression in human placenta. Placenta 22:256–258
10. Daniels GH (2001) Amiodarone-induced thyrotoxicosis. J Clin Endocrinol Metab 86:3–8
11. Laurie AJ, Lyon SG, Lasser EC (1992) Contrast material iodides: potential effects on radioactive iodine thyroid uptake. J Nucl Med 33:237–238
12. Bogazzi F, Bartalena L, Gasperi M et al (2001) The various effects of amiodarone on thyroid function. Thyroid 11:511–519
13. Sarkar SD, Kalapparambath T, Palestro CJ (2002) Comparison of I-123 and I-131 for whole body imaging in thyroid cancer. J Nucl Med 43:632–634
14. Ward LS, Santarosa PL, Granja F et al (2003) Low expression of sodium iodide symporter identifies aggressive thyroid tumors. Cancer Lett 200:85–91
15. Bertagna F, Treglia G, Piccardo G et al (2012) Diagnostic and clinical significance of F-18-FDG-PET/CT thyroid incidentalomas. J Clin Endocrinol Metab 97:3866–3875
16. Castellana M, Trimboli P, Piccardo A, Giovanella L, Treglia G (2019) Performance of 18F-FDG PET/CT in selecting thyroid nodules with indeterminate fine-needle aspiration cytology for surgery. A systematic review and a meta-analysis. J Clin Med 8:1333
17. Moog F, Linke R, Manthey N et al (2000) Influence of thyroid stimulating hormone levels on uptake of FDG in recurrent and metastatic differentiated thyroid carcinoma. J Nucl Med 41:1989–1995
18. Akamizu T, Satoh T, Isozaki O et al (2012) Diagnostic criteria, clinical features, and incidence of thyroid storm based on nationwide surveys. Thyroid 22:661–679
19. Kim YH, Chang Y, Kim Y, Kim SJ, Rhee EJ et al (2019) Diffusely increased 18F-FDG uptake in the thyroid gland and risk of thyroid dysfunction: a cohort study. J Clin Med 8:443
20. Padma V, Ramakrishnan C (2019) Malignancy in solitary thyroid nodules: a study on incidence & evaluation of risk. Indian J Public Health Res Dev 10:4253-4255
21. Kishan AM, Prasad K (2018) Prevalence of solitary thyroid nodule and evaluation of the risk factors associated with occurrence of malignancy in a solitary nodule of thyroid. Int Surg J 5(6):2279–2285
22. Guth S, Theune U, Aberle J, Galach A, Bamberger CM (2009) Very high prevalence of thyroid nodules detected by high frequency (13 MHz) ultrasound examination. Eur J Clin Investig 39:699–706
23. Jiang H, Tian Y, Yan W, Kong Y, Wang H, Wang A et al (2016) The prevalence of thyroid nodules and an analysis of related lifestyle factors in Beijing communities. Int J Environ Res Public Health 13:1-11
24. Holm LE, Blomgren H, Lowhagen T (1985) Cancer risks in patients with chronic autoimmune thyroiditis. N Engl J Med 312:601–604
25. Belfiore A, La Rosa GL, La Porta GA, Giuffrida D, Milazzo G, Lupo L et al (1992) Cancer risk in patients with cold thyroid nodules: relevance of iodine intake, sex, age, and multinodularity. Am J Med 93:363–369
26. Fabrizio Monaco F (2003) Classification of thyroid diseases: suggestions for a revision. J Clin Endocrinol Metabol 88:1428–1432

27. Fernandez-Soto L, Gonzalez A, Escobar-Jimenez F et al (1998) Increased risk of autoimmune thyroid disease in hepatitis C vs hepatitis B before, during, and after discontinuing interferon therapy. Arch Intern Med 158:1445–1448

28. Dang AH, Hershman JM (2002) Lithium-associated thyroiditis. Endocr Pract 8:232–236

29. Amino N, Tada H, Hidaka Y et al (1999) Screening for postpartum thyroiditis. J Clin Endocrinol Metab 84:1813

30. Stagnaro-Green A (2002) Postpartum thyroiditis. J Clin Endocrinol Metab 87:4042–4047

31. Premawardhana LDKE, Parkes AB, John R et al (2004) Thyroid peroxidase antibodies in early pregnancy: utility for prediction of postpartum thyroid dysfunction and implications for screening. Thyroid 14:610–615

32. Mandac JC, Chaudhry S, Sherman KE, Tomer Y (2006) The clinical and physiological spectrum of interferon-alpha induced thyroiditis: toward a new classification. Hepatology 43(4):661–672

33. Oppenheim Y, Ban Y, Tomer Y (2004) Interferon induced autoimmune thyroid disease (AITD): a model for human autoimmunity. Autoimmun Rev 3:388–393

34. Bliddal S, Nielsen CH, Feldt-Rasmussen U (2017) Recent advances in understanding autoimmune thyroid disease: the tallest tree in the forest of poly-autoimmunity. F1000Research 6:1776. https://doi.org/10.12688/f1000research.11535.1

35. Vestergaard P, Rejnmark L, Weeke J et al (2002) Smoking as a risk factor for Graves' disease, toxic nodular goiter, and autoimmune hypothyroidism. Thyroid 12:69–75

36. Fountoulakis S, Tsatsoulis A (2004) On the pathogenesis of autoimmune thyroid disease: a unifying hypothesis. Clin Endocrinol 60:397–409

37. Li Y, Teng D, Shan Z et al (2008) Antithyroperoxidase and antithyroglobulin antibodies in a five-year follow up survey of populations with different iodine intakes. J Clin Endocrinol Metab 93:1751–1757

38. Nygaard B, Knudsen JH, Hegedus L et al (1997) Thyrotropin receptor antibodies and Graves' disease, a side-effect of I-131 treatment in patients with non-toxic goiter. J Clin Endocrinol Metab 82:2926–2930

39. Surks MI, Ortiz E, Daniels GH et al (2004) Subclinical thyroid disease: scientific review and guidelines for diagnosis and management, vol 291. JAMA, pp 228–238

40. Weetman AP (2000) Graves disease. N Engl J Med 343:1236–1248

41. Ahmed A, Craig W, Krukowski ZH (2012) Quality of life after surgery for Graves' disease: comparison of those having surgery intended to preserve thyroid function with those having ablative surgery. Thyroid 22:494–500

42. Burch HB, Burman KD, Cooper DS (2012) A 2011 survey of clinical practice patterns in the management of Graves' disease. J Clin Endocrinol Metab 97:4549–4558

43. La Vecchia C, Malvezzi M, Bosetti C, Garavello W, Bertuccio P, Levi F, Negri E (2015) Thyroid cancer mortality and incidence: a global overview. Int J Cancer 136:2187–2195

44. Tumino D, Grani G, Di Stefano M, Di Mauro M, Scutari M et al (2020) Nodular thyroid disease in the era of precision medicine. Front Endocrinol 10:907

45. Elgazzar AH, Alenezi S, Alshammari JM, Ghanem M, Asa'Ad S (2015) Value of oblique view in nodular thyroid disease; revisiting fundamentals. World J Nucl Med 14:125

46. Soto GD, Halperin I, Squarcia M, Lomeña F, Domingo MP (2010) Update in thyroid imaging. The expanding world of thyroid imaging and its translation to clinical practice. Hormones 9:287–298

47. Sarkar SD (2006) Benign thyroid disease: what is the role of nuclear medicine? Semin Nucl Med 36:185–193

48. Bath SC, Steer CD, Golding J, Emmett P, Rayman MP (2013) Effect of inadequate iodine status in UK pregnant women on cognitive outcomes in their children: results from the Avon longitudinal study of parents and children (ALSPAC). Lancet 382:331–337

49. Liu Y (2009) Clinical significance of thyroid uptake on F18-fluorodeoxyglucose positron emission tomography. Ann Nucl Med 23:17–23

50. Akerstrom G, Rudberg C, Grimelius L et al (1986) Histologic parathyroid abnormalities in an autopsy series. Hum Pathol 17:520–527

51. Hynes KL, Otahal P, Burgess JR, Oddy WH, Hay I (2017) Reduced educational outcomes persist into adolescence following mild iodine deficiency in utero, despite adequacy in childhood: 15-year follow-up of the gestational iodine cohort investigating auditory processing speed and working memory. Nutrients 9:pii:E135477

52. Abel MH, Caspersen IH, Meltzer HM, Haugen M, Brandlistuen RE, Aase H, Alexander J, Torheim LE, Brantsaeter AL (2017) Suboptimal maternal iodine intake is associated with impaired child neurodevelopment at 3 years of age in the Norwegian mother and child cohort study. J Nutr 147:1314–1324

53. Levie D, Korevaar TIM, Bath SC, Dalmau-Bueno A et al (2018) Thyroid function in early pregnancy, child IQ, and autistic traits: a meta-analysis of individual participant data. J Clin Endocrinol Metabol 103:2967–297

54. Taterra D, Wong LM, Vikse J, Sanna B, Pękala P, Walocha J, Cirocchi R, Tomaszewski K, Henry BM (2019) The prevalence and anatomy of parathyroid glands: a meta-analysis with implications for parathyroid surgery. Langenbeck's Arch Surg 404(1):63-70.55

55. Alenezi SA, Asa'ad SM, Elgazzar AH (2015) Scintigraphic parathyroid imaging: concepts and new developments. Res Rep Nuclear Med 5:9–18

56. Quiros RM, Warren W, Prinz RA (2004) Excision of a mediastinal parathyroid gland with use of video-assisted thoracoscopy, intraoperative 99mTc-

sestamibi scanning, and intraoperative monitoring of intact parathyroid hormone. Endocr Pract 10:45–48

57. Taterra D, Wong LM, Vikse J, Sanna B, Pękala P, Walocha J et al (2019) The prevalence and anatomy of parathyroid glands: a meta-analysis with implications for parathyroid surgery. Langenbeck's Arch Surg 404:63–70

58. Akerstrom G, Grimelius L, Johansson H, Lundquist H, Pertoft H, Bergstrom R (1981) The parenchymal cell mass in normal human parathyroid glands. Acta Pathol Microbiol Immunol Scand 89(A):367

59. Heath H III (1991) Clinical spectrum of primary hyperparathyroidism: evolution with changes in medical practice and technology. J Bone Miner Res 6:S63–S70

60. Bilezikian JP, Bandeira L, Khan A, Cusano NE (2018) Hyperparathyroidism. Lancet 391(10116):168–178

61. Silva BC, Cusano NE, Bilezikian JP (2018) Primary hyperparathyroidism. Best Pract Res Clin Endocrinol Metab 32(5):593–607

62. Yeh MW, Ituarte PHG, Zhou HC et al (2013) Incidence and prevalence of primary hyperparathyroidism in a racially mixed population. J Clin Endocrinol Metab 98(3):1122–1129

63. Ljunghall S, Hellman P, Rastad J, Akerström G (1991) Primary hyperparathyroidism: epidemiology, diagnosis and clinical picture. World J Surg 15(6):681–687

64. Herfarth KK, Wells SA (1997) Parathyroid glands and the multiple endocrine neoplasia syndromes and familial hypocalciuric hypercalcemia. Semin Surg Oncol 13:114–124

65. Duh QY, Hybarger CP, Geist R, Gamsu G, Goodman PC, Gooding GA, Clark OH (1987) Carcinoids associated with multiple endocrine neoplasia syndromes. Am J Surg 154:142–148

66. Beus KS, Stack BC (2004) Synchronous thyroid pathology in patients presenting with primary hyperparathyroidism. Am J Otolaryngol 25:308–312

67. Sarkar SD, Afriyie MO, Palestro CJ (2001) Recombinant human thyroid-stimulating-hormone-aided scintigraphy: comparison of imaging at multiple times after I-131 administration. Clin Nucl Med 26:392–395

68. Sidhu S, Campbell P (2000) Thyroid pathology associated with primary hyperparathyroidism. Aust NZJ Surg 70:285–287

69. Hedman IL, Tisell LE (1984) Associated hyperparathyroidism and non-medullary thyroid carcinoma: the etiological role of radiation. Surgery 95:392–397

70. Lau WL, Obi Y, Kalantar-Zadeh K (2018) Parathyroidectomy in the management of secondary hyperparathyroidism. Clin J Am Soc Nephrol 13(6):952–961

71. Thompson NW, Eckhauser FE, Harness JK (1982) The anatomy of primary hyperparathyroidism. Surgery 92:814–821

72. Simeone DM, Sandelin K, Thompson NW (1995) Undescended superior parathyroid gland: a potential cause of failed cervical exploration for hyperparathyroidism. Surgery 118:949–956

73. Wang CA (1977) Parathyroid re-exploration: a clinical and pathological study of 112 cases. Ann Surg 186:140

74. Assalia A, Inabnet WB (2004) Endoscopic parathyroidectomy. Otolaryngol Clin N Am 37:871–886

75. O'Doherty MJ, Kettle AG (2003) Parathyroid imaging: preoperative localisation. Nucl Med Commun 24:125–131

76. Mitchell BK, Merrell RC, Kinder BK (1995) Localization studies in patients with hyperparathyroidism. Endocr Surg 75:483–498

77. Kao A, Shiau YC, Tsai SC, Wang JJ, Ho ST (2002) Technetium-99-m-methoxyisobutylisonitrile imaging for parathyroid adenoma: relationship to P-glycoprotein or multidrug resistance-related protein expression. Eur J Nucl Med Mol Imaging 29:1012–1015

78. Goris ML, Basso LV, Keeling C (1991) Parathyroid imaging. J Nucl Med 32:887–889

79. O'Doherty MJ, Kettle AG, Wells P, Collins RE, Coakley AJ (1992) Parathyroid imaging with technetium 99m-sestamibi: preoperative localization and tissue uptake studies. J Nucl Med 33:313–318

80. Takebayashi S, Hidai H, Chiba T, Takaga Y, Nagatani Y, Matsubara S (1999) Hyperfunctional parathyroid glands with Tc-99m MIBI scan: semiquantitative analysis correlated with histologic findings. J Nucl Med 40:1792–1797

81. Naddaf S, Anim JJ, Farghaly MM, Behbehani AE, Alshomar KA, Elgazzar AH (2004) Ultrastructure of hyperfunctioning parathyroid glands: does it explain various patterns of sestamibi uptake. Proceedings of the 9th annual Health science poster day and conference, Kuwait, April 19–21, pp61

82. Parikh AM, Suliburk JW, Morón FE (2018) Imaging localization and surgical approach in the management of ectopic parathyroid adenomas. Endocr Pract 24(6):589-598.97

83. Takahashi H et al (2013) Fusion images of MIBI SPECT and MDCT improve diagnostic performance of localization study in hyperparathyroidism with multigland disease. J Nucl Med 54:44

84. Zeng M, Liu W, Zha X, Tang S, Liu J, Yang G et al (2019) 99mTc-MIBI SPECT/CT imaging had high sensitivity in accurate localization of parathyroids before parathyroidectomy for patients with secondary hyperparathyroidism. Ren Fail 41(1):885–892

85. Beggs AD, Hain SF (2005) Localization of parathyroid adenomas using ^{11}C-methionine positron emission tomography. Nucl Med Commun 26:133–136

86. Broos WA, Wondergem M, Knol RJ, van der Zant FM (2019) Parathyroid imaging with 18 F-fluorocholine PET/CT as a first-line imaging modality in primary hyperparathyroidism: a retrospective cohort study. EJNMMI Res 9:1–7

87. Lynn MD, Gross MD, Shapiro B, Bassett D (1986) The influence of hypercholesterolemia on the adrenal uptake and metabolic handling of I-13 16β-iodomethyl-19-norcholesterol(NP-59). Nucl Med Commun 1:631–635

88. Hedeland H, Ostberg G, Hokfelt B (1968) On the prevalence of adrenocortical adenomas in an autopsy material in relation to hypertension and diabetes. Acta Med Scand 184:211–214

89. Copeland PM (1983) The incidentally discovered adrenal mass. Ann Intern Med 98:940–945

90. Vos EL, Grewal RK, Russo AE, Reidy-Lagunes D, Untch BR, Gavane SC et al (2020) Predicting malignancy in patients with adrenal tumors using 18F-FDG-PET/CT SUVmax. J Surg Oncol 122(8):1821–1826

91. Volpe C, Enberg U, Sjögren A et al (2008) The role of adrenal scintigraphy in the preoperative management of primary aldosteronism. Scand J Surg 97:248–253

92. Evangelista L, De Falco T, di Nuzzo C et al (2008) Utility of adrenal cortical scintigraphy with I-6-$-methyl-131n or cholesterol in a case of mismatch between morphological and functional PET imaging. Thyroid Sci 3:CR1–CR3

93. Huether SE, Tomky D (1998) Alterations of hormonal regulation. In: Mc Cance KL, Huether SE (eds) Pathophysiology, the biologic basis for disease in adults and children, 3rd edn. Mosby, St Louis, p 700

94. Spencer RP (1998) Tumor-seeking radiopharmaceuticals: nature and mechanisms. In: Murray IP, Ell PJ (eds) Nuclear medicine in clinical diagnosis and treatment, 2nd edn. Churchill Livingstone, HongKong, p 764

95. Elgazzar AH, Gelfand MJ, Washburn LC, Clark J, Nagaraj N, Cummings D, Hughes J et al (1995) I-123MIBG scintigraphy in adults, are port of clinical experience. Clin Nucl Med 20:147

96. Gelfand MJ, Elgazzar AH, Kriss VM, Masters PR, Golsch GJ (1994) Iodine-123MIBG SPECT versus planar imaging in children with neural crest tumors. J Nucl Med 35:1753–1756

97. Parisi MT, Sandler ED, Hattner RS (1992) The biodistribution of metaiodobenzylguanidine. Semin Nucl Med 22:46–48

98. Okuyama C, Ushijima Y, Kubota T, Yoshida T, Nakai T, Kobayashi K, Nishimura T (2003) 123I-Metaiodobenzylguanidine uptake in the nape of the neck of children: likely visualization of brown adipose tissue. J Nucl Med 44:1421–1425

99. Shapiro B, Copp JE, Sisson JC, Eyre PL, Wallis J, Beierwaltes WH (1985) Iodine-131metaiodobenzylguanidine in the locating of suspected pheochromocytoma:experiencein400cases. J Nucl Med 26:576

100. Paltiel HJ, Gelfand MJ, Elgazzar AH, Washburn LC, Harris RE, Masters PR, Golsch GJ (1994) Neural crest tumors: I-123MIBG imaging in children. Radiology 190:118

101. Liu B, Servaes S, Zhuang H (2018) SPECT/CT MIBG imaging is crucial in the follow-up of the patients with high-risk neuroblastoma. Clin Nucl Med 43(4):232–238

102. Aboian MS, Huang SY, Hernandez-Pampaloni M, Hawkins RA, VanBrocklin HF, Huh Y et al (2021) 124I-MIBG PET/CT to monitor metastatic disease in children with relapsed neuroblastoma. J Nucl Med 62(1):43–47

103. Samim A, Tytgat GA, Bleeker G, Wenker S, Chatalic KL, Poot AJ et al (2021) Nuclear medicine imaging in neuroblastoma: current status and new developments. J Personal Med 11(4):270

104. Shalaby-Rana E, Majd M, Andrich MP, Movassaghi N (1997) In-111 pentetreotide scintigraphy in patients with neuroblastoma. Comparison with I-131MIBG,N-Myconcogene amplification, and patient outcome. Clin Nucl Med 22:315–319

105. Kropp J, Hofmann M, Bihl H (1997) Comparison of MIBG and pentetreotide scintigraphy in children with neuroblastoma. Is the expression of somatostatin receptors a prognostic factor? Anticancer Res 17:1583–1588

106. Tenenbaum F, Lumbroso J, Schlumberger M, Mure A, Plouin PF, Caillou B, Parmentier C (1995) Comparison of radiolabeled octreotide and metaiodobenzylguanidine (MIBG) scintigraphy in malignant pheochromocytoma. J Nucl Med 36:1–6

107. Pashankar FD, O'Dorisio MS, Menda Y (2005) MIBG and somatostatin receptor analogs in children: current concepts on diagnostic and therapeutic use. J Nucl Med 46(Suppl1):55S–61S

108. Manil L, Edeline V, Jlumbroso J, Lequen H, Zucker JM (1996) Indium-111-pentetreotide scintigraphy in children with neuroblast-derived tumors. J Nucl Med 37:893–896

109. Krausz Y, Keidar Z, Kogan I, Even-Sapir E, Bar-Shalom R, Engel A, Rubinstein R et al (2003) SPECT/CT hybrid imaging with ^{111}In-pentetreotide in assessment of neuroendocrine tumours. Clin Endocrinol 59:565–573

110. Andersson P, Forssel-Aronsson E, Johanson V, Wangberg B, Nilsson O, Fjalling M, Ahlman H (1996) Internalization of indium-111 into human neuroendocrine tumor cells after incubation with indium-111-DTPA-D-Phe1-octreotide. J Nucl Med 37:2002–2006

111. Trampal C, Engler H, Juhlin C, Bergstrom M, Langstrom B (2004) Pheochromocytomas: detection with C-11 hydroxyephedrine PET. Radiology 230:423–428

112. Ruf J, Hueck F, Schiefer J, Denecke T, Elgeti F et al (2010) Impact of multiphase 68Ga-DOTATOC-PET/CT on therapy management in patients with neuroendocrine tumors. Neuroendocrinology 91:101–109

113. Ilias I, Yu J, Carrasquillo JA, Chen CC, Eisenhofer G, Whatley M, McElroy B et al (2003) Superiorityof6-[18F]-fluorodopamine positron emission tomography versus[131I]-metaiodobenzylguanidine scintigraphy in the localization of metastatic pheochromocytoma. J Clin Endocrinol Metab 88:4083–4087

114. Brunt LM, Moley JF (2001) Adrenal incidentaloma. World J Surg 25:905–913

115. Andersson P, Forssel-Aronsson E, Johanson V, Wangberg B, Nilsson O, Fjalling M, Ahlman H

(1996) Internalization of indium-111 into human neuroendocrine tumor cells after incubation with indium-111-DTPA-D-Phe 1-octreotide. J Nucl Med 37:2002–2200

116. Mantero F, Masini AM, Opocher G, Giovagnetti M, Arnaldi G (1997) Adrenal incidentaloma: an overview of hormonal data from the National Italian Study Group. Horm Res 47:284–289

117. Minn H, Salonen A, Friberg J, Roivainen A, Viljanen T, Langsjo J, Salmi J et al (2004) Imaging of adrenal incidentalomas with PET using C-11metomidate and 18F-FDG. J Nucl Med 45:972–979

118. Khan TS, Sundin A, Juhlin C, Langstrom B, Bergström M, Eriksson B (2003) 11C-metomidate PET imaging of adrenocortical cancer. Eur J Nucl Med Mol Imaging 30:403–410

119. Akkuş G, Güney IB, Ok F, Evran M, Izol V et al (2019) Diagnostic efficacy of 18F-FDG PET/CT in patients with adrenal incidentaloma. Endocr Connect 8:838–845

7.1 Anatomic and Physiologic Considerations

7.1.1 Major Structures

The urinary system consists of a pair of kidneys, which filter the blood, form urine, and help regulate various metabolic processes; a pair of tubular ureters, which transport urine away from the kidneys; a saclike urinary bladder, which serves as urine reservoir; and a tubular urethra, which conveys urine to the outside of the body.

Kidneys are paired bean-shaped retroperitoneal organs situated in the posterior part of the abdomen on each side of the vertebral column against the psoas major muscle. The upper pole of each kidney lies at the level of the twelfth thoracic vertebra, and the lower pole lies opposite the third lumbar vertebra. The right kidney is usually slightly more caudal in position. Each kidney's weight ranges from 120 to 170 g in the adult male and from 115 to 155 g in the adult female. It is approximately 11 × 6 × 2.5 cm in dimension. Each kidney's concave medial surface has a slit-like aperture called the hilum, through which the renal pelvis, the renal artery and vein, the lymphatics, and a nerve plexus pass into the kidney (Fig. 7.1). A tough fibrous capsule surrounds the organ.

On cut sections, two distinct regions can be identified: a pale outer region, the cortex, and a darker inner region, the medulla. In humans, the medulla is divided into 4–18 striated conical masses, the renal pyramids (average 8). Each pyramid's base is positioned at the corticomedullary boundary, and the apex extends toward the renal pelvis to form a papilla (Fig. 7.1). On the tip of each papilla are 10–25 small openings representing the distal ends of the collecting ducts. A funnel-shaped minor calyx caps the apex of each medullary pyramid. The minor calyx receives the urine from the kidney and passes it to the extrarenal collecting system.

Since renal blood flow of approximately 400 ml/100 g—1.0 and 1.2 liters per minute per 1.73 m^2 of body surface area—is much higher than that of any other well-perfused organs such as the heart and brain, kidney tissue is prone to be exposed to a significant amount of any potentially harmful circulating substances [1].

Additionally, glomerular capillaries are vulnerable to hemodynamic injury, in contrast to other capillary beds because glomerular filtration is dependent on high intra- and trans-glomerular pressure. The nephron's microvasculature organization facilitates the spreading of glomerular injury to the tubulointerstitial compartment in disease, exposing tubular epithelial cells to abnormal ultrafiltrate. Accordingly, the concept of the nephron as a functional unit (Fig. 7.2) applies not only to renal physiology but also to the pathophysiology of renal diseases.

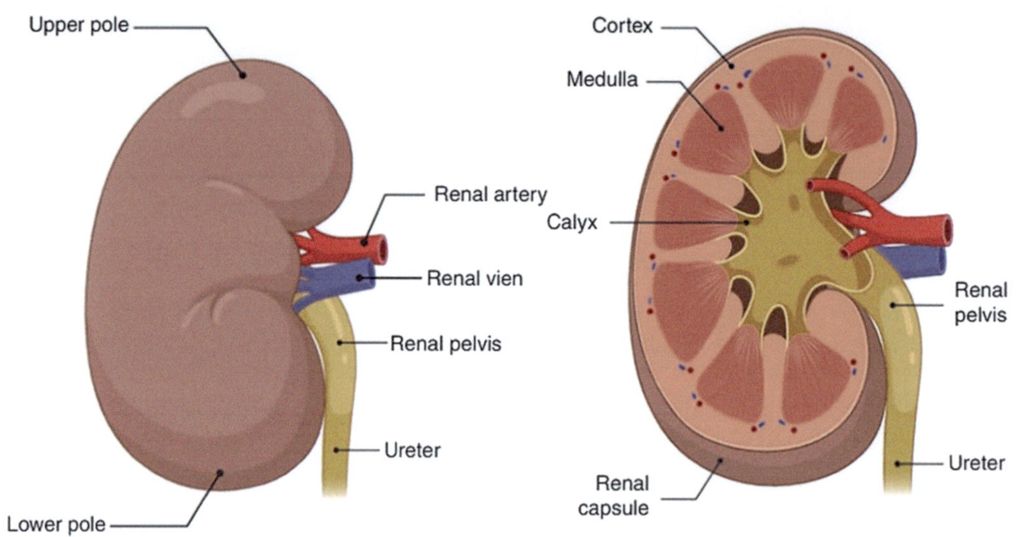

Fig. 7.1 A diagram illustrating the kidney surface anatomy and the main anatomic structures on cut surface

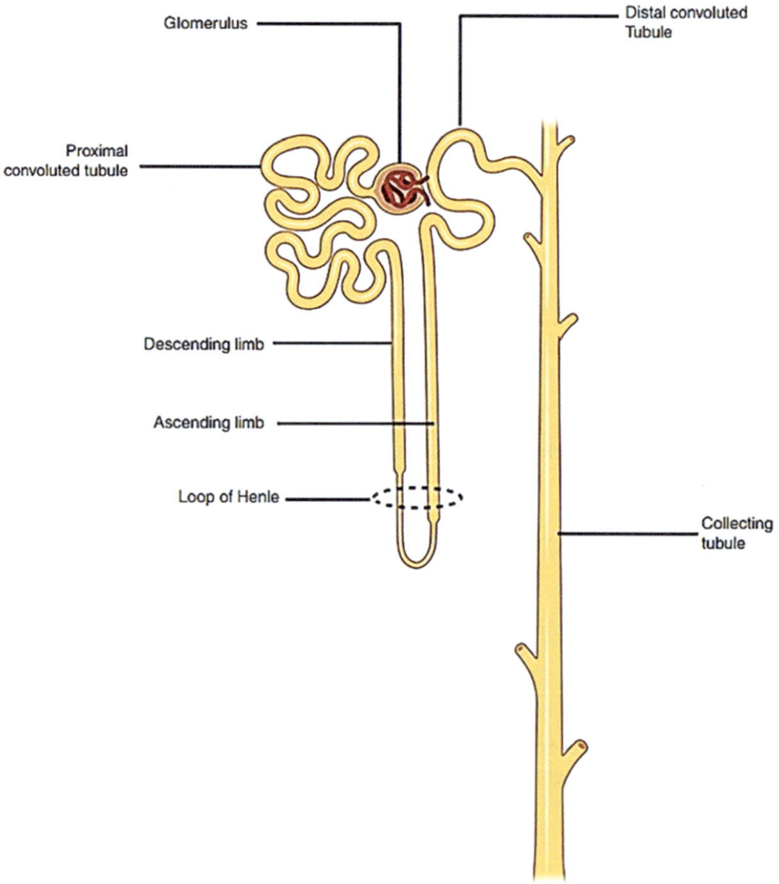

Fig. 7.2 The components of the nephron

7.1.2 Renal Vasculature

Each kidney is supplied normally by a single renal artery in the human body. However, one or more accessory renal arteries are not uncommon, which may occur in 30% of the population [2]. The renal artery enters through the hilum of the kidney and branches successively into the interlobar arteries, arcuate arteries, interlobular arteries, and afferent arterioles. Each afferent arteriole eventually branches into the glomerular capillaries. The distal glomerular capillaries merge to form the efferent arteriole. Efferent arterioles subdivide to form peritubular capillaries in the cortex or the vasa recta in the medulla. Changes in the afferent or efferent arteriolar tone play an important role in regulating the GFR.

7.1.3 Juxtaglomerular Apparatus

The afferent arteriole has specialized smooth muscle cells called juxtaglomerular (JG) cells that store renin and stretch receptors that respond to arteriolar pressure changes. Renin is released as a result of decreased stretch of the arteriolar wall when arteriolar pressure is decreased. Another stimulus for renin comes from the macula densa, which consists of specialized cells in the first part of the distal tubule, located close to the JG cells. The macula densa signals the JG cells to release renin when the sodium and chloride content of this part of the tubule is low. Finally, the sympathetic nervous system can stimulate renin release in response to systemic baroreceptor stimuli.

7.1.4 Renal Function

The main functions of the kidneys are the maintenance of water, electrolyte, acid–base balance, elimination of waste products, and blood pressure regulation. The functional unit of the kidney is the nephron, which consists of a glomerulus and a tubule. The *glomerulus* consists of a network of capillaries derived from the afferent glomerular arteriole. They can be broadly divided

into several portions: the proximal tubule, loop of Henle, distal tubule, and collecting tubule.

Urine is formed as a result of glomerular filtration, tubular reabsorption, and tubular secretion [3]. The glomerular capillary tuft acts as a filter for plasma. Two epithelial layers encase it, the inner layer becoming part of the outer capillary wall and the outer layer lining Bowman's space (capsule), which receives the filtered fluid. The glomerular filtration rate (GFR) mainly depends on the hydrostatic and colloid osmotic pressure in the glomerular capillaries and the hydrostatic pressure in Bowman's space. Filtered fluid from Bowman's space enters the *tubule*. The *proximal tubule* plays a crucial role in reabsorbing filtered solutes. About half to two-thirds of the sodium, chloride, and potassium are reabsorbed in this segment. Reabsorption of solutes is accompanied by passive osmotic diffusion of water. The *loop of Henle*, consisting of a descending limb and an ascending limb, is the reabsorption site of about 25% of the filtered solutes. Reabsorption occurs primarily in the "thick" ascending limb, where the epithelial cells are thick and metabolically very active. In this section, "loop" diuretics such as furosemide exert their effects (see later). The reabsorbed solutes enter the medullary interstitium and contribute to its hypertonicity.

The *distal tubule* transports sodium, chloride, and potassium, but not water, from its proximal part, similar to the loop of Henle. The terminal distal tubule shares similar functions with the collecting tubules (see later). At the very beginning of the distal tubule is the *macula densa*, a region of specialized cells in the vicinity of the juxtaglomerular (JG) cells in the afferent arteriole that store renin. In response to sodium and chloride concentration changes in this portion of the tubule, the macula densa sends signals to the JG cells to release renin that mainly increases arterial blood pressure.

7.2 Renal Radiopharmaceuticals

Renal radiopharmaceuticals can be described in two broad classes: those excreted rapidly into the urine and those retained for prolonged periods in the renal parenchyma.

7.2.1 Rapidly Excreted Radiopharmaceuticals

The rapidly excreted radiopharmaceuticals are used in dynamic imaging studies to assess individual renal function and include [2, 4–6]:

^{99m}Tc-mercaptoacetyltriglycine (MAG$_3$), the agent of choice, is 90% protein bound and excreted almost exclusively by the renal tubules. High renal-to-background count ratios provide excellent images and permit visualization of poorly functioning kidneys.

^{99m}Tc-diethylenetriamine penta-acetic acid (DTPA) was the most popular radiopharmaceutical in its category prior to the introduction of ^{99m}Tc-MAG$_3$. It shows little protein binding (about 5%) and is excreted exclusively by glomerular filtration. Renal uptake of ^{99m}Tc-DTPA is limited because the glomeruli filter only 20% of the renal blood flow. The 20% extraction fraction is considerably lower than that of ^{99m}Tc-MAG$_3$ and yields lower renal-to-background uptake ratios. However, it is less costly and may be used as an alternative to ^{99m}Tc-MAG$_3$, particularly if a quantitative estimate of GFR is in question. Functional assessment with ^{99m}Tc-MAG and ^{99m}Tc-DTPA generally is concordant. However, differences may be noted with glomerular-tubular dissociation in some cases of tubulointerstitial disease. Orthoiodohippurate is about 70% protein bound. Approximately 15–20% of the radiotracer is excreted by glomerular filtration and the remainder by tubular secretion. The use of 131 I-OIH for scintigraphy has been largely abandoned because of the limitations of higher radiation exposure [7] and poor image quality related to a lower administered dose (1/15 that of ^{99m}Tc-MAG3). Radiation exposure with 123 I-labeled OIH is lower, and better images can be obtained using larger amounts of the radiotracer. However, this radiopharmaceutical is expensive and not readily available. The extraction fraction of OIH, while not optimum (since it is not completely extracted by the kidneys), is the highest among the radiopharmaceuticals in use today. Therefore, it can be used for the quantification of renal blood flow.

7.2.2 Slowly Excreted Radiopharmaceuticals

The slowly excreted radiopharmaceuticals include ^{99m}Tc-dimercaptosuccinic acid (DMSA) and ^{99m}Tc-glucoheptonate. Prolonged cortical retention of these radiopharmaceuticals allows the assessment of parenchymal morphology. Since accumulation occurs only in functioning tubules, uptake can be quantified to accurately assess the differential renal function [2, 4]. The preferred agent, Technetium-99 m-DMSA, is 90% protein bound and accumulates in functioning tubules. Since very little of the radiotracer is excreted, interference from collecting system activity, particularly on delayed images, is minimal. A total of about 40% of the administered amount is accumulated in the renal cortex.

7.3 Renal Scintigraphy

According to the types of renal radiopharmaceuticals, renal scintigraphy can be of dynamic or static nature.

- **Dynamic studies** are obtained using rapidly excreted radiopharmaceuticals, while static studies are obtained utilizing slowly excreted tracers. Dynamic studies start by rapidly acquiring image frames upon injection of the tracer to follow activity passing through the blood vessels until reaching the kidneys to evaluate the blood flow. This phase is followed by another series of imaging frames every 10–20 s of the kidneys for approximately 30 min to evaluate the renal functional handling of the radiotracer.
- **Static studies** using slowly secreted radiopharmaceuticals, particularly Tc99m DMSA, are acquired 3 h after intravenous injection of the radiotracer and optionally up to 24 h based on the individual case and the kidney function. These studies are predominantly used to determine the split renal function accurately and in cases of urinary tract infections to evaluate the pathologic changes, including cortical scars.

7.3.1 Principles of Interpretation

7.3.1.1 Dynamic Studies

Assessment of function on dynamic studies is based on several criteria, including initial cortical uptake of the radiotracer, cortical retention, first visualization of the collecting system, and time-to-peak cortical activity. These parameters, however, may be affected by the state of hydration. Prolonged radiotracer uptake, reduced excretion, and cortical retention can be noted in cases of dehydration [8, 9]. An adequate assessment of renal function should include analysis of both the scintigraphic images and the time–activity curves.

7.3.1.1.1 Cortical Uptake

The first minute after radiotracer administration represents the vascular delivery phase. The next 2 min constitutes the parenchymal phase. Uptake in the kidney during this interval (between 1 and 3 min after radiotracer injection) is proportional to its function, using either tubular or glomerular agents.

7.3.1.1.2 Cortical Retention

The cortical retention of the radiotracer, quantified by expressing renal counts at 20–30 min on the time–activity curve as a percentage of the peak uptake, is a measure of the rapidity with which the kidney excretes the radiotracer. As renal function deteriorates, the percentage of retained radiotracer increases. This index can help monitor patients with renal transplants or assess renovascular hypertension [10]. An apparent increase in retention may occur with urine stasis in the collecting system.

7.3.1.1.3 First Visualization of Collecting System

The interval between radiotracer administration and excretion of activity into the collecting system (pelvis and/or calyces) is a measure of *cortical* function. This interval is obtained from the sequential images. The delayed appearance of the collecting system is associated with impaired function.

7.3.1.1.4 Time to Peak

This parameter is easily measured from the time–activity curve. However, an accurate estimate may not be possible in the absence of a peak, which is often the case in significant renal dysfunction. Prolonged values for the time to peak can be seen in physiologic retention of the tracer in the renal calyces or pelvis [11].

7.3.1.2 Static Studies

Scintigraphy with ^{99m}Tc-DMSA and ^{99m}Tc-glucoheptonate is done between 3 and 24 h after radiotracer administration. It is usually used to detect renal parenchymal defects associated with pyelonephritis, scars, and infarcts. Since only functioning tubular cells accumulate these radiopharmaceuticals, the total renal uptake is a measure of individual renal function. Relative renal function can also be measured as with the rapidly excreted radiopharmaceuticals.

7.4 Major Relevant Genitourinary Diseases

7.4.1 Renovascular Hypertension (RVH)

Approximately 5% of hypertension is renovascular in origin. It accounts for about 5.4% as a cause of secondary hypertension in adults [12–14]. Renal artery stenosis is generally due to atherosclerotic plaques or fibromuscular dysplasia, the latter occurring in younger individuals. Significant stenosis that would trigger the activation of the renin–angiotensin system and lead to the development of renovascular hypertension has been defined as a reduction in intraluminal diameter by 50% or greater. However, the degree of anatomically defined renal artery stenosis does not always correlate with the presence of renovascular hypertension.

7.4.1.1 Pathophysiology

The renin–angiotensin system serves as maintenance of systemic blood pressure in such conditions as hypotension and shock. However, with significant renal artery stenosis, the renin–angiotensin system limits a fall in GFR but causes systemic (renovascular) hypertension. Systemic blood pressure is maintained primarily by the increase in vascular tone and sodium and water retention. At the same time, a sharp reduction in GFR is prevented by the increase in the glomerular capillary hydrostatic pressure.

Glomerular capillary hydrostatic pressure is modulated by the tone of the afferent and efferent glomerular arterioles. Increased tone in the efferent arteriole or decreased tone (increased flow) in the afferent arteriole raises capillary hydrostatic pressure and GFR. In contrast, the decreased tone in the efferent arteriole or increased tone (decreased flow) in the afferent arteriole lowers GFR.

The first step in the activation of the renin–angiotensin system is the release of *renin* by the renal JG cells by several mechanisms through [15, 16] (1) signals from *baroreceptors* ("stretch" receptors) in the afferent arteriole modulated by prostaglandins, (2) chemoreceptor signals from the *macula densa* (located in the initial portion of the distal tubule) related to decreased sodium and chloride in the distal tubule and modulated by prostaglandins and adenosine, and (3) increased *sympathetic activity* due to activation of systemic cardiopulmonary and carotid sinus baroreceptors by hypotension.

Renin released due to these stimuli converts circulating *angiotensinogen*, an alpha$_2$ globulin produced by the liver, to *angiotensin I*, a decapeptide. Angiotensin I is then converted to the active octapeptide form, *angiotensin II*, by *angiotensin-converting enzyme* (ACE), found in vascular endothelium. The bulk of this conversion occurs in the pulmonary vascular bed. Angiotensin II is also produced in the kidney. Angiotensin II is a powerful vasoconstrictor that raises systemic blood pressure primarily by increasing vascular tone and stimulating the synthesis and secretion of aldosterone from the zona glomerulosa of the adrenal cortex, which promotes sodium and water reabsorption from the renal tubules.

The intrarenal effects of angiotensin II help counter a fall in GFR due to decreased afferent arteriolar and glomerular capillary hydrostatic pressure [15–18]. First, angiotensin II raises GFR by preferential constriction of the efferent glomerular arteriole. Second, angiotensin II increases tubular reabsorption of sodium and water directly and indirectly (increased tone in

efferent arteriole decreases hydrostatic pressure in peritubular capillaries with a resultant increase in sodium and water reabsorption). GFR remains unchanged in the contralateral normal kidney in unilateral renal artery stenosis because the increased efferent arteriolar tone is offset by an increase in afferent arteriolar tone in response to higher systemic blood pressure. The effects of angiotensin II eventually lead to inhibition of renin release. In unilateral renovascular disease, sodium retention is offset by pressure natriuresis (decreased sodium chloride reabsorption in the proximal tubule) by the normal kidney. The process limits the expansion in blood volume, so the pressure in the afferent arteriole of the stenotic kidney remains low. In bilateral renovascular disease, however, blood volume expansion may be sufficient to increase afferent arteriolar pressure and decrease (but not necessarily normalize) renin secretion. Angiotensin II also has a direct inhibitory effect on the JG cells.

7.4.1.2 Scintigraphy for RVH

7.4.1.2.1 Basis
The scintirenographic diagnosis of renovascular hypertension is based on the demonstration of renal physiology changes following the administration of an ACE inhibitor [19–21]. As noted above, angiotensin II, formed by the activation of the renin–angiotensin system, helps maintain GFR by increasing the tone of the efferent glomerular arteriole, raising the glomerular capillary hydrostatic pressure. These changes are reversed by ACE inhibitors, which block the conversion of angiotensin I to angiotensin II. Consequently, there is a sharp drop in GFR and proximal tubular urine flow.

Decreased GFR and tubular flow after administering an ACE inhibitor will decrease uptake and prolonged cortical retention of ^{99m}Tc-DTPA. Since renal blood flow generally is not significantly changed, ^{99m}Tc-MAG$_3$ shows only prolonged cortical retention without decreased uptake. Rarely, uptake of ^{99m}Tc-MAG$_3$ may decrease, presumably due to a fall in blood pressure below a critical level required to maintain perfusion in the stenotic kidney. The general principles of ACE inhibitor renography also apply to patients receiving chronic treatment with angiotensin II (AT1) receptor antagonists [22].

7.4.1.2.2   Interpretation

Scintigraphic studies are generally interpreted by comparing a baseline examination with the one performed after the ACE inhibitor administration. Visual analysis of the time–activity curves of both kidneys using a grading system as shown in Fig. 7.3 can be a valuable method to define the degree of suspicion of renal artery stenosis [23]. Both the images and the time–activity curves are evaluated using the traditional parameters of function discussed earlier, and the following changes after ACE inhibition are considered significant for renovascular hypertension [21–24]:

1. Increase in cortical retention by at least 15% or a change ≥ 2 in the renogram grade, i.e., 0 to 2 or 1 to 3.
2. Delay in collecting system visualization by at least 2 min.
3. Decrease in initial cortical uptake by at least 10%.
4. Increase in time to peak by at least 2 min.

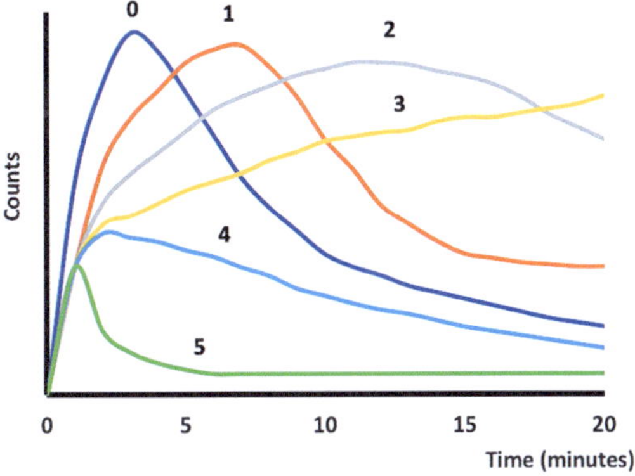

Fig. 7.3 Renographic curve patterns with the grading of suspicion for renovascular hypertension: 0, normal; 1, minor abnormalities; 2, delayed excretion rate with preserved washout phase; 3, delayed excretion rate without washout phase; 4, renal failure pattern with measurable kidney uptake; 5, renal failure pattern without measurable kidney uptake (blood-background type curve). [Adapted from 25]

7.4.1.2.3   Factors Influencing ACE Inhibitor Scintigraphy

ACE inhibitor renography is subject to several variables that may result in false-positive or false-negative studies.

1. Hypotension or a marked change in blood pressure after ACE inhibitor administration is often associated with *bilateral symmetrical* renal retention of the radiotracer.
2. Dehydration with or without diuretics. An additional oral fluid load of 5–10 mL/kg of body weight 30–60 minutes before the procedure is advised to ensure proper hydration [25].
3. Chronic ACE inhibitor therapy may potentially lower scintigraphic sensitivity and should be discontinued before the test. Alternatively, if the ACE inhibitor cannot be discontinued, scintigraphy may be performed while the patient is on therapy. If renal function appears symmetrical, renovascular hypertension is unlikely, and a baseline study need not be done. However, if the function is asymmetrical, the ACE inhibitor should be discontinued before the baseline study.
4. Aspirin and other nonsteroid anti-inflammatory agents such as indomethacin may decrease the sensitivity of the test. These drugs decrease prostaglandin activity and, therefore, indirectly decrease renin–angiotensin activity. This is particularly true with the use of DTPA, and hence MAG_3 is preferred in patients who take nonsteroidal anti-inflammatory drugs [24, 26].
5. Calcium channel blocking drugs are commonly used in renovascular hypertension. Although their effect on GFR is not as pronounced as that of ACE inhibitors, these drugs have been implicated as a cause of false-positive studies [27]. The mechanisms responsible for this finding are not entirely clear. It appears that the effect of angiotensin II on efferent arteriolar constriction requires the presence of extracellular calcium and, therefore, can be attenuated by calcium channel blockers. Perhaps a marked decrease in GFR resulting from the combined effect of calcium channel blockers and captopril may explain the above findings.

7.4.2 Urine Outflow Obstruction

Urinary tract obstruction may be complete or partial, and it may occur at various locations, including the ureteropelvic junction (UPJ), ureterovesical junction (UVJ), and bladder outlet. The clinical consequences are quite dramatic and predictable in an acute and complete obstruction, but not in a partial and chronic one, exemplified by UPJ obstruction in children. Chronic UPJ obstruction, however, may eventually lead to renal cortical atrophy.

Hydronephrosis may be due to obstruction or non-obstructive conditions such as vesicoureteral reflux, urinary tract infection, and congenital dysmorphism. It may be temporary with spontaneous resolution in infants and young children, intermittent, or progressive with eventual stabilization.

7.4.2.1 Diuretic Renography

Furosemide, used for the scintigraphic evaluation of urine outflow for diagnosis of urinary tract obstruction, and other loop diuretics block the reabsorption of sodium, chloride, and potassium in the thick ascending limb of the loop of Henle. Increased tubular sodium decreases water reabsorption by an osmotic effect. Additionally, decreased sodium reabsorption into the medullary interstitium reduces its osmolarity, which in turn reduces water reabsorption from the collecting tubules.

Diuretic renography is based on the principle that increased urine flow resulting after furosemide administration causes rapid "washout" of radiotracer from the unobstructed collecting system (Fig. 7.4), but delayed washout is noted if obstruction is present (Fig. 7.5). While furo-

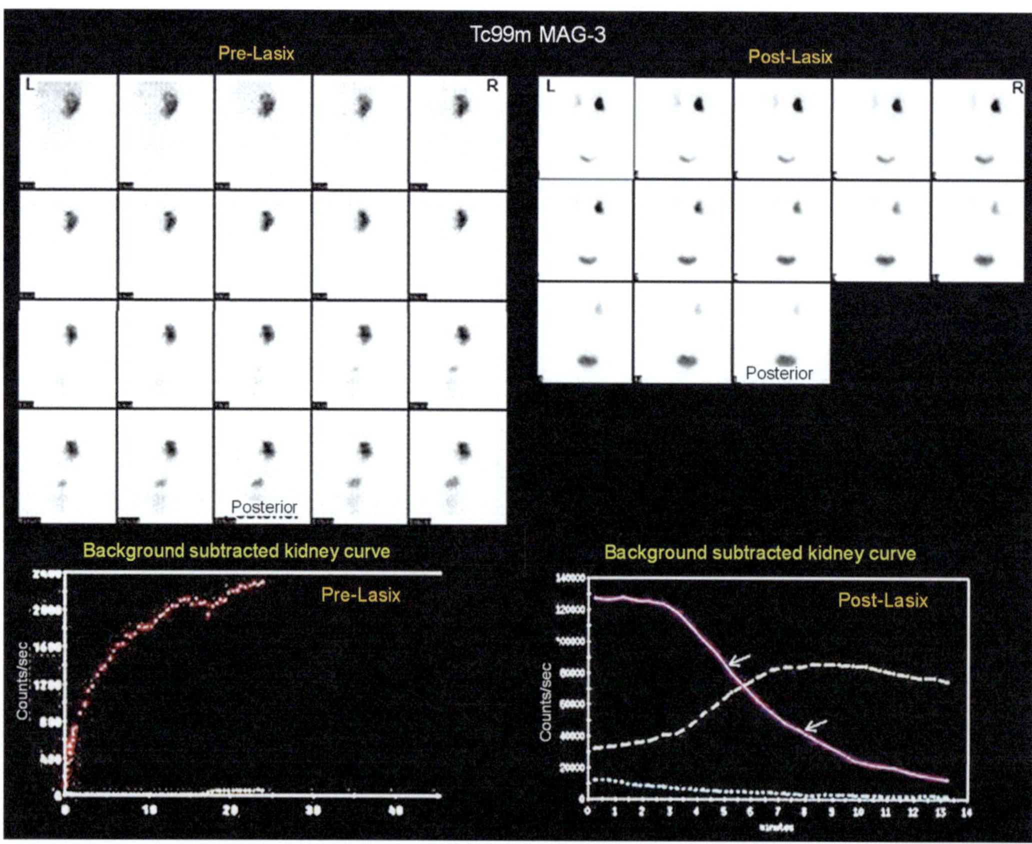

Fig. 7.4 A radionuclide diuretic renography study is illustrating hold-up activity in the right functioning kidney by the end of the pre-Lasix study with rapid washout on post Lasix study, which is clearly illustrated on the time-activity curve (*arrows*). These exemplify the non-obstructed pattern

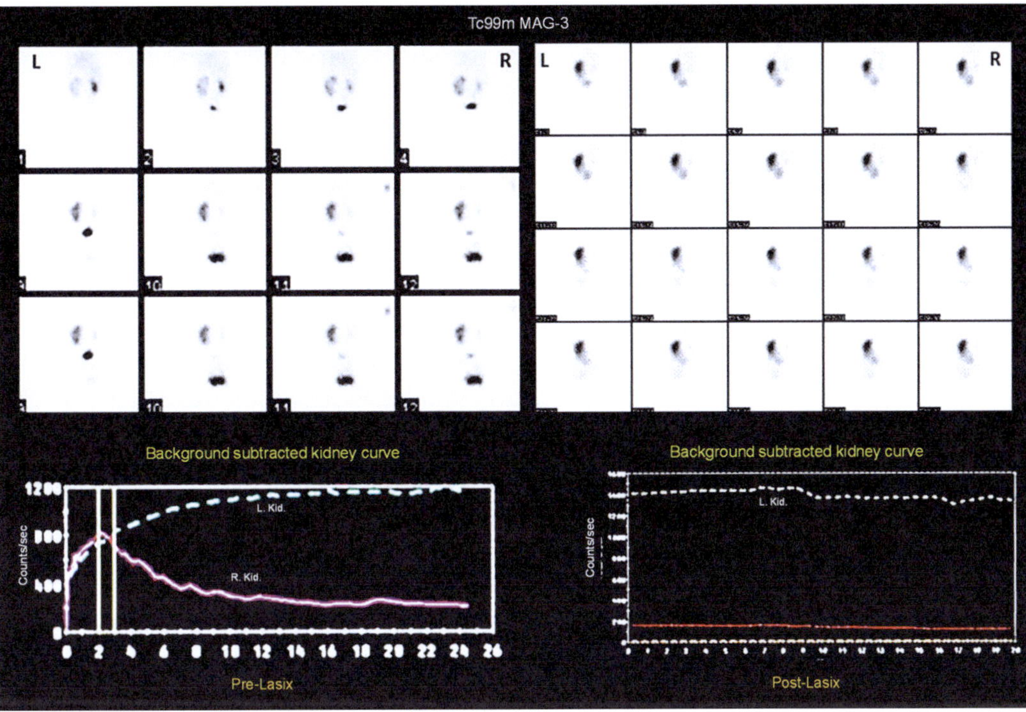

Fig. 7.5 A diuretic renography study in an adult patient illustrating obstructive pattern on the left side. Note the left kidney time activity curve, which shows no clearance before Lasix and no response to Lasix

semide generally is administered intravenously after filling the pelvicalyceal system, administration at the time of or before radiotracer administration has also been used. The standard adult dose of furosemide is 0.5 mg/kg or 40 mg, producing maximal diuresis within 3–6 minutes in patients with normal renal function [28–31]. A higher dose of furosemide may be required in patients with impaired renal function to achieve an adequate diuretic response [32]. The washout half-time following diuretic injection is determined from the time–activity curve. A half-time of 10 min or less is considered normal, 10–20 min equivocal, and more than 20 min abnormal. However, over-reliance on the washout half-time may not be justified because many factors may influence the diuretic renogram, including renal dysfunction, dehydration, inadequate furosemide dosage, atonic pelvis (redundant tissue).

Some steps may be taken to optimize the radionuclide evaluation of urinary tract obstruction. Since renal function preservation is the overriding concern, it has been suggested that renal cortical function evaluation should be the primary focus of scintigraphic assessment. Additionally, since renal impairment or its progression is unpredictable, a single study in the infant with UPJ obstruction is of limited value. Instead, *periodic scintigraphic assessments* at intervals of 3 months are more desirable. Undue reliance on a single post-diuresis washout half-time also appears unwarranted for the reasons noted earlier. If the methodology is standardized, periodic evaluation for functional assessment may improve the predictive ability of the washout parameter as well. An increasing washout time probably is more meaningful than a single "positive" study [28].

7.4.3   Urinary Tract Infection

7.4.3.1 Pathophysiology

Urinary tract infections (UTIs) are particularly important in the pediatric age group as it is one of the most common diseases in children. UTIs' overall incidence in children ranges between 1.5% and 2% [29–31]. In the neonatal period, UTIs are relatively rare and are usually caused by bacteria from the bloodstream. The incidence in newborns is higher for boys, while girls are affected (1%) more than boys (0.3%) between the ages of 1 and 5 years [29–31]. The incidence increases up to 5% among girls of school age. The most common age for UTIs in girls is 7–11 years, resulting from bacterial infection—usually a pathogenic strain of *Escherichia coli*—ascending the urethra.

Many predisposing factors affect the incidence and the severity of the disease in different age groups. These factors include individual susceptibility, bacterial virulence, and the host's anatomical abnormalities such as the presence of vesicoureteral reflux (VUR), obstruction, stasis, or stones (Table 7.1). However, UTIs may also occur in healthy children with an anatomically normal urinary tract. Individual susceptibility may be variable and can be related to familial or hereditary factors.

Chronic pyelonephritis is a result of recurrent or untreated acute pyelonephritis. It occurs almost exclusively in patients with major anatomic anomalies, including urinary tract obstruction, renal dysplasia, or, most commonly, vesicoureteral reflux (VUR) in young children.

Table 7.1 Factors predisposing to and affecting the severity of UTI in children

Individual susceptibility
Bacterial virulence
High-grade vesicoureteral reflux
Obstruction and stasis
Hydronephrosis with or without pelvic ureteric junction obstruction
Horseshoe kidney
Crossed renal ectopia
Renal duplication with ectopic ureters
Urethral polyps or diverticula
Posterior urethral valves or ureterocele
Lack of circumcision (boys)
Sexual activity (girls)
Indwelling urinary catheter
Trauma to the urinary tract
Diabetes

Although pseudomonas infection is common in UTIs following reflux, particularly the severe cases [33], the usual pathogenesis of UTIs is the proliferation of E. coli in the colon. This bacterial proliferation allows the movement of the bacteria into the periurethral mucosa. To be able to multiply, bacteria that reach the urinary tract must overcome the tendency to be washed away by urine flow and bladder voiding. Accordingly, prolonged intervals between voiding, increased storage pressure, or significant residual urine volume favor bacteria's growth and allowed even relatively nonpathogenic bacteria to cause significant infections. Vaginal filling secondary to high voiding velocity and turbulent urine flow related to a dysfunctional voiding pattern is an important factor in bacterial contamination and urinary infections in girls [34].

Urinary tract infections are divided into lower and upper infections. Lower UTI or infection of the bladder (cystitis) results in mucosal inflammation and congestion, which causes hyperactivity of the detrusor muscle and decreases the bladder capacity [35]. This also can lead to urine reflux up the ureter. This reflux can send bacteria to the kidney, leading to acute or chronic pyelonephritis, which may cause renal abscesses or scarring. Acute pyelonephritis requires more vigorous treatment than lower urinary tract infection and, if left untreated, can lead to scarring and renal insufficiency. Consequently, identifying renal involvement is critical in children with suspected urinary tract infection and parenchymal scintigraphy with the tubular agent, Tc-99 m-dimercaptosuccinic acid (DMSA), can play an important role in their diagnostic evaluation.

Ascending infection from the lower urinary tract is the usual cause of pyelonephritis (Fig. 7.6). The infection appears to originate in the urethra or the vaginal introitus, colonized by enteric flora, predominantly *Escherichia coli*. It is more common in females, presumably due to their shorter urethra. The ascending infection eventually reaches the renal calyces, from which micro-organisms enter the parenchyma through the papillae by intrarenal reflux.

Severe long-term sequelae, such as hypertension and renal failure, may develop if urinary

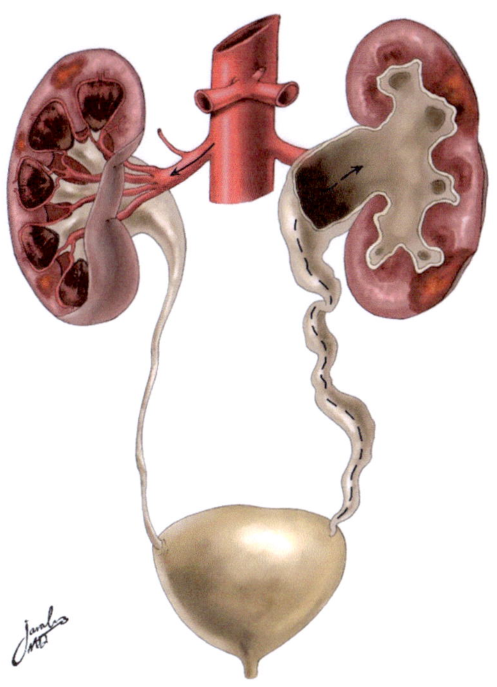

Fig. 7.6 A Diagram illustrating the routes of inducing urinary tract infection. The *left-hand side* represents the hematogenous route, while the *right-hand side* represents the retrograde route such as with vesicoureteral reflux

infection leads to acute pyelonephritis and subsequently to renal scarring. The pathophysiology of renal scarring is still obscure. Numerous factors may contribute to tissue damage following acute infection. It was found that patients with increased transforming growth factor-beta1 (TGF-beta1), a potent proinflammatory and fibrogenic cytokine known to have a key role in regulating the renal tissue fibrosis, may be at higher risk for renal damage following reflux [36].

Nonsecretor status of blood type antigen has also been associated with a higher risk of urinary tract infection (UTI) in women. A study has shown that the nonsecretor status significantly correlated with the presence of focal renal scarring (41% vs. 22% for children with and without scarring, respectively) as determined by Tc99m DMSA renal scan [37].

Scarring of the renal parenchyma is a common cause of hypertension and, if sufficiently extensive, can lead to progressive renal insufficiency and end-stage renal disease. Vesicoureteral reflux, particularly of a higher grade, is frequently associated with scarring.

The upper UTIs cannot be easily differentiated clinically from cystitis based only on symptoms. However, differentiation between upper and lower UTI is important since the former is often associated with renal parenchymal damage. It is particularly difficult in infants, who usually develop nausea, vomiting, diarrhea, or jaundice. In children, fever, frequency, urgency, enuresis or incontinence in a previously dry child, abdominal pain, foul-smelling urine, and sometimes hematuria are the most common clinical presentations. It is estimated that up to 40% of children with UTI are asymptomatic [38].

7.4.3.2 UTI Scintigraphy

Imaging strategies in pediatric urinary tract infections are controversial. The recent literature illustrates the complementary roles of ultrasound, computed tomography (CT), and nuclear medicine [39–41].

Imaging renal parenchyma with ^{99m}Tc-DMSA offers a simple and accurate method for detecting acute pyelonephritis in a child with urinary tract infection. ^{99m}Tc-DMSA localizes in functioning proximal tubular cells and is not excreted in significant amounts. Imaging at 3–24 h after radiopharmaceutical administration reveals primarily cortical uptake without interfering activity in the collecting system. A cortical defect due to pyelonephritis is characterized by the preservation of renal contour, whereas scarring (from a previous infection) typically results in organ volume contraction (Fig. 7.7).

In addition to imaging during the acute phase of the disease, follow-up studies are done to confirm the resolution of the pyelonephritic defect(s) and the absence of cortical scarring. Patients with scars are followed periodically with imaging and relative function measurements to assess for progressive renal insufficiency.

The importance of tc99m DMSA for patients with urinary tract infections for initial evaluation and follow-up of children with UTI was re-emphasized by many studies [42–45].

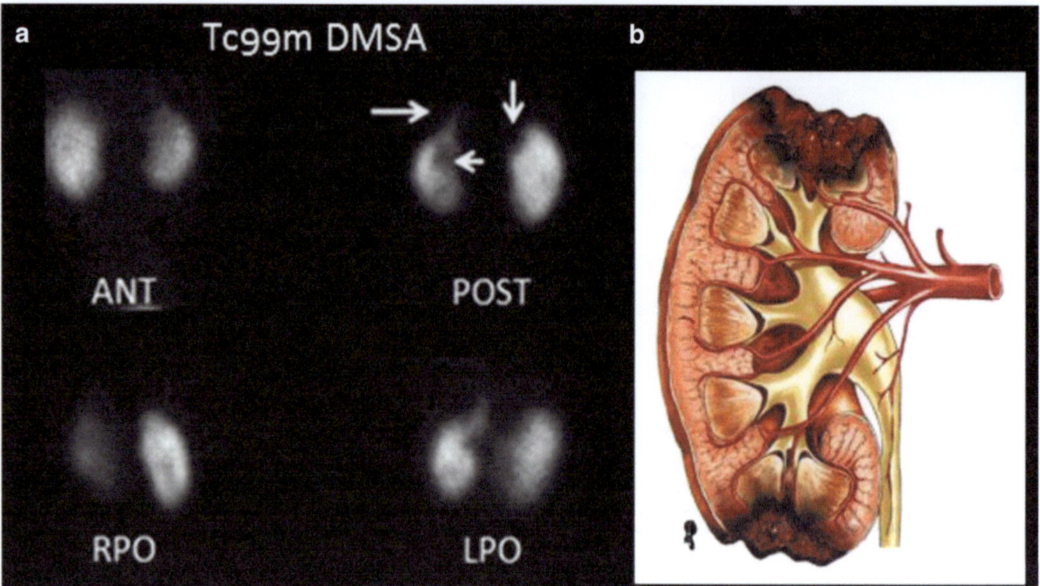

Fig. 7.7 Tc99m DMSA (**a**) study demonstrating bilateral upper pole defects and a mid-left kidney defect (arrows). A diagram (**b**) illustrates how scars affect the kidney contour

Ultrasonography is recommended by newer guidelines to be used more than before; spiral CT and magnetic resonance imaging (MRI) are other modalities that may help evaluate pyelonephritis [40, 41].

7.4.4 Renal Transplantation Complications

Renal transplantation surgery has shown significant improvement in graft survival and an increase in the number of transplantations. Graft survival is best when the donor is an HLA-identical sibling and better for living-related than cadaver donors with similar HLA matches. Other factors, including harvesting and transplantation technique, cold ischemia time (between harvest and transplantation), donor/recipient age, recurrence of primary renal disease, and race, also play an important role in graft survival. Several complications, surgical and/or medical (Table 7.2), occur following transplantation and need to be detected and evaluated to avoid graft failure and outcome.

Table 7.2 Renal Transplantation Complications

Surgical complications
Urine extravasation, ureteral obstruction
Hematoma, lymphocele
Renal artery stenosis
Medical complications
Acute tubular necrosis
Rejection
Antibody-mediated rejection
Hyperacute rejection
Accelerated acute rejection
Acute/active rejection
Chronic/sclerosing allograft nephropathy
Nephrotoxicity of drugs

7.4.4.1 Surgical Complications

7.4.4.1.1 Urine Extravasation, Ureteral Obstruction

Extravasation of urine ("urinoma") may result from ischemic injury related to devascularization during harvesting or leakage at the ureterovesical anastomosis. It may predispose to infection and therefore requires a timely diagnosis. While routine renal scintigraphy performed after transplantation may detect urine extravasation, it is often used to confirm a leak suspected clinically or sonographically. The scintigraphic appearance is an area of increased radiotracer activity, although such increase may not be apparent for up to 2–3 h after radiotracer administration in some instances.

Ureteral obstruction is thought to be usually due to ischemia or postischemic scarring. Extrinsic compression by a lymphocele or hematoma is another cause. If needed, dilatation of the ureter or stent placement/reoperation may be done. Scintigraphy, with the aid of furosemide-induced diuresis in some cases, maybe helpful in the diagnosis and post-treatment evaluation of this condition.

7.4.4.1.2 Hematoma, Lymphocele

Hematomas are generally perinephric or intravesical in location. Scintigraphy can be positive, demonstrating a photopenic region, i.e., with activity less than the background. Hematomas are usually self-limited.

Lymphoceles are extrarenal collections of lymphatic fluid from the kidney, occurring most frequently about 2–3 months after transplantation. They may be exacerbated by rejection, which increases renal lymph flow. Most lymphoceles are inconsequential, though some may be associated with ureteral compression, as noted earlier, or iliac vein compression resulting in lower extremity edema. Treatment consists of sclerotherapy, drainage, or the creation of a peritoneal window. The characteristic scintigraphic finding with lymphoceles is a perinephric photopenic region, which is easier to visualize if a high-intensity image is obtained at the end of the study to accentuate the body background. However, it should be noted that lymphoceles occasionally may become isointense with the background or exceed background activity on later images.

7.4.4.1.3 Renal Artery Stenosis

Hypertension is usually due to pathology in the native kidneys, transplant rejection, or cyclosporine/tacrolimus treatment, and, less frequently, renal artery stenosis. The stricture is generally at the anastomotic site or distal to it. The patho-

physiological consequences of renal artery stenosis in the transplanted kidney are somewhat different from unilateral stenosis in patients with two kidneys. In the latter, the elimination of sodium is decreased on the stenosed side, but increased sodium excretion by the normal kidney helps keep the blood volume from increasing. In a transplanted kidney with renal artery stenosis, a normal kidney is not available to eliminate excess sodium. Therefore, depending on the level of salt intake, the initial renin-dependent hypertension develops into volume-dependent hypertension. Consequently, the fall in GFR in response to an ACE inhibitor may be less than expected and inapparent on the scintigraphic study. However, most of these patients are on diuretics and/or a salt-restricted diet, which will help to limit the rise in blood volume.

7.4.4.2 Medical Complications

7.4.4.2.1 Acute Tubular Necrosis

Acute tubular necrosis (ATN), characterized by ischemic necrosis of the tubular epithelial cells and decreased GFR, is frequently associated with cadaver renal transplants. Possible causes are hypotension/hypovolemia in the donor and the prolonged interval between harvest and transplantation. Urine output usually starts to decrease within the first 24 h or so and improves spontaneously after a few days, although ATN may occasionally last a few weeks. It is often difficult to make a clinical distinction between ATN and rejection in the post-transplantation period. A clear scintigraphic distinction between these two conditions also has remained elusive for two reasons. First, the scintigraphic diagnosis of ATN rests on the premise that graft perfusion is preserved despite decreasing function (Fig. 7.8), in contrast to rejection, where both perfusion and function decrease in parallel (Fig. 7.9). However, depending on the severity/stage of ATN, graft perfusion may vary. Second, ATN and acute rejection may coexist. From a clinical standpoint, a cadaver transplant with impaired function is assumed to have ATN. An aggressive search/treatment for rejection is initiated if the expected recovery in graft function

Fig. 7.8 Acute tubular necrosis following renal transplantation. The perfusion (**a**) is preserved, while on sequential iamges (**b**), the function is decreased with parenchymal retention as noted on the time-activity curve (**c**)

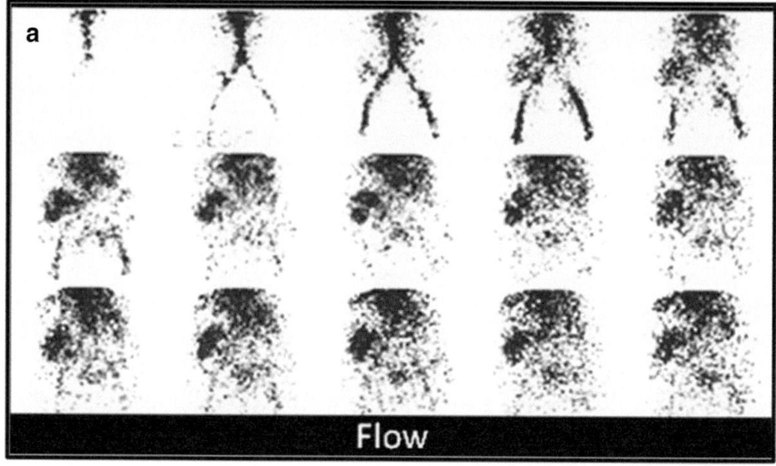

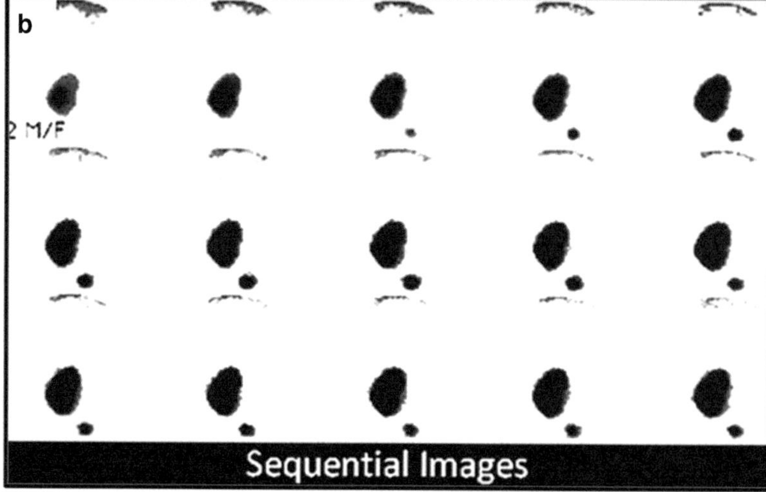

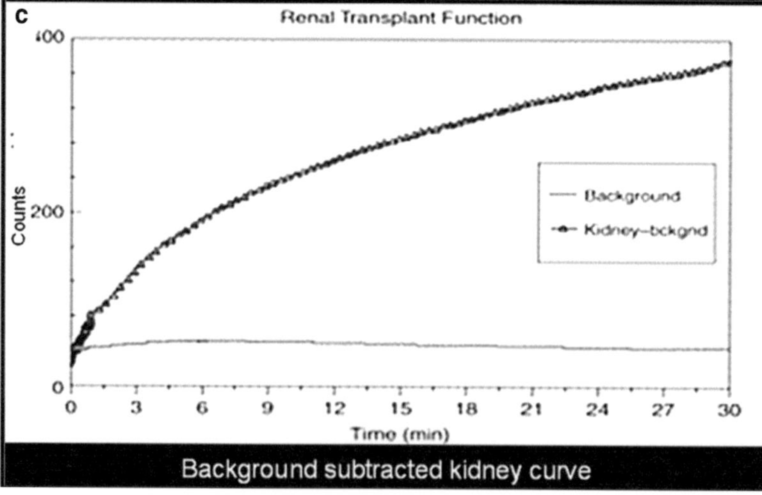

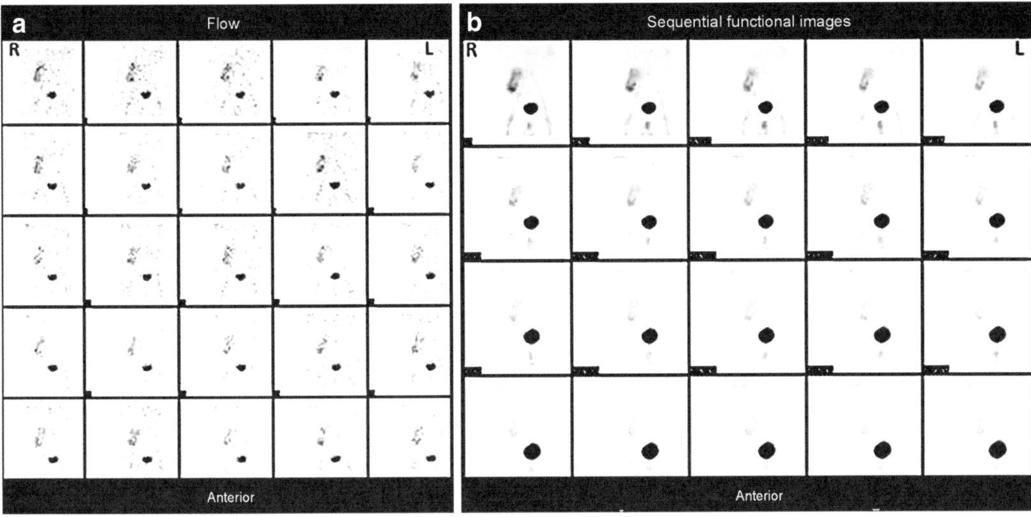

Fig. 7.9 Tc 99 m MAG-3 study for a patient with renal transplantation showing decreased perfusion (**a**) and function (**b**) of the graft illustrating the scintigraphic findings of rejection

fails to occur. Such recovery can best be ascertained by serial scintigraphy, a sensitive measure of graft function, although the two may be indistinguishable.

7.4.4.2.2   Rejection

The histopathological criteria for the diagnosis and classification of rejection have improved significantly in recent years and continue to evolve [46–48]. From a large body of literature, a consensus referred to as the *Banff Classification* has emerged. The new classification shifts the focus from diagnosis of rejection to prognosis to facilitate patient management. The distinction is made between rejection with *tubulointerstitial* changes, milder disease, and rejection with *vasculitis*, where the outcome is poorer. The types of rejection are discussed below.

1. Antibody-mediated rejection:

    Two types of antibody-mediated rejection are described, immediate or hyperacute and delayed or accelerated acute. *Hyperacute rejection* is caused by preformed anti-donor antibodies and is characterized by intense vasculitis, fibrin-platelet thrombi, and infarction of the renal cortex, with graft loss. Rejection may begin within minutes or hours and is usually apparent during surgery. Scintigraphy shows a *photopenic* region corresponding to the avascular graft. Fortunately, hyperacute rejection is rare nowadays and largely preventable by appropriate screening tests.

    Accelerated acute rejection may be considered a "slow" variant of hyperacute rejection, mediated primarily by anti-donor antibodies. It usually occurs on the second or third day following transplantation, after allograft function has been established. Clinical manifestations include fever, pain, swelling, tenderness in the transplant region, hypertension, oliguria, or anuria. Scintigraphy generally shows poor radiotracer uptake in the graft.

2. Acute/active rejection:

    Acute rejection is the most frequent type of rejection confronting the nuclear medicine physician. It is most common in the first 4 weeks following transplantation but may occur at any time between 3 days and 10 or more years. Clinical findings generally are not as dramatic as in accelerated rejection. Acute rejection is predominantly a cell-mediated process with mononuclear cell infiltration and tubulitis, although the more severe forms are associated with a humoral component with various degrees of vasculitis. Accordingly, the Banff system grades acute rejection from I to III, with subdivisions for the severity of changes. The lowest grade represents interstitial infiltration and moderate tubulitis, while the highest grade is associated with transmural arteritis and/or arterial fibrinoid change and necrosis of medial smooth muscle cells.

3. Chronic/sclerosing allograft nephropathy:

This type generally occurs 6 months to years after transplantation. It may be related to many causes, including chronic rejection, hypertension, infectious/noninfectious inflammatory process, and medications' effects (see below). If present, rejection may respond to treatment, though the diagnosis may not be apparent on biopsy. Histopathological changes in the condition also can be graded, depending on the severity of interstitial fibrosis and tubular atrophy.

7.4.4.2.3 Nephrotoxicity of Drugs

Cyclosporine and, more recently, tacrolimus (FK506) have been used routinely as immunosuppressive agents. Clinically, nephrotoxicity resulting from these drugs may be difficult to distinguish from rejection, and the conditions may be superimposed. Toxicity is generally associated with elevated blood levels of the drug, improving after dose reduction. Histopathological findings of microvascular injury, with fibrin thrombi in the glomerular arterioles and capillaries, have been noted but, unfortunately, are not diagnostic for cyclosporine or tacrolimus toxicity [49–51].

7.4.5 Vesicoureteral Reflux

7.4.5.1 Pathophysiology

VUR is the retrograde flow of the urine from the bladder into the ureter. Normally, urine is propelled from the kidney to the urinary bladder through the ureter in only one direction. The valvular role of the ureterovesical junction depends on the anatomical relationship between the ureter and the bladder. The ureter follows a retroperitoneal course from the kidney to the bladder. After penetrating the bladder wall, the ureter is securely anchored to

it throughout its entire transmural course. A specific arrangement serves to maintain a competent one-way valve at the ureterovesical junction with a mechanism that is best described as a flap valve.

VUR allows the infected urine to be repeatedly returned to the kidneys from the bladder, and the reflux drains back into the bladder at the end of each voiding. Pyelonephritis, especially in children younger than 3 years, is often a result of combined reflux and infection. VUR occurs more frequently in girls by a ratio of 10:1, and the incidence is approximately 1 in 1000 children. Reflux may be unilateral or bilateral and is commonly classified by the international radiologic grading system (Table 7.3). The international radiologic grading includes five grades using detailed anatomy, such as the characterization of the fornices that are impossible to achieve by scintigraphic studies. Accordingly, a more simplified scintigraphic grading attempt classifies reflux into three grades (Table 7.4 and Fig. 7.10) grades: mild (I), moderate (II), and severe(III) [52].

The flap mechanism of the ureterovesical junction depends on several anatomical relationships and physiological parameters. Any condition that alters these relationships can lead to reflux. Examples include abnormal obliquity of the ureter during its intramural course, conditions that weaken the bladder's muscular support to the ureter, and sphincter dyssynergia. VUR may be primary or secondary [53].

Primary reflux results from a congenitally abnormal or ectopic insertion of the ureter into

Table 7.3 Radiologic grading of vesicoureteral reflux

I Reflux into a non-dilated ureter
II Reflux into the upper collecting system without dilatation
III Reflux into mildly dilated ureter and pelvicalyceal system
IV Reflux into a grossly dilated ureter and pelvicalyceal system
V Massive reflux with marked ureteral dilatation and tortuosity and marked dilatation of the pelvicalyceal system

Table 7.4 Scintigraphic grading of vesicoureteral reflux

Grade I Reflux into the ureter
Grade II Reflux into the pelvicalyceal system
Grade III Reflux into the pelvicalyceal system with apparently dilated pelvis or both pelvises and ureters

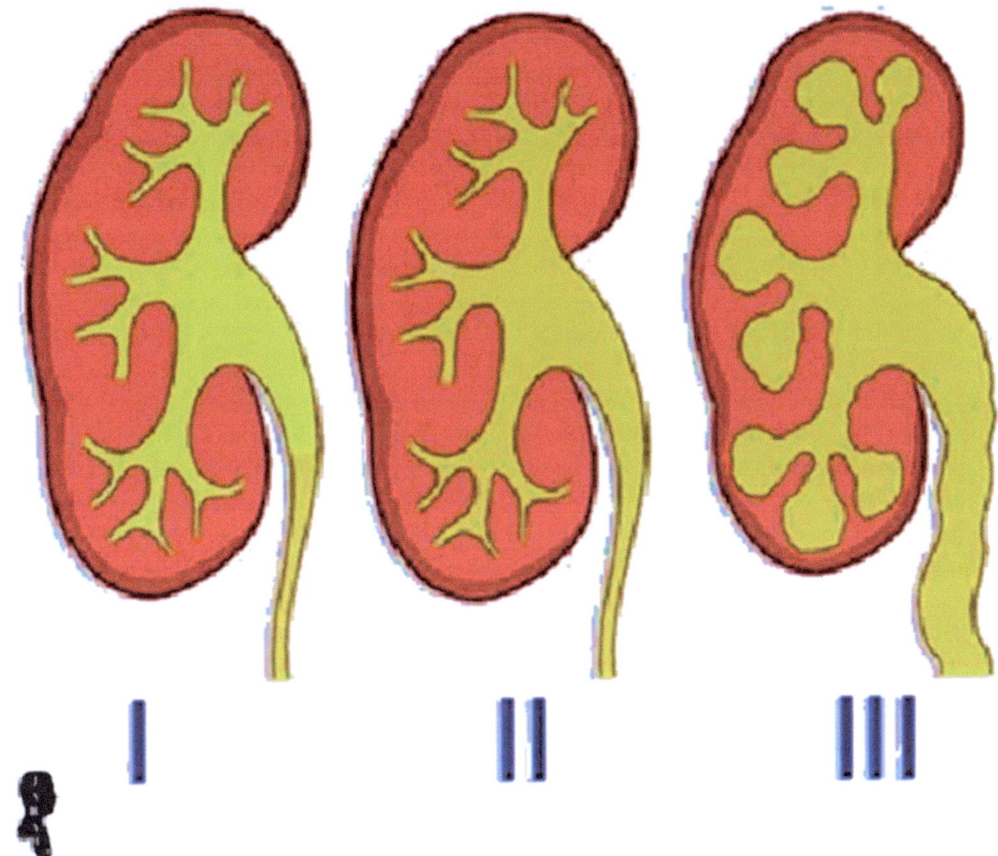

Fig. 7.10   Grades of vesicoureteral reflux used for radionuclide studies

the bladder. Occasionally, the condition is hereditary [54]. Siblings of patients with vesicoureteral reflux (VUR) are at greater risk of reflux than the general population, and screening in this group is widely accepted. In a recent study, at 48 months after diagnosis, 75% of mild reflux cases (I–III) and 37% of severe reflux (IV–V) of prenatally detected primary VUR had resolved, indicating a relatively benign clinical course [55].

Secondary reflux is more serious and may be transient or persistent [35]. It develops in association with infection, malformations of the uretero-vesical junction, increased intravesical pressure, and surgery to the ureterovesical junction.

The interstitial cells of Cajal (ICCs) are pacemaker cells that create and coordinate peristaltic motility. It was recently found that refluxing ureteral endings significantly lack these pacemaker cells, implying a malfunctioning valve mechanism permitting

VUR. Connexin 43 (gap junction protein) immunoreactivity was significantly decreased in all refluxing ureteral specimens, whereas it was homogeneously distributed in normal controls. A substantial decrease in gap junctions in this region adversely affects intercellular signaling, aggravating coordinated peristalsis, which is essential for a competent anti-reflux mechanism [53].

7.4.5.2 Reflux Scintigraphy

Voiding radionuclide cystography is a sensitive procedure for the early detection and monitoring of VUR. Early diagnosis of VUR with subsequent follow-up helps to prevent cortical scarring. It is especially attractive because of its excellent sensitivity and low absorbed radiation dose compared with the radiographic MCUG. It was estimated that its radiation exposure is less than 1/20 of the conventional contrast-enhanced micturating cystourethrogram (MCU) [53]. The sensitivity of indirect voiding urosonography without contrast media and without filling the bladder through a catheter to detect vesicoureteral reflux (VUR) in children is inadequate; its overall sensitivity is only 49% [56].

Approximately 20% of patients with vesicoureteral reflux diagnosed before 6 months of age demonstrated dysfunctional voiding after the age of toilet training [57]. Accordingly, follow-up of patients is important. The duration and methods of follow-up of VYR patients are controversial. Voiding cystography, however, may not be used in certain groups of patients for routine follow-up. For instance, follow-up of uncomplicated ureteral reimplantation in children is usually done by ultrasonography. Additionally, in this group of patients, follow-up for more than 1 year postoperatively is not warranted, and ultrasonography can be eliminated beyond the year [57].

Similarly, ultrasonography is used for screening for siblings of patients with vesicoureteral reflux who are at higher risk than the general population. If ultrasonography is abnormal, the gold-standard test, the radionuclide voiding cystography, is performed [58].

Conversely, follow-up of newborns with prenatally detected VUR might require voiding cystourethrogram (VCUG) and DMSA scan. In a study [59], 58% of such infants had bilateral VUR. Severe reflux (grades IV and V) was more common and present in 54% of infants. Renal damage was detected in 34% of the kidneys on the first renal scan, with a significant correlation between severe reflux and renal damage scars [59].

Generally, voiding cystourethrograms are associated with significant trauma to patients and should not be used routinely according to the recent guidelines. VCUG is indicated if renal and bladder ultrasonography reveals hydronephrosis, scarring, or other findings that would suggest either high-grade vesicoureteral reflux (VUR) or obstructive uropathy, as well as in other atypical or complex clinical circumstances [40, 41].

7.4.6 Testicular Torsion

7.4.6.1 Pathophysiology

Testicular torsion occurs when the spermatic cord is twisted, and it has been argued that the correct term should be spermatic cord torsion [60, 61]. Although various factors may predispose to torsion [62], a narrow mesenteric attachment from the spermatic cord to the testis and epididymis is regarded as the dominant cause, i.e., a slender attachment occurring as a result of a narrowed testicular bare area. This bare area may reach nearly one-third of the testicular circumference, allowing the testis to fall forward within the cavity of the tunica vaginalis and to rotate like a bell-clapper; the intravaginal type of torsion [63].

Other forms of testicular torsion are recognized. In neonates, the gubernaculum is not attached to the scrotal wall, and the testis is susceptible to torsion. This is termed extravaginal torsion, as the entire testis, epididymis, and tunica vaginalis twist in a vertical axis on the spermatic cord. Some vestigial testicular appendages are susceptible to torsion. There are four testicular appendages: the paradidymis (organ of Giraldés), the appendix testis (hydatid of Morgagni), the appendix epididymis, and the vas aberrans of Haller (divided into superior and inferior components). The appendix testis was most consistently present in 92% of autopsies and found to be multiple in 8% [63, 64].

Two factors are critical in testicular torsion: the extent of spermatic cord twist and the torsion duration. The degree of torsion can vary from 90° to three complete turns of the vascular pedicle. Not surprisingly, blood flow may be variably compromised. The initial disruption will be to the venous and lymphatic drainage, rather than to the arterial input of the testis, and venous infarction occurs earlier and at lesser levels of torsion [65].

Experimentally, complete cessation of blood flow to the testis occurs with the spermatic cord twisting 720° [66]. A 450° twist consistently produced no flow and testicular infarction in the normal rabbit testis, whereas a 360° twist resulted in decreased flow [67].

In patients with torsion, a twist between 360° and 720° is found. Experimental studies have shown that testicular infarction begins to appear within 2 h of complete occlusion of the testicular artery [67]; irreversible ischemia occurs after 6 h [68–70], and complete infarction is established by 24 h.

With complete vascular occlusion, the testis appears grossly swollen and hemorrhagic. Microscopically, the picture is that of hemorrhagic infarction. The degree of necrosis depends upon the duration of occlusion. If this has been longer than 10 h, the necrosis of the seminiferous epithelium is usually complete and irreversible. With incomplete occlusion, necrosis may be delayed. Torsion that lasts less than 6 h probably will not cause a testicular infarct. If torsion lasts longer than 24 h, the testis almost certainly will infarct [60, 61]. Although exceedingly rare, testicular torsion can be asynchronously bilateral [71].

The condition may be acute (symptoms last less than 6 weeks) or chronic (more than 3 months). Acute epididymitis is almost always unilateral. Gram-negative bacilli commonly cause acute epididymitis in children or following urinary tract instrumentation. The epididymis is sometimes the site of metastatic infection, such as tuberculosis.

7.4.6.2 Diagnosis

Testicular torsion results in acute pain and ischemia. The most common signs and symptoms include red, swollen scrotum, and acutely painful testicle, often in the absence of trauma. Nausea and vomiting are common. The most common conditions in the differential diagnosis include epididymitis, strangulated inguinal hernia, traumatic hematoma, testicular tumor, or testicular fracture. Physical examination techniques such as scrotal elevation can help differentiate between epididymitis and testicular torsion. However, clinical examination of the scrotum is difficult due to the small size of the testes and the epididymis in infants and young children, and eliciting patients' history is challenging. Epididymitis has been considered uncommon in childhood, but its

frequency has increased among children admitted with acute scrotum diagnosis [72].

The long-term prognosis for a functional, non-atrophied testicle is improved the sooner the torsion is diagnosed and treated. Therefore, confirming the diagnosis and quick management is crucial. Accordingly, imaging of the scrotum in children suspected of having the condition bears great importance [73, 74].

7.4.6.3 Scrotal Imaging

The classification of scrotal disorders in children into three typical clinical manifestations, namely acute scrotal disorders, scrotal masses, and cryptorchidism, is a helpful and practical basis for choosing the most suitable imaging modality available and commonly used modalities. These include sonography, scintigraphy, and magnetic resonance (MR) imaging. Either scintigraphy or sonography may be used as the first imaging study, and both can help distinguish among the disorders to different degrees. Although sonography provides superior anatomic details to scintigraphy, it may not be as accurate as it is thought to diagnose the most serious emergency reason for scrotal pain [74]. Scrotal masses are also best depicted with sonography with MRI as an adjunctive modality. In suspected cryptorchidism with equivocal clinical findings, both sonography and MR imaging are useful, but sonography is usually the initial study [75].

This strategy for imaging for acute scrotal disorders most relevant to nuclear medicine is not uniform and varies between the institutions based on the experience. In most institutions, Doppler ultrasound is used most commonly as the standard imaging technique of choice to confirm the diagnosis in most cases.

7.4.6.4 Scrotal Scintigraphy

Scintigraphy is used when color Doppler is inadequate, the diagnosis remains unclear, or if complications occur during the course of the disease. Radionuclide testicular scintigraphy is also used more commonly after the acute phase of the first 12 hours, and vascular compromise has prolonged [76–78]. Recent studies comparing both modalities indicate similar sensitivity; the two studies may provide complementary information in indeterminate cases [79–81].

A study on 41 boys with suspected testicular torsion scintigraphy and Doppler ultrasound was performed and compared. There was no statistically significant difference in the sensitivity of both modalities. Specificity was 77% for color Doppler US and 97% for scintigraphy ($P = 0.05$). Due to the higher specificity, scintigraphy can help avoid unnecessary surgery when color Doppler US shows equivocal flow [80]. In another two studies of 21 and 37 patients, respectively, scintigraphy was more accurate than Doppler ultrasonography. It also has the advantage of being simple, fast, and accurate but without any detrimental effect on the human body [79, 81].

Findings on a normal scan are symmetrical perfusion with little uptake in the blood pool images. In acute torsion (early), there will be decreased perfusion on flow images, and the blood pool images will show no activity in the affected side (Fig. 7.11).

In missed (late) torsion, there will be a halo of activity surrounding the torsion (a doughnut shape) due to increased perfusion to the surrounding tissue through the pudendal vessels (Fig. 7.12). There will be increased perfusion and hyperemia in acute epididymitis in the affected side (Fig. 7.13) due to vascular changes associated with the inflammation [82].

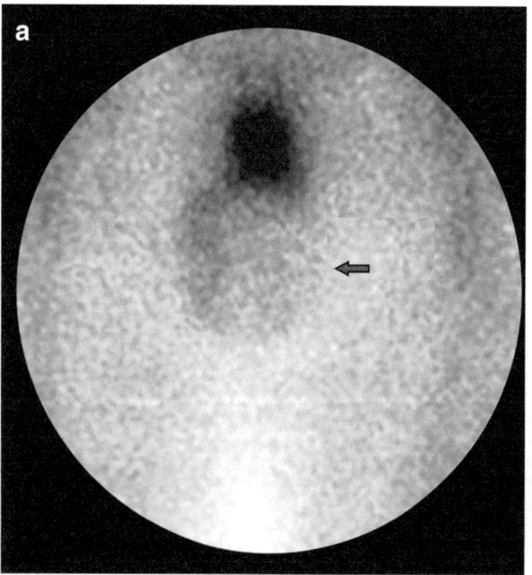

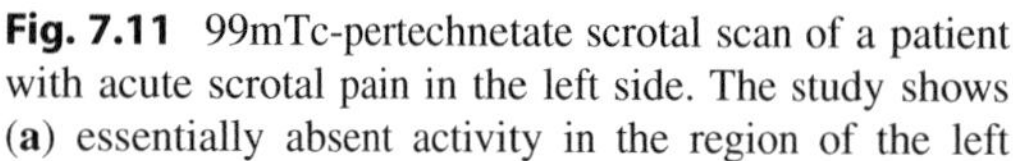

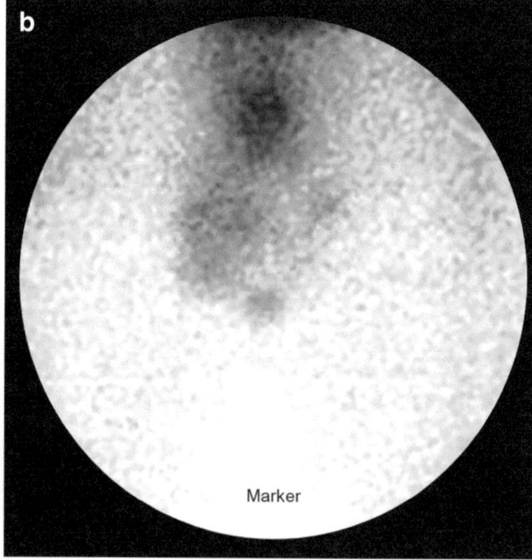

Fig. 7.11 99mTc-pertechnetate scrotal scan of a patient with acute scrotal pain in the left side. The study shows (**a**) essentially absent activity in the region of the left hemi-scrotum corresponding to the left testicle by palpation markers (**b**). This case illustrates a pattern of acute testicular torsion

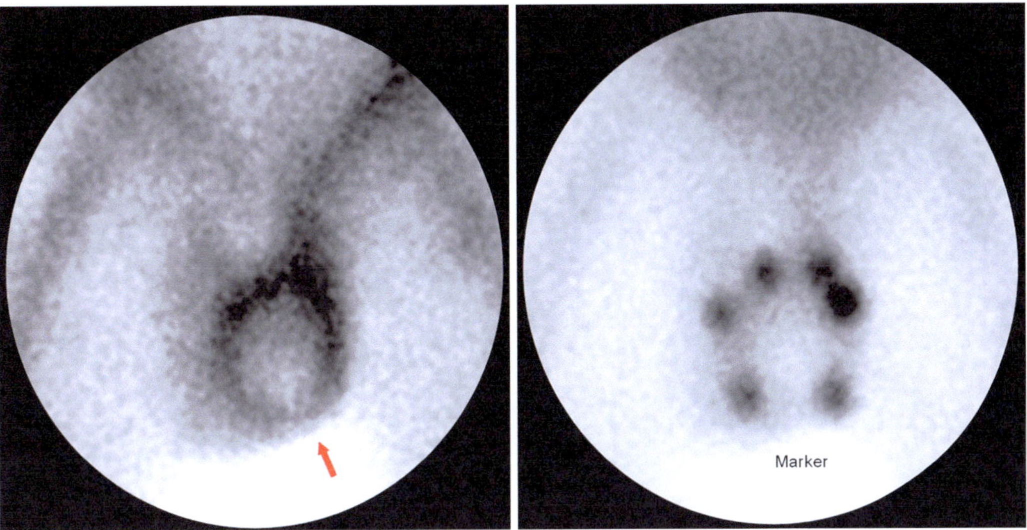

Fig. 7.12 99mTc-pertechnetate testicular imaging study showing the rim of increased uptake around the area of decreased uptake, illustrating the classic pattern of missed torsion of the left testis (arrow)

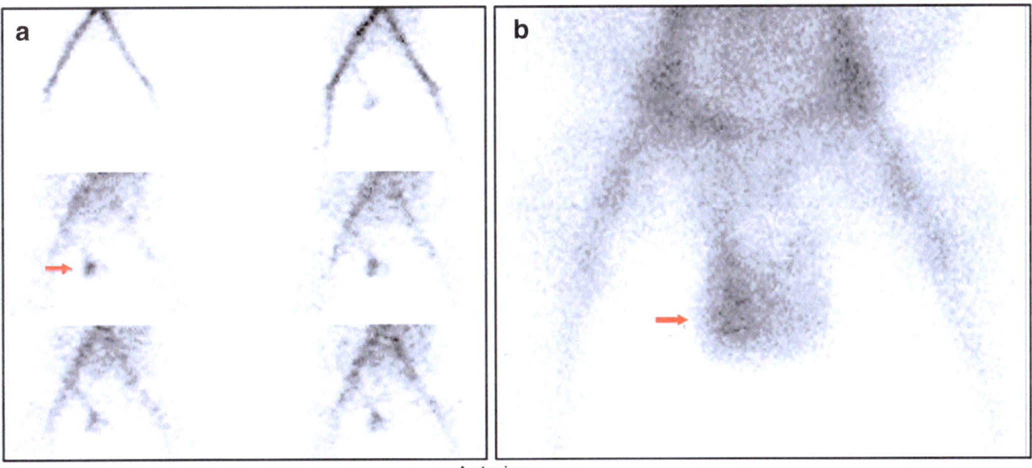

Fig. 7.13 A 14-year-old male was referred for a testicular scan to rule-out testicular torsion. The patient presented with 4 hour-history of right-sided acute testicular pain and swelling. The pain was dull in nature, with no radiation, and was associated with nausea and vomiting. There was no history of fever or any urinary Symptoms. The patient denied any history of trauma. On examination: Temperature was 37.4 C. Left testis was grossly nor-mal, and the right testis was tender and swollen. Lab investigations showed leucocytosis at 14,400. Testicular scan was performed, using l7-mCi Tc-99 m Pertechnetate given äs a bolus intravenous injection. The scan shows increased flow (**a**) and blood pool (**b**) activity in the right hemi-scrotum (arrows) in comparison to the left testis, indicating an inflammatory process in the right hemi-scrotum consistent with right epididymitis

References

1. Field M, Harris D, Pollock C (2010) 5-glomerular filtration and acute kidney injury. In: Field M, Pollock C, Harris D (eds) The renal system, 2nd edn. Churchill Livingstone/Elsevier, pp 57–67

2. Chung AA, Millner PR (2020) Accessory renal artery stenosis and secondary hypertension. Case Rep Nephrol 2020:8879165. https://doi.org/10.1155/2020/8879165

3. Chang A, Laszik ZG (2020) The kidney. In, Robbins pathologic basis of disease, 10th edn WB Saunders Company

4. Eshima D, Fritzberg AR, Taylor A Jr (1990) 99mTc renal tubular function agents: current status. Semin Nucl Med 20(1):28–40. https://doi.org/10.1016/s0001-2998(05)80174-6

5. Blaufox MD (1991) Procedures of choice in renal nuclear medicine. J Nucl Med 32(6):1301–1309

6. Rutland MD (1985) A comprehensive analysis of renal DTPA studies. I. Theory and normal values. Nucl Med Commun 6(1):11–20. https://doi.org/10.1097/00006231-198501000-00003

7. Jafri RA, Britton KE, Nimmon CC, Solanki K, Al-Nahhas A, Bomanji J, Fettich J, Hawkins LA (1988) Technetium-99m MAG3, a comparison with iodine-123 and iodine-131 orthoiodohippurate, in patients with renal disorders. J Nucl Med 29(2):147–158

8. Stabin M, Taylor A Jr, Eshima D, Wooter W (1992) Radiation dosimetry for technetium-99m-MAG3, technetium-99m-DTPA, and iodine-131-OIH based on human biodistribution studies. J Nucl Med 33(1):33–40

9. Raber SA, Schraml FV, Silverman ED (1997) Renal cortical retention of Tc-99m MAG3 in hypertension. Clin Nucl Med 22(3):190–192. https://doi.org/10.1097/00003072-199703000-00016

10. Levey CS, Schraml FV, Abreu SH, Silverman ED (1999) False-positive result of a captopril-enhanced radionuclide renogram in a child secondary to dehydration. Clin Nucl Med 24(1):6–8. https://doi.org/10.1097/00003072-199901000-00002

11. Taylor A Jr, Nally JV (1995) Clinical applications of renal scintigraphy. AJR Am J Roentgenol 164(1):31–41. https://doi.org/10.2214/ajr.164.1.7998566

12. El-Maghraby TA, de Fijter JW, van Eck-Smit BL, Zwinderman AH, El-Haddad SI, Pauwels EK (1998) Renographic indices for evaluation of changes in graft function. Eur J Nucl Med 25(11):1575–1586. https://doi.org/10.1007/s002590050338

13. Olin JW, Piedmonte MR, Young JR, DeAnna S, Grubb M, Childs MB (1995) The utility of duplex ultrasound scanning of the renal arteries for diagnosing significant renal artery stenosis. Ann Intern Med 122(11):833–838. https://doi.org/10.7326/0003-4819-122-11-199506010-00004

14. Chrysochou C, Kalra PA (2009) Epidemiology and natural history of atherosclerotic renovascular disease. Prog Cardiovasc Dis 52(3):184–195. https://doi.org/10.1016/j.pcad.2009.09.001

15. Noilhan C, Barigou M, Bieler L, Amar J, Chamontin B, Bouhanick B (2016) Causes of secondary hypertension in the young population: a monocentric study. Annales de cardiologie et d'angeiologie 65(3):159–164. https://doi.org/10.1016/j.ancard.2016.04.016

16. Safian RD, Textor SC (2001) Renal-artery stenosis. N Engl J Med 344(6):431–442. https://doi.org/10.1056/NEJM200102083440607

17. Martinez-Maldonado M (1991) Pathophysiology of renovascular hypertension. Hypertension (Dallas, Tex : 1979) 17(5):707–719. https://doi.org/10.1161/01.hyp.17.5.707

18. Sparks MA, Crowley SD, Gurley SB, Mirotsou M, Coffman TM (2014) Classical renin-angiotensin system in kidney physiology. Compr Physiol 4(3):1201–1228. https://doi.org/10.1002/cphy.c130040

19. Herrmann SM, Textor SC (2019) Renovascular Hypertension. Endocrinol Metab Clin N Am 48(4):765–778. https://doi.org/10.1016/j.ecl.2019.08.007

20. Fine EJ, Sarkar S (1989) Differential diagnosis and management of renovascular hypertension through nuclear medicine techniques. Semin Nucl Med 19(2):101–115. https://doi.org/10.1016/s0001-2998(89)80005-4

21. Hricik DE, Browning PJ, Kopelman R, Goorno WE, Madias NE, Dzau VJ (1983) Captopril-induced functional renal insufficiency in patients with bilateral renal-artery stenoses or renal-artery stenosis in a solitary kidney. N Engl J Med 308(7):373–376. https://doi.org/10.1056/NEJM198302173080706

22. Blaufox MD, De Palma D, Taylor A, Szabo Z, Prigent A, Samal M, Li Y, Santos A, Testanera G, Tulchinsky M (2018) The SNMMI and EANM practice guideline for renal scintigraphy in adults. Eur J Nucl Med Mol Imaging 45(12):2218–2228. https://doi.org/10.1007/s00259-018-4129-6

23. Picciotto G, Sargiotto A, Petrarulo M, Rabbia C, De Filippi PG, Roccatello D (2003) Reliability of captopril renography in patients under chronic therapy with angiotensin II (AT1) receptor antagonists. J Nucl Med 44(10):1574–1581

24. Fommei E, Ghione S, Hilson AJ, Mezzasalma L, Oei HY, Piepsz A, Volterrani D (1993) Captopril radionuclide test in renovascular hypertension: a European multicentre study. European Multicentre Study Group. Eur J Nucl Med 20(7):617–623. https://doi.org/10.1007/BF00176558

25. Taylor A, Nally J, Aurell M, Blaufox D, Dondi M, Dubovsky E, Fine E, Fommei E, Geyskes G, Granerus G, Kahn D, Morton K, Oei HY, Russell C, Sfakianakis G, Fletcher J (1996) Consensus report on ACE inhibitor renography for detecting renovascular hypertension. Radionuclides in Nephrourology Group.

Consensus group on ACEI renography. J Nucl Med 37(11):1876–1882

26. Mustafa S, Elgazzar AH (2013) Effect of the NSAID diclofenac on 99mTc-MAG3 and 99mTc-DTPA renography. J Nucl Med 54(5):801–806. https://doi.org/10.2967/jnumed.112.109595

27. Ludwig V, Martin WH, Delbeke D (2003) Calcium channel blockers: a potential cause of false-positive captopril renography. Clin Nucl Med 28(2):108–112. https://doi.org/10.1097/01.RLU.0000048679.45832.F3

28. Prigent A, Cosgriff P, Gates GF, Granerus G, Fine EJ, Itoh K, Peters M, Piepsz A, Rehling M, Rutland M, Taylor A Jr (1999) Consensus report on quality control of quantitative measurements of renal function obtained from the renogram: International Consensus Committee from the Scientific Committee of Radionuclides in Nephrourology. Semin Nucl Med 29(2):146–159. https://doi.org/10.1016/s0001-2998(99)80005-1

29. Sarkar SD (1992) Diuretic renography: concepts and controversies. Urol Radiol 14(2):79–84. https://doi.org/10.1007/BF02926908

30. Fine EJ (1999) Interventions in renal scintirenography. Semin Nucl Med 29(2):128–145. https://doi.org/10.1016/s0001-2998(99)80004-x

31. Pohl HG, Rushton HG, Park JS, Belman AB, Majd M (2001) Early diuresis renogram findings predict success following pyeloplasty. J Urol 165(6 Pt 2):2311–2315. https://doi.org/10.1097/00005392-200106001-00024

32. Heyman S (1994) Radionuclide studies of the genitourinary tract. In: Miller J, Gelfand M (eds) Pediatric nuclear imaging. Saunders, Philadelphia, pp 195–211

33. Taylor AT, Brandon DC, de Palma D, Blaufox MD, Durand E, Erbas B, Grant SF, Hilson A, Morsing A (2018) SNMMI procedure standard/EANM practice guideline for diuretic renal scintigraphy in adults with suspected upper urinary tract obstruction 1.0. Semin Nucl Med 48(4):377–390. https://doi.org/10.1053/j.semnuclmed.2018.02.010

34. Ring P, Huether SE (2017) Alteration of renal and urinary tract function in children. In: McCance KL, Huether SE (eds) Pathophysiology, 8th edn. Mosby, Philadelphia, pp 1278–1295

35. Strand WR (1999) Urinary infection in children: pathogenesis, bacterial virulence, and host resistance. In: Bauer SB, Gonzales E (eds) Pediatric urology practice. Lippincott Williams & Wilkins, Philadelphia, pp 433–461

36. Kaefer M, Diamond D (1987) Vesicoureteral reflux. In: Retik A, Cukier J (eds) Pediatric urology. Williams and Wilkins, Baltimore, pp. 463–486

37. Solari V, Owen D, Puri P (2005) Association of transforming growth factor-beta1 gene polymorphism with reflux nephropathy. J Urol 174(4 Pt 2):1609–1611. https://doi.org/10.1097/01.ju.0000179385.64585.dc

38. Kanematsu A, Yamamoto S, Yoshino K, Ishitoya S, Terai A, Sugita Y, Ogawa O, Tanikaze S (2005) Renal scarring is associated with nonsecretion of blood type antigen in children with primary vesicoureteral reflux. J Urol 174(4 Pt 2):1594–1597. https://doi.org/10.1097/01.ju.0000176598.60310.90

39. Shaikh N, Osio VA, Wessel CB, Jeong JH (2020) Prevalence of asymptomatic bacteriuria in children: a meta-analysis. J Pediatr 217:110–117.e4. https://doi.org/10.1016/j.jpeds.2019.10.019

40. Mahyar A, Ayazi P, Mavadati S, Oveisi S, Habibi M, Esmaeily S (2014) Are clinical, laboratory, and imaging markers suitable predictors of vesicoureteral reflux in children with their first febrile urinary tract infection? Korean J Urol 55(8):536–541. https://doi.org/10.4111/kju.2014.55.8.536

41. Subcommittee on Urinary Tract Infection (2016) Reaffirmation of AAP clinical practice guideline: the diagnosis and management of the initial urinary tract infection in febrile infants and young children 2-24 months of age. Pediatrics 138(6):e20163026. https://doi.org/10.1542/peds.2016-3026

42. National Institute for Health and Clinical Excellence (NICE) (2018) clinical guideline 54—Urinary tract infection in under 16s: diagnosis and management

43. Pokrajac D, Sefic-Pasic I, Begic A (2018) Vesicoureteral reflux and renal scarring in infants after the first febrile urinary tract infection. Med Arch (Sarajevo, Bosnia and Herzegovina) 72(4):272–275. https://doi.org/10.5455/medarh.2018.72.272-275

44. Roupakias S, Sinopidis X, Tsikopoulos G, Spyridakis I, Karatza A, Varvarigou A (2017) Dimercaptosuccinic acid scan challenges in childhood urinary tract infection, vesicoureteral reflux and renal scarring investigation and management. Minerva Urol Nefrol 69(2):144–152. https://doi.org/10.23736/S0393-2249.16.02509-1. Epub 2016 Jun 29

45. Breinbjerg A, Jørgensen CS, Frøkiær J et al (2021) Risk factors for kidney scarring and vesicoureteral reflux in 421 children after their first acute pyelonephritis, and appraisal of international guidelines. Pediatr Nephrol

46. Ramos CD, Onusic DM, Brunetto SQ, Amorim BJ, Souza TF, Saad S, Lima M (2019) Technetium-99m-dimercaptosuccinic acid renal scintigraphy and single photon emission computed tomography/computed tomography in patients with sickle cell disease. Nucl Med Commun 40(11):1158–1165. https://doi.org/10.1097/MNM.0000000000001086

47. Vasco M, Benincasa G, Fiorito C, Faenza M, De Rosa P, Maiello C, Santangelo M, Vennarecci G, Napoli C (2021) Clinical epigenetics and acute/chronic rejection in solid organ transplantation: an update. Transplant Rev (Orlando) 35(2):100609. https://doi.org/10.1016/j.trre.2021.100609

48. Hruba P, Madill-Thomsen K, Mackova M, Klema J, Maluskova J, Voska L, Parikova A, Slatinska J,

Halloran PF, Viklicky O (2020) Molecular patterns of isolated tubulitis differ from tubulitis with interstitial inflammation in early indication biopsies of kidney allografts. Sci Rep 10(1):22220

49. Callemeyn J, Ameye H, Lerut E, Senev A, Coemans M, Van Loon E, Sprangers B, Van Sandt V, Rabeyrin M, Dubois V, Thaunat O, Kuypers D, Emonds MP, Naesens M (2020) Revisiting the changes in the Banff classification for antibody-mediated rejection after kidney transplantation. Am J Transplant Off J Am Soc Transplant Am Soc Transplant Surg. https://doi.org/10.1111/ajt.16474. Advance online publication

50. Randhawa PS, Tsamandas AC, Magnone M, Jordan M, Shapiro R, Starzl TE, Demetris AJ (1996) Microvascular changes in renal allografts associated with FK506 (Tacrolimus) therapy. Am J Surg Pathol 20(3):306–312. https://doi.org/10.1097/00000478-199603000-00007

51. Asher J, Vasdev N, Wyrley-Birch H, Wilson C, Soomro N, Rix D, Jaques B, Manas D, Torpey N, Talbot D (2014) A prospective randomised paired trial of sirolimus versus tacrolimus as primary immunosuppression following non-heart beating donor kidney transplantation. Curr Urol 7(4):174–180. https://doi.org/10.1159/000365671

52. Munib S, Ahmed T, Ahmed R, Najam-Ud-Din (2021) Renal allograft biopsy findings in live-related renal transplant recipients. J Coll Physicians Surg Pak 31(2):197–201. https://doi.org/10.29271/jcpsp.2021.02.197

53. Lebowitz RL, Olbing H, Parkkulainen KV, Smellie JM, Tamminen-Möbius TE (1985) International system of radiographic grading of vesicoureteric reflux. International reflux study in children. Pediatr Radiol 15(2):105–109. https://doi.org/10.1007/BF02388714

54. Williams G, Fletcher JT, Alexander SI, Craig JC (2008) Vesicoureteral reflux. J Am Soc Nephrol: JASN 19(5):847–862. https://doi.org/10.1681/ASN.2007020245

55. Rodriguez MM (2004) Developmental renal pathology: its past, present, and future. Fetal Pediatr Pathol 23(4):211–229. https://doi.org/10.1080/15227950490923453

56. Jana S, Blaufox MD (2006) Nuclear medicine studies of the prostate, testes, and bladder. Semin Nucl Med 36(1):51–72. https://doi.org/10.1053/j.semnuclmed.2005.09.001

57. Kopac M, Kenig A, Kljucevsek D, Kenda RB (2005) Indirect voiding urosonography for detecting vesicoureteral reflux in children. Pediatr Nephrol (Berlin, Germany) 20(9):1285–1287. https://doi.org/10.1007/s00467-005-1961-2

58. Charbonneau SG, Tackett LD, Gray EH, Caesar RE, Caldamone AA (2005) Is long-term sonographic followup necessary after uncomplicated ureteral reimplantation in children? J Urol 174(4 Pt 1):1429–1432. https://doi.org/10.1097/01.ju.0000173128.73742.bc

59. Giel DW, Noe HN, Williams MA (2005) Ultrasound screening of asymptomatic siblings of children with vesicoureteral reflux: a long-term followup study. J Urol 174(4 Pt 2):1602–1605. https://doi.org/10.1097/01.ju.0000176596.87624.a3

60. Penido Silva JM, Oliveira EA, Diniz JS, Bouzada MC, Vergara RM, Souza BC (2006) Clinical course of prenatally detected primary vesicoureteral reflux. Pediatr Nephrol (Berlin, Germany) 21(1):86–91. https://doi.org/10.1007/s00467-005-2058-7

61. Muschat M (1932) The pathological anatomy of testicular torsion: explanation of its mechanism. Surg Gynaecol Obstet 54:758–763

62. Allan WR, Brown RB (1966) Torsion of the testis: a review of 58 cases. Br Med J 1(5500):1396–1397. https://doi.org/10.1136/bmj.1.5500.1396

63. Scorer CG, Farrington GH (1971) Congenital deformities of testis and epididymis, 1st edn. Butterworth, London

64. Corriere JN Jr (1972) Horizontal lie of the testicle: a diagnostic sign in torsion of the testis. J Urol 107(4):616–617. https://doi.org/10.1016/s0022-5347(17)61093-0

65. Skoglund RW, McRoberts JW, Ragde H (1970) Torsion of testicular appendages: presentation of 43 new cases and a collective review. J Urol 104(4):598–600. https://doi.org/10.1016/s0022-5347(17)61790-7

66. Rencken RK, du Plessis DJ, de Haas LS (1990) Venous infarction of the testis—a cause of non-response to conservative therapy in epididymo-orchitis. A case report. S Afr Med J = Suid-Afrikaanse tydskrif vir geneeskunde 78(6):337–338

67. Kogan SJ (2002) Swellings of the Intrascrotal contents. In: Gillenwalter JY (ed) Adult and pediatric urology, 4th edn. Lippincott Williams & Wilkins, Philadelphia

68. Frush DP, Babcock DS, Lewis AG, Paltiel HJ, Rupich R, Bove KE, Sheldon CA (1995) Comparison of color doppler sonography and radionuclide imaging in different degrees of torsion in rabbit testes. Acad Radiol 2(11):945–951. https://doi.org/10.1016/s1076-6332(05)80693-2

69. Luker GD, Siegel MJ (1994) Color doppler sonography of the scrotum in children. AJR Am J Roentgenol 163(3):649–655. https://doi.org/10.2214/ajr.163.3.8079863

70. Herbener TE (1996) Ultrasound in the assessment of the acute scrotum. J Clin Ultrasound : JCU 24(8):405–421. https://doi.org/10.1002/(SICI)1097-0096(199610)24:8<405::AID-JCU2>3.0.CO;2-O

71. Patriquin HB, Yazbeck S, Trinh B, Jéquier S, Burns PN, Grignon A, Filiatrault D, Garel L, Dubois J (1993) Testicular torsion in infants and children: diagnosis with Doppler sonography. Radiology 188(3):781–785. https://doi.org/10.1148/radiology.188.3.8351347

72. Olguner M, Akgür FM, Aktuğ T, Derebek E (2000) Bilateral asynchronous perinatal testicular torsion: a case report. J Pediatr Surg 35(9):1348–1349. https://doi.org/10.1053/jpsu.2000.9330

73. Pogorelić Z, Mustapić K, Jukić M, Todorić J, Mrklić I, Messštrović J, Jurić I, Furlan D (2016) Management of acute scrotum in children: a 25-year single cen-

ter experience on 558 pediatric patients. Can J Urol 23(6):8594–8601

74. Laher A, Ragavan S, Mehta P, Adam A (2020) Testicular torsion in the emergency room: a review of detection and management strategies. Open access Emerg Med: OAEM 12:237–246. https://doi.org/10.2147/OAEM.S236767

75. Hörmann M, Balassy C, Philipp MO, Pumberger W (2004) Imaging of the scrotum in children. Eur Radiol 14(6):974–983. https://doi.org/10.1007/s00330-004-2248-x

76. Shin J, Jeon GW (2020) Comparison of diagnostic and treatment guidelines for undescended testis. Clin Exp Pediatr 63(11):415–421. https://doi.org/10.3345/cep.2019.01438

77. Lavallee ME, Cash J (2005) Testicular torsion: evaluation and management. Curr Sports Med Rep 4(2):102–104. https://doi.org/10.1097/01.csmr.0000306081.13064.a2

78. Ring N, Staatz G (2017) Bildgebende Diagnostik beim akuten Skrotum [diagnostic imaging in cases of acute scrotum]. Aktuelle Urol 48(5):443–451. https://doi.org/10.1055/s-0043-100497

79. Saleh O, El-Sharkawi MS, Imran MB (2012) Scrotal scintigraphy in testicular torsion: an experience at a tertiary care centre. IIUM Med J Malaysia 11:1. https://doi.org/10.31436/imjm.v11i1.540

80. Yuan Z, Luo Q, Chen L, Zhu J, Zhu R (2001) Clinical study of scrotum scintigraphy in 49 patients with acute scrotal pain: a comparison with ultrasonography. Ann Nucl Med 15(3):225–229. https://doi.org/10.1007/BF02987836

81. Nussbaum Blask AR, Bulas D, Shalaby-Rana E, Rushton G, Shao C, Majd M (2002) Color Doppler sonography and scintigraphy of the testis: a prospective, comparative analysis in children with acute scrotal pain. Pediatr Emerg Care 18(2):67–71. https://doi.org/10.1097/00006565-200204000-00001

82. Wu HC, Sun SS, Kao A, Chuang FJ, Lin CC, Lee CC (2002) Comparison of radionuclide imaging and ultrasonography in the differentiation of acute testicular torsion and inflammatory testicular disease. Clin Nucl Med 27(7):490–493. https://doi.org/10.1097/00003072-200207000-00005

Respiratory System 8

8.1 Anatomic and Physiologic Considerations

The pulmonary system consists of the lungs, airways, pulmonary and bronchial circulation, and chest wall. The lungs consist of lobes, three in the right (upper, middle, and lower) and two in the left lung (upper and lower). Each lobe is again divided into segments and lobules (Fig. 8.1). The airway system consists of upper airways (nasopharynx and oropharynx) and lower airways (trachea, bronchi, bronchioles, and alveolar ducts) connected by the larynx (Fig. 8.2).

8.1.1 Respiratory Airways

The *upper airways* are lined by a ciliated mucosa, richly supplied with blood, which warm and humidify the inspired air and help get rid of foreign particles. The air normally flows by way of the nose, nasopharynx, and oropharynx to the lower airways. When the nose is obstructed or additional flow of air is needed, during exercise, air flows via the mouth and oropharynx to the lower airways. Foreign particle removal and humidification are not efficient with mouth breathing as compared with the usual breathing through the nose.

The *lower airways* are formed of a conducting system and a gas exchange system (Fig. 8.2). The trachea divides into two main bronchi at the carina, and each bronchus enters the corresponding lung at the hilum along with the pulmonary blood vessels and lymphatic channels. The trachea measures up to 25 cm in length and 2.5 cm in diameter. The right main bronchus extends to the right lung more vertically than the left bronchus to the left lung. This explains the more frequent aspiration of foreign material on the right side. At the hila, the bronchi divide into lobar bronchi, then segmental and subsegmental bronchi, and then into smaller bronchioles, and at the 16th division, the tracheobronchial tree ends in the tiny terminal bronchioles which form the ends of the conducting airways and are followed by the gas exchange airways. The lung segments are individual units with their bronchovascular supply; hence, they can be individually resected. The airways responsible for conducting air from outside the body into the lungs are lined by ciliated mucous membranes. The cilia, which are hairlike projections, act as sweepers to prevent dust and foreign particles from passing distally into the lungs. Damage to the respiratory epithelium and its cilia allows bacteria and viruses to proliferate and induce infection.

The gas exchange airways start where the terminal bronchioles divide further into smaller, respiratory bronchioles which include increasing numbers of alveoli as the division progresses. By the 23rd division, the respiratory bronchioles end in alveolar ducts that lead to alveolar sacs, which are made up of numerous alveoli. The alveoli are

Fig. 8.1 Diagram of the lobes and segments of the lungs

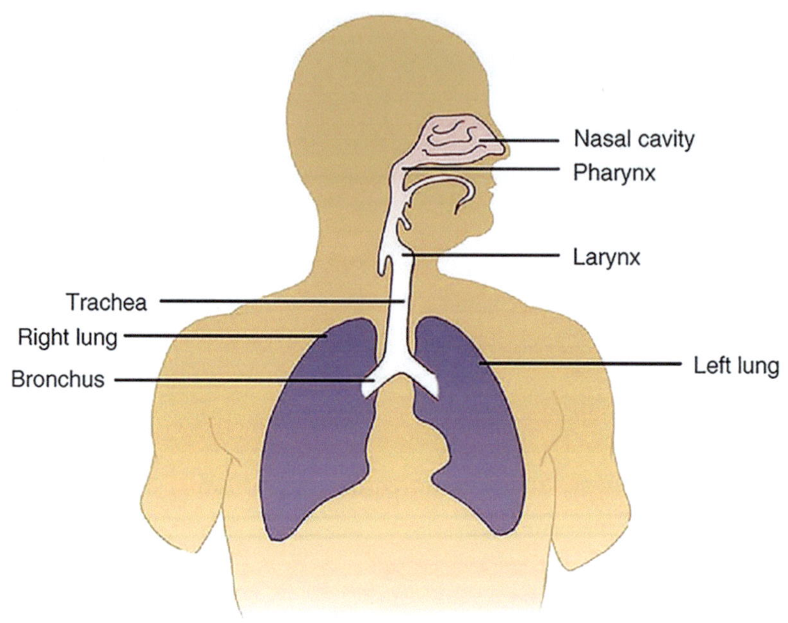

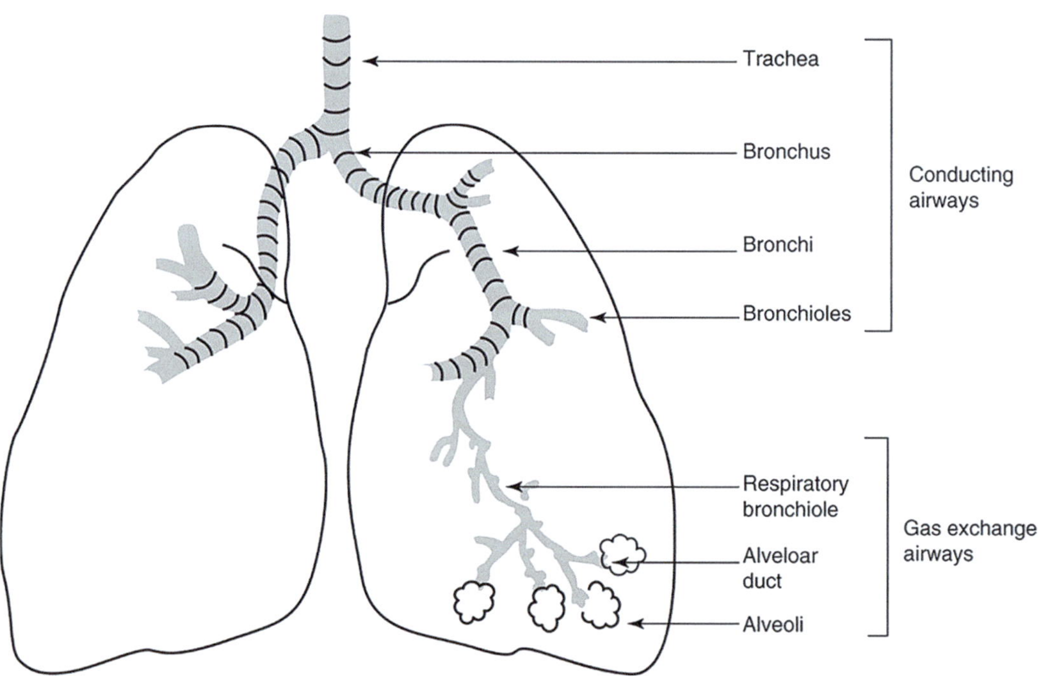

Fig. 8.2 The trachea, bronchi, and bronchioles form the tracheobronchial tree, so called since it resembles an inverted tree. The conducting system is composed of the trachea, bronchi, and bronchioles up to the 16th division and is lined by ciliated mucosa. The gas exchange system consists of the more distal bronchioles (respiratory) and the alveoli that are lined by nonciliated mucus membrane

extremely thin-walled sacs surrounded by capillaries and are the primary site of gas exchange. At birth there are approximately 25 million alveoli; this increases to 300 million in adults. The alveoli are lined by type I alveolar cells that provide structure to the alveolar wall and type II cells that secrete a lipoprotein, the surfactant which coats the alveolar inner surface and aids its expansion during inspiration [1].

Ventilation describes the process by which air flows in and out of the gas exchange airways. Ventilation is involuntary most of the time and is controlled by the sympathetic and parasympathetic autonomic nervous systems, which adjust the caliber of the airway via contraction and relaxation of the bronchial smooth muscle and control the depth and rate of ventilation.

The nose and trachea trap most particles of more than 10 μm in diameter, while the cilia of the bronchi and bronchioles pick up particles 2–10 μm in diameter that are deposited in these airways. Smaller particles remain airborne till they are deposited in the alveoli and removed by macrophages. Extremely small particles behave as a gas and are breathed out. This is the basis of scintigraphic ventilation studies using radioactive aerosols and gases. The flow of oxygen through the ^{99m}Tc-DTPA reservoir should create small aerosol particles to be airborne and deposited distally in the alveoli. Larger particles are deposited in the more proximal airways and influence the quality of ventilation studies. This also explains the longer biologic clearance of aerosols compared with radioactive gases, which are breathed out without deposition.

8.1.2 Pulmonary Vasculature

The lung is supplied by two different blood circulations. Pulmonary circulation is a low-pressure, low-resistance system through which oxygen enters and carbon dioxide is removed. Bronchial circulation is a part of the high-pressure systemic circulation that supplies oxygenated blood to the lung tissue itself.

The pulmonary circulation contains the vast majority of blood present in the lung, and since it has lower pressure than systemic circulation, its vessels have a thinner muscle layer. The mean pulmonary artery pressure is 18 mmHg, compared with 90 mmHg for the aorta. The gas exchange airways are served by this pulmonary circulation, which is considered a separate division of the circulatory system. The pulmonary circulation is carried through the pulmonary artery, which branches out to two main pulmonary arteries, one to each lung, entering the hilum. It then divides progressively into smaller branches, following the branches of the bronchial tree to the smallest, precapillary arterioles, which divide to form a capillary network surrounding the alveoli. The membrane that surrounds the alveoli and contains the capillaries is called the alveolocapillary membrane [2].

The precapillary arterioles are approximately 35 μm in diameter and number approximately 300 million in adults. The capillaries, 7–10 μm in diameter, number 300 billion in adults. The more proximal terminal arterioles have a diameter of approximately 100 μm. This basic anatomical fact is important in determining the size of particles injected for perfusion studies; they should be less than 100 μm to prevent blocking of the terminal arterioles [3].

Although the pulmonary circulation is innervated by the autonomic nervous system, vasodilation and vasoconstriction are controlled mainly by local and humoral factors, particularly arterial oxygenation and acid–base balance. Vasoconstriction of the pulmonary arterial system occurs secondary to alveolar hypoxia and acidemia and by the presence of inflammatory mediators such as histamine, bradykinin, serotonin, and prostaglandin.

The bronchial circulation, on the other hand, carries approximately 5% of the blood coming to the lungs and is part of the systemic circulation. In contrast to the pulmonary circulation, it does not participate in gas exchange. It supplies the tracheobronchial tree, large pulmonary vessels, and other structures of the lungs, including the pleurae, with blood.

8.1.3   Respiratory Function

The major function of the respiratory system is to oxygenate the blood and remove waste products from the body in the form of carbon dioxide. Oxygen in the inhaled air diffuses from the alveoli into the surrounding blood in the capillaries, where it attaches to hemoglobin molecules and red blood cells and is carried to the various tissues of the body. Carbon dioxide, on the other hand, as a waste product of cellular metabolism, diffuses in the opposite direction, from the blood in capillaries into the alveoli, and is removed from the body during expiration.

Respiration is controlled by the respiratory center in the medulla at the base of the brain. The respiratory center in the brain stem sends impulses to respiratory muscles to contract and relax. The respiratory center also receives impulses from two main types of peripheral receptors, neuro- and chemoreceptors. Neuroreceptors (lung receptors) monitor the mechanical aspects of ventilation such as the need to expel unwanted substances and expansion of the lungs. The chemoreceptors in the brain circulatory system monitor the pH status of the cerebrospinal fluid and arterial oxygen content (PO_2) to regulate ventilation accordingly.

Any change in the carbon dioxide in the blood will affect the rate and depth of respiration. A slight increase in carbon dioxide concentration in the blood increases the rate and depth of respiration, such as when the individual exercises, since the accumulated waste gas must be removed from the body.

This increase in respiratory rate and depth is secondary to the stimulation of the muscles of respiration, which include the diaphragm and the intercostal muscles, by the respiratory center. Contraction of these muscles causes the volume of the chest cavity to increase, with a consequent drop in the pressure within the lungs, and forces air to move into the tracheobronchial tree. When these respiratory muscles relax, the volume of the chest cavity decreases, the pressure increases, and the air is pushed out of the lungs. When breathing is difficult, or in patients with obstructive airway disease, special muscles of expiration, abdominal and internal intercostal muscles, may be additionally needed.

8.1.4   Distribution of Ventilation and Perfusion

Normally, the lower zones of the lungs are better perfused and ventilated because of the effect of gravity. This gradient is more pronounced in perfusion than in ventilation (Fig. 8.3). This physiological fact will usually cause the perfusion to

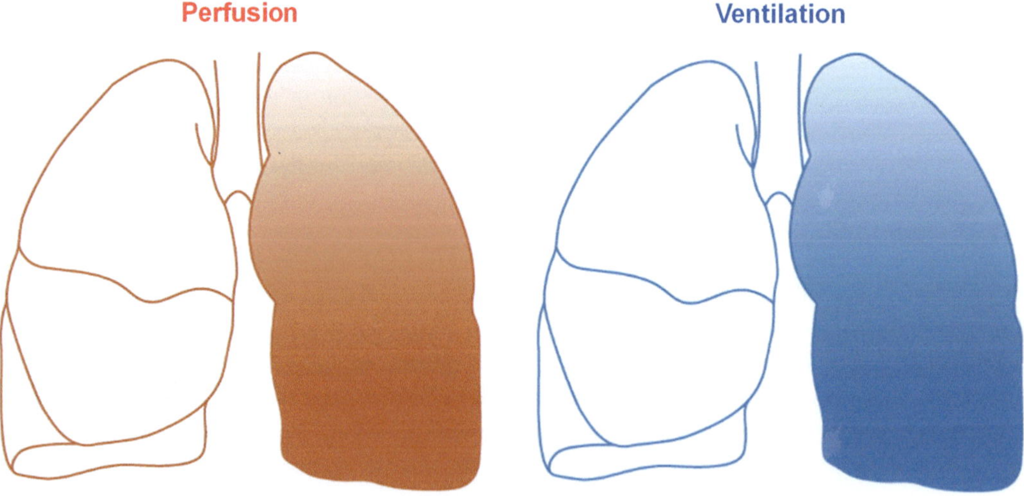

Fig. 8.3 The gradient pattern in perfusion and ventilation of the lungs (From Elgazzar et al. with permission)

appear less than the ventilation in the lung apices on scintigraphy. This should not be confused with a mismatching pattern. ^{99m}Tc-macroaggregated albumin (MAA) is injected for perfusion imaging while the patient is in the supine position to minimize the gradient. Injection while the patient is taking a deep breath also helps.

8.2 Pulmonary Embolic Disease

Venous thromboembolism, clinically presenting as DVT or PE, is the third most frequent acute cardiovascular syndrome globally with around 10 million cases per year worldwide [5, 6]. The true incidence of PE is unknown, but in the United States, it is estimated that nearly one-third of hospitalized patients are at risk of developing venous thromboemboli and up to 600,000 cases of VTE are diagnosed per year [7].

Pulmonary embolism is potentially fatal and the most common pathological condition involving the lungs of hospitalized patients. The majority of fatal emboli are not recognized or suspected prior to death.

8.2.1 Pathogenesis and Risk Factors

The vast majority of pulmonary emboli are thromboemboli originating from deep veins mostly from the lower extremity [8, 9].

Fat, air, or tumor emboli are rare [10]. Fat emboli are reported with long bone fractures and liposuction, while air emboli occur in cardiac and neurosurgeries. Renal cell carcinoma with invasion reaching inferior vena cava is a clinical setting that may lead to tumor emboli. Data indicate that 90% of pulmonary thromboemboli originate from the lower extremities and pelvis. The remainder comes from thrombi that occur in the right side of the heart or in bronchial or cervical veins. Embolization and symptomatology are proportional to how proximal is the vein that contains the thrombus. The vast majority of pulmonary thromboemboli originating from thrombi of the lower extremities come more frequently from the thigh and pelvis (75%) than from smaller veins of the calf and feet [9, 11, 12]. Only 6% of the time upper extremity DVTs cause PE [13]. Septic embolus refers to an infected thromboembolus that occurs either on-site or secondary to detachment of an infected vein thrombus of the lower extremities. The risk of pulmonary embolus is also directly related to the presence of a residual clot at the site of a venous thrombus [14].

Recently a common, yet not novel, risk factor for thromboembolism and PE is established with the Corona Virus Disease (COVID 2019) infection. Early in COVID-19 pandemic, multiple clinical, pathological, laboratory, and imaging reports demonstrated an association between COVID-19 infection and coagulopathies. These coagulopathies manifested as PE or venous, arterial, and/or microvascular thrombosis which are associated with severe viral injury of lung endothelium. In the available early and limited data, coagulopathy was reported in up to 50% of patients with severe COVID-19 manifestations. Deep vein thrombosis and PE was reported in up to 40% of patients. Current evidence is limited by small retrospective studies, and the true prevalence of thrombosis in COVID-19 is yet to be evaluated.

Pathogenesis of viral coagulopathy in the previously known various coronavirus infections has been extensively investigated. Some of the mechanisms proven include platelets consumption, thrombin generation, and increased fibrin degradation product (FDP) leading to disseminated intravascular coagulation (DIC)-like syndrome.

The specific mechanisms increasing the risk of thrombotic complications in a patient with COVID-19 are currently under extensive investigation. Many factors are considered including the high levels of D-dimer and FDPs, the high levels of proinflammatory cytokines, and the endothelial dysfunction associated with the infection. It is hypothesized that an imbalance between coagulation and inflammation may result in COVID-19 hypercoagulable state. It is also suggested that COVID-19 coagulopathy is distinct from sepsis-induced DIC and it reflects dysregulated hemostasis [15–20].

8.3   Pulmonary Embolic Disease

Pulmonary embolism is potentially fatal and the most common pathological condition involving the lungs of hospitalized patients. The majority of fatal emboli are not recognized or suspected prior to death.

8.3.1   Pathogenesis and Risk Factors

The vast majority of pulmonary emboli are thromboemboli originating from deep veins. Fat, air, or tumoremboli are rare [5]. Fat emboli are reported with long bone fractures and liposuction, while air emboli occur with cardiac- and neurosurgeries. Renal cell carcinoma with invasion reaching inferior venacava may lead to tumor emboli. Data indicate that 90% of pulmonary thromboemboli originate from the lower extremities and pelvis. The remainder comes from thrombi that occur in the right side of the heart or in bronchial or cervical veins. Embolization and symptomatology are proportional to how proximal is the vein that contains the thrombus. The vast majority of pulmonary thromboemboli originating from thrombi of the low extremities come more frequently from the thigh and pelvis (75%) than from smaller veins of the calf and feet [6, 7]. Septicembolus refers to an infected thromboembolus which occurs either onsite or secondary to detachment of an infected vein thrombus of the lower extremities. The risk of pulmonary embolus is also directly related to the presence of a residual clot at the site of a venous thrombus [8].

8.3.2   Deep Venous Thrombosis

The best solution to the problem of embolism is to prevent it. However, prevention requires identification of those at risk. Perhaps the most important step in defining who is at risk for this disorder has been the recognition that pulmonary emboli arise from the sites of deep venous thrombosis, almost exclusively in the lower extremity veins. Therefore, those at risk for deep venous thrombosis are those at risk for pulmonary embolism. The classical risk triad elucidated by Virchow in the nineteenth century includes venous stasis, intimal injury, and alteration in coagulation. These are the primary factors in the pathogenesis of venous thrombosis. Deficiencies of antithrombin III, protein C, protein S, and protein Z are clearly important, as is the presence of lupus anticoagulant. There are other rarer conditions such as homocystinuria and deficiencies of the fibrinolytic system. More factors are being identified, but at the present time, up to 90% of all patients with thromboembolism have no identifiable coagulopathy. Thus, in most patients, some clinical states associated with venous stasis, intimal injury, or both are the basis for an increased risk of deep venous thrombosis. These clinical states include injury to the pelvis or lower extremities, surgery involving the lower extremities, all surgical procedures requiring prolonged (at least 30 min) general anesthesia, burns, pregnancy and the postpartum state, previous venous thrombosis with residual obstruction, right ventricular failure of any cause, occupations in which prolonged venous stasis is involved, and any cause of immobility. Other risk factors are age (particularly above 70 years), obesity, cancer and the use of estrogen-containing medications, neoplasm, infection in the immediate area of veins, and hypercoagulability (Table 8.1).

An important point to note is that risk factors should be regarded as cumulative, not independent. These factors allow the establishment of a "risk profile" for a given patient, a profile that conditions the intensity of prophylactic initiatives. The anatomical location of the deep venous thrombosis affects as well the likelihood of extending into a pulmonary embolism as noted earlier.

Venous thrombi appear to begin either in the vicinity of a venous valve, where eddy current arises, or at the site of intimal injury. Platelet aggregation and release of mediators initiate the

Table 8.1 Risk factors for deep vein thrombosis and pulmonary thromboembolism*

Inherited factors
1. Antithrombin deficiency
2. Protein C deficiency
3. Protein S deficiency
4. Factor V Leiden
5. Prothrombin gene mutation

Acquired factors
1. Postoperative state especially following operations on the abdomen and pelvis
2. Trauma, including fractures, particularly of the lower extremities
3. Neoplasms
4. Prior history of thromboembolic disease
5. Venous stasis
6. Vascular spasm
7. Intimal injury
8. Hypercoagulability states
9. Immobilization
10. Infection of the area in the immediate veins
11. Heart disease, especially:
    Myocardial infarction
    Atrial fibrillation
    Cardiomyopathy
    Congestive heart failure
12. Pregnancy
13. Polycythemia
14. Hemorrhage
15. Obesity
16. Old age
17. Extensive Varicose veins
18. Certain drugs such as oral contraceptives, estrogens
19. Following cerebrovascular accidents
20. Smoking
21. Central venous instrumentation within the past 3 months
22. Homocystinemia
23. Homocystinuria
24. Hyperlipidemia
25. Hypertension
26. COVID-19

[7, 15–21]

sequence. With stasis, there is a local accumulation of coagulation factors; the coagulation cascade is activated, and the characteristic red fibrin thrombus develops. Pathologically there will be a platelet nidus from which a large fibrin thrombus extends.

Regarding natural history, one of three events can happen after the formation of the thrombus. First, the red thrombus grows explosively and obstructs the vein completely. This can happen even within a few minutes. Second, partial venous obstruction may occur. Blood flow, therefore, continues over the thrombus surface. Under this circumstance, thrombus growth tends to occur by the progressive layering of platelets and fibrin on the clot surface, pathologically seen as the lines of Zahn. Third, probably the most common scenario, a small thrombus is swept away before it reaches an appreciable size. It lodges in the pulmonary vasculature without symptoms.

Unless fibrinolytic resolution is prompt, organization of the thrombus begins within hours of formation. The thrombus is slowly replaced by granulation tissue. This process anchors the thrombus to the venous wall.

The dynamic battle between fibrinolysis and thrombus formation is fought out over a period of 7–10 days, at the end of which time either complete resolution has occurred or an endothelialized residual is present. At any time during this period, a portion or all of the thrombus can detach as an embolus. This risk is highest early, before significant dissolution or organization occurs [12].

8.3.3 Pulmonary Thromboembolism

8.3.3.1 Consequences

Pulmonary thromboemboli occur more commonly in the lower lobes because of the preferential blood flow to these regions. This also applies to the right lung because of the straighter course of the pulmonary artery. Immediately after acute embolism, there is a decrease of perfusion distal to the occluded vessel along with a transient decrease of ventilation to the affected segment. The blood flow is diverted to the other portions of the lung, and pulmonary artery pressure may increase, although cardiac output usually remains stable. The resultant tissue ischemia disturbs certain metabolic functions of the lung such as the production of surfactants. Reduction of the surfactant concentration reduces the alveolar surface tension and may cause the atelectasis that often accompanies embolism. If the embolus completely occludes an artery or an arteriole and the collateral bronchial circulation is insufficient to sustain tissue viability, infarction occurs over 24–48 h. Pulmonary infarction with coagulative necrosis results in an area of radiographic opacity that requires an average of 20 days to resolve but occurs in less than 10–15% of patients with pulmonary embolism. There is a significant inflammatory component in pulmonary infarcts which is the basis behind the reported significant FDG uptake in recent lung infarcts and can cause false-positive interpretation for lung malignancy [22]. More frequently, incomplete infarction with hemorrhage but without necrosis occurs. This type of injury resolves quickly and produces only transient radiographic opacities. Infarction always involves the pleural surface of the lung (peripheral) and more frequently involves the lower lobes than other sites.

The regional decrease in ventilation is due to local bronchoconstriction with a tendency for redistribution of ventilation away from the hypoperfused segment. This probably occurs due to decreased regional alveolar and airway carbon dioxide tension, which is the usual stimulus for bronchodilation. This hypocapnia is corrected quickly, since patients inhale carbon dioxide-rich tracheal "dead space air" into the alveolar zones after the embolic event, raising the alveolar pCO_2 [12]. The release of neurohumoral factors, most importantly serotonin and thromboxane A_2, also causes bronchoconstriction. These factors are released after embolization by activated platelets and mediate bronchospasm of small airways through their effects on the smooth muscles [23]. The ventilation of the hypoperfused areas returns to normal within several hours after acute embolism [24, 25]. This concept is the pathophysiological basis for the scintigraphic interpretation of ventilation and perfusion scans, which show segmental perfusion defects with preserved ventilation as a typical scintigraphic pattern for pulmonary embolism. Those showing only regions of matched perfusion and ventilation defects carry a low probability of pulmonary embolism if no chest X-ray abnormalities are noted at the same sites, since this pattern is more likely associated with nonembolic conditions and is more typical of parenchymal lung disease. Because

patients with pulmonary emboli usually arrive at the hospital after normalization of the ventilation at the site of pulmonary emboli, the mismatching pattern is typical of pulmonary emboli. However, inpatients may have their V/Q scans within a short time after presentation and matching abnormalities may be associated with pulmonary emboli. This has to be borne in mind, and the duration of symptoms should be a factor in decision-making regarding the management of pulmonary embolism.

Some degree of arterial hypoxemia may also occur, one reason being the widening of the arteriovenous oxygen difference caused by acute right ventricular failure. Another reason is the enhanced perfusion of poorly ventilated or nonventilated lung zones. Loss of pulmonary surfactant may add to hypoxemia. Hyperventilation almost always occurs and may partly explain the normal levels of oxygen arterial pressure seen in 10–25% of patients with pulmonary emboli.

An increase in the resistance of the pulmonary arterial circulation, due primarily to mechanical blockage by numerous small emboli in the pulmonary vasculature and also to humorally mediated vasoconstriction, may follow pulmonary emboli. These hemodynamic consequences may include increased pulmonary arterial resistance with elevated pulmonary arterial and right ventricular systolic pressures and hypoxemia. When pulmonary hypertension occurs, it indicates at least 25% obstruction of pulmonary vascular tree as assessed by angiography [26]. The higher the degree of obstruction, the more severe the abnormalities of the cardiopulmonary hemodynamics become. When over 50% of the pulmonary vasculature is included (massive pulmonary embolism), acute pulmonary hypertension and/or right ventricular failure (cor pulmonale) occurs [26]. Systemic hypoxemia results from pulmonary arteriovenous shunting and from perfusion of hypoventilated lung segments (V–P imbalances). The AV shunting accounts for the clinical observation that administration of 100% oxygen will only partially correct hypoxemia induced by pulmonary emboli [27].

The physiological consequences of a pulmonary embolism depend on the size of the embolic mass and the general status of the pulmonary circulation. In young individuals with good cardiovascular function and good collateral circulation, thrombi of a large central vessel may be associated with only minimal functional impairment if any. On the other hand, in patients with cardiovascular or severely debilitating diseases, pulmonary embolism may lead to infarction.

8.3.3.2 Resolution

Pulmonary emboli may, spontaneously or with treatment, fragment into smaller portions that travel distally and block smaller arterioles (Fig. 8.4). This may create new, smaller perfusion defects that are more peripherally located in comparison to the original defect caused by the original embolus. This pattern should not be mistaken for recurrent pulmonary emboli on a follow-up scan. If this pattern is the only interval change with no other defects seen in areas other than those in the vicinity of the distribution of the original embolus, it does not suggest recurrent emboli [26].

Resolution of pulmonary thromboembolus may start within hours. It can be seen on perfusion scans as early as 24 h and is progressively noted up to 3 months, with insignificant change after 6 months (Fig. 8.5). This is the basis of the recommendation that follow-up ventilation and

perfusion scans are performed 3 months after the initial incident for evaluation of resolution and function as a baseline for future incidents to differentiate between acute and unresolved old emboli. This resolution is dependent on the age of the patient, with complete resolution in young age groups and less complete and less significant resolution in older age groups [26, 27]. Other factors include age of the thromboembolus or length of time between formation of the embolus and the institution of proper anticoagulation. This is the basis behind the relatively recent trend of starting anticoagulant therapy in most patients with pulmonary emboli who have no contraindication for anticoagulation immediately when a pulmonary thromboembolus is suspected before finishing the workup for the condition. Anticoagulant therapy may then be stopped if the condition is excluded.

8.3.3.3 Chronic Pulmonary Thromboembolism

Incomplete resolution of acute pulmonary embolism is frequently observed and may rarely result in chronic thromboembolic pulmonary hypertension [29]. Chronic thromboembolic disease is characterized by intraluminal thrombus organization and fibrous stenosis or complete obliteration

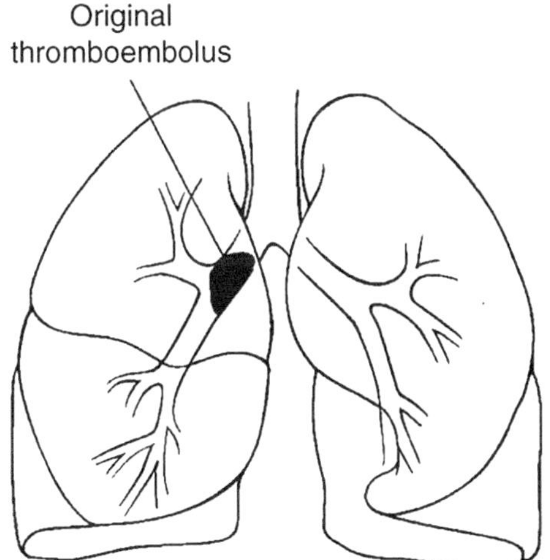

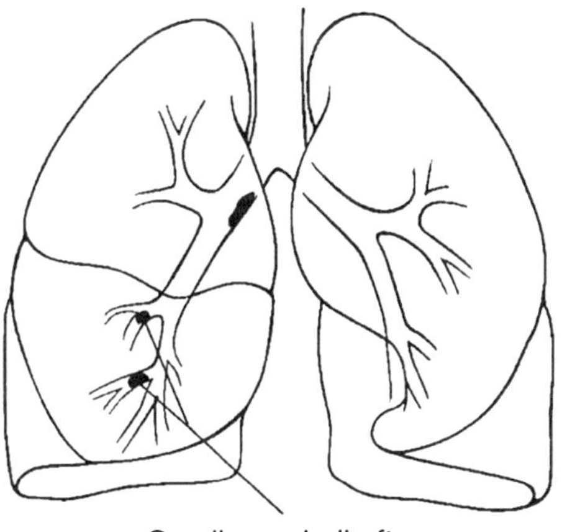

Fig. 8.4 The phenomenon of fragmentation of the thromboemboli (From Elgazzar [4] with permission)

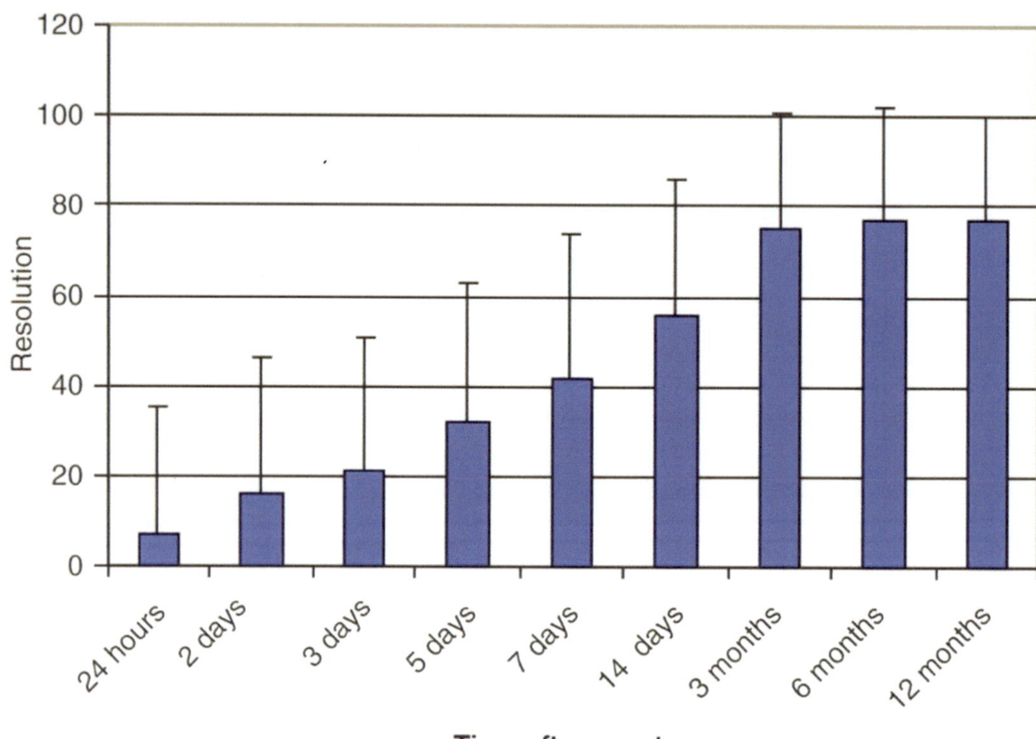

Fig. 8.5 Histogram illustrating the percent resolution of pulmonary emboli. Note that there is a progressive increase of the percentage over time until 3 months after the event with no significant increase afterward (Data are based on the Urokinase Study [27, 28])

of pulmonary arteries. The consequence is increased pulmonary vascular resistance resulting in pulmonary hypertension and progressive right heart failure. Pulmonary endarterectomy is the preferred treatment [30].

8.3.3.4 Recurrence

Pulmonary thromboemboli recur in up to 50% of patients [31], although the incidence in treated PIOPED patients was only 8.3% [32]. The vast majority of deaths among pulmonary embolism patients are due to recurrent emboli. In the PIOPED study population, it was found that nine of ten people who died had recurrent pulmonary embolus [33]. Recurrence has been reported to occur at the same site as the original thromboembolus [34].

8.3.3.5 Diagnosis

The clinical diagnosis of pulmonary thromboembolism is difficult and unreliable, due to the non-

specificity of its symptoms and signs as well as the laboratory and chest X-ray findings [35, 36]. Chest X-ray, however, must be obtained since it may show many parenchymal diseases and must be available for lung scan interpretation. Pulmonary embolism may also be asymptomatic. In the literature, only 24% of fatal emboli were diagnosed as antemortem (Table 8.2) [37–46]. Furthermore, the presentation is commonly more difficult and atypical in older age groups compared to younger patients [47, 48]. Accordingly, only 24% of fatal emboli were diagnosed as antemortem (Table 8.2). Data indicate that the mortality of pulmonary embolism is more than 30% if untreated. Promptly diagnosed and treated, emboli have a mortality of 2.5–8% [27, 28, 33]. The mortality of PE was found to vary among patients with or without cardiac disease. Paraskos et al. [49] reported survival rates at a mean follow-up period of 29 months of 19% among patients with prior congestive heart failure and

Table 8.2 Antemortem diagnosis of PE

Author	Year	No. (%) of cases with antemortem PE diagnosis
Stein and Henry [37]	1995	6/20 (30)
Morgenthaler and Ryu [38]	1995	29/92 (32)
Morpurgo and Schmid [39]	1991	26/92 (28)
Sperry et al. [40]	1990	275/812 (34)
Karwinski and Svendsen [41]	1989	267/1450 (18.4)
Gross et al. [42]	1988	7/18 (39)
Dismuke and Wagner [43]	1986	41/203 (20)
Goldhaber et al. [44]	1982	16/54 (30)
Rubio-Jurado, et al. [45]	2020	9/66 (14)
Total		675/2807(24)

86% for those with no prior congestive heart failure. Pulmonary angiography is the most accurate modality for the diagnosis of pulmonary emboli with an accuracy of 96% [50]. However, angiography is invasive and is not suitable as a screening imaging modality.

D-dimer is a fibrin degradation product present in the blood after a thrombus is degraded through fibrinolysis. The blood test to determine D-dimer concentration helps diagnose thrombosis. Although a negative result practically rules out thrombosis, a positive result can indicate thrombosis but does not rule out other potential causes. Its main use, therefore, is to exclude thromboembolic disease where the clinical probability is low. On the other hand, the positive predictive value of elevated D-dimer levels is low and D-dimer testing is not useful for confirmation of PE. D-dimer is also more frequently elevated in patients with cancer [51], in hospitalized patients [51–53], in severe infection or inflammatory disease, and during pregnancy [54].

8.3.3.5.1   Imaging

Scintigraphy remains the most cost-effective noninvasive screening modality. The major advantages include its ability to provide regional and quantitative information useful for the diagnosis, as well as for mapping to guide selective angiography if needed for the diagnosis. SPECT V/P scan has been strongly recommended as it is more accurate than planar imaging in establishing the diagnosis of PE even in the presence of diseases like COPD, heart failure, and pneumonia. Furthermore, adding low-dose CT(SPECT/CT) improves the scan specificity, especially in patients with other lung diseases [55].

CTPA is useful in detecting central emboli which has become the most commonly used modality in many centers at the expense of scintigraphy although data are still controversial for peripheral emboli [56–59]. Multislice CT was found to have no added value in patients with high-probability V/Q scans and has a comparable diagnostic value with SPECT V/Q scans [60]. CT also as a single study is not cost effective [61]. It also requires the use of iodinated contrast media with its risk of renal failure and ionizing radiation with its risk of cancer induction [62, 63]. And it was also found to result in overdiagnosis of pulmonary emboli [58]. MRI pulmonary angiography will play a greater role [64]; however, the use of contrast media is still a shortcoming. In an experimental study, reversible PE was induced by inflating a nondetachable silicon balloon in the left pulmonary artery of five New Zealand white rabbits. MR V/Q scans were obtained prior to, during, and after balloon deflation. High-resolution contrast-enhanced MR pulmonary angiography was also used to confirm the occlusion of the pulmonary artery. Similar to radionuclide ventilation/perfusion technique, acute PE produced a mismatched defect in the MR V/Q scan. MRA verified the occlusive filling defect in the left pulmonary artery. The study suggests that high-resolution MRA and MR V/Q imaging of the lung is feasible and allows comprehensive assessment of pulmonary embolism in one imaging session [64]. Recently, non-contrast MRI has been studied in the diagnosis of PE [65]. There are growing evidence-based outcome data that Contrast-enhanced pulmonary MRA is a safe and accurate and radiation-free examination for the exclusion of clinically significant PE [66].

Scintigraphy is also valuable in pregnancy. When indicated low activity of 1 mCi (37 MBq) is used for perfusion, if the perfusion study is abnormal, then ventilation and chest X-ray (if not obtained earlier) are obtained as needed. Based upon the available data, there are no apparent short- or long-term consequences to the fetus from the radiation received as a result of diagnostic ventilation/perfusion scintigraphy. For a V/Q scan, fetal dose would mostly come from tracer accumulating in the bladder, with some internal scatter from the lungs. Either Xenon133 or 99mTc agents can be used safely for the ventilation portion of the exam. Xenon103 has the advantage of not being excreted via the urine.

8.3.3.5.2 Scintigraphic Agents

Ventilation Agents

Several agents have been used for ventilation (Table 8.3). Every agent has certain advantages and limitations. Xenon 133 (Fig. 8.6) is useful in evaluating obstructive airway disease. Krypton-81 (Fig. 8.7), 99mTc-DTPA (Fig. 8.8), and Technegas (Fig. 8.9) provide the ability to perform ventilation studies after the perfusion, particularly krypton-81. 99mTc-macroaggregated albumin is used for perfusion. For proper interpretation of lung perfusion/ventilation study, chest X-ray must be available and should be obtained within 12 h of the time of the scans.

99mTc-DTPA aerosol is commonly used for ventilation studies worldwide. Using an aerosol delivery system that generates submicronic particles, 30 mCi of Tc-DTPA in 3 ml of saline (3–5 min of rebreathing on the system with the oxygen at 8–10 l/min) delivers about 500–750 μCi of tracer to the lungs. This dose yields 100 K count images in about 2 min on a standard gamma camera with a low-energy general purpose collimator. The typical radiation exposure to the lungs is about 100 mrads. This is less than the several hundred milliard exposures from a typical Xe133 rebreathing

Table 8.3 Ventilation agents

Agent	Advantages and limitations
Aerosols	
99mTc-DTPA aerosol	Lung half-clearance time = 58 min
	Pre- or post-perfusion
	Multiple projections
99mTc-pyrophosphate aerosol	Post-perfusion
	Suitable for SPECT
Technegas	Multiple projections Pre- or post perfusion
	Good peripheral deposition
Gases	
Xenon-133	Ability to obtain single breath, equilibrium, and washout images
	Very sensitive to obstructive airway disease
	Only a posterior view is possible in most patients
	Low energy of 81 keV
	Pre-perfusion acquisition
Krypton-81m	Expensive—Available only in some areas
	Energy: 190 keV
	Half-life: 13 s
	Multiple views
	Pre- or post-perfusion

ventilation exam. The dose to the lungs is also less than that from a Kr-81. Images should be acquired for 100 K counts or 5 min. Exposure to personnel is usually less than that delivered in a Xenon study.

Technegas is a ventilation aerosol agent that gained popularity recently. It is ultrafine labeled carbon particles produced by heating 99mTc-pertechnetate to very high temperatures of approximately 2500 °C in the presence of 100% argon gas. An ash material is produced that acts like a

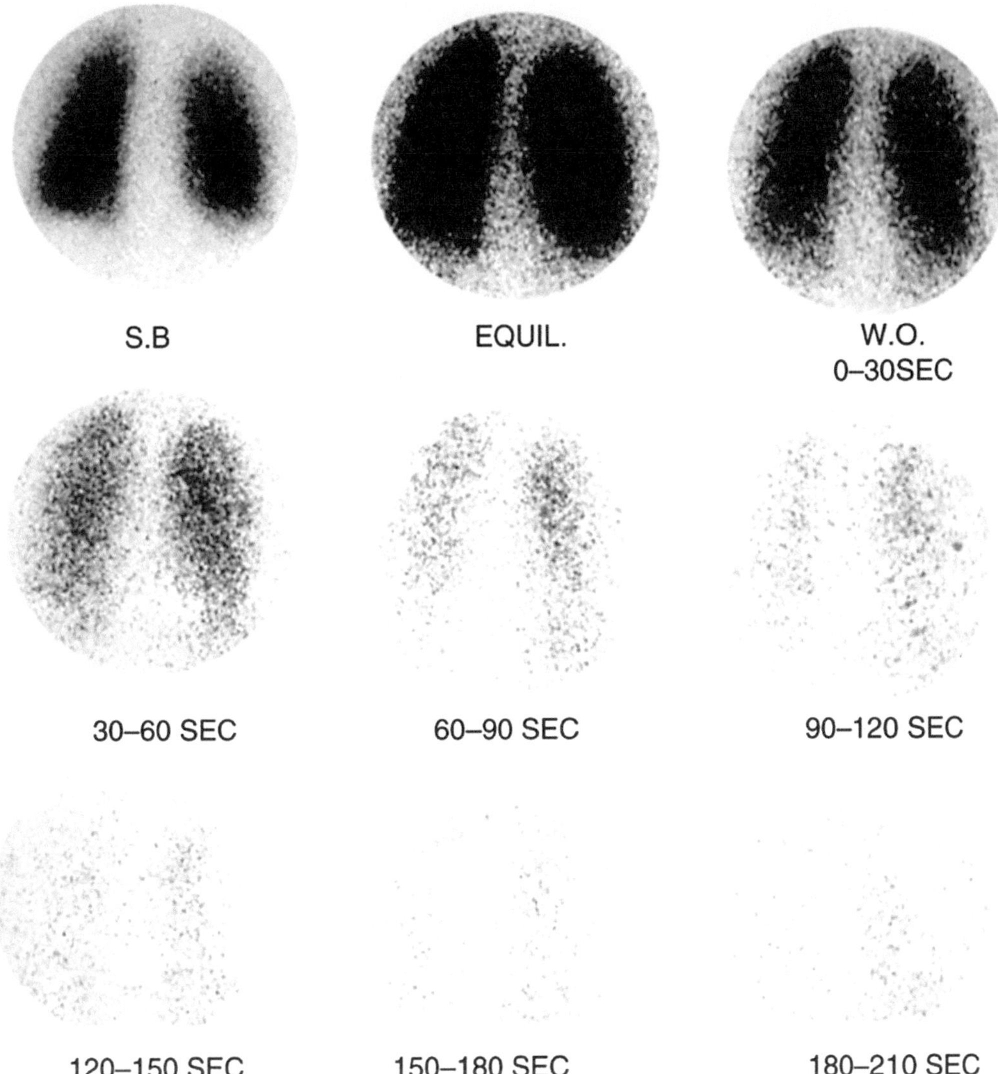

Fig. 8.6 Xenon-133 ventilation normal study with uniform distribution of the radiotracer in both lungs on a single breath and equilibrium images. The washout images reveal prompt clearance with no significant retained activity

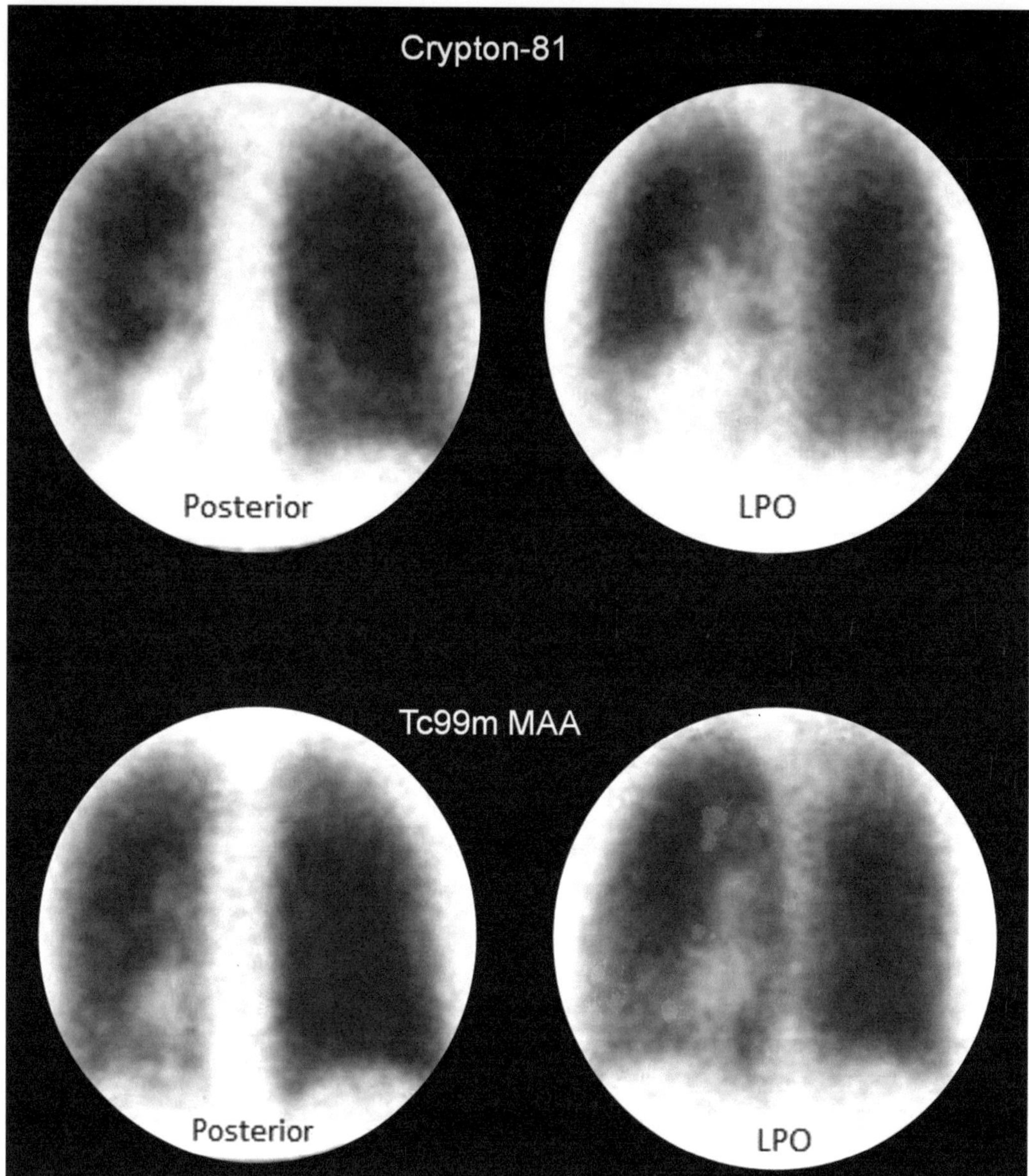

Fig. 8.7 Representative images of krypton-81 ventilation study obtained post-perfusion. Note the good quality of the images. The shown anterior and left posterior oblique (LPO) images illustrate the ability to evaluate the ventilation status at the regions of the perfusion abnormalities seen on the same projections

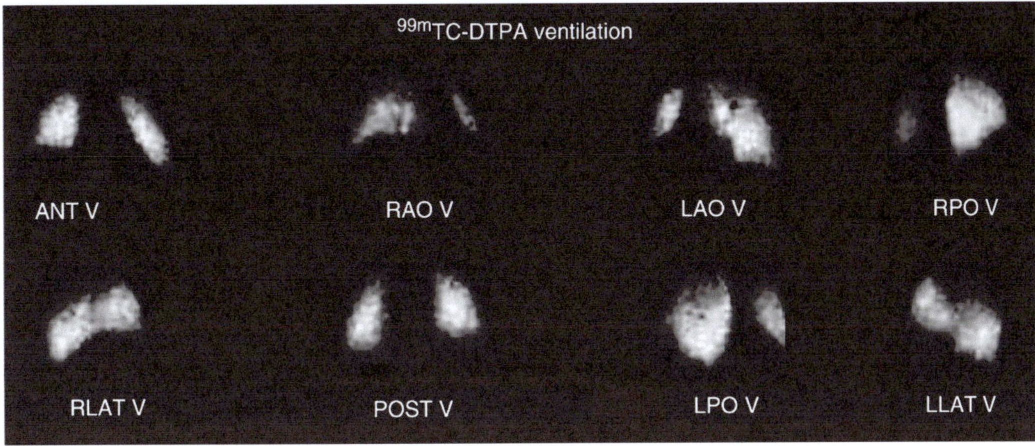

Fig. 8.8 ^{99m}Tc-DTPA aerosol ventilation study. Images show no abnormalities. Observe the activity in the esophagus and stomach due to swallowed activity

Fig. 8.9 ^{99m}Tc-Technegas ventilation study for a patient suspected of having pulmonary embolism. The study shows no abnormalities and illustrates the good quality of ventilation studies obtained using this agent. The perfusion, on the other hand, reveals perfusion defects in both lungs and no matching ventilation or X-ray abnormalities, indicating a high probability of pulmonary embolism

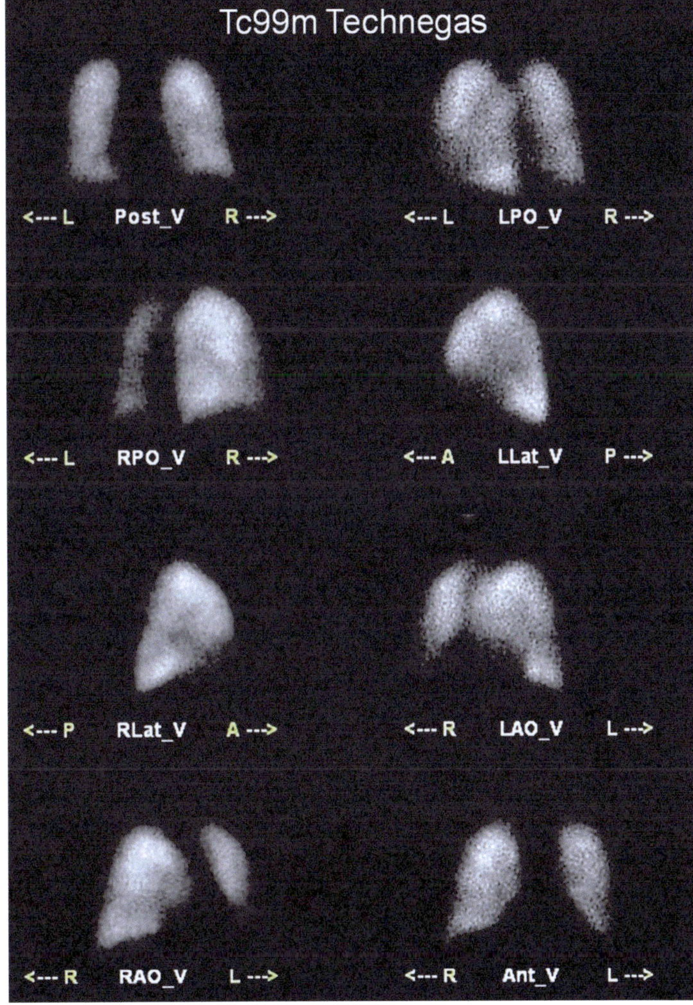

gas with good peripheral deposition because the particles are so small, with a median size of 0.05–0.15 μm. Technegas has a half-clearance time of 4–6 h. Since the material produced is not filtered and contains up to 50% of the initial radioactivity, a large number of appropriately sized particles are inhaled with each breath. Thus, only a few inspirations (typically 2–10) are needed to reach an adequate dose. Usually about 1 mCi is deposited in the lung. Extrapulmonary activity in the oropharynx, trachea, and stomach can be seen in about 30% of patients. The exam may be technically inadequate in up to 15% of patients, particularly in severely ill patients that cannot be instructed for inhalation or in patients with very shallow or rapid breathing. If the Technegas portion of the exam is performed following the perfusion study, a counting rate of at least two times the count rate of the perfusion exam is considered adequate.

Another agent, pertechnegas, which is a vapor of pertechnetate, is prepared similarly but, in the presence of 2–5% oxygen, has a shorter clearance time and shows excellent deposition in the lungs.

Perfusion Agents

^{99m}-Tc macro aggregated albumin (^{99m}MAA) is the standard agent for lung perfusion studies. The particle size of ^{99m}Tc-MAA) is generally between 10 and 90 μm (90% of particles), and no particles should be larger than 150 μm. ^{99m}Tc-MAA is injected slowly IV and lodges in precapillary arterioles, obstructing approximately 0.1% of their total number. The particles clear by enzymatic hydrolysis and are phagocytized by RE cells (the agent has a biological half-life in the lungs of between 6 and 8 h). Normally, only 3–6% of the injected ^{99m}Tc-MAA will bypass the pulmonary vasculature. The critical organ is the lungs which receive a dose of about 1 rad (1 cGy) from a typical 5 mCi dose. The kidneys and bladder receive moderate exposure largely from the excretion of degraded albumin. Table 8.4 summarizes the essential information relevant to its use in obtaining adequate perfusion scan.

Table 8.4 Characteristics of ^{99m}Tc-macroaggregated albumin (^{99m}Tc-MAA)

Size	10–90 μm (mostly 20–50)
Minimum number of particles to be used in adults	100,000 unless pulmonary hypertension or right to left shunt is present
Ideal number of particles	200,000–500,000
Biologic half-life	4–8 h
Injection	Slow intravenous. Care should be taken not to cause particle aggregates that can produce hot spots
Safety	Particles block <1/1000 of the capillaries and precapillary arterioles

8.3.3.5.3 Interpretation of V/Q Scan

For proper interpretation of lung perfusion/ventilation study, chest X-ray must be available and should be obtained within 12 h of the time of the scans.

A normal perfusion study (Fig. 8.10) rules out any clinically significant pulmonary emboli. Since the ventilation and perfusion lung scans lack specificity (Table 8.5), probabilities have been used for the interpretation of abnormal studies. Based on the pathophysiological changes and scintigraphic observations, several scintigraphic features of perfusion abnormalities are known to affect the probability of a scan for pulmonary emboli (Table 8.6). One of the important features is the size of segmental perfusion defects. A small defect occupies up to 25% of the segment, a moderate defect between 25 and 75%, while a large defect takes up 75% or more. Using these features, several retrospective and prospective studies were conducted to refine the interpretation of ventilation and perfusion scans and assess their value in managing patients suspected of having embolic disease [67–71]. PIOPED study [32] established the value of normal and high-probability scans in excluding and diagnosing pulmonary embolism. It validated the segment equivalent concept (Fig. 8.11) and clarified the use of Bayesian analysis utilizing

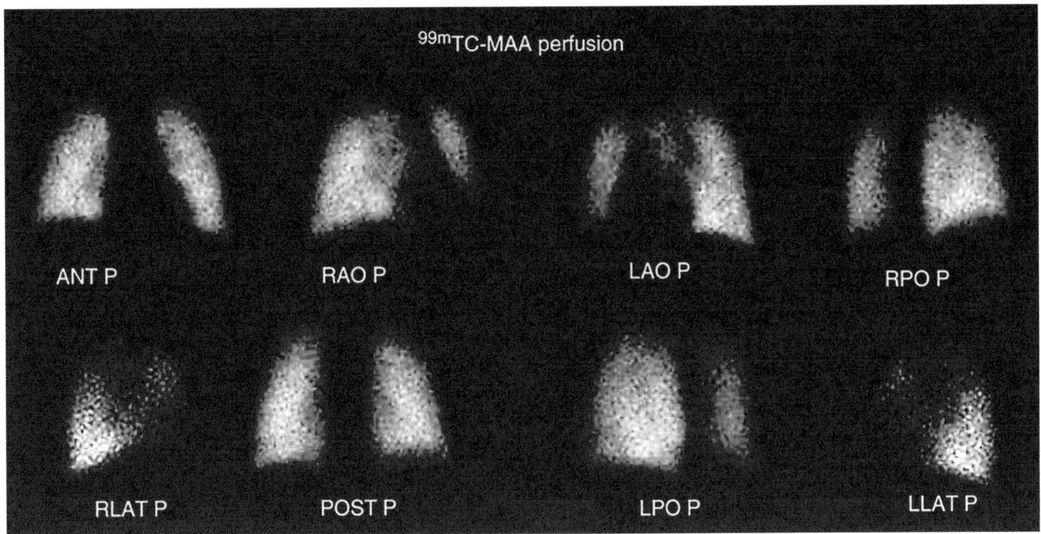

Fig. 8.10 Normal perfusion study. A ^{99m}Tc-MAA perfusion scan of a patient suspected of having pulmonary embolism. The perfusion study reveals uniform perfusion throughout both lungs with no defects. Note the parallel medial borders of both lungs on the posterior view and the sharp delineation of the costophrenic angles

Table 8.5 Causes of abnormal perfusion lung scintigraphy

Emphysema
Inflammatory diseases
Pneumonia
Abscess
Granulomatous disease (sarcoidosis, tuberculosis)
Pulmonary fibrosis
Bronchial obstruction
Infection
Neoplasm
Acute and chronic asthma
Mucus plug
Foreign body
Rib fractures (reduced lung excursion)
Congenital hypoplasia or absence of the pulmonary arteries
Peripheral pulmonary artery stenosis
Thromboembolic disease
Thrombus
Tumor embolism
Fat embolism
Air embolism
Extrinsic vessel compression (tumor, inflammation)
Left ventricular failure
Mitral valve disease
Veno-occlusive disease
Prior lung resection
Radiation

Table 8.6 Features of perfusion defects associated with a higher probability of pulmonary emboli

Size	Moderate and large
Larger relative size compared with that of chest X-ray densities	
Location	Pleural-based defects
Lower lobes	
Shape	Wedge shaped
Type	Segmental
Relation to ventilation pattern	Mismatching
Number	Multiple

the clinical pre-scan and scan probabilities to figure the post-scan or diagnostic probability. The study showed clearly that when the clinical odds agree with the scan probability in the low- and high-probability categories, pulmonary embolism can be ruled out or confirmed with a high degree of certainty.

Based on the modifications of PIOPED criteria and other validated criteria, a simplified set is shown in Table 8.7. Small perfusion defects indicate a low probability of pulmonary emboli as well as matching perfusion and ventilation defects regardless of size with no matching X-ray abnormalities (Fig. 8.12). Nonsegmental

Fig. 8.11 The segment equivalent concept (From Elgazzar [31] with permission)

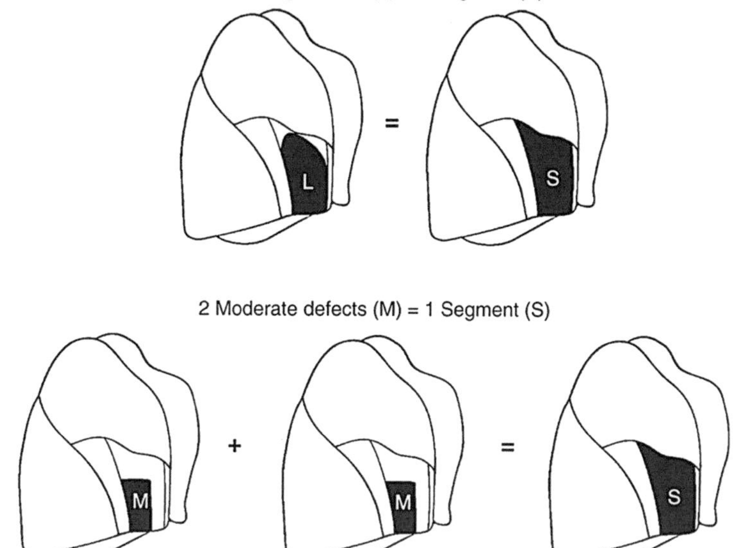

Table 8.7 Criteria for the interpretation of ventilation/perfusion lung scans

Category	Pattern on V/Q images
Normal	No perfusion defects. Allow for impressions explained by enlarged heart or other hilar structures as seen on chest X-ray
Near normal	Nonuniform uptake with no definite segmental or subsegmental perfusion defects
Low	Nonsegmental perfusion defects other than those explained by cardiomegaly or other prominent hilar structures
	Matching V/Q defects with no corresponding CXR abnormalities
	Any number of only small defects regardless of ventilation and CXR patterns
	Stripe sign
	Perfusion defect substantially smaller than CXR abnormality
High	Two or more large mismatching defects or their equivalent (4 moderate or 1 large plus 2 moderate defects) with no corresponding CXR abnormalities
	Perfusion defect substantially larger than CXR abnormality[a]
Intermediate	Perfusion defect matching chest X-ray abnormality and of the same approximate size
	Single moderate up to less than two segmental mismatching defects with no corresponding chest X-ray abnormalities
	Difficult to categorize as low or high

[a]1.5 in patients with no prior cardiopulmonary disease can be considered high probability

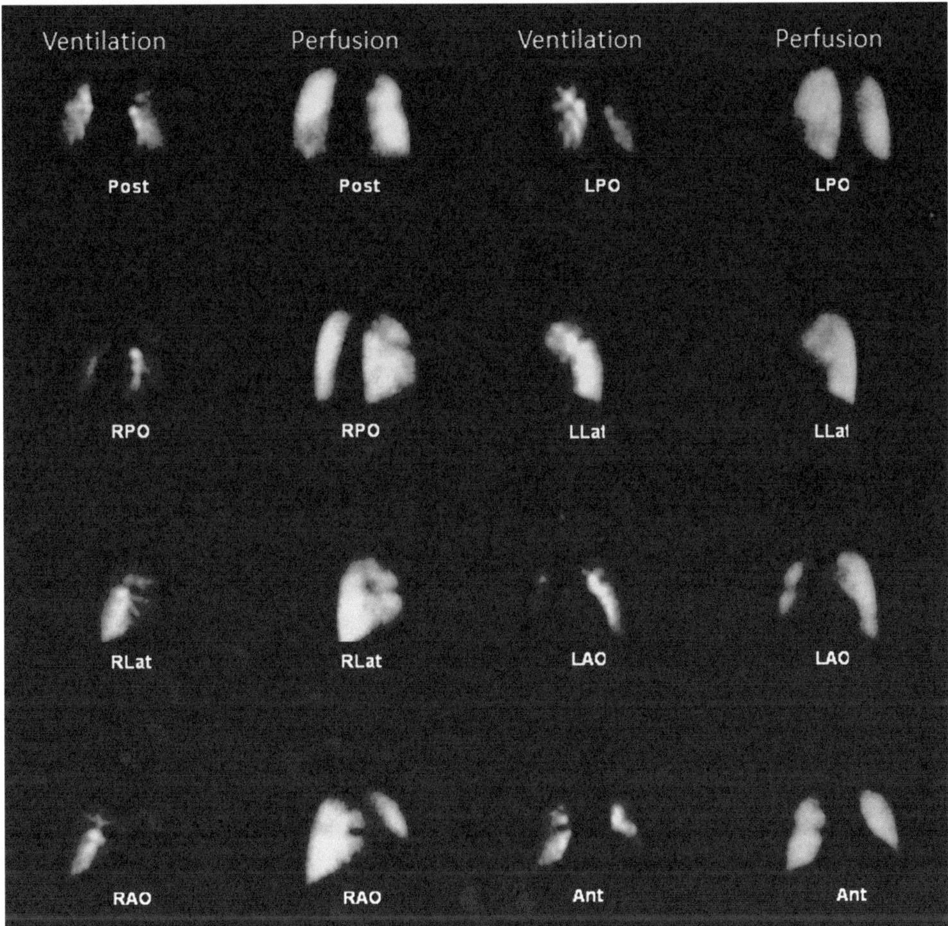

Fig. 8.12 ^{99m}Tc-DTPA aerosol ventilation and ^{99m}Tc-MAA perfusion studies of a patient suspected of having a pulmonary embolism. The X-ray was normal. The perfusion study shows multiple small perfusion defects matching the ventilation pattern indicating a low probability of pulmonary emboli

defects also indicate low probability. When perfusion defects match the X-ray abnormalities, it may indicate low, intermediate, or high probability based on the relative size of perfusion compared to the X-ray densities. When the perfusion defect is of the same approximate size as the matching X-ray density (Fig. 8.13), it indicates intermediate probability (approximately 25%).

The minimum number of mismatching perfusion defects is two segment equivalent defects with no matching chest X-ray abnormalities to make a high-probability interpretation (Fig. 8.14). However, a study analyzing PIOPED data indicated that defects equivalent to 1.5 segments are indicating a high probability among patients with no prior cardiopulmonary diseases [72].

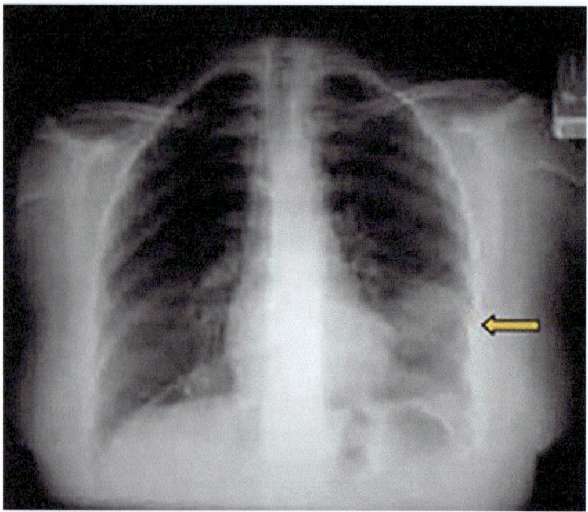

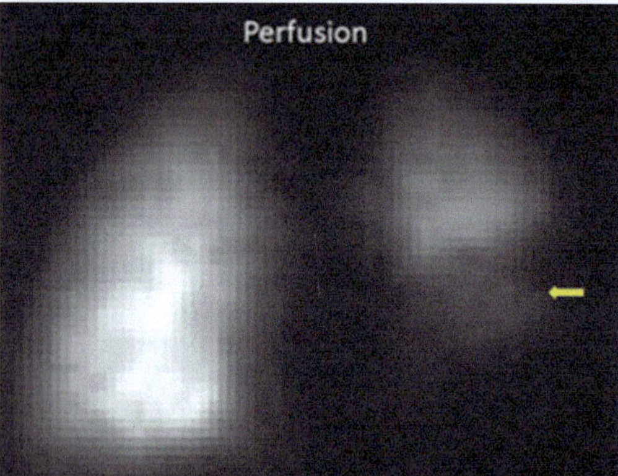

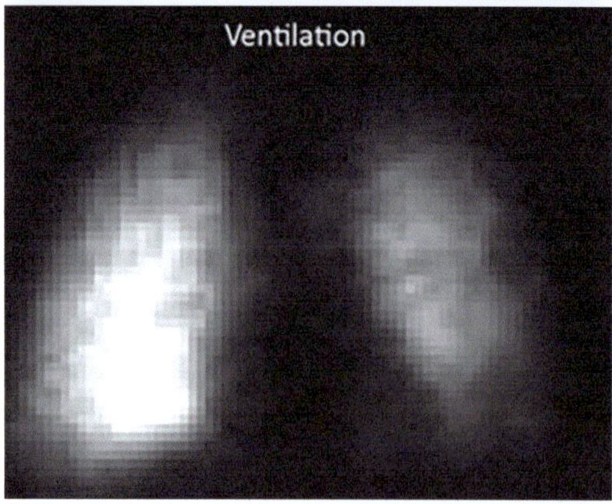

Fig. 8.13 Chest X-ray of a patient referred to rule out pulmonary embolism with a density in the left lower lobe (*arrow*) matching the perfusion defect on 99 m Tc-MAA scan and is of the same approximate size (arrow) indicating intermediate probability of pulmonary emboli

To improve interpretation, SPECT is being used more frequently in V/Q scans. SPECT scintigraphy has been reported to be strongly preferred to V/Q planar as it provides more accurate diagnosis of PE even in the presence of comorbid diseases such as COPD and pneumonia [64, 65, 73, 74].

Recently, trinary interpretative system for V/Q scans has been proposed and validated in some studies. This system is similar to the interpretative strategy for CT. V/Q scans were interpreted as "PE present," "PE absent," or "nondiagnostic." According to this system, the normal, very low (near normal), and low probabilities are grouped together and reported as PE absent. The high-probability pattern is reported as PE present, while the intermediate patterns are reported as nondiagnostic [75].

This approach can simplify the scan report for the referring physicians since the probability system still causes confusion. This leads to a decrease in the utilization of V/Q scans although recent data show increasing evidence that lung scintigraphy is not only safe but also accurate enough to be quite useful clinically in patients with suspected PE. It is available conveniently in the clinical setting. Additionally, using the scintigraphic diagnostic strategy results in an important reduction of radiation dose, particularly for the female breast [76].

Many algorithms have been developed to diagnose PE utilizing D-dimer test, echocardiography, Doppler ultrasound, scintigraphy, and multislice CT. None of these algorithms have gained uniform acceptance, and many variations were found in practice patterns among physicians, geographic locations, available resources, and experience [77].

Till further development, proper utilization of V/Q scans along with DVT imaging and laboratory tests, and CT solves most diagnostic problems and minimizes the need for angiograms (Table 8.7) [78].

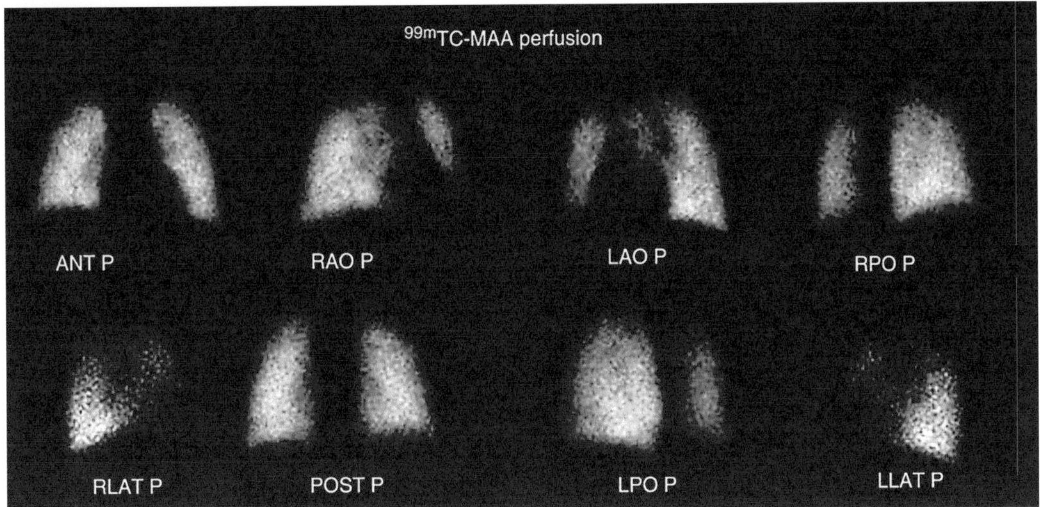

Fig. 8.14 Ventilation and perfusion scans of a 74-year-old man with a history of fracture of left femur 3 days earlier treated with internal fixation. Patient was referred to rule out pulmonary emboli because of acute onset of shortening of breath. Perfusion study shows multiple perfusion defects equivalent to more than two segments with no matching abnormalities on ventilation study and no corresponding changes in the chest X-ray which was normal. This illustrates a typical pattern of high probability of pulmonary emboli on ventilation/perfusions scans

8.4 Pulmonary Hypertension

Normal pulmonary artery systolic pressure at rest is 18–25 mmHg, with a mean pulmonary pressure ranging from 12 to 16 mmHg. This low pressure is due to the large cross-sectional area of the pulmonary circulation, which results in low resistance. An increase in pulmonary vascular resistance or pulmonary blood flow results in pulmonary hypertension. It is defined as a pulmonary artery systolic pressure higher than 30 mmHg or a pulmonary artery mean pressure higher than 20 mmHg.

Pulmonary hypertension may have no cause (primary) which is rare or may follow cardiac or pulmonary disorders (secondary). Pathophysiologically, three predominant mechanisms may be involved in the pathogenesis of secondary pulmonary hypertension, (1) hypoxic vasoconstriction, (2) decreased area of the pulmonary vascular bed, and (3) volume/pressure overload.

Chronic hypoxemia such as COPD causes pulmonary vasoconstriction by a variety of actions on pulmonary artery endothelium and smooth muscle cells.

A variety of causes may decrease the cross-sectional area of the pulmonary vascular bed, primarily due to disease of the lung parenchyma. Examples of these conditions include collagen vascular diseases particularly systemic scleroderma or CREST (calcinosis cutis, Raynaud phenomenon, esophageal motility disorder, sclerodactyly, and telangiectasia) syndrome and acute and chronic pulmonary emboli [29, 30].

Disorders of the left heart may cause secondary pulmonary hypertension, resulting from volume and pressure overload. Pulmonary blood volume overload is caused by left-to-right intracardiac shunts, such as in patients with atrial or ventricular septal defects. Left atrial hypertension causes a passive rise in pulmonary arterial systolic pressure in order to maintain a driving force across the vasculature.

8.5 *Pneumocystis carinii (jiroveci)* Pneumonia

Pneumocystis carinii (*jiroveci*) is an opportunistic pathogen currently classified as a fungus [79]. It is a significant cause of morbidity and mortality in human immunodeficiency virus and nonhuman immunodeficiency virus-associated immunosuppressed patients [80, 81] although it also occurs in non-immunocompromised patients [82–85]. Highly effective active antiretroviral therapy in industrialized nations, however, has led to dramatic declines in the incidence of AIDS-associated complications, including PCP, but no decline has occurred in developing countries [80, 81]. The organism attaches to the alveolar macrophages through a mechanism that involves fibronectin. The trophozoite develops into cysts that produce daughter trophozoites. As the number of organisms increase, the permeability of the alveolar capillary endothelium increases, producing respiratory distress. Typically, infection with *P. carinii* (now called *P. jiroveci*) produces a patchy or lobar interstitial pneumonia or, rarely, a bronchopneumonia pattern. Severe infections produce diffuse alveolar damage. The classical histological findings consist of alveolar exudates having a granular or foamy appearance that represent nonstaining clusters of the cysts and trophozoites of *P. carinii* within an eosinophilic staining background of the organism's filopodia and host cellular debris. Atypical pulmonary reactions include the formation of granulomas, focal pulmonary infection, and cavitary lesions. In extremely immunosuppressed persons, the inflammatory reaction may be minimal and consist only of sparse collections of alveolar macrophages. Since clinical manifestations of *P. carinii* pneumonia (PCP) in AIDS patients may precede X-ray changes by at least 2 weeks and as long as 18 months, ^{67}Ga has an important role in the diagnosis of early PCP. ^{67}Ga is more sensitive than chest X-ray for early PCP and is more accurate in measuring the extent of inflammation. The pattern of uptake is typically diffuse and bilateral, although other patterns may be noted [84, 85]. Localized lung uptake and perihilar uptake patterns can be seen in addition to the diffuse pattern, which may be further classified into homogeneous and heterogeneous diffuse patterns. The heterogeneous pattern has the highest positive predictive value, which is even more specific when it is of high-grade uptake and when accompanied by normal chest radiograph.

8.6 Idiopathic Pulmonary Fibrosis

Idiopathic pulmonary fibrosis is a rare disease characterized by chronic, progressive irreversible interstitial lung fibrosis along with inflammatory changes of unknown cause. Clinically, the condition is often diagnosed at an advanced stage, carry a poor prognosis. The median estimated survival time from the time of diagnosis is 2–5 years. Recently several subtypes have been clearly identified with different outcomes [86, 87]. Idiopathic pulmonary fibrosis is characterized by parenchymal inflammation and interstitial fibrosis that may eventually be fatal. The inciting factors in the development of IPF remain unknown [88]. A widely held hypothesis is that this disorder occurs in susceptible individuals following some unknown stimuli.

The major histopathological findings vary from active alveolitis and minimal fibrosis in early cases to severe fibrosis and honeycombing with minimal alveolitis in late stages. The alveolitis is characterized by an outpouring of mononuclear cells, macrophages, and lymphocytes into the alveolar space, with relatively intact alveolar walls which will be deranged by edema, fibrinous exudate, mononuclear cell infiltration, and fibroblast proliferation [89]. Connective tissue alteration occurs later in the process. ^{67}Ga has an important role in evaluating the activity of the disease and in following up the response to treatment. The degree of ^{67}Ga uptake correlates with the degree of interstitial and alveolar cellularity as seen on lung biopsies. Accordingly, it helps evaluate the extent and activity of the disease by visual assessment and/or quantitation of the uptake.

8.7 Pulmonary Sarcoidosis

Sarcoidosis, a multisystem granulomatous disorder, occurs most commonly in young adults, more commonly in blacks and in temperate areas. A second peak is known to occur in older age group (over age 60 years) [90]. The exact etiology of the disease is unknown, but it is believed to be due to exaggerated cellular immune response on the part of helper/inducer T lymphocytes to exogenous or autoantigens. It presents most frequently as bilateral hilar adenopathy, pulmonary infiltrates, and skin and eye lesions. It may be acute or chronic. Current evidence points to genetic predisposition and exposure to yet unknown transmissible agent(s) and/or environmental factors as etiological agents . Recently, it has been recognized to be a Th1-mediated disease as it is dominated by gene signatures associated with IFNȳ signaling [91].

The acute variant has an abrupt onset and may commonly show spontaneous remission within 2 years; the response to steroids is excellent. The chronic variant has an insidious onset and is more likely to cause progressive disease with fibrosis. The disorder is characterized by the presence of epithelioid (correct spelling) granuloma in affected organs that may lead to fibrosis and organ dysfunction. Granulomas of sarcoidosis often exist diffusely throughout the body despite the lack of clinical evidence of disease. Histological features are usually quite typical, but not specific. The architecture of the lesion is that of multiple similar granulomas, consisting of whorls of elongated cells (fibroblasts and epithelioid cells) with mononuclear inflammatory cells at their periphery. Giant cells are located within the granulomas (Fig. 8.15), and multinucleated cellular inclusion bodies are frequently found. Scarring with

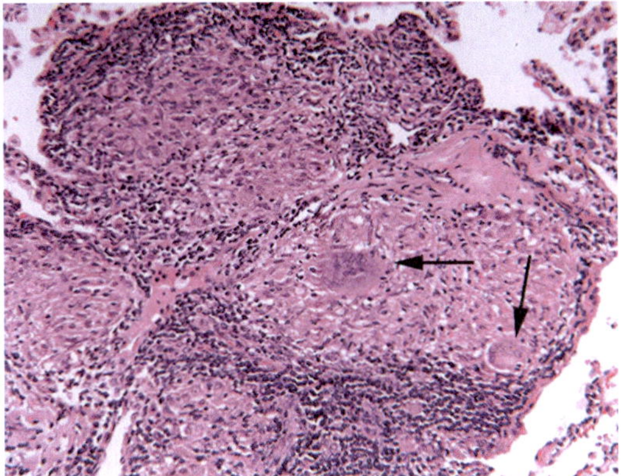

Fig. 8.15 Microphotograph of a noncaseating granuloma of a case of sarcoidosis. Note multinucleated giant cells (*arrows*)

fibrosis suggests chronicity. Epithelioid cells secrete a number of cytokines and other mediators including angiotensin-converting enzyme (ACE) which is suggested to reflect the granuloma burden in sarcoidosis and may play a role in its pathophysiology. Lung is involved in more than 90% of cases. Pulmonary sarcoidosis starts as diffuse interstitial alveolitis, followed by the characteristic granulomas. Granulomas are present in the alveolar septa as well as in the walls of the bronchi and pulmonary arteries and veins. The center of the granuloma contains epithelioid cells derived from mononuclear phagocytes, multinucleated giant cells, and macrophages. Lymphocytes, macrophages, monocytes, and fibroblasts are present at the periphery of the granuloma [92].

The diagnosis is based on a compatible clinical and/or radiologic picture, histopathological evidence of noncaseating granulomas in tissue biopsy specimens, and exclusion of other diseases capable of producing similar clinical or histopathological appearances. Patients with pulmonary sarcoidosis may have no symptoms and are discovered by chest X-ray obtained for nonpulmonary reasons. When symptomatic, dyspnea, chest pain, and cough are the most common chest symptoms [94]. The distinction between sarcoidosis and tuberculosis can be difficult at times, and the two diseases may coexist in the same patient. Similar granulomas may occur in a wide variety of other diseases, such as with malignancy or immune deficiencies, berylliosis, and foreign body reactions. [67]Ga is useful in evaluating the activity of the disease and the response to therapy. Diffuse lung uptake and bilateral hilar uptake (Fig. 8.16) are the most common patterns seen, but they lack specificity [94]. The major value of ^{67}Ga is in evaluating the activity of the disease, in detecting extrathoracic sites of involvement, and in evaluating the response to therapy. FDG uptake in sarcoidosis (Figs. 8.17 and 8.18) is nonspecific in both intensity and pattern and is not generally useful in making an initial diagnosis. FDG PET/CT, however, can be useful in monitoring disease progression or remission [95].

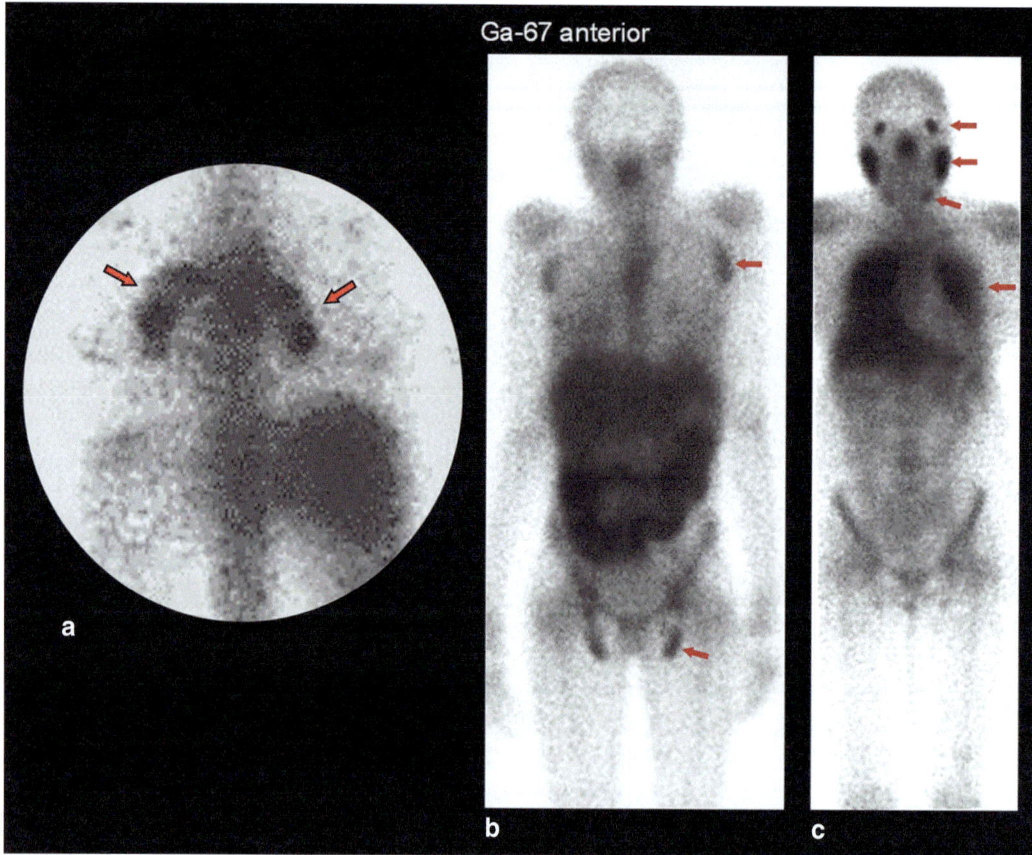

Fig. 8.16 Forty-eight hour Ga-67 posterior image of a patient with sarcoidosis Ga-67 illustrating uptake in the axillary and inguinal lymph nodes as we as mild diffuse accumulation in the lungs (**a**). Another patient (**b**) with diffuse lung uptake (arrow) and intense Ga-67 uptake in the parotids, sub-mandibular salivary glands and lacrimal gland (arrows) illustrating another typical uptake patterns of Sarcoidosis

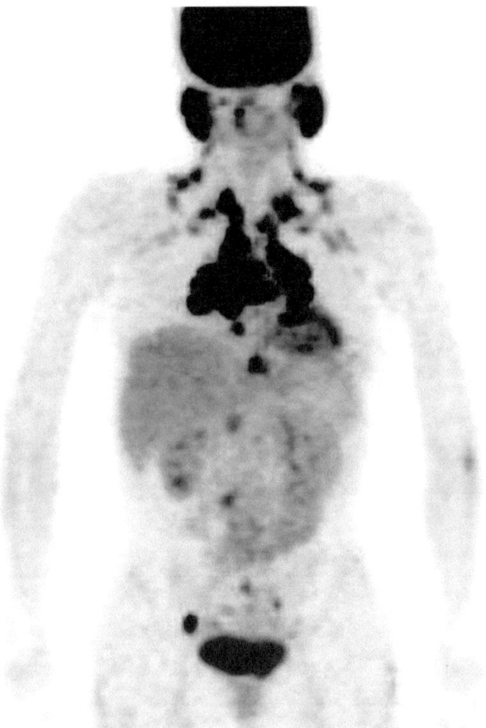

Fig. 8.17 F-18 FDG image of a 35-year-old female with proven sarcoidosis. The study shows uptake in the areas of active inflammation in mediastinum, pulmonary hilus, salivary glands, and cervical, supraclavicular, axillary, para-aortic, iliac, and inguinal lymph nodes (Courtesy of Professor Osama Sabry)

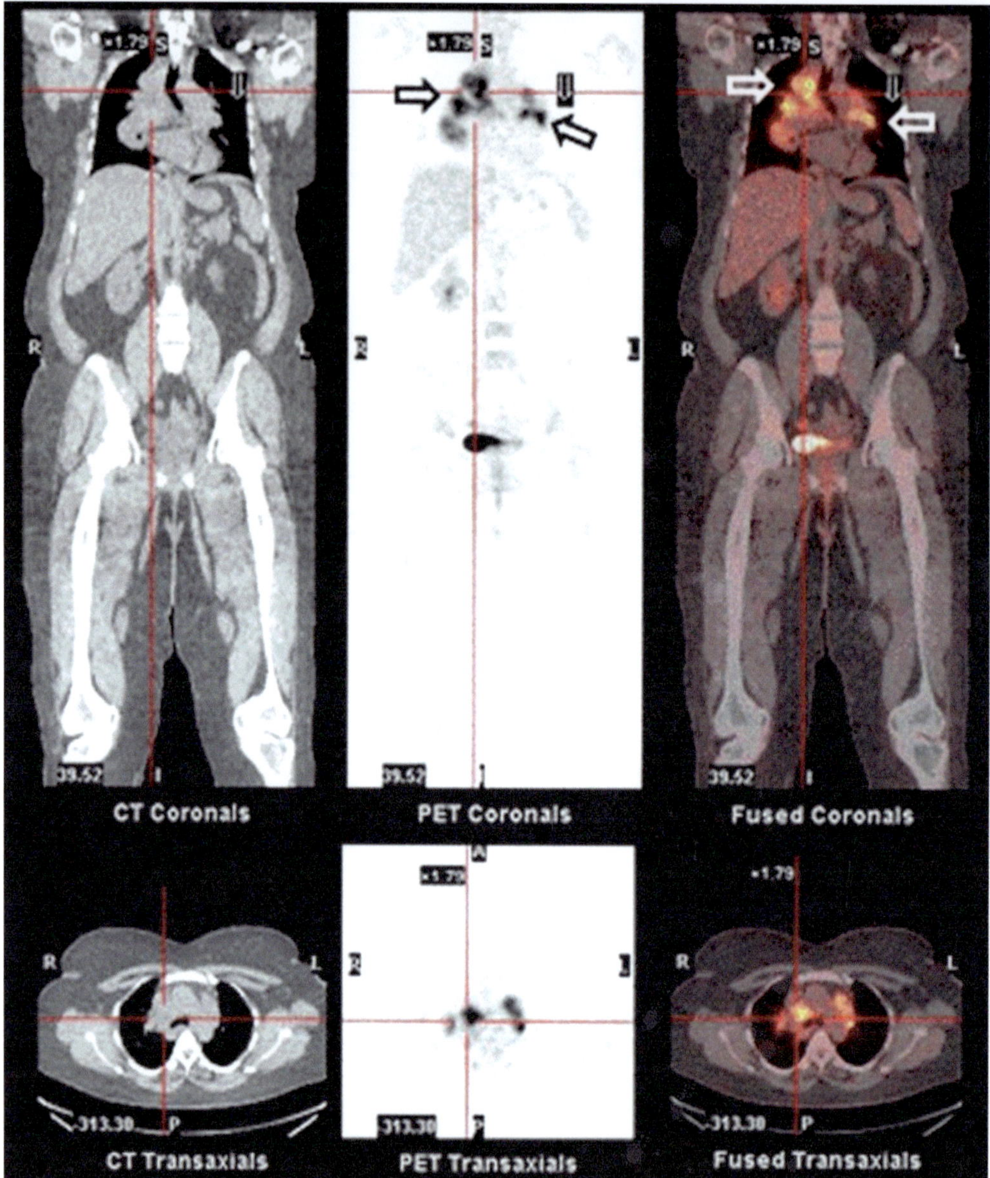

Fig. 8.18 F-18 FDG PET/CT study of a patient with pulmonary sarcoidosis illustrating bilateral hilar hypermetabolic activity (arrows)

8.8 Obstructive Airway Disease

Chronic bronchitis, emphysema, and bronchial asthma are collectively known as obstructive airway disease. Chronic bronchitis and emphysema are common among smokers but are also caused by air pollutants. In chronic bronchitis, the walls of the bronchi and bronchioles are inflamed with edema, cellular infiltrates, fibrosis, and an increase in the mucus glands and bronchial secretions and thickening of the bronchial walls. All these changes result in progressive narrowing of the lumina of the bronchi and bronchioles.

Emphysema indicates irreversible dilation of the alveoli, and destruction of their septa can occur alone or, commonly, in association with chronic bronchitis as part of chronic obstructive airway disease. Hyperinflation of the alveoli and septal destruction may lead to the formation of large air spaces (bullae). Air spaces formed adjacent to the pleura are called blebs.

Bronchial asthma is characterized by episodes of airflow obstruction, which affect both large and small airways. Decreased ventilation and perfusion can be seen on ventilation and perfusion scans within moments of the asthma attack.

Obstructive airway disease can cause an abnormal ventilation scan with or without abnormal perfusion. Xenon-133 is the most sensitive agent for detecting ventilation abnormalities, particularly in the washout phase [96]. ^{99m}Tc-DTPA aerosol studies show nonuniformity with varying degrees of central deposition of the particles, depending on the severity of bronchial narrowing. The associated perfusion abnormalities range from minimal nonuniformity to complete absence of perfusion, matching the ventilation defects.

8.9 Pleural Effusions

Many etiologies can cause pleural effusion, including inflammatory, traumatic, and neoplastic diseases, and disturbance in organ functions. Pulmonary embolism is not uncommonly associated with pleural effusion. Based on the underlying cause, pleural effusion may consist of transudate, exudate, pus, or blood. With pleural effusions, there is diminished ventilation and perfusion, which is proportional to the amount of effusion [97]. Elevated hemidiaphragm causes a similar pattern. The appearance of pleural effusion may change with the position of the patient when effusion is freely mobile or may not change when the effusion is loculated or encapsulated.

8.10 Pneumonia

Pneumonia is an acute inflammation of the lung parenchyma, which often impairs gas exchange. The condition is prevalent in infants, old individuals, and immunocompromised patients. It is the leading secondary cause of death in the United States. Three major types can be recognized: lobar, lobular (bronchopneumonia), and interstitial. Lobar pneumonia is usually bacterial and involves the alveoli of one lobe or more, but not the bronchi. Chest X-ray and other imaging modalities show varying degrees of abnormalities based on the amount of inflammatory exudate. X-ray will show opacities of different degrees, while nuclear medicine procedures such as labeled WBC or ^{67}Ga show abnormalities correlating in size and intensity with the severity of inflammation and its duration (see Chap. 4). Lobular pneumonia (bronchopneumonia) shows inflammation of bronchi, bronchioles, and alveoli in a patchy manner. Interstitial pneumonia, also called pneumonitis or viral pneumonia, is a milder form that usually accompanies other viral conditions such as measles. Typically, no exudates are present in the alveoli.

8.11 Bronchial Obstruction

Bronchial obstruction may be caused by obstruction from within or from outside the bronchi. It may be acute, such as obstruction due to a foreign body or mucus plug, or gradual, as in some patients with bronchial compression by an adjacent mass. Depending on the level and severity of obstruction, ventilation and perfusion are affected. Usually, the ventilation is affected more severely than the perfusion and may be totally absent with complete obstruction (Fig. 8.19).

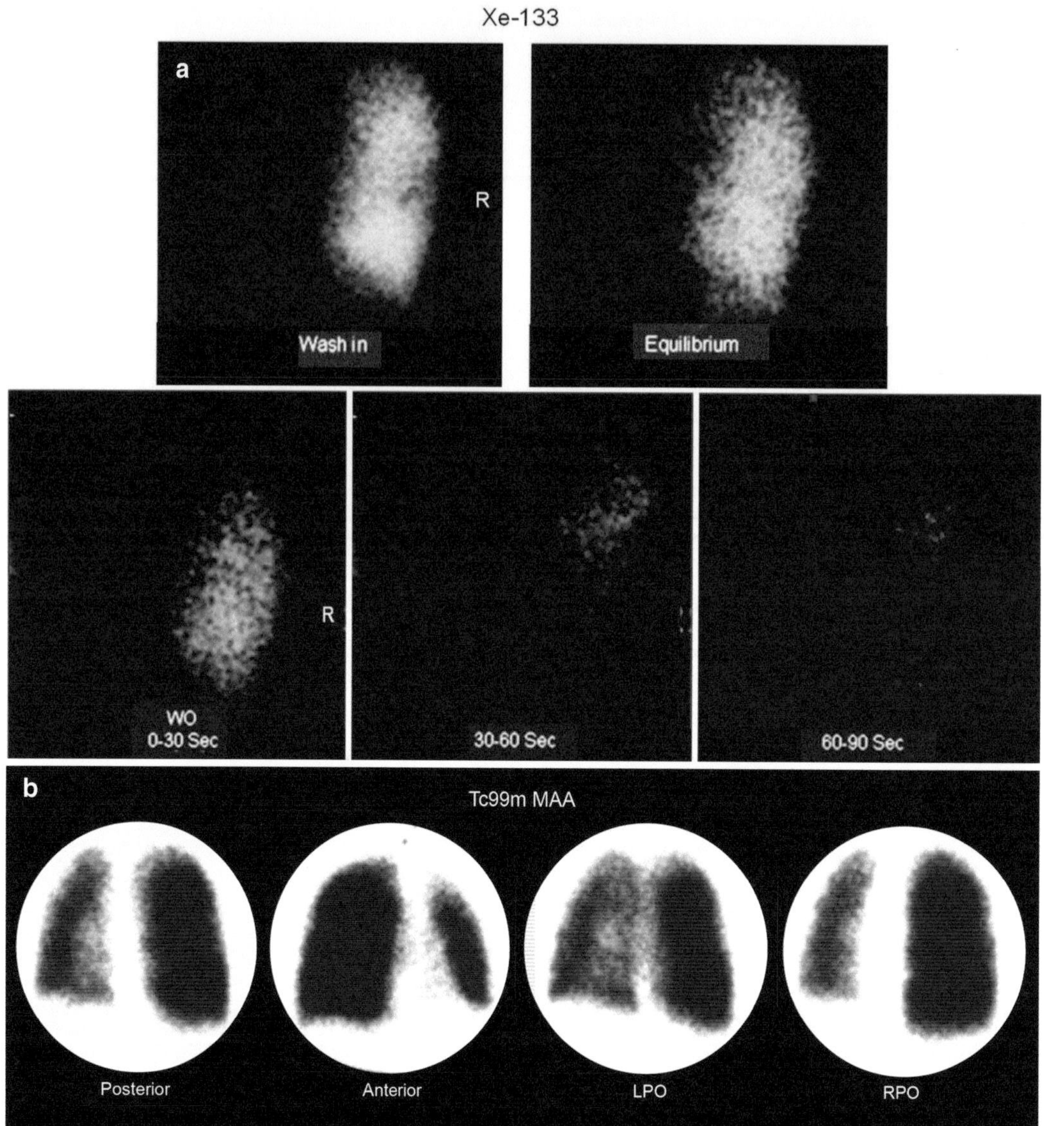

Fig. 8.19 (**a, b**) Xenon-133 washout images of a patient complaining of severe shortness of breath. The images reveal a nonvisualized left lung. ^{99m}Tc-MAA perfusion study of the same patient shows decreased perfusion to same lung diffusely. This pattern suggests bronchial obstruction with reflex vasoconstriction. The patient has a mucus plug obstructing the left main bronchus

8.12 Lung Cancer (see Chap. 12)

Lung cancer is the second most common cancer in both men and women (second to prostate and breast cancers). It is, however, the leading cause of cancer death in both men and women [98].

FDG PET/CT is useful for imaging lung cancer since the tumor cells have both an increased uptake of glucose due to a higher number of Glut-1 surface proteins as well as a higher rate of glycolysis compared to nonneoplastic cells [99].

Histologically, lung cancer may be squamous (epidermoid), adenocarcinoma (bronchogenic carcinoma), small cell carcinoma, adenosquamous carcinoma, and anaplastic carcinoma. The role of nuclear medicine particularly PET/

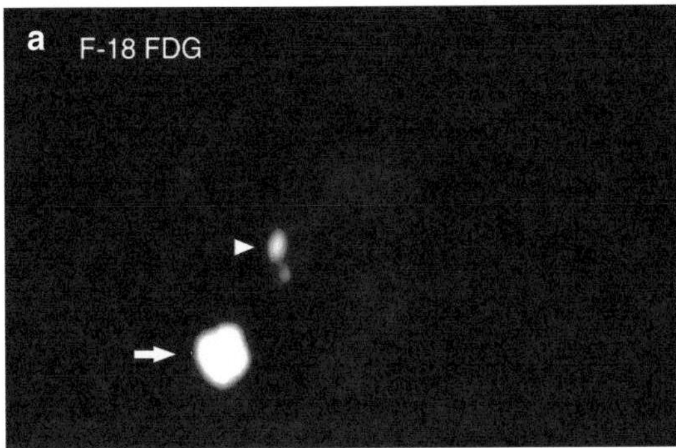

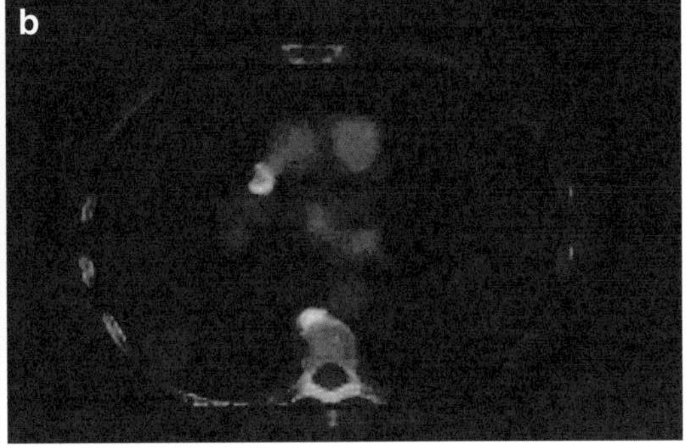

Fig. 8.20 (**a**, **b**) FDG PET study (**a**) illustrating right lung nodule (*arrow*) with intense uptake and a mediastinal involvement (*arrow head*) corresponding to lesions seen on CT scan (**b**). These represent non-small cell lung cancer. The example demonstrates the value of FDG in determining the nature of morphologic findings of nodules and in staging the disease

CT (Fig. 8.20) lies in the detection of the primary tumor in some patients, and more importantly, staging of the tumor determines the best treatment choice, evaluating the response to therapy and sometimes predicting its success [100]. When pneumonectomy is planned for lung cancer, postoperative lung function can be predicted with optimal accuracy by a preoperative perfusion scan in the upright or supine positions. The ventilation scan is less accurate [101]. When pneumonectomy is planned for lung cancer, postoperative lung function can be predicted with optimal accuracy by a preoperative perfusion scan in the upright or supine positions. The ventilation scan is less accurate.

References

1. Brashers BL, Davey SS (1998) Structure and function of the pulmonary system. In: McCance KL, Huether SE (eds) Pathophysiology, the biologic basis for disease in adults and children, 3rd edn. Mosby, St Louis, pp 1131–1157
2. Thibodeau GA, Patton KI (1996) Anatomy and physiology, 3rd edn. Mosby, St Louis
3. De Nardo GL, De Nardo SJ (1984) The lungs. In: Freeman LM, Johnson PM (eds) Clinical radionuclide imaging, 3rd edn. Grune and Stratton, Orlando, pp 1051–1139
4. Elgazzar AH (1997) Scintigraphic diagnosis of pulmonary embolism: unraveling the confusion seven years after PIOPED. Nucl Med Ann:69–101
5. Raskob GE, Angchaisuksiri P, Blanco AN, Buller H, Gallus A, Hunt BJ, Hylek EM, Kakkar A, Konstantinides SV, McCumber M, Ozaki Y, Wendelboe A, Weitz JI (2014) Thrombosis: a major contributor to global disease burden. Arterioscler Thromb Vasc Biol 34:23632371
6. Anderson FA, Zayaruzny M Jr, Heit JA, Fidan D, Cohen AT (2007) Estimated annual numbers of US acute-care hospital patients at risk for venous thromboembolism. Am J Hematol 82:777–782
7. Turetz M, Sideris AT, Friedman OA, Triphathi N, Horowitz JM (2018) Pulmonary embolism: epidemiology, pathophysiology, and natural history of pulmonary embolism. In: Seminars in interventional radiology, vol 35. Thieme Medical Publishers, New York, p 92
8. Kucher N, Tapson VF, Goldhaber SZ, DVT FREE Steering Committee (2005) Risk factors associated with symptomatic pulmonary embolism in a large cohort of deep vein thrombosis patients. Thromb Haemost 93:494–498. https://doi.org/10.1160/TH04-09-0587
9. Stein PD, Matta F, Musani MH, Diaczok B (2010) Silent pulmonary embolism in patients with deep venous thrombosis: a systematic review. Am J Med 123(05):426–431
10. Frieman DG, Suyemoto J, Wessler S (1965) Frequency of pulmonary thromboembolism in man. N Engl J Med 272:1278–1280
11. McLachlin J, Patterson JC (1961) Some basic observations on venous thrombosis and pulmonary embolism. Surg Gynecol Obstet 93:1–8
12. Moser KM (1990) Venous thromboembolism: state-of-the-art. Am Rev Respir Dis 141:235–249
13. Muñoz FJ, Mismetti P, Poggio R et al (2008) Clinical outcome of patients with upper-extremity deep vein thrombosis: results from the RIETE Registry. Chest 133(01):143–148
14. Palevsky HI, Alavi A (1991) Noninvasive strategy for management of patients suspected of pulmonary embolism. Semin Nucl Med 21:325–331
15. Miesbach W, Makris M (2020) COVID-19: coagulopathy, risk of thrombosis, and the ratio-

nale for anticoagulation. Clin Appl Thromb Hemost 26:1076029620938149. https://doi.org/10.1177/1076029620938149

16. Kipshidze N, Dangas G, White CJ, Kipshidze N, Siddiqui F, Lattimer CR, Carter CA, Fareed J (2020) Viral coagulopathy in patients with COVID-19: treatment and care. Clin Appl Thromb Hemost 26:1076029620936776. https://doi.org/10.1177/1076029620936776

17. Salabei JS, Fishman TJ, Asnake ZT, Ali A, Iyer UG (2021) COVID-19 coagulopathy: current knowledge and guidelines on anticoagulation. Heart Lung 50:357–360

18. Colling ME, Kanthi Y (2020) COVID–19-associated Coagulopathy: an exploration of mechanisms. Vasc Med 25:471–478

19. Malas MB, Naazie IN, Elsayed N, Mathlouthi A, Marmor R, Clary B (2020) Thromboembolism risk of COVID-19 is high and associated with a higher risk of mortality: A systematic review and meta-analysis. EClinical Med 29–30:100639

20. Akel T, Qaqa F, Abuarqoub A, Shamoon F (2020) Pulmonary embolism: A complication of COVID-19 infection. Thromb Res 193:79–82

21. Bělohlávek J, Dytrych V, Linhart A (2013) Pulmonary embolism, part I: epidemiology, risk factors and risk stratification, pathophysiology, clinical presentation, diagnosis and nonthrombotic pulmonary embolism. Exp Clin Cardiol 18(2):129–138

22. Kamel E, Mckee T, Calcagni M, Schmidt S, Markl S, Bischof Delaloye A (2005) Occult lung infarction may induce false interpretation of F19 FDG PET in primary staging of pulmonary malignancies. Eur J Nucl Med Mol Imaging 32:641–646

23. Manny J, Hechtman HB (1985) Vasoactive humoral factors. In: Goldhaber SZ (ed) Pulmonary embolism and deep venous thrombosis. Saunders, Philadelphia, p 283

24. Dass H, Hcekscher T, Anthonisen NR (1967) Regional pulmonary gas exchange in patients with pulmonary embolism. Clin Sci 33:355–364

25. Smith R, Alderson PO (1987) Ventilation perfusion scintigraphy in pulmonary embolism in pulmonary nuclear medicine. In: Loken MK (ed) Pulmonary nuclear medicine. Appleton and Lange, Norwalk, pp 51–79

26. Wolfe MW, Skibo LK, Goldhaber SZ (1993) Pulmonary embolic disease: diagnosis, pathophysiologic aspects and treatment with thrombolytic therapy. Curr Probl Cardiol 18:587–633

27. National Heart, Lung and Blood Institute (1970) Urokinase pulmonary embolism trial—phase I results. JAMA 214:2163–2172

28. National Heart, Lung and Blood Institute (1974) Urokinase pulmonary embolism trial—phase II results. JAMA 229:1606–1613

29. Elgazzar AH, Jobalia R, Subramanian P, Ryan J, Hughes JA (1994) Multiple ventilation and perfusion (V/Q) scans in patients with and without pulmonary emboli (PE). J Nucl Med 35:239

30. Klok FA, Mos IC, van Kralingen KW, Vahl JE, Huisman MV (2012) Chronic pulmonary embolism and pulmonary hypertension. Semin Respir Crit Care Med 33:199–204

31. Hoeper MM, Mayer E, Simonneau G, Rubin LJ (2006) Chronic thromboembolic pulmonary hypertension. Circulation 110:2011–2020

32. PIOPED Investigators (1990) Value of the ventilation/perfusion scan in acute pulmonary embolism: results of the prospective investigation of pulmonary embolism diagnosis (PIOPED). JAMA 263:2753–2759

33. Carson JL, Kelley MA, Duff A, Weg JG, Fulkerson WJ, Palevsky HI, Schwartz JS, Thompson BT, Popovich J Jr, Hobbins TE et al (1992) The clinical course of pulmonary embolism. N Engl J Med 326:1240–1245

34. Schober B (1980) Do pulmonary emboli lodge preferentially in prior foci? J Nucl Med 21:659–661

35. Hoffman JM, Lee A, Grafton S, Bellamy P, Hawkins RA, Webner M (1994) Clinical signs and symptoms in pulmonary embolism. A reassessment. Clin Nucl Med 19:803–808

36. Stein PD, Terrin ML, Hales CA, Palevsky HI, Saltzman HA, Thompson BT, Weg JG (1991) Clinical, laboratory, roentgenographic, and electrocardiographic findings in patients with acute pulmonary embolism and no pre-existing cardiac or pulmonary disease. Chest 100:598–603

37. Stein PD, Henry JW (1997) Prevalence of acute pulmonary embolism in central and subsegmental pulmonary arteries and relation to probability interpretation of ventilation/perfusion lung scans. Chest 111:1246–1248

38. Morgenthaler TI, Ryu JH (1995) Clinical characteristics of fatal pulmonary embolism in a referral hospital. Mayo Clin Proc 70:417–424

39. Morpurgo M, Schmid C (1995) The spectrum of pulmonary embolism. Clinicopathologic correlations. Chest 107:18S–20S

40. Sperry KL, Key CR, Anderson RE (1990) Towards a population-based assessment of death due to pulmonary embolism in New Mexico. Hum Pathol 21:159–165

41. Karwinski B, Svendsen E (1989) Comparison of clinical and postmortem diagnosis of pulmonary embolism. J Clin Pathol 42:135–139

42. Gross JS, Neufeld RR, Libow LS, Gerber I, Rodstein M (1988) Autopsy study of the elderly institutionalized patient: review of 234 autopsies. Arch Intern Med 1:173–176

43. Dismuke SE, Wagner EH (1986) Pulmonary embolism as a cause of death. JAMA 225:2039–2042

44. Goldhaber SZ, Hennekens CH, Evans DA, Newton EC, Goldleski JJ (1982) Factors associated with correct antemortem diagnosis of major pulmonary embolism. Am J Med 73:822–826

45. Rubio-Jurado B, Albores-Arguijo RC, Guerra-Soto A, Plasencia-Ortiz T, Tavarez-Macías G, Huerta-Hernández J, Riebeling-Navarro C, Nava-Zavala AH (2020) Concordance between clinical diagnosis of pulmonary thromboembolism at hospital discharge and anatomopatho-

logical diagnosis. Int J Immunopathol Pharmacol 34:2058738420942390

46. Timmons S, Kingston M, Hussain M, Kelly H, Liston R (2003) Pulmonary embolism: differences in presentation between older and younger patients. Age Ageing 32:601–605

47. Berman AR, Arnsten JH (2003) Diagnosis and treatment of pulmonary embolism in the elderly. Clin Geriatr Med 19:157–175

48. Paraskos JA, Adelstein SJ, Smith RE, Rickman FD, Grossman W, Dexter L, Dalen JE (1973) Late prognosis of acute pulmonary embolism. N Engl J Med 239:55–58

49. Stein PD, Athanasoulis C, Alavi A, Greenspan RH, Hales CA, Saltzman HA, Vreim CE, Terrin ML, Weg JG (1992) Complications and validity of pulmonary angiography in acute pulmonary embolism. Circulation 85:462–468

50. Righini M, Le Gal G, De Lucia S, Roy PM, Meyer G, Aujesky D, Bounameaux H, Perrier A (2006) Clinical usefulness of D-dimer testing in cancer patients with suspected pulmonary embolism. Thromb Haemost 95:715719

51. Douma RA, Mos IC, Erkens PM, Nizet TA, Durian MF et al (2011) Prometheus study group. Performance of 4 clinical decision rules in the diagnostic management of acute pulmonary embolism: a prospective cohort study. Ann Intern Med 154:709718

52. Miron MJ, Perrier A, Bounameaux H, de Moerloose P, Slosman DO, Didier D, Junod A (1999) Contribution of noninvasive evaluation to the diagnosis of pulmonary embolism in hospitalized patients. Eur Respir J 13:13651370

53. Chabloz P, Reber G, Boehlen F, Hohlfeld P, De Moerloose P (2001) TAFI antigen and D-dimer levels during normal pregnancy and at delivery. Br J Haematol 115(1):150–152

54. Bajc M, Schümichen C, Grüning T, Lindqvist A, Le Roux PY, Alatri A, Bauer RW, Dilic M, Neilly B, Verberne HJ, Delgado Bolton RC, Jonson B (2019) EANM guideline for ventilation/perfusion single-photon emission computed tomography (SPECT) for diagnosis of pulmonary embolism and beyond. Eur J Nucl Med Mol Imaging 46(12):2429–2451

55. Schoepf UJ, Goldhaber SZ, Costello P (2004) Spiral computed tomography for acute pulmonary embolism. Circulation 109:2160–2167

56. Radan L, Mor M, Gips S, Schlang-Eisenberg D, Lurie Y, Dickstein K, Bitterman H, Ben-Haim S (2004) The added value of spiral computed tomographic angiography after lung scintigraphy for the diagnosis of pulmonary embolism. Clin Nucl Med 29:255–261

57. Wiener RS, Schwartz LM, Woloshin S (2013) When a test is too good: how CT pulmonary angiograms find pulmonary emboli that do not need to be found. BMJ 347:3368

58. Aviram G, Levy G, Fishman JE, Blank A, Graif M (2004) Pitfalls in the diagnosis of acute pulmonary embolism on spiral computed tomography. Curr Probl Diagn Radiol 33:74–84

59. Perrier A (2001) Pulmonary embolism: from clinical presentation to clinical probability assessment. Semin Vasc Med 1:147–154

60. Kanne JP, Lalani TA (2004) Role of computed tomography and magnetic resonance imaging for deep venous thrombosis and pulmonary embolism. Circulation 109(1):115–121

61. Mitchell AM, Kline JA (2007) Contrast nephropathy following computed tomography angiography of the chest for pulmonary embolism in the emergency department. J Thromb Haemost 5:50–54

62. Smith-Bindman R, Lipson J, Marcus R et al (2009) Radiation dose associated with common computed tomography examinations and the associated lifetime attributable risk of cancer. Arch Intern Med 169:2078–2086

63. Altes TA, Mai VM, Munger TM, Brookeman JR, Hagspiel KD (2005) Pulmonary embolism: comprehensive evaluation with MR ventilation and perfusion scanning with hyperpolarized helium-3, arterial spin tagging, and contrast-enhanced MRA. J VascInterv Radiol 16:999–1005

64. Mudge CS, Healey TT, Atalay MK, Pezzullo JA (2013) Feasibility of detecting pulmonary embolism using noncontrast MRI. Radiology 2013:1–5

65. Benson DG, Schiebler ML, Repplinger MD, François CJ, Grist TM, Reeder SB, Nagle SK (2017) Contrast-enhanced pulmonary MRA for the primary diagnosis of pulmonary embolism: current state of the art and future directions. Br J Radiol 90(1074):20160901. https://doi.org/10.1259/bjr.20160901. Epub 2017 Apr 12

66. Biello DR, Mattar AG, McKnight RC, Siegel BA (1979) Ventilation-perfusion studies in suspected pulmonary embolism. AJR Am J Roentgenol 103:1033–1037

67. Hull RD, Hirsh J, Carter CJ, Jay RM, Dodd PE, Ockelford PA, Coates G, Gill GJ, Turpie AG, Doyle DJ, Buller HR, Raskob GE (1983) Pulmonary angiography, ventilation lung scanning, and venography for clinically suspected pulmonary embolism with abnormal perfusion lung scan. Ann Intern Med 98:891–899

68. Onyedika C, Glaser JE, Freeman LM (2010) Pulmonary embolism: role of ventilation-perfusion scintigraphy. Semin Nucl Med 43(2):82–87

69. Freeman LM, Glaser JE, Haramati LB (2012) Planar V/Q imaging for pulmonary embolism: the case for "outcomes" medicine. Semin Nucl Med 42(1):3–10

70. Burns SK, Haramati LB (2012) Diagnostic imaging and risk stratification of patients with acute pulmonary embolism. Cardiol Rev 20:15–24

71. Stein PD, Coleman ER, Gottscalk A, Saltzman H, Terrin ML, Weg JG (1991) Diagnostic utility of ventilation/perfusion lung scans in acute pulmonary embolism is not diminished by pre-existing cardiac or pulmonary disease. Chest 100:604–606

72. Harris B, Bailey D, Miles S, Bailey E, Rogers K, Roach P, Thomas P, Hensley M, King GG (2007)

Objective analysis of tomographic ventilation–perfusion scintigraphy in pulmonary embolism. Am J Respir Crit Care Med 175:1173–1180

73. Bajc M, Neilly JB, Miniati M, Schuemichen C, Meignan M, Jonson B (2009) EANM guidelines for ventilation/perfusion scintigraphy. Part 1. Pulmonary imaging with ventilation/perfusion single photon emission tomography. Eur J Nucl Med Mol Imaging 36:1056–1070

74. Glaser JE, Chamarthy M, Haramati LB, Esses D, Freeman LM (2011) Successful and safe implementation of a trinary interpretation and reporting strategy for V/Q lung scintigraphy. J Nucl Med 52:1508–1512

75. Sostman HD, Pistolesi M (2011) Scintigraphy for pulmonary embolism: too old to rock 'n' roll, too young to die? J Nucl Med 52:11A–12A

76. Bhargavan M, Sunshine JH, Lewis RS, Jha S, Owen JB, Vializ J (2010) Frequency of use of imaging tests in the diagnosis of pulmonary embolism: effects of physician specialty, patient characteristics, and region. AJR Am J Roentgenol 194:1018–1026

77. The Task Force for the Diagnosis and Management (2008) Guidelines on the diagnosis and management of acute pulmonary embolism. Eur Heart J 29:2276–2315

78. Wazir JF, Ansari NA (2004) Pneumocystis carinii infection: update and review. Arch Pathol Lab Med 128:1023–1027

79. Feldman C (2005) Pneumonia associated with HIV infection. Curr Opin Infect Dis 18:165–170

80. Morris A, Lundgren JD, Masur H, Walzer PD, Hanson DL, Frederick T, Huang L, Beard CB, Kaplan JE (2004) Current epidemiology of pneumocystis pneumonia. Emerg Infect Dis 10:1713–1720

81. Medrano FJ, Montes-Cano M, Conde M, de la Horra C, Respaldiza N, Gasch A, Perez-Lozano MJ, Varela JM, Calderon EJ (2005) Pneumocystis jirovecii in general population. Emerg Infect Dis 11:245–250

82. Al Soub H, Taha RY, El Deeb Y, Almaslamani M, Al Khuwaiter JY (2004) Pneumocystis carinii pneumonia in a patient without a predisposing illness: case report and review. Scand J Infect Dis 36:618–621

83. Kramer EL, Sanger JJ (1989) Detection of thoracic infections by nuclear medicine techniques in the acquired immunodeficiency syndrome. Radiol Clin N Am 27:1067–1075

84. Woolfenden JM, Carrasquillo JA, Larson SM, Simmons JT, Masur H, Smith PD, Shelhamer JH, Ognibene FP (1987) Acquired immunodeficiency syndrome: ga-67 citrate imaging. Radiology 162:383–387

85. Raghu G, Collard HR, Egan JJ, Martinez FJ, Behr J et al (2011) An official ATS/ERS/JRS/ALAT statement: idiopathic pulmonary fibrosis: evidence-based guidelines for diagnosis and management. Am J Respir Crit Care Med 183:788–824

86. Travis WD, Costabel U, Hansell DM, King TE Jr, Lynch DA et al (2013) An official American Thoracic Society/European Respiratory Society statement: update of the international Mul-tidisciplinary classification of the idiopathic interstitial pneumonias. Am J Respir Crit Care Med 188:733–748

87. Noble PW, Homer RJ (2004) Idiopathic pulmonary fibrosis: new insights into pathogenesis. Clin Chest Med 25:749–758

88. Line BR, Fulmer JD, Reynolds HY, Roberts WC, Jones AE, Harris EK, Crystal RG (1978) Gallium-67 citrate scanning in the staging of idiopathic pulmonary fibrosis: correlation with physiologic and morphologic features and bronchoalveolar lavage. Am Rev Respir Dis 118:355–365

89. Baughman RP (2004) Pulmonary sarcoidosis. Clin Chest Med 25:521–530

90. Culver DA, Valeyre D (2016) Emerging ideas about sarcoidosis pathophysiology. Curr Opin Pulm Med 22:466–468. https://doi.org/10.1097/MCP.0000000000000310]

91. Mandel J, Weinberger SE (2001) Clinical insights and basic science correlates in sarcoidosis. Am J Med Sci 321:99–107

92. ACCESS Research Group (1999) Design of a case control etiologic study of sarcoidosis (ACCESS). J Clin Epidemiol 52:1173–1186

93. Scadding JG (1961) Prognosis of intrathoracic sarcoidosis in England. Br Med J 4:1165–1172

94. Gupta RG, Beckerman C, Silcian L et al (1982) Gallium citrate scanning and serum angiotensin converting enzyme levels in sarcoidosis. Radiology 144:895–899

95. Prabhakar HB, Rabinowitz CB, Gibbons FK, O'Donnell WJ, Shepard JA, Aquino SL (2008) Imaging features of sarcoidosis on MDCT, FDG PET, and PET/CT. AJR Am J Roentgenol 190:s1–s6

96. Elgazzar AH, Silberstien EB, Hughes J (1995) Perfusion and ventilation scans in patients with diffuse obstructive airway disease: utility of single breath (wash in) xenon-103. J Nucl Med 36:64–67

97. Anthonisen NR, Martin RR (1977) Regional lung function in pleural effusion. Am Rev Respir Dis 116:201–207

98. American Cancer Society (2013) Cancer fact & figures. American Cancer Society, Atlanta, p 2013

99. Higashi K, Ueda Y, Sakuma T et al (2001) Comparison of [(18)F]FDG PET and (201)Tl SPECT in evaluation of pulmonary nodules. J Nucl Med 42:1489–1496

100. Tümkaya E, Büyükdereli G (2013) The role of F-18-FDG PET and PET/CT in lung cancer. Arch Med Rev J 22:470–485

101. Kristersson S (1974) Prediction of lung function after lung surgery. A Xe-133 radiospirometric study and in lung cancer. Arch Med Rev J 22:470–485

9.1 The Heart

9.1.1 Anatomical Considerations

The heart consists of muscles, valves, specialized tissues, coronary arteries, and pericardium. In the embryo, during the first month of gestation, a primitive straight cardiac tube is formed. The tube comprises the sinoatrium, the bulbus cordis, and the truncus arteriosus. In the second month of gestation, this tube doubles over on itself to form two parallel pumping systems, each with two chambers and a great artery. The two atria develop from the sinoatrium; the right and left ventricles develop from the bulbus cordis. Differential growth of myocardial cells causes the straight cardiac tube to bear to the right, and the ventricular portion of the tube doubles over on itself, bringing the ventricles side by side (Fig. 9.1) [1].

The coronary arteries originate from the left and right coronary sinuses of the aorta (Fig. 9.2). The left main coronary artery, which comes off the left coronary sinus, continues for a variable distance before it divides into two major arteries, the left anterior descending and circumflex arteries [2]. The left anterior descending artery (LAD) descends in the anterior interventricular groove and, most of the time, continues to the apex, supplying the apical and inferior apical portions. The LAD gives off septal branches that course deep into the interventricular septum. The septal

branches vary in size and number. The anterior two-thirds of the septum derive their supply from the septal LAD branches, while the rest of the septum is supplied by the perforator branches from the posterior descending branch of the right coronary artery. The LAD provides also diagonal branches, which run on the epicardial surface diagonally to supply the lateral wall of the left ventricle. Usually, the first one or two diagonal branches are large enough for angioplasty or bypass consideration.

The left circumflex artery (LCx) branches off from the left main artery and runs in the left atrioventricular groove. It then continues to the left and posteriorly. It supplies several posterolateral ventricular branches, which in turn supply the posterior lateral surface of the left ventricle and parallel the diagonal branches of the LAD. In most cases, the LCx continues as a small terminal posterior left ventricular branch.

The right coronary artery (RCA) arises from the right coronary sinus and descends in the right atrioventricular (AV) groove. Its first supply is to the proximal pulmonary conus and right ventricular outflow region. Normally, there are also two or three large right ventricular branches that course diagonally over the right ventricle and supply the right ventricular myocardium. Most of the time the RCA continues along the diaphragmatic surface of the heart in the AV groove to reach the crux. At the crux, the RCA divides into a posterior descending artery (PDA) and a poste-

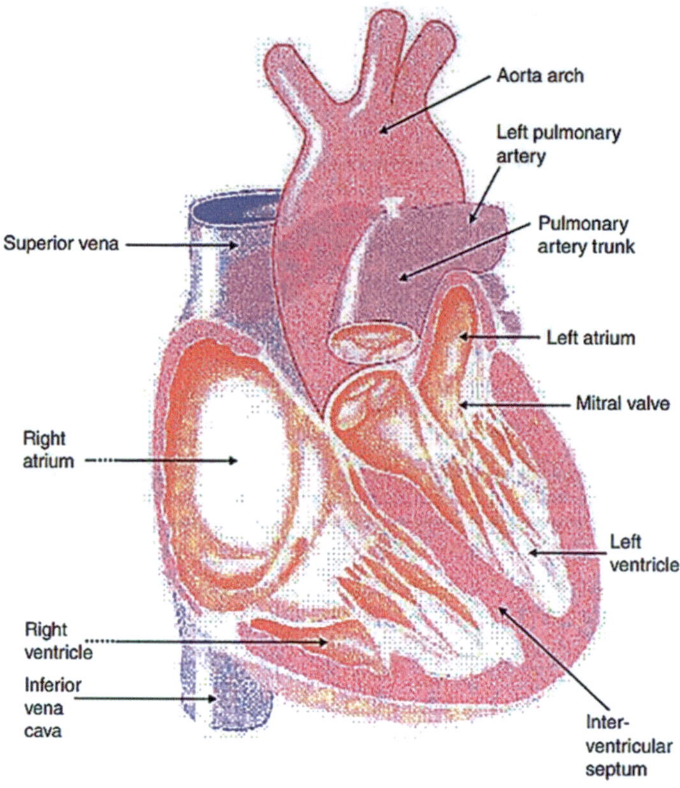

Fig. 9.1 Cutaway view of the heart

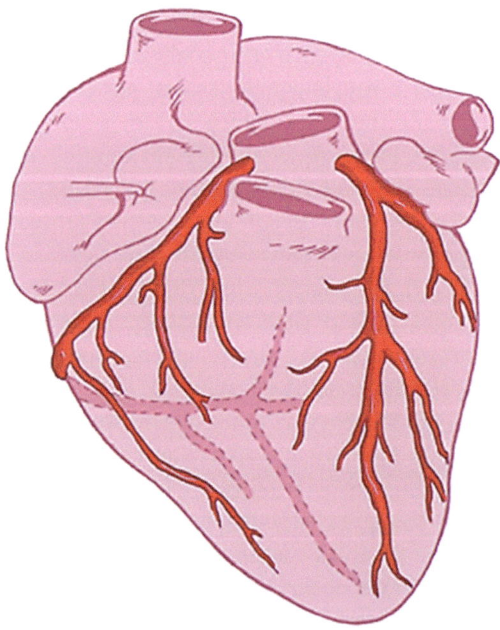

Fig. 9.2 Heart showing the origination of the coronary arteries from the left and right coronary sinuses of the aorta

rior left ventricular branch. The PDA branch is usually a large artery that runs in an anterior direction in the inferior interventricular groove. The PDA supplies the inferior third of the septum. The PDA septal branches can provide a rich collateral pathway via septal perforating arteries of the LAD. The other terminal branch of the RCA, the posterior left ventricular branch, continues in the AV groove and communicates with the terminal branch of the Cx.

9.1.2 Physiological Considerations

9.1.2.1 Physiology of Coronary Blood Flow

The heart is continuously filled with blood throughout the whole life although blood within the cardiac chambers does not significantly contribute to the function, viability, and maintenance of cardiac tissue. A specialized separate coronary circulation provides the myocardial tissue with

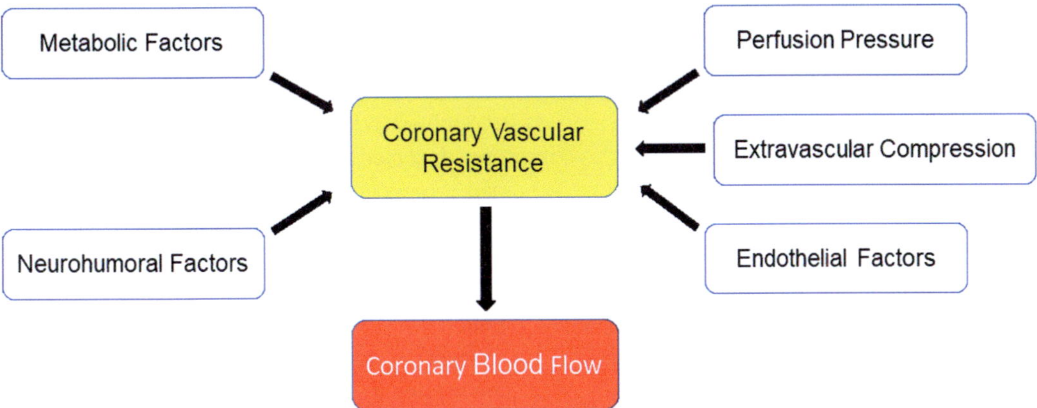

Fig. 9.3 Diagram illustrating factors affecting coronary vascular resistance, the main determinant of coronary blood flow

oxygen and substrates to ensure normal function and viability.

Based on the demands for operating a constantly functioning contractile organ, the heart has the highest per gram oxygen consumption of any organ (50–100 µl O_2/min/g) and hence it extracts 70%–80% of delivered oxygen even under resting conditions compared to skeletal muscle which utilizes only about 30%–40% of delivered oxygen at rest [3–5].

Coronary blood supply depends on coronary vascular resistance. Coronary vascular resistance depends on several factors (Fig. 9.3) and is continuously regulated to deliver sufficient quantities of oxygen supply to meet any change in the metabolic demand of the myocardial tissue (metabolism-perfusion matching) [4, 6–8].

Regional myocardial blood flow can be currently measured noninvasively in units of milliliters of blood per minute per gram myocardium. These noninvasive measurements are achieved by Positron Emission Tomography (PET) and can also be done using MRI and CT. Flow estimates with these different imaging modalities were found in animal experimental studies to correlate well with invasive flow estimates by the arterial blood sampling-microsphere technique which is considered the "gold standard" of blood flow measurements [9, 10].

Changes in myocardial work and, consequently, in energy demand, are accompanied by proportional changes in coronary blood flow. This flow increase is initiated by a metabolically mediated decrease in microvascular resistance with vascular smooth muscle relaxation and hence to adjust the vessel diameter [9, 10].

Seven to 15% of patients with acute coronary syndrome have nonobstructed coronary arteries and myocardial infarction is not accompanied by obstructed coronary arteries [11, 12]. Quantitative measurements of myocardial blood flow identify functional rather than structural disturbances that may reflect adverse effects of coronary risk factors on endothelial function or early stages of developing coronary artery disease.

The most useful application of measuring myocardial blood flow is in cases with coronary disease confined to microvasculature with angiographically nonidentifiable coronary disease. In other words, there is coronary disease affecting microvessels with no apparent macrovascular alterations. This condition may also show diffuse luminal narrowing without discreet coronary stenosis [6, 10]. This condition is now known to be associated with several conditions such as diabetes and cardiomyopathy (Table 9.1) [13–16]. In addition to normal angiography or a finding of diffuse narrowing, myocardial perfusion studies can also be normal even in the presence of symptoms [6, 10]. However, myocardial blood flow is typically diminished in response to vasodilator stress, although it is most likely in the range of normal resting status.

Table 9.1 Major causes of microvascular coronary disease

Diabetic microangiopathies
Hypertrophic cardiomyopathy
Systemic vasculopathies associated with inflammatory disorders
Transplant vasculopathies

9.1.2.2 Myocardial Contractility

Cardiac muscle has two essential properties: electrical excitability and contractility.

9.1.3 Electrical Excitation

The conduction system is composed of modified cardiac cells. The sinoatrial and atrioventricular nodes have cells with high electrical impulse automaticity, while the His bundle and the Purkinje system cells have higher rapid impulse conductivity. The contraction of the heart is normally initiated by an impulse in the sinoatrial node and then spreads over the atrial muscles to the atrioventricular node. The impulse then runs through the His bundle and the Purkinje system to reach all areas of both ventricles at approximately the same time [17].

9.1.3.1 Contraction

The ability of myocardial muscles to shorten and generate the force necessary to maintain blood circulation is a fascinating property of the heart. This is achieved primarily through the unique contractile function of two proteins of the sarcomere (actin and myosin) of the syncytially arranged myocardial fibers. The two main mechanisms that can alter cardiac muscle performance are a change in initial muscle length (Frank-Starling mechanism) and a change in contractile state. In the intact heart, these are determined by preload status, afterload status, the contractile state under a given set of loading conditions, and the heart rate. There is a passive exponential relationship between the length and the tension of muscle fibers. Cardiac muscle tissue, like other body tissues, is not entirely elastic. Thus, this relationship does not exist beyond certain muscle stretch limits. Additionally, there is an active pro-

portional relationship between the initial length of myocardial muscle and the force generated by this muscle, again up to certain length limits [17].

Unlike skeletal muscles, cardiac muscle cells are connected to each other by intercalated disks and do not run the length of the whole muscle. Also, heart muscle has a rich supply of the high-energy phosphate needed for the contraction. Therefore, it may not easily develop an oxygen deficit as skeletal muscle does when its work exceeds its oxygen supply. Cardiac sarcomeres are limited by the fact that they can be extended only to a certain limit (the optimum length of 2.2 µm), whereas sarcomeres of skeletal muscles can be stretched out beyond that. Finally, cardiac muscle has all-or-none twitch contraction and cannot be physiologically tetanized as skeletal muscle can.

9.1.3.2 Assessment of Left Ventricular Performance

9.1.3.2.1 Left Ventricular Function Curve

The left ventricular function curve usually refers to plotting of some of the LV performance measurements such as stroke volume or work against some of the preload indices such as pulmonary capillary wedge pressure [18]. This analysis requires invasive measurements and is useful not only for providing prognostic information in acute cardiac conditions but also for monitoring responses to therapeutic interventions.

9.1.3.2.2 Ejection Fraction

The ejection fraction is the most useful single number of the LV performance, defined as the stroke volume divided by the end-diastolic volume. This functional index can be measured by both invasive and noninvasive techniques. Ejection fraction is closely related to the LV function curve; however, it is very sensitive to loading conditions [18].

9.1.3.2.3 Pressure–Volume Relationship Measurement

By studying the pressure–volume relationship, a stroke work index can be obtained [18]. This is defined as stroke volume X (mean LV systolic ejection pressure—mean LV diastolic pressure). It is a very sensitive index since it is affected by all factors that may alter LV performance.

9.1.3.2.4 Regional Wall Motion Assessment

The assessment of regional wall motion is extremely useful in confirming and locating the site of coronary artery disease (CAD). As with LV ejection fraction measurement, it can be studied using both invasive and noninvasive methods.

9.1.3.2.5 Diastolic Function

Diastolic function is usually assessed by studying the relationship between LV passive pressure and volume and by examining the rate of relaxation after contraction. Several important measurements have been derived from various invasive and noninvasive techniques that can be used for both evaluating and monitoring the changes in diastolic function [18].

9.2 Pathophysiological Considerations

9.2.1 Heart Failure

Heart failure is considered a pathophysiological condition rather than a specific disease. In such a condition, the heart fails to supply enough blood to meet the metabolic demand of the tissues. Most cases of heart failure are due to primary myocardial dysfunction or intrinsic abnormalities, which include hypertensive myocardial hypertrophy, ischemic heart disease, valvular heart disease, pulmonary hypertension, pericardial disease, and other cardiomyopathies (Table 9.2). Various extrinsic abnormalities can cause heart failure as well, despite normal ventricular function, referred to as secondary heart failure. These include hypovolemia, anemia, and distributive (vaspdilatory) shock [19, 20]. Heart failure in this situation could have many reasons: inadequate blood volume as in hemorrhage, inadequate oxygen delivery as in anemia, inadequate venous return as in tricuspid stenosis,

Table 9.2 Major causes of heart failure

A. Systolic dysfunction
1. Ischemic heart disease (e.g., chronic ischemia and myocardial infarction)
2. Valvular heart disease (e.g., mitral regurgitation and aortic regurgitation)
3. Dilated cardiomyopathy (idiopathic and nonidiopathic)
4. Chronic uncontrolled arrhythmia
B. Diastolic dysfunction
1. Hypertension
2. Ischemic heart disease (e.g., acute ischemia)
3. Infiltrative myocardial disease (e.g., amyloid)
4. Left ventricular outflow tract obstruction (e.g., hypertrophic obstructive cardiomyopathy and aortic stenosis)
5. Uncontrolled arrhythmia

profound capillary vasodilatation as in toxic shock, and peripheral vascular abnormalities as in arteriovenous shunts.

Under normal conditions, the heart receives blood at low pressure in diastole, then ejects it at higher pressure during systole. Heart failure occurs when the heart fails to maintain adequate cardiac output (CO) to meet the body's metabolic demands. CO is the ejected amount of blood by the ventricle per minute. It is equal to the stroke volume (SV) multiplied by the heart rate (HR), i.e., $CO = SV \times HR$. Stroke volume is the amount of blood ejected from the ventricle during systole, which is equal to the end-diastolic volume (EDV) minus end-systolic volume (ESV). SV depends on three determinants; preload, afterload, and contractility. Preload is the ventricular pressure at the end of diastole, while afterload is the pressure during ventricular systolic contraction. Myocardial contractility accounts for the change in contraction intensity. Ventricular SV increases when there is an increase in preload, a decrease in afterload, or enhanced contractility [21].

Chronic heart failure occurs when the afterload increases or ventricular contractility is reduced, a condition termed "systolic dysfunction." Essential causes of increased afterload are systemic hypertension and severe aortic stenosis. Significant causes of impaired contractility are coronary atherosclerosis, mitral regurgitation, aortic regurgitation, and dilated cardiomyopathies. Chronic heart failure may also result from impaired ventricular filling and diastolic relaxation which is known as "diastolic dysfunction." Accordingly, heart failure has been categorized into two groups; heart failure with reduced EF, i.e., systolic dysfunction and heart failure with normal EF, i.e., diastolic dysfunction [22, 23].

All the physiological principles described in heart failure are essentially applied to both left- and right-sided failure. However, the right ventricle is highly compliant compared to the left ventricle and therefore can accept larger volumes of blood with little changes in its filling pressure [21].

Compensatory mechanisms in heart failure include the Frank-Starling mechanism. When LV contractile function is impaired, this results in incomplete emptying and increased LV pressure. Myocardial fibers act through the Frank-Starling mechanism, increase stretch to induce a greater stroke volume which helps to empty the enlarged LV and maintain a normal cardiac output. The second compensatory mechanism is neurohormonal activation which comprises increased adrenergic activation, renin–angiotensin–aldosterone system, and increased antidiuretic hormone. The third (space)mechanism includes ventricular hypertrophy and remodeling. All such compensatory mechanisms can be beneficial within limits, but eventually fail to maintain adequate cardiac output [24, 25].

9.2.2 Systemic Hypertension

Blood pressure (BP) is the result of cardiac output (CO) and peripheral resistance (PR), i.e., BP = CO X PR. There are four structures that are responsible for regulation of BP. These include the heart or the pump that creates the ejecting pressure; blood vascular tone which is responsible for peripheral resistance; the kidneys which control the intravascular volume; and neurohormones that moderate the previous three structures. However, a fourth short-term regulatory mechanism of BP is through the baroreceptor reflex, which plays a significant role in momentary changes in BP. Such receptors are present in the walls of the aortic arch and carotid sinuses. Whenever BP rises, baroreceptors are stimulated and transmit impulses to the brain stem medulla, which sends negative feedback signals through the autonomic nervous system, causing inhibition of the sympathetic nervous system and stimulation of the parasympathetic system with a consequent fall in BP. Contrarily, baroreceptors transmit fewer impulses to the medulla following a transient fall in BP, resulting in the restoration of BP [26].

Hypertension increases the workload of the heart and damages the systemic arterial vasculature. It increases the afterload and can cause systolic dysfunction, left ventricular hypertrophy, which if uncontrolled, can eventually end in diastolic dysfunction. All of such effects can lead to left ventricular failure. Increased afterload will, in turn, increase the myocardial oxygen demands, which can lead to chronic myocardial ischemia. In addition, hypertension causes vascular endothelial damage, the most significant triggering mechanism for the initiation of atherosclerosis [27]. Hence, the role of hypertension as a risk factor for atherosclerosis cannot be overstated. In addition to its atherogenic role, hypertension contributes to many arterial pathological complications, which include tissue ischemia, thrombosis, embolism, aneurysm, and hemorrhage. Such effects may influence important and vital target organs, such as the heart, brain, kidneys, and eyes.

The increased arterial peripheral resistance raises the pressure inside the LV with increased afterload. As a compensatory mechanism, LV hypertrophy ensues in the form of concentric hypertrophy, mostly without dilatation. Increased LV muscular rigidity results in diastolic dysfunction [28]. In such conditions, HF is manifested with a normal ejection fraction (EF).

9.2.3 Pulmonary Hypertension

The degree of pulmonary blood flow is affected mainly by the lumen size of the pulmonary vessels [29]. Further, pulmonary vascular resistance is defined as the difference between mean alveolar pressure and left atrial (LA) pressure divided by pulmonary blood flow. A change in any of these factors may therefore give rise to pulmonary hypertension. Pulmonary hypertension can be either primary or secondary to many other causes. In congenital heart diseases, increased medial thickening and atherosclerotic changes of the pulmonary vasculature are observed [30]. The sudden rise of PA pressure with irreversible RV failure and the usual significant decrease in LV systolic function association in acute pulmonary embolization are the cause of high mortality within the first hour in these patients [31]. Conversely, intimal fibrosis due to thrombus organization is the reason behind the cor pulmonale in chronic pulmonary embolization [32].

Pulmonary hypertension can also develop due to a rise in pulmonary venous pressure caused by LV diastolic dysfunction or high LA pressure. If such a condition persists long enough, medial thickening and arterialization of pulmonary veins will develop, which results in pulmonary fibrosis and destruction of alveolar capillaries [29]. The most common chronic lung disease associated with cor pulmonale is chronic bronchitis. The increased pulmonary vascular resistance in this case is caused by a reduction in the total area of the pulmonary vascular tree as well as mild thickening of the pulmonary arterioles [33, 34].

Unlike the LV, the RV is a high-volume, low-pressure pump. Consequently, as pulmonary vascular resistance increases, a decrease in RV stroke volume and EF is observed [22, 35].

9.2.4 Atherosclerosis

Currently, atherogenesis is largely viewed as a chronic inflammatory process. Several decades back, it was regarded as a simple imbibition of elevated plasma lipoproteins through permeable vascular endothelium. The evolution of early atheromatous lesions, i.e., fatty streaks, may commence as early as during infancy [36]. Atherogenesis is a complex and incompletely understood multifactorial procedure. There are

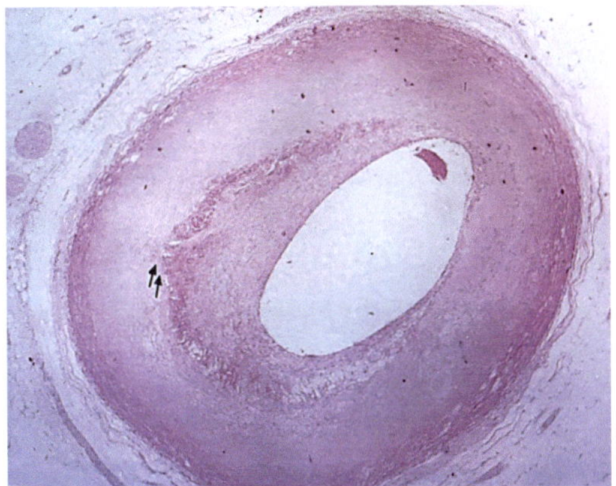

Fig. 9.4 Coronary atherosclerotic plaque showing an organized thrombus (arrows) building up the atheromatous growth

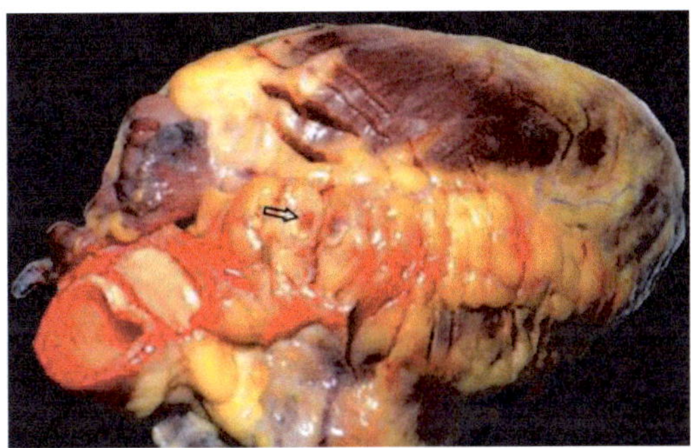

Fig. 9.5 Picture of a heart from a postmortem autopsy illustrating intracoronary thrombosis (arrow) (Courtesy of Prof. M. Elfawal)

two adopted theories of atherogenesis; the first is the response to Injury, which probably contributes to the build-up of atherosclerotic lesions during the early stages of the disease. The second, thrombogenic theory, possibly participates in the progression of a pre-existing plaque that undergoes thrombotic formation (Figs. 9.4, 9.5, and 9.6), with healing by organization and reendothelialization, and further progressive narrowing of the arterial lumen. The current view of atherogenesis incorporates elements of both theories and includes the recognized modifiable and unmodifiable risk factors [37, 38].

The response to injury theory entails dynamic interaction between (1) endothelial dysfunction, (2) subendothelial inflammation, and (3) vascular smooth muscle cell response [39].

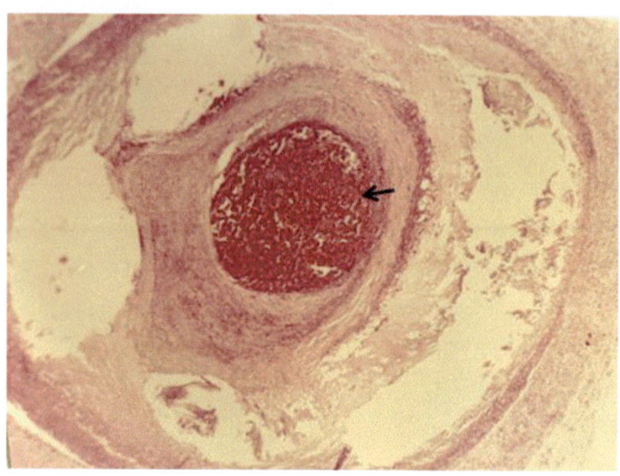

Fig. 9.6 Occluding recent thrombus (arrow) in a severely narrowed coronary artery by a predominantly fatty concentric atherosclerotic plaque

Endothelial dysfunction can be initiated by a number of risk factors, which include sheer mechanical stress related to hypertension, oxidized low-density lipoprotein (OxLDL), diabetes mellitus, smoking, elevated homocysteine levels, infectious agents, among others. Such physical and chemical stressors impair endothelial permeability, promote the release of inflammatory cytokines, increase monocyte adhesion, alter the release of vasoactive substances (e.g., prostacyclin and nitric oxide), and interfere with normal antithrombotic properties. Dysfunctional endothelium leads to (a) increased permeability to lipoproteins and (b) promoting passage of monocytes across the endothelium. The low-density lipoprotein (LDL) trapped in the subendothelium undergoes oxidation (OxLDL). The resultant inflammatory reaction involves incorporation of OxLDL in the subendothelium into the modified macrophages, forming foam cells that represent the earliest lesions known as fatty streaks or the precursor lesions. Fatty streaks are observed in the aorta and coronary arteries of most individuals by 20 years of age. The intimal thickening in fatty streaks is due to the accumulation of monocyte-derived macrophages filled with lipid (cholesterol esters) forming foamy cells [40, 41].

Some fatty streaks, especially those involving the coronary arteries, have been shown to progress to the classic atherosclerotic plaques, because of progressive lipid accumulation and migration and proliferation of smooth muscle cells. Some fatty streaks may regress, while others remain unchanged.

The pathogenesis of the atherosclerotic plaque involves the entry of LDL into the intima, where it binds to receptors of macrophages to form foam cells as described before. Once within the intima, LDL becomes chemoattractant to more blood monocytes and also causes macrophage aggregation, as well as further injury to the endothelium [40, 42, 43].

Monokines from the activated macrophages also attract migration of smooth muscle cells from the media into the intima where they proliferate under the influence of platelet-derived growth factor (PDGF) and other cytokines released by endothelial cells, activated macrophages, and the smooth muscle cells themselves [44, 45].

Smooth muscles then modify into collagen fibers to form the fibrous component of the atheromatous plaque. In this fashion, fatty streaks progress into fibrofatty lesions or plaques. Instead of following a sequential pathway, the cells constantly interact and modify each other's behavior, forming plaques in one of many possible configurations.

The proportion of fibrous and fatty elements within the plaque varies from one lesion to another, i.e., some lesions are predominantly soft and fatty (with a thin fibrous cap and necrotic core), while others are largely hard and fibrous (with a thick fibrous cap). Beneath the cap is an accumulation of smooth muscle cells and macrophages containing lipid (foamy cells), as well as areas of necrosis (due to the toxic effects of oxidized extracellular lipid) and pools of lipid consisting of soluble cholesterol (cholesterol crystals). There is usually an associated chronic inflammatory infiltrate of lymphocytes and plasma cells. In large arteries (e.g., aorta), the lesions may appear as isolated or confluent plaques which eventually cover the entire intimal surface. In smaller arteries, however, e.g., coronary and cerebral, the involvement of the intima may be eccentric, reducing and pushing the lumen to one side, or it may be circumferential and concentric with a narrowed central lumen depending on the extent of intimal thickening. It is noteworthy that eccentric plaques may undergo outward plaque remodeling, which can partly compensate for progressive growth of atherosclerotic lesions. However, such outward remodeling can possibly conceal angiographic diagnosis of large-sized plaques, and may be associated with an increased risk of plaque rupture [46, 47].

Advanced or complicated plaques may show ulceration, superimposed thrombosis (Fig. 9.5), or dystrophic calcification within the necrotic material in the intima. The size of the plaque determines the extent to which blood flow in the vessel is reduced. In the coronary artery, a plaque occupying >75% of cross-sectional area of the vessel (or >50% reduction of the lumen diameter) would cause significant interference with blood flow manifested as chronic ischemia in stable angina. Dynamic changes within the plaque may trigger fissuring or "rupture" of a thin fibrous cap (as in the vulnerable soft lipid plaque), thus exposing the circulating blood to potentially thrombogenic contents of the plaque. The clinical consequence of coronary plaque rupture depends upon a variety of elements. The site, i.e., proximal or distal, and caliber of the ruptured artery are crucial factors. Type of coronary circulation, i.e., right or left dominant circulation, will also influence the outcome. The nature of the composition of the ruptured plaque, i.e., soft fatty or hard fibrous, is another significant determinant factor. Finally, the presence of adequate collateral circulation in the area supplied by the ruptured vessel plays a very important role in such a context.

Ruptured plaque may result in luminal thrombus formation, with partial occlusion manifested by unstable angina, or total (or near total) occlusion leading to myocardial infarction or sudden death. Alternatively, a ruptured cap may admit blood inside the plaque causing intimal hemorrhage and/or intimal (intramural) thrombosis. Either of these may lead to rapid plaque enlargement, with the potential to occlude the lumen, partially, or completely, as a result of pressure from inside the plaque. Ruptured plaque and subsequent intraluminal thrombosis may be also followed by organization of the thrombus and its

incorporation within the plaque with further progressive arterial stenosis (thrombogenic theory). Furthermore, plaque erosion, or a small plaque fissuring may predispose to sudden coronary spasm without thrombosis, and the recognized manifestations of variant or Prinzmetal angina.

Extracellular matrix fortifies the fibrous cap(space) and (space) separates the thrombogenic plaque (space) core (space) from coagulating substrates within the circulation [48, 49]. Macrophages, T-cells, and their mediators play an important role in the pathogenesis of plaque rupture. Inflammatory signals alter collagen metabolism by reducing the synthesis and promoting the breakdown of collagen throughout the overproduction of matrix metalloproteinases (MMPs). In such conditions, the consequent thin and friable fibrous cap renders the plaque vulnerable to rupture and thrombotic complications. These inflammatory signals not only alter collagen synthesis and breakdown but also increase the potential for thrombosis through excessive production of tissue-factor procoagulants. Such dual actions elucidate the strong association between inflammation and thrombosis in atherosclerosis [50, 51].

Meanwhile, favorable effects of lipid lowering include reduction of the inflammatory signaling in plaques, with consequent reduction of the expression of MMPs, and increasing endothelial nitric oxide synthase. Coupled with the well-known anti-inflammatory effects of statins, low lipid levels seem to have a beneficial impact in stabilizing atherosclerotic plaques and reducing thrombotic potential [52].

Although it is essentially an intimal disease, atherosclerosis is frequently associated with thinning, atrophy, and weakening of the media. This is due to indirect consequences of the intimal changes and can predispose to aneurysm formation. This is best seen in large arteries, e.g., abdominal aorta and iliac arteries. The adventitia also demonstrates neovascularization, arising from vasa vasorum, in addition to chronic inflammatory changes as a response to oxidized lipids within the plaque.

In summary, one or more of the risk factors, such as hypertension, diabetes mellitus, smoking, dyslipidemia, and others, can induce injury to the arterial endothelium, which promotes entry of LDL and monocyte-derived macrophages into the intima. This initial step is followed by a cascade of events that lead to the formation of atherosclerotic plaque. Further evolution of changes within the plaque leads to increased intimal thickening with further arterial stenosis and chronic ischemic effects, or acute plaque events resulting in acute ischemic episodes. Stages of atheroma include fatty streaks, atheromatous plaque, and complicated lesions, namely ulceration, thrombosis, and calcification. Diseases commonly associated with atherosclerosis result either from acute ischemia, e.g., myocardial infarction, stroke, and sudden death, or prolonged ischemic effects such as angina, chronic ischemic heart failure, vascular dementia, chronic renal ischemia, intermittent claudication, gangrene, among other chronic health impediments. Consequences of large-size arterial lesions, e.g., aorta, include aneurysm formation, which may lead to rupture or thromboembolic complications.

9.2.5 Ischemic Heart Disease

Ischemic heart disease (IHD) is a group of closely related syndromes due to myocardial ischemia, which means an imbalance between coronary blood supply and metabolic demands of the heart for oxygenated blood. In normal individuals, if the myocardial metabolic requirements are increased, even following forceful physical exertion, the oxygen supply to the heart matches such an upsurge, in order to maintain this balance [53].

Myocardial oxygen demand is proportionate to both the heart rate and myocardial contractility; when demand is increased both the rate and the contractility are increased as well. Commonly referred to as coronary artery disease (CAD), IHD in the vast majority of cases, probably more than 98%, is due to advanced coronary atherosclerosis. Other minor causes include congenital ostium stenosis, arteritis, aneurysm, and thromboembolism. Two factors influence coronary

artery flow: (a) coronary perfusion pressure and (b) coronary vascular resistance. The greatest coronary perfusion occurs during diastole, i.e., during myocardial relaxation to allow adequate coronary filling, which is unlike other arterial systems in the body. Hence, conditions that impair the aortic pressure, such as hypotension and aortic regurgitation, can have a negative impact on coronary perfusion.

Normally, physical or mental stress is associated with coronary vasodilatation. This is regulated by activation of the sympathetic nervous system, with enhanced blood flow and release of endothelial-derived vasodilators, such as nitric oxide (NO). The relaxation effect of NO seems to outweigh the direct constricting effect of catecholamines on arterial smooth muscle. Risk factors for atherosclerosis, such as hypertension, diabetes mellitus, smoking, and hypercholesterolemia, are associated with the diminished release of NO into the arterial wall, either because of impaired synthesis or due to excessive oxidative degradation. Diminished NO bioactivity may cause constriction of coronary arteries during physical or mental stress, thus contributing to myocardial ischemic injury.

In patients suffering from atherosclerosis, coronary perfusion is influenced by fluid mechanics, as well as the anatomy of the affected arteries. Fluid mechanics are essentially determined by the degree of coronary stenosis. From the anatomical point of view, distal intramural small-caliber arteries are less affected by atherosclerosis, compared to proximal epicardial large coronaries, which display more frequent extents of atherosclerotic narrowing. Nevertheless, such small coronary vessels can play a significant compensatory role, by vasodilatation, in cases of proximal atherosclerotic narrowing. Thus, the hemodynamic impact of coronary stenosis is dependent upon the degree of epicardial proximal coronary stenosis, as well as the vasodilatation capability of the distal arteries. However, remodeling of plaques with outward expansion of the arterial wall allows sizable atheromatous lesions to reside in the walls of affected arteries without causing significant narrowing of the lumen. Thus, such plaques are undetectable on

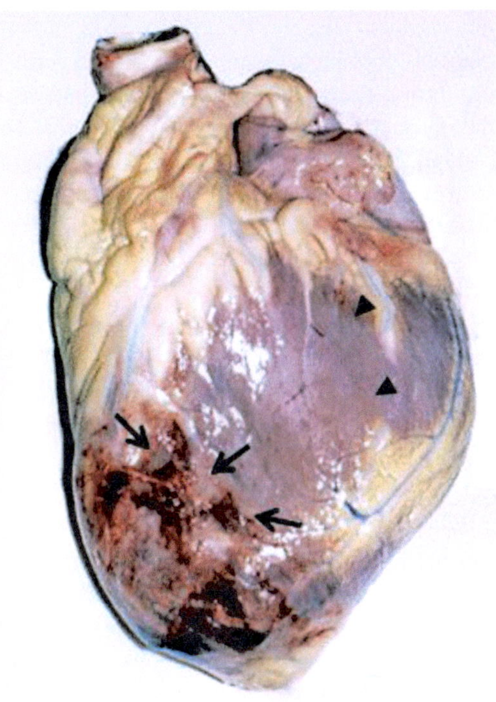

Fig. 9.7 Acute MI (Arrows) note the discoloration of the cardiac muscle with bloody spots compared to the adjacent viavle muscle (arrowheads)

arteriograms and conceal warning symptoms or signs to both the patients and clinicians [52].

Although atherosclerotic plaques are usually developed over many years or even decades, they frequently produce clinical manifestations suddenly and without warnings. IHD may be manifested by a variety of presentations. The most popular form is through chest pain or "angina" (Angina Pectoris = chest pain). Angina pectoris in its broad term is an uncomfortable feeling in the chest and neighboring anatomic structures produced by myocardial ischemia. Clinical presentation of coronary atherosclerosis can be gradual, as a result of progressive flow-limiting stenosis and exertional angina, or dramatic, with plaque rupture and thrombosis triggering unstable angina, myocardial infarction (Fig. 9.7) or even sudden death. "Stable angina" is associated with stable coronary plaques of more than 75% cross-sectional stenosis and without acute coronary pathology, e.g., plaque rupture or thrombus formation. In such patients, pain occurs following physical exertion, i.e., increased demands.

"Unstable angina," on the other hand, is a consequence of acute coronary lesions, mainly plaque rupture, and subsequent thrombosis. However, myocardial ischemia in such patients is not severe enough to cause permanent death of the myocardial cells. The third, less common form of anginal chest pain, is due to transient ischemia as a result of short-term coronary spasm and is known as "variant" or "Prinzmetal angina." A more severe clinical form of IHD is "acute myocardial infarction" (MI). This follows severe, commonly occlusive, coronary thrombosis that results in everlasting myocardial cell necrosis. Therefore, plaque rupture underlies most unstable angina, myocardial infarction, and sudden death due to IHD. Chronic IHD with CHF is the consequence of either chronic myocardial ischemia, in which there is scattered focal myocardial fibrosis following focal necrosis, or secondary to the healing of an acute MI with replacement fibrosis [48].

9.2.6 Cardiomyopathies

Cardiomyopathy entails a diverse group of disorders with a primary myocardial dysfunction. Secondary myocardial changes, e.g., ischemic, hypertensive, and valvular, can lead to extrinsic cardiomyopathy, i.e., myocardial dysfunction with the primary pathology is not within the myocardium.

9.2.6.1 Dilated Cardiomyopathy

Dilated cardiomyopathy (DCM) is the most common form and accounts for almost 90% of cases. The etiology can be idiopathic and is possibly related to genetic, viral, or immunologic factors. DCM may also follow viral myocarditis with Coxsackie B virus, childbirth, and exposure to toxins or drugs, e.g., cocaine, cobalt, or alcohol. The four cardiac chambers are markedly dilated, although areas of ventricular hypertrophy may be shown. Ventricular dysfunction is systolic as a result of impaired contractility. Thromboembolic complications are not uncommon. Functional mitral and tricuspid regurgitation are frequent consequences due to valve annular dilatation [54, 55].

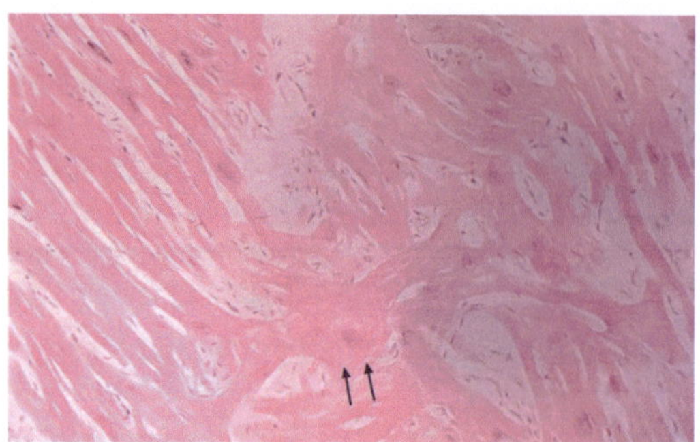

Fig. 9.8 Microphotograph of the myocardium illustrating the disarray of hypertrophied myocytes (arrows) in a case of HCM

9.2.6.2 Hypertrophic Cardiomyopathy

Hypertrophic cardiomyopathy (HCM) is almost exclusively genetic [56, 57].

It is characterized by asymmetric myocardial hypertrophy, particularly of the left ventricle. Thickness of the interventricular septum exceeds that of the left ventricle free wall, and may cause obstruction of the blood flow in one-third of the cases; a condition termed hypertrophic obstructive cardiomyopathy (HOCM). Diastolic dysfunction is due to ventricular stiffness and impaired compliance [58].

Microscopically, the hallmark is the disorganized alignment or disarray of hypertrophied myocardial fibers (Fig. 9.8). Massive ventricular hypertrophy, high left ventricular pressure and intramural coronary dysplasia (medial thickening and luminal narrowing), can lead to ischemic effects with anginal pain in the absence of coronary atherosclerosis.

9.2.6.3 Restrictive Cardiomyopathy

Restrictive cardiomyopathies are less common than DCM and HCM. The ventricles are abnormally rigid, but not necessarily thickened. This results in impaired cardiac filling with diastolic dysfunction, although the systolic function is usually normal [59].

There are two forms of restrictive cardiomyopathy; the first comprises a group of rare endomyocardial diseases that are of poorly understood etiology, including endomyocardial fibrosis (EMF), hypereosinophilic syndrome, and endocardial fibroelastosis (EFE). In EMF, the endocardium and the subendocardial layer of the myocardium display thickening with fibrotic plaques of variable extents. The second form is infiltrative cardiomyopathy, with infiltration of the myocardium by an abnormal substance. The commonest cause of this form is amyloidosis. Other causes include sarcoidosis, radiation fibrosis, and hemochromatosis.

9.2.7 Pericardial Effusion

The pericardium is a sac surrounding the heart, composed of two layers, a layer on the heart (visceral pericardium), which is mesothelium, while the external portion (parietal pericardium) is mesothelium internally and fibrous externally. Normally, 15–35 ml of serous fluid surrounds the heart. The pericardium prevents the displacement of the heart and large vessels, prevents sudden dilatation of the heart, and the spread of infection or cancer from the pleura or lung as well as minimizes friction between the heart and surrounding structures [60]. Pericardial effusion is considered to be present when the amount of fluid in the pericardial space exceeds 50 ml. It may be presented as an incidental finding to a life-threatening emergency. Pericardial effusion can be associated with generalized processes not related to the pericardium, as the pericardium may be involved in a large number of systemic diseases (space) such as congestive heart failure, hypoalbuminemia, volume overload, and pulmonary hypertension or may be diseased, as an isolated process. The numerous causes of pericardial effusion can generally be divided into inflammatory and non-inflammatory etiologies (Table 9.3) [63].

Table 9.3 Causes of pericarditis

A. Infectious
Viral (common), bacterial, parasitic, or fungal
B. Non-infectious
Autoimmune diseases
Cancer
Metabolic conditions (e.g., end-stage renal disease)
Trauma, direct and indirect (e.g., post-myocardial infarction, post-pericardiotomy, and penetrating injury)
Drugs (e.g., chemotherapy)
Miscellaneous: Amyloidosis, chronic heart failure.
Idiopathic

Adopted from [61, 62]

The most common causes are neoplastic, uremic, infectious, and idiopathic pericarditis. The hemodynamic consequences of pericardial effusion depend on the rate at which the effusion is developing and the compliance of both the pericardium and the ventricles. With a significant increase in the pericardial fluid pressure, the filling pressure of both ventricles may decrease, which subsequently leads to a decrease in cardiac output. This condition is called pericardial tamponade and in severe cases is associated with a high mortality. Echocardiography is an excellent tool for the diagnosis and follow-up of pericardial effusion. The condition is also invariably seen with equilibrium radionuclide angiography (ERNA); however, an effusion of more than 400 ml is usually needed to be well recognized. The identification of pericardial effusion is important to be able to start an appropriate workup for this potentially lethal condition.

9.2.8 Correlative Scintigraphic Evaluation of Cardiac Diseases

9.2.8.1 Evaluation of Ventricular Function

Radionuclide techniques including first-pass, equilibrium blood pool, and gated myocardial SPECT provide both accurate and noninvasive means of evaluating cardiac function with simple indices, such as left ventricular volumes and ejection fraction (LVEF). It provides diagnostic and prognostic implications in the spectrum of cardiac diseases [64].

Although most ventricular function studies are performed with the patient at rest, exercise functional studies can also be done to assess regional and global myocardial contraction changes with stress. The cardiac information obtained by these methods is summarized in Table 9.4 [65, 66].

Nuclear medicine techniques are accurate and reproducible for cardiac function evaluation. They provide much important information that is useful in the diagnosis and management of the following clinical situations: Assessment and prognosis of congestive heart failure, monitoring drug therapy and exposure to cardiotoxins, and were also used for diagnosis of coronary artery

Table 9.4 Information obtained by radionuclide evaluation of ventricular function

1. Global left and right ventricular ejection fraction
2. Regional right and left ventricular function
3. Absolute ventricular volumes
4. Systolic emptying and diastolic filling rates
5. Detection and quantitation of cardiac shunts

disease. Echocardiography made the utilization of gated blood pool studies more limited [67, 68].

The left ventricular (LV) ejection fraction is the preferred parameter applied for the noninvasive evaluation of LV systolic function in clinical practice. It has an established and important extensive role in the clinical management of numerous cardiac conditions.

9.2.8.2 Equilibrium Radionuclide Angiography

Studies with radiopharmaceuticals require the use of an intravascular tracer that equilibrates within the blood pool. The ease with which ^{99m}Tc-pertechnetate can be attached to the patient's own red blood cells (RBCs) makes labeled RBCs the preferred technique over labeled pooled human serum albumin. The usual adult dose is about 30 mCi. Three methods of labeling the RBCs are commonly used: in vivo, modified in vitro, and in vitro. The characteristics of each method are described below. All three methods allow the ^{99m}Tc to bind irreversibly to the hemoglobin and remain in the intravascular space, allowing serial studies to be performed for up to 6–8 h following labeling of the RBCs [69].

RBCs from patients receiving heparin therapy are sometimes difficult to label, and in such cases the use of ACD as an anticoagulant is preferred to increase the labeling efficiency. Inadequate anticoagulation or too aggressive shaking of cells may cause thrombus formation and result in hot spots in the lungs. Likewise, stannous pyrophosphate can be oxidized by water in glucose solutions, and this may lead to poor RBC labeling.

Assessing ejection fraction and regional wall motion requires measurement of volume changes and wall motion at different intervals throughout the cardiac cycle. Acquisition of multiple timed images of the blood pool activity in the heart will then be triggered by each R-wave (Fig. 9.9). The duration of

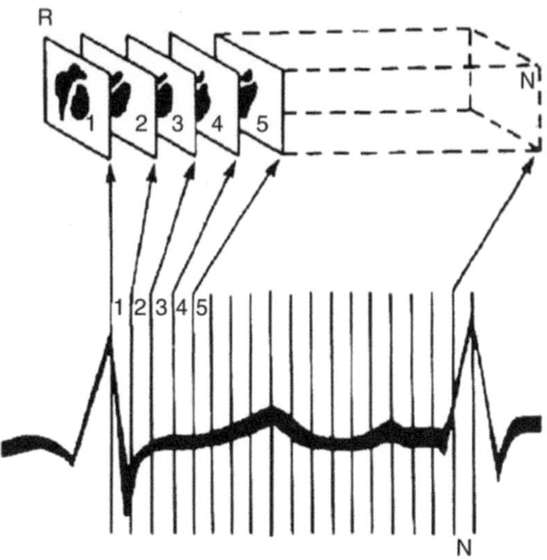

Fig. 9.9 Method by which the computer generates multiple gated images. The cardiac cycle is divided into a preselected number of frames of equal duration. Scintigraphic data from successive beats are placed into separate parts of the computer memory, depending on the temporal relation of the scintigraphic data to the R-wave marker (*R*). For each frame (*1…N*), scintigraphic data from successive beats are accumulated either until a preset time is reached (e.g., 2 min for exercise scintigraphy) or until the average cardiac image contains a predetermined number of counts (e.g., 200,000 counts for typical resting studies) (Reproduced with permission from Berman et al. [70].

every frame maybe 1–60 ms. Multiple beats are acquired to obtain adequate counts in each frame, and typically a complete radionuclide ventriculographic study will consist of 200–800 summed beats for each of the three planar views [65] (Fig. 9.10).

There are three possible modes of acquiring ERNA: list, frame, and dynamic arrhythmia filtration. Each method has its advantages and disadvantages, as described below and summarized in Table 9.5.

9.2.8.2.1 ECG-Gated Myocardial Perfusion SPECT

Gated myocardial perfusion SPECT studies provide information on both myocardial perfusion and ventricular function. Quantification of gated SPECT images provides a global LVEF, plus indices of regional wall motion and wall thickening, useful in evaluation of ventricular function and LV dyssynchrony that occurs with primary contractile dysfunction [71] (see later). Recently

a low-dose SPECT(as low as 8 mci) gated blood-pool SPECT for quantification of LV function was used [72–74]. The low-dose ^{99m}Tc-RBC imaging method was proved to provide precise quantification of LV function and resulted in the most consistent assessment of LV function compared with the gold standard high-dose ERNA method, along with excellent inter-observer reproducibility with a greater than 67% reduction in radiation dose [72].

The advantages of this technique over the usual planarmethod include the ability to visualizeeach cardiac chamber without count contamination from adjacent structures.Regional wall motion can be also viewed in any projection. Additionally, the need for customizing the camera position to obtain the various planar views is overcome as patient has to be positioned once in the SPECT technique. Unlike planar ERNA studies, accurate computation of RVEF may be possible with SPECTERNA due to the removal of chamber overlap and the 3D nature of SPECT. Finally, ERNASPECT can be performed in approximately half the time used to acquire a 3-view planar ERNA series [33, 34].

9.2.8.3 First-Pass Radionuclide Angiography

Examination of the initial transit of a radio nuclide bolus through the different major vascular compartments can provide information about the function of each chamber. This is probably the most accurate method of calculating RV ejection fraction and it is excellent for calculating LV ejection fraction as well. Optimal performance is achieved using a high count rate gamma camera interfaced to a high-speed computer. Multicrystal gamma camera systems offer the highest count rate capabilities but are not widely available [32]. The preferred radiopharmaceutical for rapid bolus injection is any ^{99m}Tc compound in a volume less than 1 ml and a dose of 15–30 mCi. Good-quality studies require that the radioactivity remain as a compact bolus to avoid overlapping of chambers' radioactivity at any given time. If serial studies are essential, for example, at rest and following peak exercise, the initial resting study is done using an agent cleared rapidly by the kidneys (^{99m}Tc-DTPA or glucoheptonate) or

Fig. 9.10 Example of a normal gated blood pool study. The pictures on the *left* represent end-diastolic (*ED*) frames, while the images on the *right* represent end-systolic (*ES*) frames. The main structures are identified in each projection: *AO* aorta, *RV* right ventricle, *LV* left ventricle, *RA* right atrium, *PA* pulmonary artery, *LA* left atrium

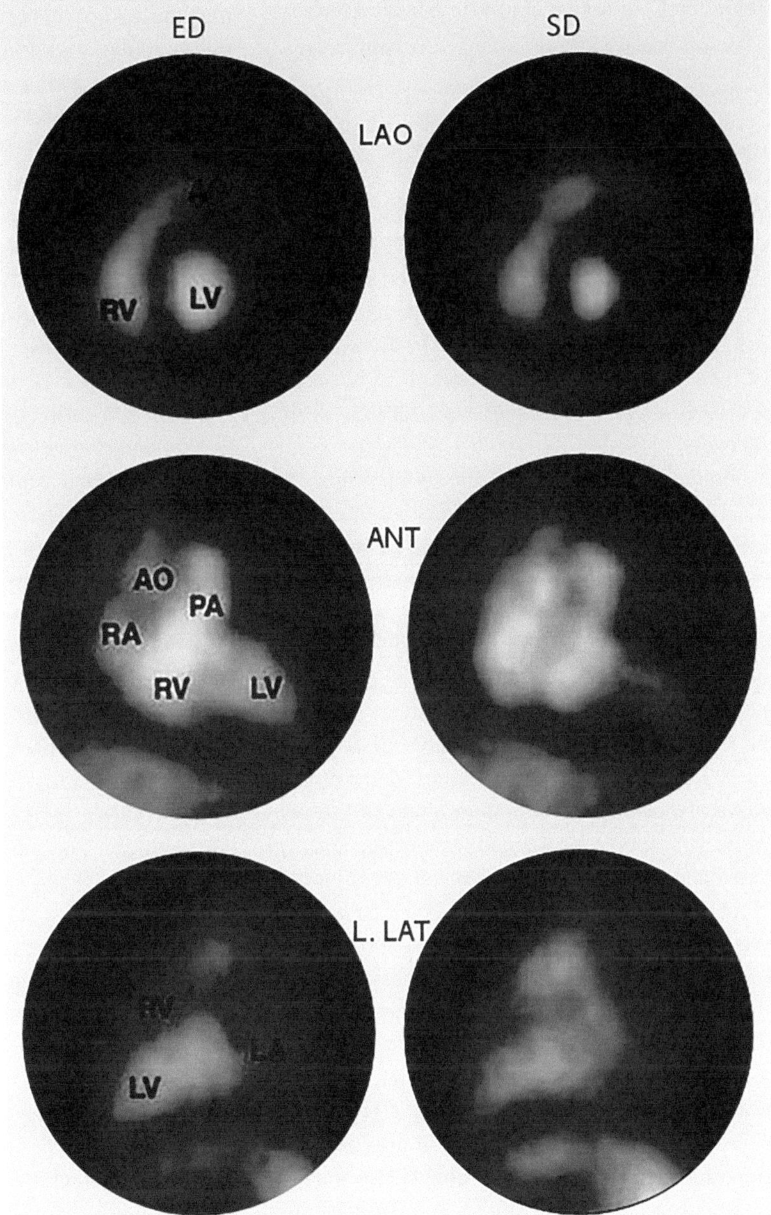

Table 9.5 Comparison between the different modes of computer acquisition

Mode of acquisition	Advantages	Disadvantages
List mode	Optimal temporal resolution	Intensive memory requirement
	Excellent arrhythmia rejection	Longer processing time
Frame mode	Easy setup	Count drop-off
	Minimum memory	Fixed temporal resolution
		Poor arrhythmia rejection
Dynamic arrhythmia (buffered beat) mode	Flexible temporal resolution and arrhythmia rejection	Longer setup for greater options
	Less memory than list	
	Accurate systole/diastole	

Table 9.6 Clinical Uses of radionuclide gated studies

Assessment and prognosis of congestive heart failure
Cardiac transplant evaluation
Cardiotoxin monitoring
Assessment and prognosis of myocardial infarction
Preoperative cardiac risk assessment
Monitoring valvular heart disease
Myocardial hypertrophy evaluation

liver (^{99m}Tc-sulfur colloid). The second study at peak exercise can then be performed using ^{99m}Tc-per technetate, which will allow in vivo labeling of the RBC pool and acquisition of ERNA views for assessment of regional wall motion during recovery.

Immediately following the bolus injection, 25–100 frames/s are acquired in the anterior or 30° RAO position. With multihead cameras, two or more projection images of the chest can be assessed simultaneously. The transit of the bolus can be evaluated either by ECG gating or continuous dynamic cine display. Using the gated first-pass technique, four to five individual beats can be summed to increase the number of counts in each frame; this provides better definition of valve planes and the lateral contours of the ventricle, which must be defined for ejection fraction calculation. Unlike equilibrium studies, cardiac chambers, especially the atria, can be studied individually with minimal interference from background or overlapping chambers. Because ERNA studies have difficulty in separating the RV from the RA due to overlap, the first-pass technique is considered the method of choice for accurate RV evaluation. Moreover, it is the only radionuclide method for detection and quantitation of left-to-right cardiac shunts [75].

Radionuclide Gated studies are accurate and reproducible for cardiac function evaluation. They provide much important information that is useful in the diagnosis, assess risk and prognosis and management of the several clinical situations (Table 9.6).

9.2.8.4 Evaluation of Myocardial Perfusion

Coronary artery disease management and follow-up can be aided by several radionuclide studies including myocardial perfusion SPECT imaging, myocardial perfusion PET imaging, exercise radionuclide angiography, and radionuclide viability studies using conventional and positron emission radiotracers.

9.2.8.5 Myocardial Perfusion SPECT Imaging

Myocardial perfusion imaging (MPI) reflects the relative distribution of coronary flow, which is normally almost uniform in the absence of prior infarction or fibrosis. In the presence of luminal narrowing, flow nonuniformity corresponds to anatomical location of the coronary stenoses and to the cumulative severity of the obstructions along the coronary arterial tree and the size of its watershed [73]. Therefore, MPI can diagnose not only the presence of coronary artery disease but also its extent, severity, and physiological impact, thereby providing great prognostic information.

Most diagnostic methods, both invasive and noninvasive, depend on detection of luminal narrowing of the coronary vessels. An increase of coronary flow caused by exercise or pharmacological stress exaggerates flow nonuniformity, through either increased metabolic demand or vasodilation. The easiest method of increasing coronary flow is physical exercise, using a motorized treadmill or a stationary bicycle. In patients who are unable to exercise adequately, pharmacological agents (adenosine, dipyridamole, dobutamine, and arbutamine) are used for transient elevation of coronary flow.

9.2.8.6 Stressors

9.2.8.6.1 Exercise

Exercise stress is the most frequently used test for noninvasive diagnosis of coronary artery disease (CAD). This form of stress is usually performed with exercise protocols using either a treadmill or bicycle. Exercise is associated with sympathetic stimulation and changes in a coronary vasomotor tone which affects coronary blood flow through dilatation of coronary arteries. Exercise results in increase in myocardial oxygen demand and coronary vasodilation allowing increased oxygen delivery which is crucial to myocardial perfusion to prevent ischemia. This hyperemic effect is behind the identification of ischemia, as stenotic vessels do not vasodilate efficiently [76]. ETT evaluates the hemodynamic changes and provides independent prognostic information including total exercise time and capacity, heart rate response, blood pressure response, and symptoms during stress [77] Systolic blood pressure is expected to increase during stress to maintain adequate cardiac output. Any drop in blood pressure during exercise may indicate the presence of coronary artery disease and, therefore, poor prognosis and outcome [78–80]. Heart rate is also expected to increase during the exercise preferably up to 85% of the maximum age-predicted heart rate (MPHR), which can be calculated by subtracting the patient age from 220 [81]. However, achievement of 85% of MPHR is not an indication for termination of the test and ETT should rather be symptom-limited Slow heart rate during exercise can be normally seen in athletes.

9.2.8.6.2 Pharmacologic Stress Testing

Patients who cannot exercise for noncardiac reasons (e.g., orthopedic, neurological, and peripheral vascular) or are unable to exercise adequately (for a meaningful period of time and/or to an adequate heart rate) are candidates for pharmacological stress testing. Pharmacological stress makes it possible evaluation of patients unable to exercise for noncardiac reasons, including sick and debilitated patients. However, physiologically useful parameters derived from an exercise test, valuable for a comprehensive evaluation, are lost. Adenosine, dipyridamole, and regadenoson are coronary vasodilators. Dobutamine and arbutamine are beta-adrenergic agonists and increase myocardial oxygen demand; they also have some direct vasodilatory effects [82] (Table 9.7).

9.2.8.6.3 Adenosine

Adenosine is an endogenous coronary vasodilator produced from ADP and AMP in myocardial and vascular smooth muscle cells. Adenosine affects two kinds of receptors: A1 and A2. Activation of the A1 receptor slows AV conduction. Activation of the A2 receptor leads to coronary vasodilation (Fig. 9.11, Table 9.7). The half-life of adenosine is extremely short (seconds only). Perfusion tracers are therefore injected during continuous adenosine infusion (140 µg/kg/min for 6 min). The half-life of adenosine is extremely short (seconds only). Perfusion tracers are therefore injected during continuous adenosine infusion (140 µg/kg/min for 6 min). Adenosine may trigger bronchospasm and should not be used in patients with bronchospastic disease, particularly those who have clinical asthma and/or are being treated with bronchodilators. Caffeine, theophylline, and their metabolites competitively block adenosine receptors. Therefore, patients should abstain from caffeine-containing beverages and medication for 12–24 h prior to the test [81].

9.2.8.6.4 Dipyridamole

Dipyridamole is an indirect vasodilator: It increases intravascular concentration of endogenously produced adenosine by blocking its cellular reuptake (Fig. 9.11). Dipyridamole has a longer half-life than adenosine and does not affect AV conduction. Dipyridamole is usually infused for 4 min. The perfusion tracer is injected at 7 min. In some laboratories, the patient is asked to perform low-level exercise or handgrip exercise to enhance its effects. Contraindications for dipyridamole use are similar to those for adenosine, although chest pain is less frequent. An effective antidote is IV aminophylline (50–

Table 9.7 Main Coronary vasodilators

	Adenosine	Dipyridamole
Effect	Direct	Indirect
Half-life	<10 s	Minutes
Onset of action	Seconds	Minutes
Time to peak effect	1 min	7 min
A-V block	3–4%	0%
Contraindications	Bronchospasm	Bronchospasm

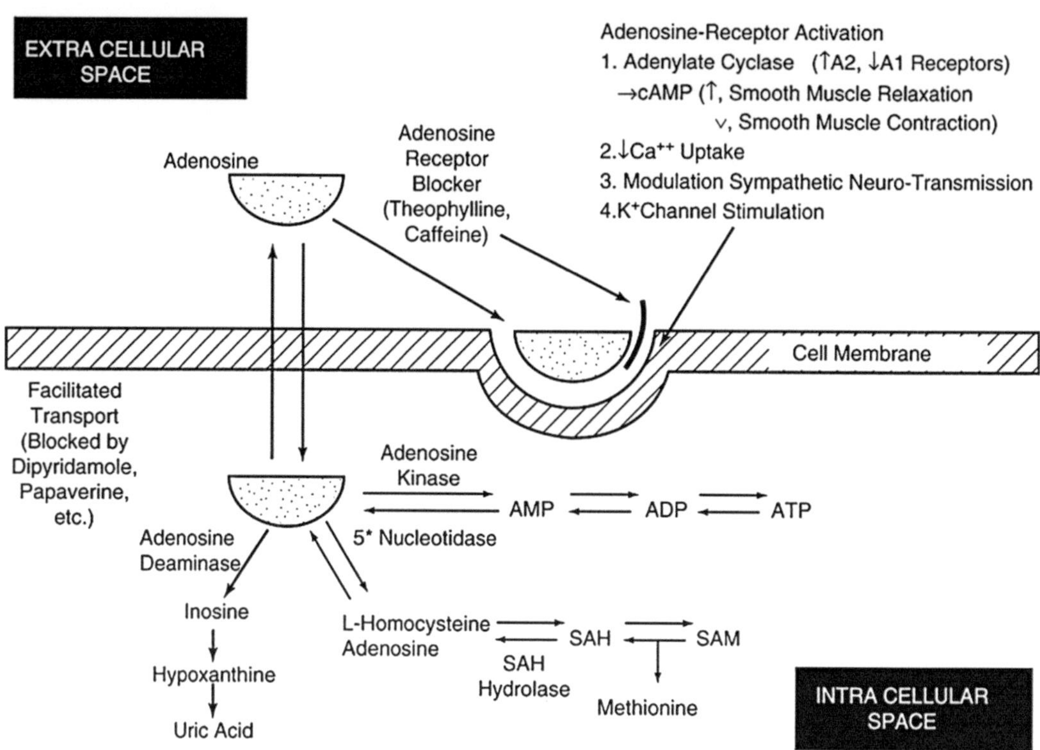

Fig. 9.11 Mechanisms of the vasodilating stress agents. Adenosine is synthesized intracellularly and leaves the cells to act on surface membrane receptors. Dipyridamole blocks adenosine reentry into the cell, increasing extracellular adenosine that can bind to the receptor. Methylxanthines, such as theophylline and caffeine, competitively block the receptor sites (Reproduced from Iskandrian et al. [83] with permission)

100 mg IV), which can be used to normalize hemodynamic changes, relieve ischemia, and/or treat side effects.

9.2.8.6.5 Dobutamine and Arbutamine

Dobutamine is a synthetic catecholamine with predominantly β1 affinity and a short plasma half-life (approximately 2 min). In the presence of significant epicardial coronary artery stenosis, the increase in oxygen demand caused by positive inotropic and chronotropic effects of dobutamine can induce myocardial ischemia. Additionally, dobutamine at higher doses induces coronary vasodilation. The infusion rate used for diagnostic imaging (40–50 μg/kg/min) is higher than the customary therapeutic infusion rate of dobutamine (10–20 μg/kg/min) used for inotropic support in the intensive care units. The side effects of dobutamine in our patient series included supraventricular and ventricular arrhythmia (6% of patients), palpitations (40%), chest

pain (20%), shortness of breath (17%), headache (15%), and GI symptoms (5%). Dobutamine was used mostly in patients who are unable to exercise and have bronchospastic disease [84], but its use has decreased since the introduction of the selective A_{2A} vasodilator agonist regadenoson.

Arbutamine is also a synthetic catecholamine which is not widely used due to complexity and cost.

9.2.8.6.6 Regadenoson

Regadenoson is an A_{2A} receptor agonist that is a coronary vasodilator with very weak affinity for A_1, A_{2B}, and A_3 receptors that are associated with adenosine's unpleasant side effects. It is supplied in prefilled syringe doses of 0.4 mg in 5 mL of solution. It is administered as a single-dose bolus (less than 10 s), which leads to increased coronary blood flow to more than twice baseline levels within 30 s, with maximal vasodilation 1–4 min after injection, and decreases to less than twice baseline within 10 min. This is accompanied by a decrease in systolic and diastolic blood pressure and an increase in heart rate [85].

9.2.8.6.7 Combined Pharmacological and Exercise Stress Testing

Many centers have found it useful to combine low-level treadmill exercise with either adenosine, regadenoson, or dipyridamole. This has been found to reduce the unpleasant side effects of flushing, headache, dizziness, or nausea due to either stressor. Image quality is also improved through a decrease in hepatic and gut uptake of the technetium-99 m perfusion tracers, which is more common with adenosine or dipyridamole, compared to exercise [86]. Combined exercise with pharmacological stress should be avoided in patients with left bundle branch block or RV pacemaker, since the likelihood of false-positive myocardial perfusion stress images is increased with exercise.

9.2.8.7 Radiopharmaceuticals for Myocardial Perfusion Imaging

Thallium-201 and the ^{99m}Tc-labeled tracers (^{99m}Tc-sestamibi and ^{99m}Tc-tetrofosmine) are used for SPECT myocardial perfusion imaging (Table 9.8). While N-13 Ammonia, Rubidium-82, Oxygen-15 Water and Fluorine-18 Flurpiridaz are the radiotracers for PET myocardial perfusion imaging (Table 9.9).

Table 9.8 Tracers for SPECT myocardial perfusion imaging

	Thallium-201	Tc-90-sestamibi	Tc-99 m-tetrofosmin
Brand name	N/a	Cardiolite	Myoview
Class	K′ analogue	Isonitrile	Diphosphine
Preparation	Cyclotron	Kit (beated)	Kit (cold)
Charge	Cation	Cation	Cation
Lipophilicity	Low	High	High
Redistribution	Yes	Minimal	Minimal
Tissue clearance(h)	5046/4	>6	>6
Excretion	Renal	Gl(renal)	Gl(renal)
Time of imaging (min)	5–10	20–60	10–45
Completion time(h)	4–6	3–4	3–4
Counts	Adequate	High	High
SPECT	Ycs	Yes	Yes
Extraction	0.85	0.39	0.24
Gating	±	Yes	Yes
Heart liver(1 h)	2.6	1.2	1.4
Tede	2.1 rem/3.5 mCi	1.1 rem/30 mCi	0.8 rem/30 mCi
Clinical use			
Diagnosis	Yes	Yes	Yes
Prognosis	Yes	Yes	Yes
Viability	Yes	Yes	Yes

Table 9.9 Positron-emitting tracers for myocardial perfusion

Tracer	Physical half-life	Mean range (mm)	Production	Scan duration	Mechanism	Require on-site cyclotron
N-13 ammonia	9.8 min	0.7	Cyclotron	20 min	Metabolic trapping in myocardium	Yes
Rubidium-82	75 s	2.4	Generator	6 min	Free diffusion, metabolically inert	No
F-18 flurpiridaz	110 min	0.2	Cyclotron	20 min	Metabolic trapping in myocardium	Yes
O-15 water	2.0 min	1.1	Cyclotron	6 min	Metabolic trapping in myocardium	No

9.3 Clinical Uses of Myocardial Perfusion Imaging

9.3.1 Uses of Myocardial Perfusion SPECT Imaging

Initially, myocardial perfusion imaging was a primarily diagnostic method for noninvasive detection of coronary artery disease (Figs. 9.12 and 9.13). Later applications have extended to evaluation of prognosis to assess the patient risk and outcome (Table 9.10).

Diagnosis: MPI is used for patients with intermediate pretest probability for the presence of coronary artery disease. The pretest probability is determined from easily obtained parameters: age, gender, symptoms, and rest ECG. MPI is inap-

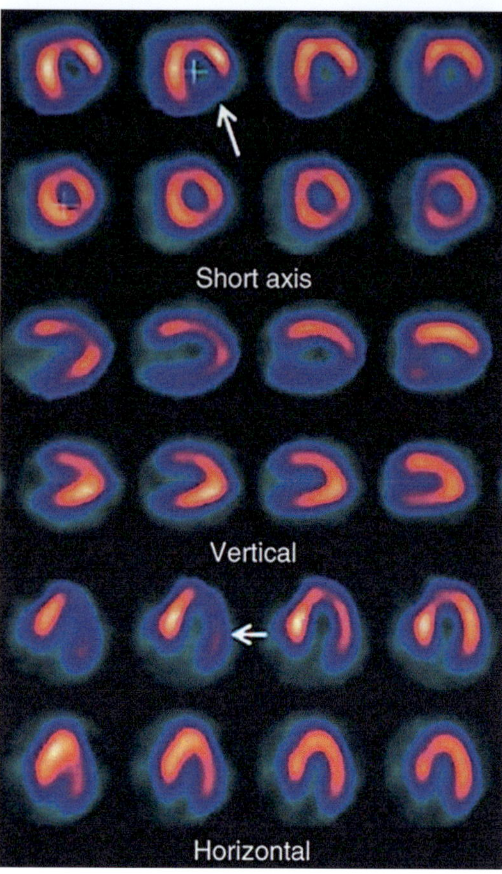

Fig. 9.13 Antero apical fixed defect (*arrows*) with no difference between stress images (*upper rows*) and resting study (*lower rows*)

Table 9.10 Candidate patients for MPI for prognostic and risk stratifications

1. Stable CAD evaluated for prognosis
2. Acute chest pain syndromes
3. Post-acute myocardial infarction
4. Post-revascularization procedures (CABG, PTCA, coronary stenting)
5. Before noncardiac surgery
6. Post-cardiac transplantation

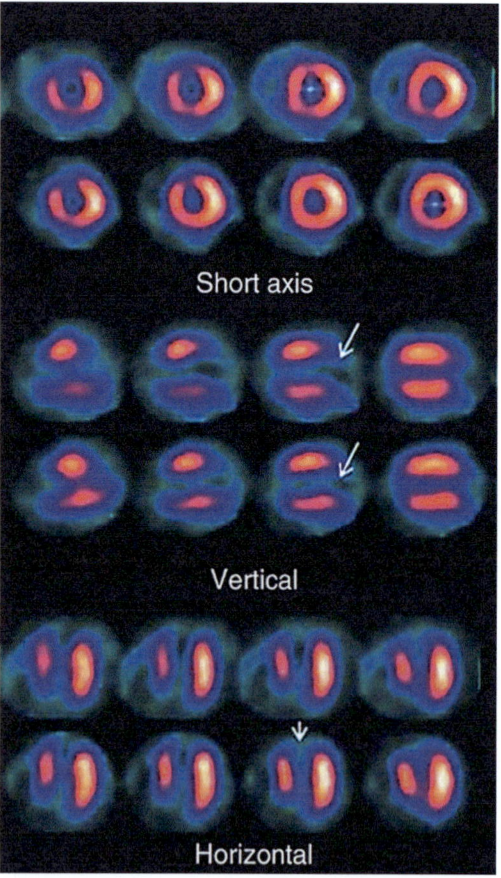

Fig. 9.12 Myocardial perfusion scan with stress-induced ischemia of the inferolateral wall (*arrows*)

propriate for patients with a low pretest probability due to the high rate of false-positive results in such patients. Patients with several risk factors for CAD and typical symptoms with a high probability of CAD do not gain so much from MPI for diagnosis, as the diagnosis is nearly certain on clinical grounds.

Prognosis: Certain groups of patients are commonly referred for MPI for prognostic assessment:

1. Prognosis for Stable CAD: MPI provides information that aids the physician in assessing different aspects of the disease. Perfusion abnormalities can be classified according to size, localization, severity, and reversibility. Left ventricular volumes, systolic wall thickening, segmental wall motion, and ejection fraction can be quantified. A normal perfusion pattern in patients with an adequate level of stress and with high-quality study is consistent with an excellent short-term prognosis, regardless of coronary anatomy [67]. The average annual cardiac event rate in patients with abnormal images is 12-fold than in patients with normal images. Both fixed and reversible defects are prognostically significant. Fixed defects are a predictor of death, whereas reversible defects are an important predictor of nonfatal myocardial infarction.

2. Prognosis for Acute Chest Pain Syndromes: Acute chest pain may be due to myocardial ischemia as a result of a coronary artery plaque rupture and may be potentially life threatening. Rapid and reliable triage is needed for speedy diagnosis of acute myocardial infarction and to prevent unnecessary hospitalizations and inappropriate discharges from the emergency room. Some centers perform MPI at rest. Abnormal results lead to hospital admission.

3. Prognosis Assessment After an Acute Myocardial Infarction; Early or predischarge MPI evaluation after an acute myocardial infarction provides assessment of the extent of sustained damage, and residual ischemia. Patients with a limited amount of ischemia after an acute myocardial infarction can be risk stratifed noninvasively and, if found to have a low-risk profile, treated medically with the same results as those treated with interventions [87].

4. Prognosis Assessment After Revascularization Procedures. MPI is an efficient means to determine the need for additional and/or repeat interventions, especially when the clinical symptoms are vague or nonspecific.

5. Risk Assessment Prior to Noncardiac Surgery: Risk stratification based on preoperative testing can help the patient and physician choose the best type and timing of surgery, perioperative care, and long-term postoperative management.

6. Prognosis Assessment After heart transplantation: Immunologically mediated obstructive coronary vasculopathy has emerged as the most devastating late complication after cardiac transplantation. Pain is absent because of denervation of the transplanted heart. MPI helps detect asymptomatic myocardial ischemia.

9.3.2 Uses of Myocardial Perfusion PET Imaging

Currently, PET is considered the gold standard for noninvasive quantitative assessment of myocardial perfusion and metabolism although the availability is still limited. Although the role of SPECT MPI in the diagnosis and management of ischemic heart disease is well established and its qualitative or semiquantitative assessment of regional perfusion is most used in clinical practice, it has limitations in determining the extent of the disease, particularly in patients with multivessel disease and its inability to delineate the extent and severity of diffuse atherosclerosis and microvascular dysfunction. On the other hand, PET enables better assessment of disease by analyzing myocardial perfusion, function, and metabolism (Table 9.11). The clinical uses of PET in Heart Diseases is increasinly seen in the diagnosis and risk stratifcation (Table 9.12).

The tracers used most commonly are 82Rb-chloride and 13 N-ammonia [88]. Less commonly used are O-15 water and F-18 flurpiridaz. Each has specific features that make one preferable over another in individual situations.

The perfusion tracer is injected intravenously at rest, followed by a PET acquisition, and again

Table 9.11 Advantages of PET imaging in heart disease

Offers reliable attenuation correction
Higher resolution
Ability to reliably detect coronary disease down to about 50% occlusion
Ability to delineate the extent and severity of diffuse atherosclerosis and microvascular dysfunction
More reliable in obese patients
Absolute perfusion quantitation
Lower radiation than SPECT MPI

Table 9.12 Clinical applications of PET in heart diseases

1. Perfusion assessment
2. Absolute quantification of myocardial blood flow
3. Assessment of myocardial viability
4. Prognostic assessment
5. Assessing ventricular function
6. Cardiovascular prosthetic infection
7. Cardiac sarcoidosis and amyloidosis

during pharmacological stress with either intravenous regadenoson, dipyridamole, adenosine, or dobutamine/arbutamine.

9.3.3 Evaluation of Myocardial Metabolism and Uses of Metabolic Imaging

While gated myocardial perfusion SPECT imaging offers invaluable diagnostic and prognostic information for the evaluation of patients with suspected or known coronary artery disease, advances in the cellular and molecular biology of the cardiovascular system lead to molecular imaging, which can play a role in the early detection of CAD at the level of the vulnerable plaque, the evaluation of cardiac remodeling, and monitoring of important new therapies including gene therapy and stem cell therapy [89, 90].

Unlike skeletal muscle, cardiomyocytes sustain an everlasting cycle of contraction and relaxation in order to supply the body with blood and maintain the homeostasis of nutrients and metabolic gases [91]. Cardiomyocytes are specialized for the aerobic metabolism of fatty acids and are packed with mitochondria performing oxidative phosphorylation and β-oxidation. Cardiac health is dependent on the heart's ability to utilize different substrates to support overall oxidative metabolism to generate ATP. In other words, it is a process that converts energy-providing fuels to ATP, the energy currency in the cell. ATP is largely used to maintain myocardial contraction and to regulate the membrane pumps and movements of ions in and out of the cell. Cardiac health is dependent on the heart's ability to utilize different substrates to support overall oxidative metabolism to generate ATP.

For a given physiologic environment, the heart consumes the most efficient metabolic fuel. In the normally oxygenated heart, fatty acids account for the majority of ATP production with glucose making only a small contribution to the ATP production, unless there is an insulin surge. During an acute increase in workload (for example, inotropic stimulation), the heart immediately mobilizes its metabolic reserve contained in glycogen (transient increase in glycogen oxidation) and meets the need for additional energy from the oxidation of carbohydrate substrates (glucose and lactate). When the oxygen supply is decreased, the heart protects itself from an oxygen-deficient state by switching its energy source to glycolysis, downregulating mitochondrial oxidative metabolism, and reducing contractile function. A substrate preference is characteristic of a variety of cardiac diseases such as diabetic heart disease, in which fatty acid metabolism predominates, and dilated cardiomyopathy, in which glucose metabolism predominates [92]. Thus, the tight coupling between metabolism and contractile function in the heart offers a unique opportunity to assess cardiac performance at different levels in vivo: coronary flow, myocardial perfusion, oxygen delivery, metabolism, and contraction [93, 94].

Based on understanding the metabolic changes of several cardiac diseases, several tracers are used for the evaluation of such diseases. Tables 9.13 and 9.14 summarize the main tracers and conditions evaluated respectively.

9.3.3.1 Quantification of Myocardial Blood Flow

In addition to qualitative and semi-quantitative grading, PET enables absolute quantification of perfusion. Absolute quantification of myocardial

Table 9.13 Main conditions evaluated by molecular imaging for evaluating metabolic alterations

Radiotracer	Condition evaluated	Basis of uptake
F-18 FDG	Myocardial viability	Glucose metabolism
C-11 palmitate	Idiopathic dilated cardiomyopathy	Fatty acid metabolism
C-11 acetate	Hypertrophic cardiomyopathy	Tricarboxylic acid flux
F-18 FTHA	CAD	Fatty acid metabolism
F-18 FTP	Diabetes type 2	Fatty acid metabolism
F-18 FCPHA	CAD	Fatty acid metabolism

Table 9.14 Clinical applications of PET in heart diseases

1. Perfusion assessment
2. Absolute quantification of myocardial blood flow
Assessment of myocardial viability
3. Prognostic assessment
4. Assessing ventricular function
5. Cardiovascular prosthetic infection
Cardiac sarcoidosis, amyloidosis

blood flow expands the scope of conventional relative MPI from identifying only end-stage epicardial IHD to the earlier identification and characterization of abnormalities in coronary endothelial function and subclinical stages of IHD (microvascular dysfunction) [95, 96]. Quantitation of myocardial perfusion offers an objective parameter that is more reproducible than visual interpretation. PET has become the noninvasive imaging modality of choice for the quantification of MBF.

In conclusion, it adds not only to diagnostic certainty but also provides prognostic value (see later).

9.3.3.2 PET in Prognosis Assessment

PET MPI, similarly to SPECT MPI, has great prognostic value in patients with known or suspected IHD. Marvick et al. noted that defect severity with PET was related to outcome [97]. Work by Yoshinaga et al. supports these findings [98]. Work by Chow et al. [99] indicates that patients with normal rubidium-82 PET MPI have a good prognosis, regardless of ECG changes during stress. Work by Nemirovsky et al. supports these findings [100]. The study by Yoshinaga et al. [98] with a mean follow-up of 3.1 years in 367 patients evaluated with dipyridamole Rb-82 PET MPI showed a significant prognostic value of PET MPI for predicting cardiac events and death. They observed significant prognostic value in patients whose diagnosis was uncertain after SPECT MPI and in obese patients.

The extent and severity of PET perfusion defect, rest left ventricular (LV) ejection fraction (LVEF), stress LVEF and LVEF reserve (stress LVEF—rest LVEF), LV volumes, and myocardial flow reserve provide valuable prognostic information [101–104]. Even in the presence of angiographically significant IHD, normal findings on stress MPI are generally associated with a low risk of CV events (around 1% per year) [105].

Myocardial flow reserve was found to independently augment clinical outcome prediction The quantification of blood flow at rest and during maximal pharmacological stress allows measurement of flow reserve in various hypertrophies and cardiomyopathies, posttransplant CAD [106], syndrome X, and other vascular endothelial disorders and to study the effects of smoking, diabetes, and various medications [107–110], and lipid control.

Multiple studies documented the greater prognostic value of PET-derived myocardial flow reserve (MFR) compared to clinical factors and perfusion defect size and severity in patients with known or suspected IHD [111–113]. The addition of PET-derived MFR, led to the correct reclassification of estimated risk categories in 35% of patients with previously intermediate risk of death [114].

Since MFR indirectly reflects microvascular disease, it also has prognostic value in diabetic patients with diabetes and in patients with chronic kidney disease [115].

In viability imaging, FDG PET has the greatest sensitivity for predicting global LV functional recovery following revascularization, compared with SPECT, dobutamine stress echocardiography and cardiac MRI [116–118].

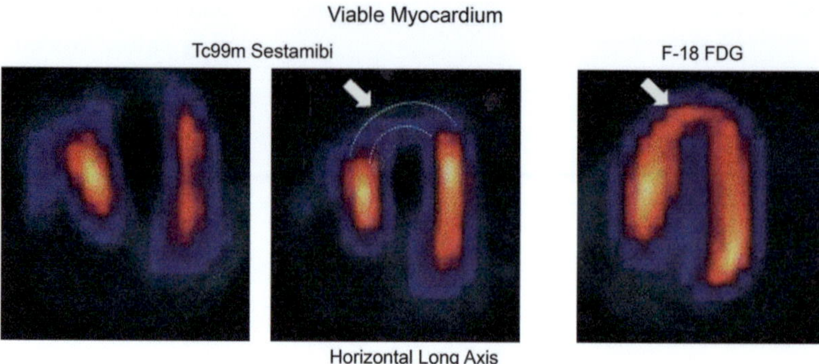

Fig. 9.14 Viable myocardium pattern

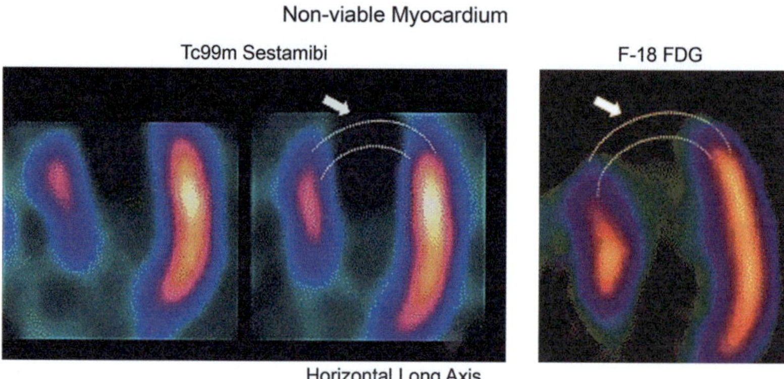

Fig. 9.15 Pattern of nonviable myocardium

9.3.3.3 PET in Assessment of Myocardial Viability

PET is very valuable in assessing viability in stunned myocardium (delayed functional recovery myocardium) and hibernating myocardium (chronically depressed function of hypoperfused myocardium). Demonstration of preserved glucose metabolism by FDG is a marker of myocardial viability (Fig. 9.14) While matching defet on perfusion and FDG indicates nonviable myocardium (Fig. 9.15). The detection of viable myocardium is accurately estimated by referencing the level of myocardial glucose metabolism to the level of MBF [119]. Sequential perfusion-metabolism imaging gives the most complete information, yielding different interpretation scenarios. See later for more details.

9.3.3.4 PET in Assessing Ventricular Function

Gated first-pass ^{18}F-FDG PET has also been introduced for assessing ventricular function [120].

9.3.3.5 PET in Endocarditis and Cardiovascular Prosthetic Infection

Infective endocarditis is among the most severe infectious diseases. Patients with damaged or artificial heart valves and heart defects are at greatest risk for endocarditis. Cardiovascular prosthetic infection is a difficult condition to diagnose. PET has a major role in the diagnosis of endocarditis and prosthetic infections (Fig. 9.16).

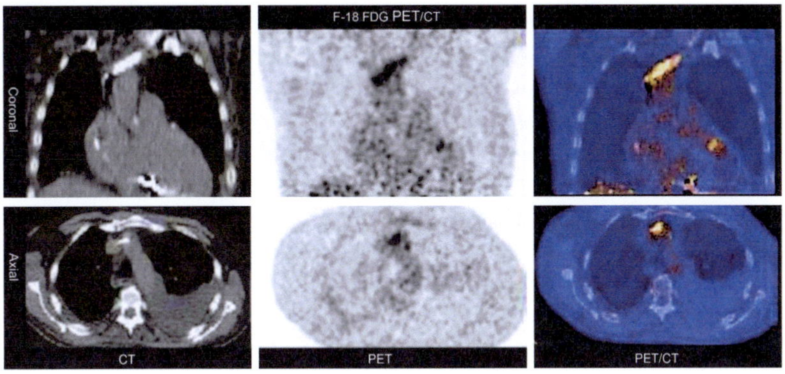

Fig. 9.16 FDG PET/CT study for a 68-year-old male with bacteremia and questionable infectious endocarditis. There is increased FDG accumulation around electrode in the left subclavian vein near superior vena cava. Findings are consistent with infection. Note successful suppression of normal cardiac uptake of FDG after 6–12 h fasting and unfractionated iv heparin administration

9.3.3.6 PET in Cardiac Sarcoidosis and Amyloidosis

Sarcoidosis and Amyloidosis are both multiorgan systemic diseases. Diagnosis of cardiac involvement is particularly important because it can be fatal. Sarcoidosis is a multisystem granulomatous disorder affecting the heart in up to 25% of patients. Cardiac involvement is often associated with a poor prognosis [121]. as it may lead to advanced heart block, cardiomyopathy, arrhythmias, or death. PET may be essential in the diagnosis, risk stratification, and patient management [122, 123]. When sarcoidosis involves the heart it affects left ventricle (multifocal or subepicardial), septum, and right ventricular free wall in >90% of cases [124]. F-18 FDG PET and 18-FDG PET/ MRI are useful in the diagnosis of cardiac involvement of sarcoidosis [125]. Cardiac sarcoidosis may be an incidental finding Cardiac MR or PET shows similar accuracy in the diagnostic workup of CS compared with autopsy studies. Combining 18F-FDG-PET/CT study with SPECT/CT perfusion is particularly useful, as the finding of multiple uptake areas associated with the matching perfusion abnormalities seen in SPECT/CT indicate a high probability of an accurate diagnosis18F-FDG-PET/CT may also be useful to assess the therapeutic and prognostic factors [126].

Amyloidosis is a clinical condition caused by the deposition of unstable misfold proteins as amyloid fibrils. Cardiac amyloidosis is the condition in which the primary interstitial protein deposition occurs in the extracellular space of the heart. Systemic amyloidosis represents a debilitating, underdiagnosed but increasingly recognized group of disorders characterized by the extracellular deposition of these misfolded proteins in one or more organs. Cardiac amyloid deposition leads to infiltrative or restrictive cardiomyopathy and is the major contributor to poor prognosis in patients with systemic amyloidosis. Many proteins can form amyloid fibrils, but the two main types that can infiltrate the heart are monoclonal immunoglobulin light-chain amyloid and transthyretin amyloid. Cardiac amyloidosis is classified into amyloid immunoglobulin light chain (AL) and amyloid transthyretin (ATTR) types [127]. These two most common types of cardiac amyloidosis have distinct therapeutic management and prognosis. Cardiac amyloidosis can be acquired in older individuals or inherited from birth. Early and accurate diagnosis of cardiac amyloidosis is crucial for the implementation of appropriate patient care and is now more important than ever given the availability of new therapies [128].

Cardiac amyloidosis is currently diagnosed more frequently than in the past owing to the advanced diagnostic modalities. Echocardiography and Cardiac MRI play a crucial role in the diagnostic workup of cardiac amyloidosis; however, the differentiation between the subtypes of cardiac amyloidosis is still difficult [126]. Scintigraphy is valuable in the diagnosis and follow-up of the disease. Radiotracers for amyloidosis include (1) bone tracers including PYP, (2) amyloid-directed molecules, (3) PET amyloid agents, and (4) I-123-MIBG. Bone tracers are particularly sensitive in detection of ATTR-type amyloidosis, whereas PET amyloid agents show a higher affinity for the AL type. An important limitation of ^{18}F-FDG is the physiologic uptake in the myocardium, which may remain in approximately 20% of patients even after proper preparation [127]. This fact limited the FDG PET scan's sensitivity for detection of cardiac involvement to 62.5% [129]. ^{11}C-Labeled Pittsburgh compound B (^{11}C-PiB), a radiolabeled derivative of thioflavin-T that is used to detect Aβ-amyloid deposition in Alzheimer's disease [130]. The findings of ^{11}C-PiB PET were found to correlate well with postmortem histopathological samples [124]. Finally, 123I-MIBG scintigraphy is capable of detecting cardiac sympathetic denervation in cardiac amyloidosis [131].

9.3.3.7 Assessment of Myocardial Viability

Nonfunctioning but viable myocardium includes stunned and hibernating myocardium and also remodeling

1. Stunned myocardium shows decreased contractility after an episode of prolonged ischemia, but intact blood flow at the time of observation. Oxygen-derived free radicals contribute to postischemic dysfunction [132]. Stunned myocardium generally improves without further intervention. In most cases of exercise-induced ischemia, this may take a few minutes or, uncommonly, several hours. Following an acute coronary occlusion and thrombolysis, most of the improvement takes place over 7–10 days, but it may take longer in the presence of residual stenosis and/or repeated stunning [78]. Patients may experience repeated episodes of ischemia, often silent, in the same territory, and the stunned

myocardium may not be able to recover, leading to a quasi-permanent state of stunning [133, 134] and progressing to hibernation. When superimposed on an already severely dysfunctional heart, it may become dangerous, and the patient may require hemodynamic support. Recovery of myocardial function is spontaneously provided that myocardial perfusion remains normal. The duration of stunning is directly proportional to the duration of the preceding ischemia.

Hibernation occurs in the myocardium that has undergone a downregulation of contractile function, thus reducing cellular demand for energy, in response to chronic or repetitive ischemia [135].

2. Hibernation may represent a spectrum, with chronic repetitive stunning showing normal or near normal resting perfusion and impaired MFR at one end and reduced rest MBF at the other. In most cases, the impairment is only detected through reduced MFR, with reduced rest MBF only being seen in the most advanced cases. Hibernation, by definition, requires the restoration of blood flow in order to improve function. Benefits also may be expected from reduced metabolic demand via hemodynamic support.
3. **Remodeling** may result in dysfunctional myocardium in the area adjacent to an infarct or hibernation also which may or may not improve with revascularization].

Studies have found that the majority (72%) of dysfunctional but viable segments are in fact due to stunning, with only a minority (28%) due to hibernation [136]. The definition of either stunning or hibernation requires the recovery of function, either spontaneously or after intervention. Other potential benefits from the reversal of stunning or hibernation, include prevention of remodeling or arrhythmias. The above definitions also ignore the possibility that the different tissue types may coexist with each other and with inducible ischemia and scarred tissue in the same or adjacent myocardial segments. Melon et al. showed that dysfunctional but "viable" myocardium is a heterogeneous condition [137]. This may partially explain the limitations in predictive abilities for all imaging techniques.

Dysfunctional but viable myocardium is not uncommon. Up to 50% of patients with previous infarction may have areas of dysfunctional viable myocardium mixed with scar tissue, even in areas with Q waves on the ECG [138].

Resting wall motion imaging identifies myocardium which is thickening and moving well and that which is not. It cannot differentiate dysfunctional viable myocardium from permanently scarred myocardium, except by documenting serial changes in function over time.

The uptake and retention of myocardial perfusion agents are good evidence of myocardial viability. However, impaired retention of perfusion tracers can be seen in dysfunctional, stunned myocardium, while decreased uptake due to decreased perfusion is often seen in hibernation [139]. Simple stress-redistribution imaging with Tl-201 has been shown to underestimate the presence of viability. Augmentation with late (12–24 h) imaging and/or resting reinjection was found to increase sensitivity for viability [131, 140–142].

Gated Tc-99 m sestamibi imaging with nitroglycerin (NTG) administration can be used successfully as an alternative to rest-redistribution Tl-201 SPECT imaging [143]. Tc-99 m tetrofosmin showed performance similar to that of Tl-201 stress-redistribution imaging and slightly lower sensitivity than rest-late redistribution Tl-201 imaging [143].

Another strategy is the addition of metabolic imaging to perfusion imaging using analogs of either free fatty acids or glucose imaging. Injured myocardium frequently demonstrates impaired oxidative metabolism, impaired free fatty acid utilization, and an excess of glucose utilization relative to flow. Myocardial perfusion can be imaged with N-13 ammonia or Rb-82 with PET imaging or Tl-201, Tc-99m sestamibi, or Tc-99m tetrofosmin imaging using SPECT (Figs. 9.17, 9.18, and 9.19).

Stunned myocardium shows relatively preserved flow and either matched or excessive FDG accumulation. Hibernation has been shown to demonstrate decreased perfusion and relatively preserved or disproportionately increased FDG accumulation [144]. Infarcted myocardium shows a matched decrease in both perfusion and FDG uptake (Figs. 9.25 and 9.26) while ischemia shows a mismatched pattern.

Table 9.15 summarizes the accuracies of different imaging procedures for viability.

A somewhat different approach uses labeled free fatty acid (FFA) analogs. Myocardial imaging with iodine-123-labeled FFAs shows uptake and rapid clearance in the normal myocardium and delayed clearance or accumulation in the presence of impaired oxidation. Thus, impaired FFA clearance represents recoverable myocardium [145, 146].

The importance of myocardial viability imaging is in its prognostic value, rather than in the mere prediction of increased LVEF after revascularization.

9.3.3.8 Cardiac Shunt Evaluation

Two distinctive types of studies can be obtained to both qualitatively and quantitatively evaluate cardiac shunts, depending on the type of shunt suspected.

9.3.3.8.1   Left-to-Right Shunt

A first-pass study should be performed to assess patients with this type of shunt. Subsequently, a time–activity curve is generated from a region of interest drawn in the lung field. The pulmonary transit time is normally shown as a narrow spike, with symmetric limbs that represent the pulmonary blood flow of the radioactivity. However, this curve, particularly the descending limb, is distorted in left-to-right shunts due to early recirculation of pulmonary blood from the shunt. Calculation of the pulmonary-to-systemic flow ratio can be obtained by subtracting the fitted shunt curve from the pulmonary one. This is a sensitive method for detecting pulmonary-to-systemic blood flow shunts between 1.2 and 3.0, provided that the patient has no pulmonary hypertension, congestive heart failure, or tricuspid regurgitation [66].

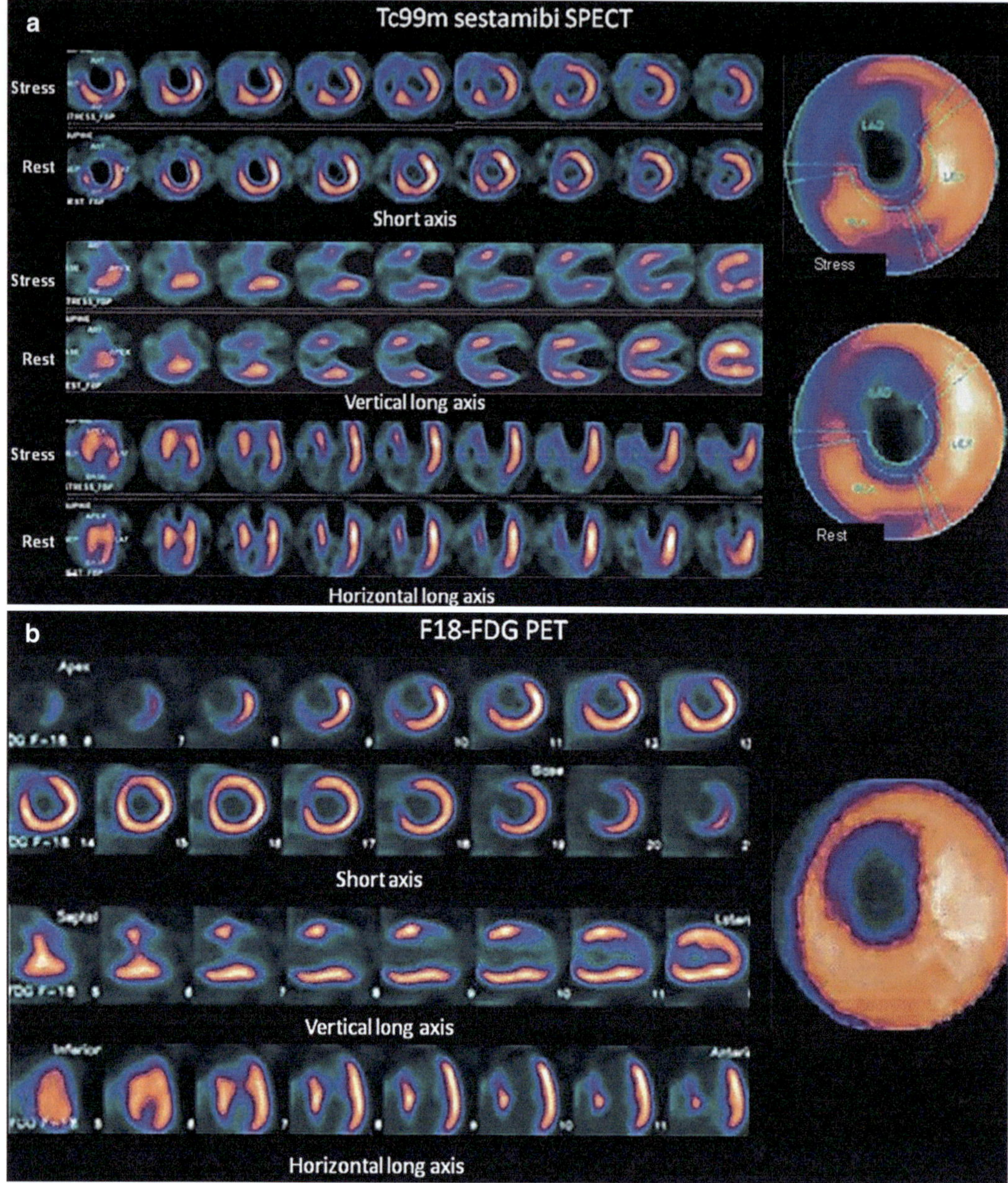

Fig. 9.17 Tc-99m sestamibi stress and rest myocardial perfusion SPECT images and polar maps (**a**) and F-18 FDG studies for a 62-year-old male with dyslipidemia, smoking, and fixed perfusion defect on myocardial perfusion SPECT. The patient was referred for viability study Tc-99m sestamibi SPECT images demonstrate a large area of fixed perfusion defect involving apex and mid anteroseptal region with stress-induced ischemia in the anteroseptal base. FDG PET images (**b**) demonstrate absent glucose metabolism in the same region. Findings are consistent with nonviable/scar tissue in the apex/mid-anteroseptal region

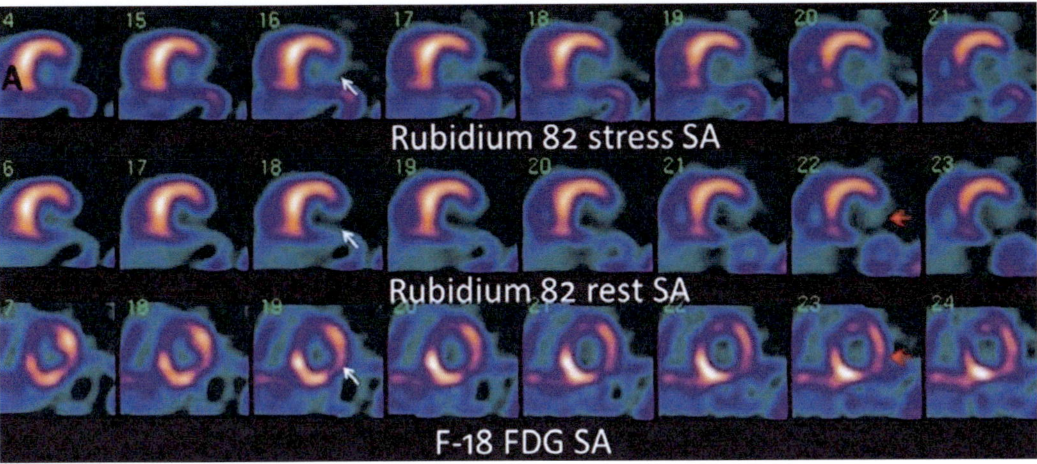

Fig. 9.18 Viable myocardium indicated by filling of the inferior-lateral defect by activity on FDG images (arrows) while is fixed on the perfusion study obtained utilizing Rubidium-82 (*SA* short axis)

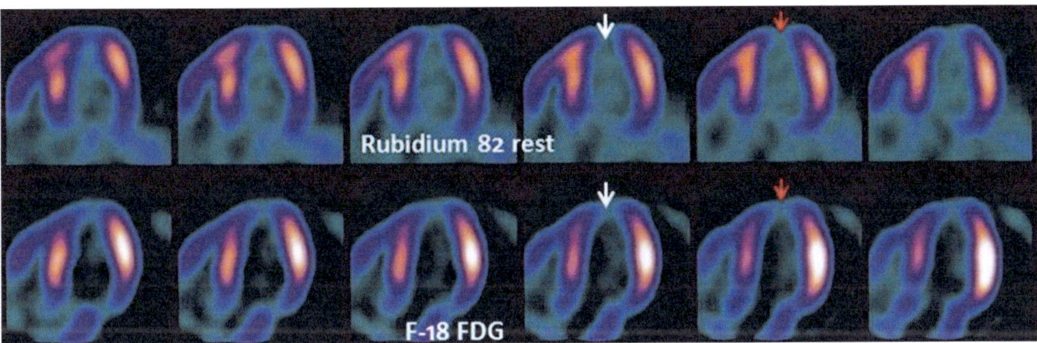

Fig. 9.19 Rubidium-82 Perfusion (upper) and metabolic (lower) images show no difference in an apical defect indicating a scar with no viability

9.3.3.9 Right-to-Left Shunt

This can be suggested from visual examination of a first-pass study, where there will be early visualization of the LV. A more accurate and quantitative method of assessing these types of shunt is to inject ^{99m}Tc-macroaggregated albumin (Fig. 9.20). The small particles of this radiopharmaceutical, used mainly in perfusion lung scan, are trapped in the capillary beds as they pass through the pulmonary arteries. However, in the presence of a right-to-left shunt, the pulmonary capillary system is bypassed and the particles enter the systemic circulation, where they are trapped in end organs such as the brain and the kidneys. Qualitative as well as quantitative analysis of activity within the body can be accurately obtained. A significant right-to-left shunt is present if the organ counts are greater than 7% of the

Table 9.15 Sensitivity and specificity of various methods of imaging for myocardial viability [55]

Method	No. of patients	Sensitivity (%)	Specificity (%)
Tc-99m MIBI	207	83	69
Tc-99m MIBI + NTG	55	91	88
Tl-201 reinjection	209	86	47
Tl-201 rest-redistribution	145	90	54
LDDE	448	84	81
F-18 FDG PET	332	88	73

Tc99m MAA

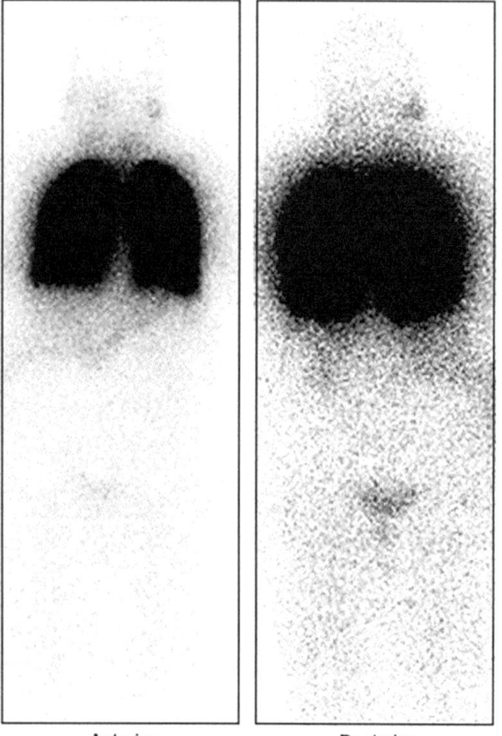

Fig. 9.20 Tc-99m MAA shunt study illustrating normal findings. There is intense activity seen in the lungs and no abnormal activity in the brain or kidney parenchyma. Mild activity in the kidneys is due to excreted activity in pelvicalyceal structures

total lung uptake [147]. Complication because of capillary blockage is not a clinical concern with this procedure, as the number of particles used is very small compared with the number of capillaries in any organ.

9.3.4 Lymphatic System

9.3.4.1 Anatomic and Physiologic Considerations

The lymphatic system is the second vascular system, after blood circulation, in mammalian species. Knowledge of the normal anatomy of the lymphatic system is crucial for predicting which lymph nodes may be the site of metastatic disease for primary tumors and for understanding the pathophysiological changes of lymphatic disorders such as lymphedema. In addition to organs, the lymphatic system is a complex microtubular system consisting of lymphatic vessels and lymph nodes (Table 9.16) that transport the ultrafiltrate of extracellular fluid back to the intravascular space.

Different investigators have classified the spleen differently as being a component of the circulatory system, hematopoietic system, mononuclear phagocytic system, and lymphatic sys-

Table 9.16 Components of the Lymphatic System

(a) Organs
I. Primary lymphoid organs
1. Bone marrow
2. Thymus
II. Secondary lymphoid organs
1. Spleen
2. Lymph nodes
3. Tonsils and adenoids
(b) Tissue
1. Peyer's patches
2. Vermiform appendix
(c) Lymphatic vessels
(d) Collecting ducts

tem. The average adult spleen measures 12 × 7 × 3.5 cm with a weight of 150 g and a volume of approximately 300 ml. A spleen longer than 14 cm is usually clinically palpable. The spleen is a functionally complex organ. One of the basic functions of the splenic blood flow is to filter blood of aging, senescent and abnormal red cells (culling), and intraerythrocytic inclusions (pitting) as well as extrinsic or foreign particles. The mechanism(s) by which these functions are actually carried out are still poorly understood.

Regardless of the mechanisms involved, it is apparent that red or other cells bound for destruction (aged cells, abnormal cells, etc.) become trapped or held within the meshwork of splenic cords, and as the splenic transit time increases, the cells become vulnerable to destruction by resident phagocytic cells. The ability of the spleen to remove intraerythrocytic inclusions while maintaining the integrity of the red cells is known as the pitting function of the spleen. This process occurs in a variety of pathological states and includes Heinz bodies (denatured hemoglobin), Howell-Jolly bodies (nuclear remnants), and Pappenheimer bodies (iron granules) [148, 149].

When these cells pass through the splenic red pulp and try to reenter the circulation through the slit-like fenestrations of the sinus endothelium, the deformable part of the red cell can negotiate and pass through the fenestrations, whereas the nondeformable inclusion is removed or held back by the macrophages [149].

The splenic macrophages are also capable of removing particulate matter from the circulating blood by their phagocytic functions.

The spleen serves important immunological functions. The presence of T- and B-lymphocytes in close proximity to the resident and circulating macrophages as well as the architecture of the splenic pulp and the splenic cord make it ideally suited to play a coordinating role both in the non-specific and the specific arms of immune responses. The nonspecific functions involve the clearance of pathogens, the clearance of opsonized red cells and platelets, the production of complement components, and perhaps surveillance against malignant cells. The spleen plays an important role in removing blood-borne pathogens such as bacteria, especially encapsulated ones, viruses, and circulating immune complexes. It is well known that asplenic or hyposplenic patients or patients—particularly children—after splenectomy are prone to develop fulminant septicemia most often involving encapsulated bacteria (e.g., pneumococci and meningococci) and overwhelming post-splenectomy sepsis (OPSI) [149].

The lymphatic capillary network wraps around the surface of the body and also lines the internal surface of the gastrointestinal and respiratory tract. Normally, some fluid is forced out of the vascular space at the arterial end of the capillary bed but is reabsorbed at the venous end. Capillary egress, however, exceeds venous reabsorption by approximately 3 l/day (approximately 10% of capillary contents), leaving behind fluid in the interstitial tissue [150]. This fluid can contain protein and often fat, especially after meals. The peripheral lymphatic capillary collection site has a single layer of overlapping endothelial cells with a poorly developed basement membrane [148]. When the volume of fluid in the interstitial space increases, the intercellular gaps between the endothelial cells widen to allow the surplus of fluid to enter [148]. Lymphatic vessels coalesce into increasingly larger vessels that eventually contain smooth muscle and one-way valves to promote forward flow back toward the vascular space via the thoracic duct or the right lymphatic duct. Fluid travels through the lymphatic system at an average rate of 120 ml/h or 2–3 l/day, encountering numerous lymph nodes which serve as filters to remove foreign elements such as tumor cells and bacteria. Lymph enters the nodes through the afferent lymphatic vessel, filtering through the sinusoids of the node and subsequently leaving through the efferent lymphatic vessel. The lymphatic system plays an important role in the dynamic control of fluid volume, protein concentration, and, consequently, the pressure in the interstitial space.

The lymphatic system is distributed throughout the entire human body, except CNS (not including the dura mater), the bone marrow, and cartilage [149], endomysium of muscle [148].

All human beings have similar lymphatic system anatomy; however, there can be considerable variation in the exact route of drainage from different locations of the body. Lymph nodes are present between the head to around the knee region. The spleen is considered the largest lymphatic organ according to the US national library of Medicine. The lymph from lymphatic vessels is emptied into collecting ducts (right and left thoracic ducts) which return lymph into bloodstream as they connect to subclavian vein. The lymphatic vessels are usually located in close proximity to the venous system. Approximately 800 lymph nodes are present in the human body, with a short axis diameter that ranges from a few millimeters to 1 cm [151]. Lymph nodes contain reticuloendothelial cells, primarily tissue phagocytes, that remove abnormal substances.

Lymphatic vessels have the capability of regeneration and can establish their own anastomoses within a short period (weeks) after organ transplantation [111, 152]. Additionally, new lymph tracts can develop and may subsequently reconnect to the main system. This occurs when small lymphatics are surgically transected or there is an attempt to circumvent flow obstruction.

Lymphatic vessels are divided into three categories according to their structural characteristics: lymph capillaries, pre-collectors, and lymph-collecting vessels [153]. The lymph capillaries (between 20 and 70 μm in diameter) do not have a valvular structure. The lymph capillary begins with a blind ending. The endothelial cells that form the lymph capillary connect with each other loosely. A fibrous structure called an anchoring filament connects the endothelial cell with the surrounding tissue [154]. When the tissue increases in volume owing to extra interstitial fluid (edema), the anchoring filaments pull the endothelial cells outward so that the junctions between the cells open up to capture the extra interstitial fluid into the lumen [149].

The lymph capillaries connect to pre-collectors (70–150 μm in diameter) which have a valvular structure that regulates the direction of lymph flow unidirectionally. The pre-collectors connect to the lymph-collecting vessels, or collectors. These collectors (between 150 and 500 μm in diameter). The lymph-collecting vessels have a three-layered wall made of endothelial cells, smooth muscle cells, and collagen fibers with fibroblasts that contracts rhythmically to propel lymph flow [149].

The lymph node barrier theory postulates that each lymphatic vessel connects to at least one lymph node before connecting to the vein. Lymph nodes are classified as regional or interval, according to their location. Regional lymph nodes are groups of lymph nodes that form lymphatic basins into which lymph drains from different skin regions or organs. The regional lymph nodes are the target of lymph node dissection in cancer treatment to halt the spread of cancer cells, with neck dissection for tongue cancer, axillary dissection for breast cancer, and inguinal dissection for lower extremity melanoma. Interval lymph nodes are located in the limbs, and the lymph vessels pass through them on the way to the regional lymph nodes. The superficial lymphatic system in the upper extremities originates in the lymph capillaries in the fingertips and palms while the superficial lymphatic system in the lower extremities originates in the lymph capillaries in the toes and soles of the feet [149].

9.3.5 Pathophysiology of Relevant Lymphatic Disorders

9.3.5.1 Lymphedema

Lymphedema is the excess accumulation of protein-rich fluid in the interstitial space. It may develop due to excess production of lymph, obstruction of lymphatic drainage, or disruption of the integrity of the lymphatic system. Excess production occurs when there is (a) obstruction of the capillary or venous system with resultant increased pressure, (b) excessive fluid migration from the vascular space due to low oncotic pressure, or (c) a leak in the system. Obstruction of lymphatic drainage occurs secondary to scarring following trauma, radiation, surgery, and infection or when there is abnormal development of the lymphatic system or compression of the main lymphatic by a mass [155]. These conditions force fluid to travel back to the vascular space via the nearest accessible lymphatic route.

Lymphedema may be primary or secondary (Table 9.17). The primary type is uncommon, may be congenital or developmental, and usually causes only minimal disturbances in lymphatic flow. Primary lymphedemas have been subclassified on the basis of their onset into congenital, peripubertal (lymphedema Praecox), and late-onset lymphedema (Tarda). Many genes have been associated with different forms of primary lymphedemas including VEGFC-VEGFR3, CCBE1, PTPN14, FOXC2, and SOX18 [156]. The more common secondary type can be due to several factors including infection, trauma, and other venous disorders. Since lymph is rich in protein, it promotes a cycle of inflammation that may be followed by fibrosis, leading to progressive scar formation, which can worsen lymphatic obstruction [155]. Lymphedema should not be confused with lipedema which is a chronically progressive accumulation of adipose tissue primarily in the lower extremities but can also affect arms. It affects almost exclusively woman and can be inherited. It is symmetrical (Lymphedema is asymmetrical) and does not involve feet (affected by Lymphema) [157].

Causes include chronic inflammation with fibrosis, malignant tumors, physical disruption, radiation damage, and certain infectious agents.

Severe edema of the upper limb may complicate the effective treatment of breast cancer. The surgical removal and irradiation of the breast and associated axillary lymph nodes results in lymphedema in 6%–30% of patients [158] *GJC2* (CX47) mutations are associated with a predisposition toward the development of postmastectomy lymphedema [159].

The most dramatic example of secondary lymphedema is seen in lymphatic filariasis, a neglected tropical disease that affects about 40 million people in the endemic areas of Africa, South America, and South-East Asia. This disease is caused by mosquito-transmitted parasitic nematodes, such as *Wuchereriabancrofti* (in 90% of the cases), which target and dwell in lymphatic vessels and LNs for years, resulting in extensive fibrosis. This may cause significant edema of the lower limbs and external genitalia that is so massive to be named elephantiasis [156].

Podoconiosis (endemic nonfilarial elephantiasis), is another tropical secondary lyphedemavisa noninfectious geochemical disease of the lower limb lymphatic vessels resulting from chronic barefoot exposure to red-clay soil derived from volcanic rock. Pathogenesis was suggested to be due to mineral particles in red-clay soils being absorbed through the skin of the foot and engulfed by macrophages in the lymphatic system of the lower limbs, inducing an inflammatory response in the lymphatic vessels resulting in fibrosis and vessel obstruction [156].

9.3.5.2 Lymph Nodes with Metastases

In general, tumors can metastasize by several routes including venous, arterial, lymphatic, and local invasion. It is believed that while most tumors initially spread through the lymphatic system, temporarily being retained at successive levels of lymph nodes by the body's defense system, some tumors may spread through both the

Table 9.17 Causes of lymphedema	Class	Pathogenesis
	Primary	Defects in genes involved in lymphatic vessel development
	Secondary	Damage or physical obstruction of lymphatic vessels or LNs due to inflammation malignancy radiation therapy filariasis surgical dissection trauma recurrent dermatitis

vascular and the lymphatic systems nearly simultaneously. Since lymph nodes are common sites of metastasis, knowledge of their involvement is crucial for patient management and prognosis. When small numbers of tumor cells (micrometastases) are found in lymph nodes, the architecture and physiological characteristics of the lymph node are not altered. Even with larger tumor loads, lymph nodes may remain normal in size, making them difficult to detect with anatomical imaging studies. Determination of focal defects within lymph nodes secondary to tumor infiltration is usually unreliable with all current imaging modalities [160].

9.3.5.3 Sentinel Node

The lymph node(s) that receives initial lymphatic drainage from a location harboring tumor has been termed the "sentinel node." There can be single or multiple nodes that may be located in one or different lymphatic beds [161]. Since determination of lymph node involvement is an integral part of tumor staging and management, lymph node excision with pathological evaluation is commonly performed. A complete nodal dissection (often involving large areas of tissue), however, can cause considerable morbidity, including lymphedema, and still fail to remove small diseased nodes [162]. If the sentinel node(s) can be identified, extensive pathological examination of the node(s) can forecast whether tumor dissemination has occurred, since it is the first filter that metastatic cells encounter. Identification of the sentinel node can be done by injections of blue dye around the tumor just before surgery or by using a radiopharmaceutical injected in a similar fashion [163, 164]. See Chap. 12.

9.3.6 Scintigraphy of Lymphatic System

9.3.6.1 The Spleen Imaging

Visualization of the spleen becomes necessary in pathological conditions associated with enlargement of this organ (splenomegaly) as well as in diseases in which splenic atrophy or asplenia occurs. The determination of spleen size by traditional radiographic techniques remains unsatisfactory and usually fails to detect minor enlargement often undetected on physical examination.

Even a moderately enlarged spleen may be difficult to palpate in obese persons. In recent years, several imaging techniques have been used very successfully for visualization of the spleen. These include ultrasonic imaging, magnetic resonance imaging (MRI), and computed tomography (CT) scan. Most or all of these procedures yield excellent structural details with little or no information about splenic function. Radionuclide imaging of the spleen, in addition, provides a major advantage in that more reliable information is obtained on the functions of the spleen.

The principle of radionuclide scintillation scanning of the spleen involves intravenous injection of radiolabeled autologous red cells of the patients, after these red cells have been subjected to certain procedures to damage them in a manner that when injected, they are rapidly removed from the circulation by the spleen. The red cells of the patient are labeled with 51 Cr, 111 In, or 99 m Tc and then heated to a temperature of 49.5 °C for precisely 20 min. These radiolabeled heated red cells are injected back into the patient, and scintillation scanning is usually done about 1 h later, but it can be performed up to 3–4 h later [165]. This procedure is very useful for mapping out the spleen size and in the diagnosis of splenomegaly, space-occupying lesions such as splenic cysts, and tumor deposits, for identifying abnormally disposed spleen and accessory splenic tissue, and for demonstrating asplenia, splenic atrophy, or the presence of residual splenunculus (Figs. 9.21 and 9.22).

Splenic activity can be measured by studying the rate of clearance of heat-damaged 51 Cr-labeled red cells from circulation. A sample of blood is collected from the patient exactly 3 min after the midpoint of the injection of heat-damaged 51 Cr-labeled red cells, and further samples are collected at 5-min intervals for 30 min, then at 45 min, and finally at 60 min. The

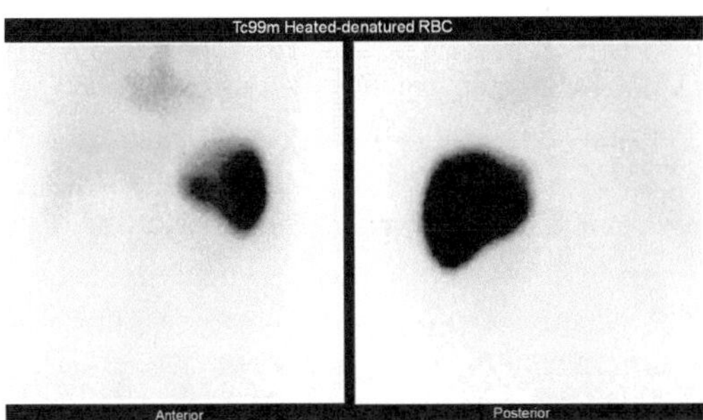

Fig. 9.21 A 47-year-old female with a history of persistent thrombocytopenia. A 99m Tc-denatured labeled RBC scan has been performed to rule out functional hyposplenia. The study shows homogeneous radiotracer distribution to the normally located splenic tissue. Findings indicate normally functioning splenic tissue

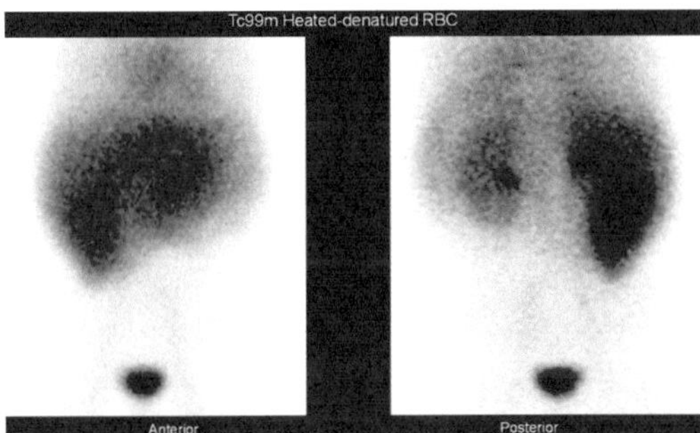

Fig. 9.22 A 99m Tc-denatured red blood cell study of a 9-year-old boy known to have sickle cell anemia with recurrent vaso-occlusive crises. A 99m Tc-sulfur colloids can previously done showed hepatomegaly with nonvisualized spleen. This denatured labeled RBC study was obtained to assess the sequestration function of the spleen. The study shows hepatomegaly with no scintigraphic evidence of sequestrating splenic tissue indicating nonfunctioning splenic tissue

radioactivity in each sample is measured and expressed as a percentage of the radioactivity in the 3-min sample. These are plotted on semilogarithmic graph paper, the radioactivity of the 3-min sample being taken as 100%. The radioactivity curve is generally exponential, and the rate of blood flow is calculated as the reciprocal of the time taken for the radioactivity to fall to 50% value ($T\frac{1}{2}$). In individuals with normal splenic activity, the $T\frac{1}{2}$ ranges from 5 to 15 min. The clearance rate is considerably prolonged in thrombocythemia and in other conditions associated with splenic atrophy such as sickle cell anemia or celiac disease [166–169].

9.3.6.2 Lymph Nodes and Lymphatic Vessels

Tracer is injected into a specific location, and imaging is then performed while the material crosses into the lymphatic system and migrates toward the vascular space. Agent movement will depend on the specific radiopharmaceutical used and the location of the injection. Particulate agents such as colloids are not transported into the peripheral collection sites as well because of their larger size. However, they are better retained in the lymph nodes because of their localization within RES cells. Nonparticulate agents travel much faster and efficiently but are not retained within a lymph node because they do not localize to any of the tissue components but are simply passing through. Because of the very rich supply of lymphatics in the skin, injections into this location will show very efficient uptake and movement of tracer, while breast injections move much slower due to a much sparser lymphatic system.

9.3.6.2.1 Detection and Follow-Up of Lymphedema

Lymphoscintigraphy can demonstrate (a) clearance of radiolabeled colloid from an interstitial injection and (b) flow to regional lymph node(s), along with some lymph node anatomical features. Several acquisition protocols can be used. The procedure usually consists of a 45-min dynamic acquisition followed by delayed imaging, usually at 90 min post-injection. For lower extremity disease, if movement of the tracer through the lymphatic system is not seen in early images, patients may be instructed to exercise their calf muscles by walking. Interpretation of images includes visual assessment of the injection sites, lymphatic tracts, lymph nodes, and time–activity curves, along with review of the early dynamic acquisition via a computer-generated cine display. Several quantitative procedures have been advocated for use in detecting lymphatic flow disturbances, with some attempting to define the cause of the disease [170].

These include determination of the timing as well as the amount of tracer uptake in the draining lymph nodes. However, care is advised when using such measures because there is a normal decrease in lymphatic flow parameters with age, and the use of different radiopharmaceuticals, different injection techniques, and additional procedures such as exercise can alter expected values.

Normally, there is rapid and fairly symmetrical transport of the radiotracer from foot injections through one or two lymphatic vessels in the calf and one lymphatic vessel in the thigh.

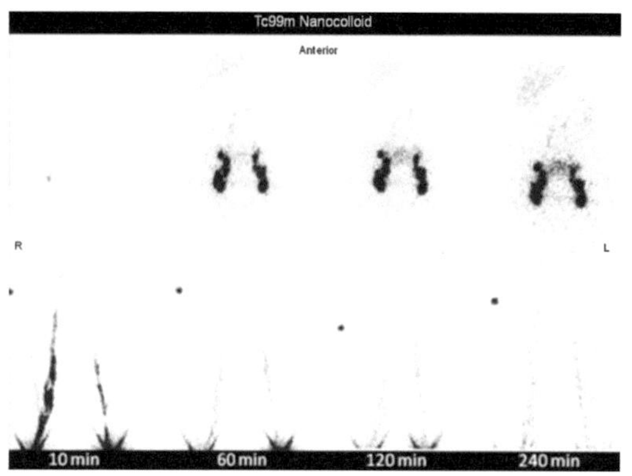

Fig. 9.23 Tc-99m nanocolloid images of the lower extremities. Anterior view images at 10, 60, 120, and 240 min. Images demonstrate normal ascend of activity throughout the lymphatic channels, particularly the medial band, and localization in the inguinal nodes bilaterally within 1 h. The lymph nodes are in symmetric appearance and similar numbers

Multiple pelvic lymph nodes should be clearly visualized within 1 h (Fig. 9.23 but may be seen within 6 min when a nonparticulate agent such as ^{99m}Tc-HSA is used [171]. Upper extremity findings in normal flow are similar (Fig. 9.24).

Scan findings in patients with lymphedema will depend on the cause of the swelling, the length of time that the process has been present, and compensatory mechanisms that have developed to circumvent the flow disturbance [172]. Figures 9.25, 9.26, and 9.27 illustrate lymphedema studies.

9.3.6.2.2 Detection of Lymph Node Metastases

Since lymph nodes have reticuloendothelial cells that phagocytose foreign material, radiocolloids are used to visualize them. Direct determination of the presence of tumor is extremely difficult, since the desired space-occupying defects caused by tumor infiltration require a significant portion of the node to be involved. When lymphatic tissue is largely replaced by tumor, lymph nodes may not be visualized because the tracer is blocked from entering. Tumor-involved nodes can even show more tracer uptake than normal nodes [161]. This may be explained by reactive changes in the lymph node, with increased numbers of RES

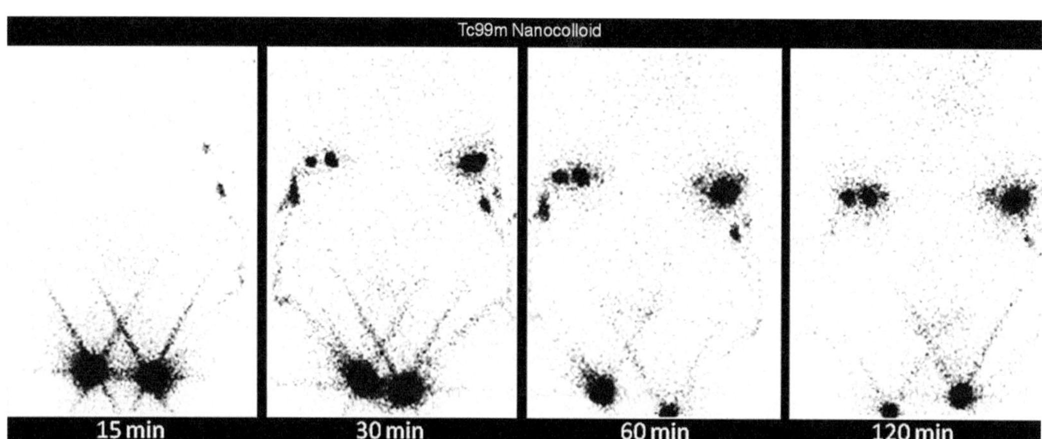

Fig. 9.24 Tc-99m nanocolloid lymphoscintigraphy images of the upper extremities. Anterior view images at 15, 30, 60, and 120 min. Normal upper extremity lymphoscintigraphy images demonstrate normal ascend of activity through lymphatic channels and localization in axillary lymph nodes bilaterally within 30 min. The lymph nodes are in symmetric appearance and similar number

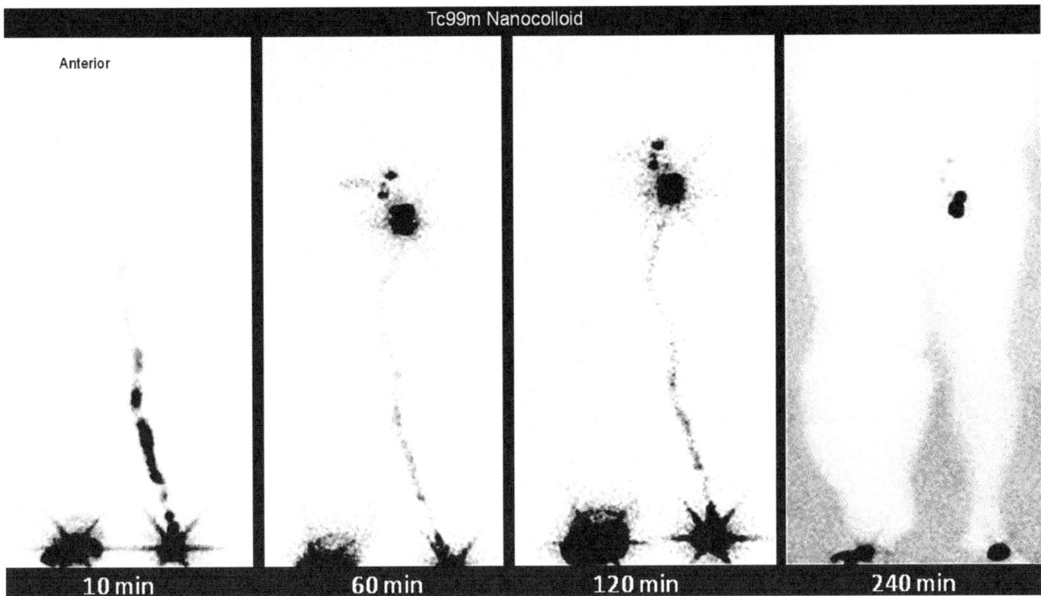

Fig. 9.25 Forty-seven-year-old male with severe right leg swelling. No lymphatic channels or lymph nodes are identified in the significantly swollen right leg and inguinal region (primary lymphedema). Findings are normal on the left side with normal visualization of lymphatic channels and inguinal lymph nodes which are in normal appearance

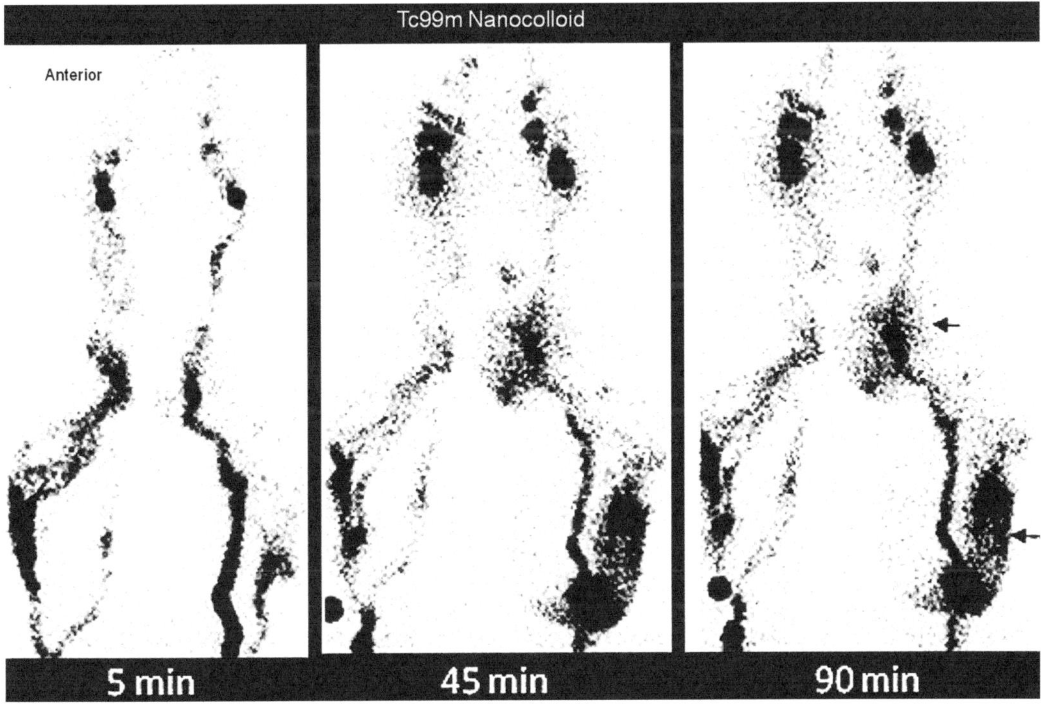

Fig. 9.26 Bilateral Lower Limb Lymphedema in a 65-five-year-old female with bilateral leg swelling for 2 years. Images were obtained at 5, 45, and 90 min and demonstrate prominent lymphatic channels and dermal backflow in the left lower and upper leg (arrows) indicating secondary lymphedema in bilateral legs

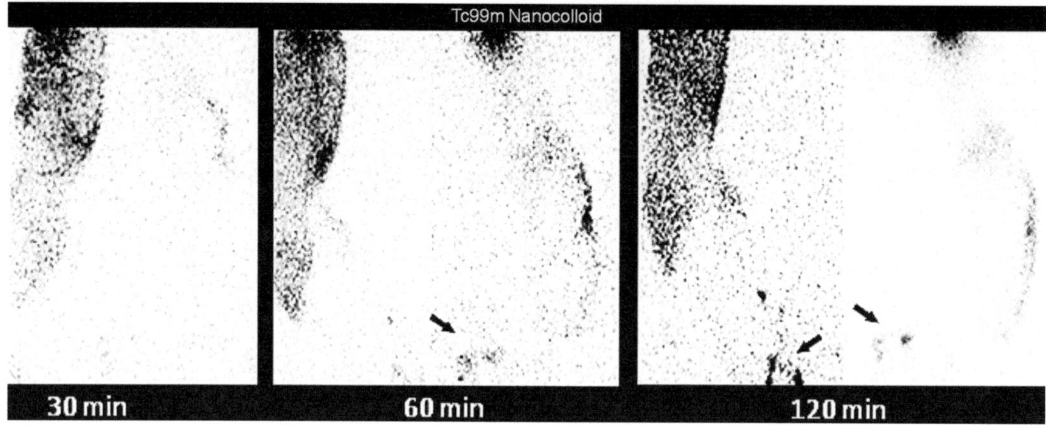

Fig. 9.27 Lymphoscintigraphy of the upper extremities for a 75-year-old woman with a history of long-standing lymphedema in upper limbs. There is dermal backflow which is significant in the right arm and mild in the left arm. No lymphatic channels are identified in both arms. There is an activity in few lymph nodes in both axilla (arrows)

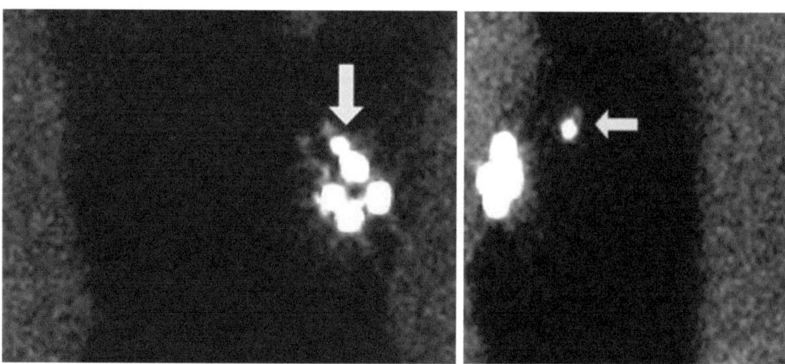

Fig. 9.28 A sentinel lymph node localization study in a patient with left breast cancer showing visualization of a sentinel lymph node in the anterior projection and more clearly in the left lateral projection (*arrows*)

cells being present, possibly in reaction to the presence of tumor antigens.

Lymphoscintigraphy with radiolabeled antitumor antibodies such as anti-CEA has been used to detect occult tumors in lymph nodes. Contrary to radiocolloid lymphoscintigraphy, which depends on phagocytosis, radiolabeled antibody localization requires attachment of the antibody directly to tumor cells. Interstitial injection of these agents has the advantage of producing a higher concentration of tracer at the tumor site in the lymph node than when the antibody is injected intravenously. However, the presence of a definitive number of metastatic cells is required for detection, depending on the agent and the imaging technique used. More recently FDG PET is being used to detect more effectively lymph node metastasis of many tumors. It has proven useful in detecting lymph node metastasis of lung cancer changing the mode of therapy in a significant number of cases [170, 173].

9.3.6.2.3 Sentinel Node Detection
Radioactive sentinel nodes can be detected using imaging with a gamma camera and/or a gamma probe at surgery. Lymphoscintigraphy using dynamic and static imaging better defines the sequence of lymphatic flow from the tumor site to draining lymph nodes, especially the sentinel node (Fig. 9.28) SPECT/CT is much better in achieving accurate localization, Fig. 9.29) (see Chap. 12).

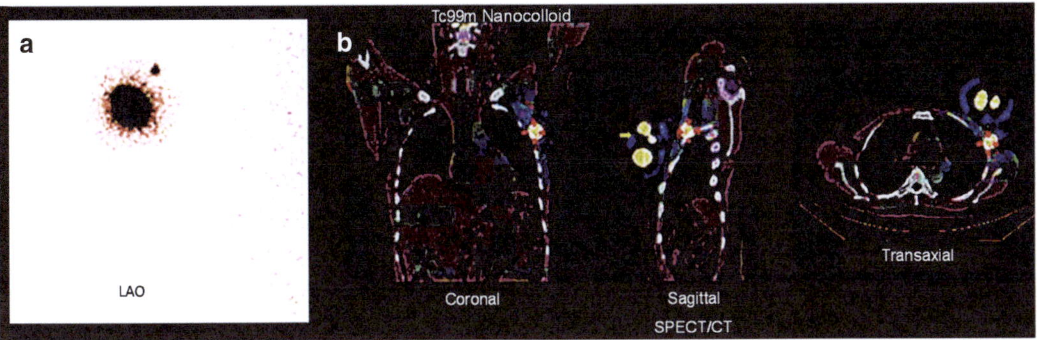

Fig. 9.29 Tc-99m nanocolloid sentinel node scintigraphy in a patient with breast cancer. Anterior oblique view of the left breast and axilla (**a**) and selected coronal, sagittal, and transaxial SPECT/CT fusion images of the chest (**b**). Images show intense activity at the injection site in the left breast as well as radiotracer accumulation in the left axillary sentinel lymph node. SPECT/CT better locates the lymph node in the axilla (level 1)

References

1. Parmley WW, Wikman-Coffelt J (1991) Physiology of cardiac muscle contraction. In: Parmley WW, Chatterjee K (eds) Cardiology. Lippincott, Philadelphia, pp 1–26
2. Parmley WW (1991) Ventricular function. In: Parmley WW, Chatterjee K (eds) Cardiology. Lippincott, Philadelphia, pp 1–20
3. Hall WD Jr, Gravanis MB (1991) Cardiac hypertrophy and hypertensive heart disease. In: Parmley WW, Chatterjee K (eds) Cardiology. Lippincott, Philadelphia, pp 118–138
4. Duncker DJ, Bache RJ (2008) Regulation of coronary blood flow during exercise. Physiol Rev 88:1009–1086
5. Tune JD (2014) Coronary circulation. Morgan & Claypool Life Sciences, San Francisco, CA
6. Izumo S, Nadal-Ginard B, Mahvadi V (1988) Proto-oncogene induction and reprogramming of cardiac gene expression produced by pressure overload. Proc Natl Acad Sci U S A 85:339
7. Ardehali A, Ports TA (1990) Myocardial oxygen supply and demand. Chest 98:699–705
8. Goodwill AG, Dick GM, Kiel AM, Tune JD (2017) Regulation of coronary blood flow. Compr Physiol 7(2):321–382
9. Levy D, Garrison RJ, Detal SD (1990) Prognostic implications of echocardiographically determined left ventricular mass in the Framingham study. N Engl J Med 322:1561
10. Schelbert HR (2010) Anatomy and physiology of coronary blood flow. J Nucl Cardiol 17:545–554
11. Harrison DG, Florentine MS, Brooks LA et al (1988) The effect of hypertension and left ventricular hypertrophy on the lower range of coronary autoregulation. Circulation 77:1108
12. Niccoli G, Scalone G, Crea F (2015) Acute myocardial infarction with no obstructive coronary atherosclerosis: mechanisms and management. Eur Heart J 36:475
13. Conrad GH, Brooks WW, Robinson KG et al (1987) Impaired myocardial function in the spontaneously hypertensive rate with heart failure. J Mol Cell Cardiol 19(Suppl 4):565
14. Gould KL, Nakagawa Y, Nakagawa K, Sdringola S, Hess MJ, Haynie M et al (2000) Frequency and clinical implications of fluid dynamically significant diffuse coronary artery disease manifest as graded, longitudinal, base-to-apex myocardial perfusion abnormalities by noninvasive positron emission tomography. Circulation 101:1931–1939
15. Cecchi F, Olivotto I, Gistri R, Lorenzoni R, Chiriatti G, Camici PG (2003) Coronary microvascular dysfunction and prognosis in hypertrophic cardiomyopathy. N Engl J Med 349:1027 1035
16. Neglia D, Michelassi C, Trivieri MG, Sambuceti G, Giorgetti A, Pratali L et al (2002) Prognostic role of myocardial blood flow impairment in idiopathic left ventricular dysfunction. Circulation 105:186–193
17. Haworth SG (1987) Pulmonary vascular disease in ventricular septal defect: structural and functional correlations in lung biopsies from 85 patients without come of intracardiac repair. J Pathol 152:157–168
18. Sharma GV, Mc Intyre KM, Setal S (1984) Clinical and hemodynamic correlates in pulmonary embolism. Clin Chest Med 5(421):37
19. Palevsky HI, Weiss DW (1990) Pulmonary hypertensions econdary to chronic thromboembolism. J Nucl Med 31:1–9
20. Hayley BD, Burwash IG (2012) Heart failure with normal left ventricular ejection fraction: role of echocardiography. Curr Opin Cardiol 27(2):169–180
21. Miranda D, Lewis GD, Fifer MA (2016) Heart failure, Chapter 9. In: Lilly LS (ed) Pathophysiology of heart disease: a collaborative project of medical students and faculty. Wolters Kluwer, Alphen aan den Rijn, pp 220–248

22. Berger HJ, Matthay RA, Lake J et al (1978) Assessment of cardiac performance with quantitative radionuclide angiocardiography: right ventricular ejection fraction with reference to findings in chronic obstructive pulmonary disease. Am J Cardiol 41:897–905

23. Gazewood JD, Turner PL (2017) Heart failure with preserved ejection fraction: diagnosis and management. Am Fam Physician 96(9):582–588

24. Grossman W (1991) Iastolic dysfunction congestive heart failure. N Engl J Med 325:1557–1567

25. Hartupee J, Mann DL (2017) Neurohormonal activation in heart failure with reduced ejection fraction. Nat Rev Cardiol 14(1):30–38

26. Patel PA, Ali N (2017) Mechanisms involved in regulation of Systemic Blood Pressure. Arch Clin Hypertension 3(1):016–020

27. Oakley CM, Gravanis MB, Ansari AA (1993) Cardiomyopathies. In: Gravanis M (ed) Cardiovascular disorders: pathogenesis and pathophysiology. Mosby, St Louis, pp 210–253

28. Corbett JR, Akinboboye OO, Bacharach SL, Borer JS, Botvinick EH et al (2006) Quality Assurance Committee of the American Society of nuclear cardiology. Equilibrium Radionuclide Angiocardiography. J Nucl Cardiol 13:e56–e79

29. Akinboboye O, Nicholes K, Wang Y, Dim UR, Reichek N (2005) Accuracy of radionuclide ventriculography assessed by magnetic resonance imaging in patients with abnormal left ventricles. J Nucl Cardiol 12:418–427

30. Haworth SG (1987) Pulmonary vascular disease in ventricular septal defect: structural and functional correlations in lung biopsies from 85 patients with outcome of intracardiac repair. J Pathol 152:157–168

31. Sharma GV, McIntyre KM, Sharma S et al (1984) Clinical and hemodynamic correlates in pulmonary embolism. Clin Chest Med 5(421):37

32. Friedman JD, Berman DS, Borges-Neto S, Hayes SW, Johnson LL, Nichols KJ, Pagnanelli RA, Port SC (2006) Quality Assurance Committee of the American Society of Nuclear Cardiology. First-pass radionuclide angiography. J Nucl Cardiol 13:e42–e55

33. Nichols KJ, Van Tosh A, Wang Y, Palestro CJ, Reichek N (2009) Validation of gated blood-pool SPECT regional left ventricular function measurements. J Nucl Med 50:53–60

34. Daou D, Coaguila C, Benada A (2006) Comparison of inter study reproducibility of equilibrium electrocardiography-gated SPECT radionuclideangiography versus planar radionuclide angiography for the quantification of global left ventricular function. J Nucl Cardiol 13:233–243

35. Schwartz RG, McKenzie WB, Alexander J et al (1987) Congestive heart failure and left ventricular dysfunction complicating doxorubicin therapy: seven-year experience using serial radionuclideangio cardiography. Am J Med 82:1109–1118

36. McGill HC Jr, McMahan CA, Herderick EE, Malcom GT, Tracy RE, Strong JP (2000) Origin of atherosclerosis in childhood and adolescence. Am J Clin Nutr 72(5 Suppl):1307S–1315S

37. Heiba SI, Jacobson AF, Cerqueira MD, Shattuc S, Sharma S (1999) The additive values of radionuclide ventriculography and extent of myocardium at risk to dipyridamole thallium-201 imaging for optimal risk stratification prior to vascular surgery. Nucl Med Commun 20:887–894

38. Tegos TJ, Kalodiki E, Sabetai MM, Nicolaides AN (2001) The genesis of atherosclerosis and risk factors: a review. Angiology 52(2):89–98

39. Shahawy S, Libby P (2016) Atherosclerosis, Chapter 5. In: Lilly LS (ed) Pathophysiology of heart disease: a collaborative project of medical students and faculty, 6th edn. Wolters Kluwer, pp 112–133

40. Grech ED (2003) Pathophysiology and investigation of coronaryartery disease. BMJ 326:1027–1030

41. Moore KJ, Sheedy FJ, Fisher EA (2013) Macrophages in atherosclerosis: a dynamic balance. Nat Rev Immunol 13(10):709–721

42. Libby P, Theroux P (2005) Pathophysiology of coronaryartery disease. Circulation 111:3481–3488

43. Borén J, Chapman MJ, Krauss RM, Packard CJ, Bentzon JF et al (2020) Low-density lipoproteins cause atherosclerotic cardiovascular disease: pathophysiological, genetic, and therapeutic insights: a consensus statement from the European Atherosclerosis Society Consensus Panel. Eur Heart J 41:2313–2330

44. He C, Medley S, Hu T, Hindstale ME, Lupu F, Virmani R, Olsen LE (2015) PDGFRβ signalling regulates local inflammation and synergizes with hypercholesterolaemia to promote atherosclerosis. Nat Commun 6:7770

45. Ramji DP, Davies TS (2015) Cytokines in atherosclerosis: Key players in all stages of disease and promising therapeutic targets. Cytokine Growth Factor Rev 26(6):673–685

46. Ray KK, Cannon C (2005) The potential relevance of the multiple lipid-independent (pleiotropic) effects of statins in the management of acute coronary syndromes. J Am Coll Cardiol 46:1425–1433

47. Ward MR, Pasterkamp G, Yeung AC, Borst C (2000) Arterial remodeling mechanisms and clinical implications. Circulation 102:1186–1191

48. DeWiner RJ, Koster RW, Stark A et al (1995) Value of myoglobin, troponinT, CK-MB mass in ruling out an acute myocardial infarction in the emergency room. Circulation 92:3401–3407

49. Wilder J, Sabatine MS, Lilly LS (2016) In: Lilly LS (ed) Ischemic Heart Disease, Chapter 6, In Pathophysiology of heart disease: a collaborative project of medical students and faculty, 6th edn. Wolters Kluwer, Alphen aan den Rijn, pp 134–161

50. Piek JJ, Becker AE (1988) Collateral blood supply to the myocardium at risk inhuman myocardial

infarction:a quantitative post-mortem assessment. J Am Coll Cardiol 1:1290–1296

51. Croce K, Libby P (2007) Intertwining of thrombosis and inflammation in atherosclerosis. Curr Opin Hematol 14:55–61

52. Libby P (2013) Mechanisms of acute coronary syndromes. N Engl J Med. 369:883–884

53. Antonopoulos AS, Goliopoulou A, Vogiatzi G, Tousoulis D (2018) Myocardial Oxygen Consumption, Chapter 2.2. In: Tousoulis D (ed) Coronary Artery Disease From Biology to Clinical Practice. Academic Press, Cambridge, pp 127–136

54. Detrano R, Gianrossi R, Froelicher VF (1989) The diagnostic accuracy of the exercise electrocardiogram: a meta-analysis of 22 years of research. Prog Cardiovasc Dis 33:173–205

55. Arbustini E, Narula J, Tavazzi J et al (2014) The MOGE(S) classification of cardiomyopathy or clinicians. J Am Coll Cardiol 64:304–318

56. Roger VL, Jacobsen SI, Pelikka PA et al (1998) Prognostic value of treadmill exercise testing. A population based study in Olmsted County. Minnesota Circulation 98:2836–2841

57. Garfinkel AC, Seidman JG, Seidman CE (2018) Genetic pathogenesis of hypertrophic and dilated cardiomyopathy. Heart Failure Clin 14:139–146

58. Maron BJ, Ommen SR, Semsarian C et al (2014) Hypertrophic cardiomyopathy: Present and future, with translation into contemporary cardiovascular medicine. J Am Coll Cardiol 64:83–99

59. Rammos A, Meladinis V, Vovas G, Patsouras D (2017) Restrictive cardiomyopathies: the importance of noninvasive cardiac imaging modalities in diagnosis and treatment-a systematic review. Radiol Res Pract 2017:2874902

60. Jung HO (2012) Pericardial effusion and pericardiocentesis: role of echocardiography. Korean Circ J 42(11):725–734

61. Cheong XP, Law L, Seow SC, Tay L, Tan HC, Yeo WT, Low AF, Kojodjojo P (2020) Causes and prognosis of symptomatic pericardial effusions treated by pericardiocentesis in an Asian academic medical centre. Singapore Med J 61(3):137–141, 49

62. Albugami S, Al-Husayni F, AlMalki A, Dumyati M, Zakri Y, AlRahimi J (2020) Etiology of pericardial effusion and outcomes post pericardiocentesis in the western region of Saudi Arabia: A single-center experience. Cureus 12:e6627

63. Vakamudi S, Ho N, Cremer PC (2017) Pericardial effusions: causes, diagnosis, and management. Prog Cardiovasc Dis 59(4):380–388

64. Vasileios Sachpekidis MD, EfstratiosMoralidis MD, Georgios Arsos MD (2018) Equilibrium radionuclide ventriculography: still a clinically useful method for the assessment of cardiac function? Hell J Nucl Med 21(3):213–220

65. Hachamovitch R, Berman DS, Kiat H et al (1996) Exercise myocardial perfusion SPECT in patients without known CAD. Incremental prognostic value and use in risk stratification. Circulation 93:905–914

66. Heiba SI, Cerqueira MD (1994) Evaluation of cardiac function. In: Cerqueira MD (ed) Nuclear cardiology. Blackwell Scientific, Cambridge, pp 53–117

67. Bateman TM (1997) Clinical relevance of a normal myocardial perfusion scintigraphic study. J Nucl Cardiol 4:172–173

68. Soufer A, Liu C, Henry ML, Baldassarre LA (2020) Nuclear cardiology in the context of multimodality imaging to detect cardiac toxicity from cancer therapeutics: Established and emerging methods. J Nuclear Cardiol 27:1210–1224

69. Iskander S, Iskandrian AE (1998) Risk assessment using single-photonemission computed tomographic technetium-99m sestamibi imaging. J Am Coll Cardiol 32:57–62

70. Berman DS, Maddahi J, Garcia EV et al (1981) Assessment of left and right ventricular function with multiple gated equilibrium cardiac blood pool scintig raphy. In: Berman DS, Mason DT (eds) Clinical nuclear cardiology. Grune and Stratton, New York

71. Scatteia A, Silverio A, Padalino R, De Stefano F, America R, Cappelletti AM, Dellegrottaglie S (2021) Non-Invasive Assessment of Left Ventricle Ejection Fraction: Where Do We Stand? J Pers Med 11(11):1153

72. Dakik HA, Kleiman NS, Farmer JA, He ZX, Wendt JA et al (1998) Intensive medical therapy versus coronary angioplasty for suppression of myocardial ischemia in survivors of acute myocardial infarction. A prospective, randomized pilot study. Circulation 98:2017–2023

73. Liu YH, Fazzone-Chettiar R, Sandoval V et al (2021) New approach for quantification of left ventricular function from low-dose gated bloodpool SPECT: Validation and comparison with conventional methods in patients. J. Nucl Cardiol 28:939–950

74. Ramon AJ, Yang Y, Wernick MN, Pretorius PH, Johnson KL, Slomka PJ, King MA (2020) Evaluation of the effect of reducing administered activity on assessment of function in cardiac gated SPECT. J Nucl Cardiol 27(2):562–572

75. Heiba SI, Cerqueira MD (1994) Evaluation of cardiac function. In: Cerqueira MD (ed) Nuclearcardiology. Blackwell Scientific, Cambridge, pp 53–117

76. Vilcant V, Zeltser R (2020) Treadmill Stress Testing. StatPearls

77. Braunwald E, Kloner RA (1982) The stunned myocardium: prolonged, post-ischemic ventricular dysfunction. Circulation 66:1146–1149

78. Ferrari R, LaCanna G, Giubbini R et al (1994) Left ventricular dysfunction due to stunning and hibernation in patients. Cardiovasc Drugs Ther 8(Suppl 2):371–380

79. Wasserman K, Hansen JE, Sue DY et al (2012) Principles of Exercise Testing and Interpretation, 5th edn. Wolters Kluwer/Lippincott Williams & Wilkins, Philadelphia, PA

80. Farell MB (2016) Myocardial Perfusion Imaging 2015: Quality, Safety, and Dose Optimization. Society of Nuclear Medicine and Molecular Imaging Technologist Section, Reston, VA

81. Heller GV, Hendel R, Mann A (2009) Nuclear Cardiology: Technical Applications. McGraw-Hill, New York, NY

82. Strauss HW, Miller DD, Wittry MD, Cerqueira MD, Garcia EV, Iskandrian AS, Schelbert HR, Wackers FJ, Balon HR, Lang O, Machac J (2008) Procedure guideline for myocardial perfusion imaging 3.3. J Nucl Med Technol 36(3):155–161

83. Iskandrian AS, Verani MS, Heo J (1994) Pharmacologic stress testing: mechanism of action, hemodynamic responses, and results in detection of coronary artery disease. J NuclCardiol 1:94–111

84. Travin MI, Wexler JP (1999) Pharmacological stress testing. Semin Nucl Med 29:298–318

85. Iskandrian AE, Bateman TM, Belardinelli L et al (2007) Adenosine versus regadenoson comparative evaluation in myocardial perfusion imaging: Results of the ADVANCE phase 3 multicenter international trial. J NuclCardiol 14:645–658

86. Vitola JV, Brambatti JC, Caligaris F et al (2001) Exercise supplementation to dipyridamole prevents hypotension, improves electrocardiogram sensitivity, and increases heart-to-liver activity ratio on Tc-99m sestamibi imaging. J NuclCardiol 8:652–659

87. Mahmarian JJ, Mahmarian AC, Marks GF et al (1995) Role of adenosine thallium-201 tomography for defning long-term risk in patients after acute myocardial infarction. J Am Coll Cardiol 25:1333–1340

88. Manapragada PP, Andrikopoulou E, Bajaj N, Bhambhvani P (2021) PET Cardiac Imaging (Perfusion, Viability, Sarcoidosis, and Infection). Radiol Clin N Am 59:835–852

89. Abraham A, Nichol G, Williams KA et al (2009) 18F-FDGPET of myocardial viability in an experienced center with access to ^{18}F-FDG and integration with clinical management teams: the Ottawa-FIVE substudy of the PARR2 trial. J Nucl Med 51:567–574

90. Russell RR III, Zaret BL (2006) Nuclear cardiology: present and future. Curr Probl Cardiol 31(9):557–629

91. Lopaschuk GD et al (2010) Myocardial fatty acid metabolism in health and disease. Physiol Rev 90:207–258

92. Luyten K, Schoenberger M (2017) Molecular imaging of cardiac metabolism, innervation, and conduction. EMJ Cardiol 5(1):70–78

93. Burt RW, Perkins OW, Oppenheim BE et al (1995) Direct comparison of fluorine-18-FDGSPECT, fluorine-18-FDGPET, and rest thallium-201 SPECT for detection of myocardial viability. J Nucl Med 36:176–179

94. Taegtmeyer H, Dilsizian V (2013) Imaging cardiac metabolism. In: Atlas of nuclear cardiology. Springer, New York, NY, pp 289–321

95. Haas F, Haehnel CJ, Picker W et al (1997) Preoperative positron emission tomographic viability assessment and perioperative and post-operative risk in patients with advanced ischemic heart disease. J Am Coll Cardiol 30:1693–1700

96. Ohira H, Dowsley T, Dwivedi G et al (2014) Quantification of myocardial blood flow using PET to improve the management of patients with stable ischemic coronary artery disease. Future Cardiol 10:611–631

97. Marwick TH, Shan K, Patel S et al (1997) Incremental value of rubidium-82 positron emission tomography for prognostic assessment of known or suspected coronary artery disease. Am J Cardiol 80:865–870

98. Yoshinaga K, Chow BJW, de Kemp R et al (2004) Prognostic value of rubidium-82 perfusion positron emission tomography: preliminary results from the consecutive 153 patients. J Am Coll Cardiol 43:338A

99. Chow BJW, Wong JW, Yoshinaga K et al (2005) Prognostic significance of dipyridamole-induced ST depression in patients with normal Rb-82 PET myocardial perfusion imaging. J Nucl Med 46:1095–1101

100. Nemirovsky D, Henzlova MJ, Machac J et al (2005) Prognosis of normal rubidium-82 myocardial perfusion study. J Nucl Cardiol 12:S118

101. Holman BL, Tanaka TT, Lesch M (1976) Evaluation of radiopharmaceuticals for the detection of acute myocardial infarction in man. Radiology 121:427

102. Huckell VF, Lyster DM, Morrison RT et al (1985) Comparison of technetium-99m pyrophosphate and technetium-99m methylene diphosphonate with variable amounts of stannous chloride in the detection of acute myocardial infarction. Clin Nucl Med 10:455–462

103. Parkey RW, Bonte FJ, Buja LM et al (1977) Myocardial infarct imaging with technetim-99m phosphates. Semin Nucl Med 7:15

104. Dorbala S, Di Carli MF, Cardiac PET (2014) perfusion: prognosis, risk stratification, and clinical management. Semin Nucl Med 44:344–357

105. Shaw LJ, Iskandrian AE (2004) Prognostic value of gated myocardial perfusion SPECT. J Nucl Cardiol 11:171–185

106. Pethig K, Heublein B, Meliss RR et al (1999) Volumetric remodeling of the proximal left coronary artery: early versus late after heart transplantation. J Am Coll Cardiol 34:197–203

107. Julius BK, Vassalli G, Mandonow L et al (1999) Alpha-adrenergic blockade prevents exercise-induced vasoconstriction of stenotic coronary arteries. J Am Coll Cardiol 33:1499–1505

108. O'Driscoll G, Green D, Maiorana A et al (1999) Improvement in endothelial function by angiotensin-converting enzyme inhibition in non-insulin-dependent diabetes mellitus. J Am Coll Cardiol 33:15–16

109. Kugiyama K, Motoyama T, Doi H, Kawano H et al (1999) Improvement of endothelial vasomotor dysfunction by treatment with alpha-tocopherol in patients with high remnant lipoproteins levels. J Am Coll Cardiol 33:1512–1518

110. Gould KL, Martucci JP, Goldberg DI, Hess MJ, Edens RP, Latifi R, Dudrick SJ (1994) Short-term cholesterol lowering decreases size and severity of perfusion abnormalities by positron emission tomography after dipyridamole in patients with coronary artery disease. A potential noninvasive marker of healing coronary endothelium. Circulation 89:1530–1538

111. Aljizeeri A, Ahmed AI, Suliman I, Alfaris MA, Elneama A, Al-Mallah MH (2023) Incremental prognostic value of positron emission tomography-derived myocardial flow reserve in patients with and without diabetes mellitus. Eur Heart J Cardiovasc Imaging 24(5):563–571. https://doi.org/10.1093/ehjci/jead023. PMID: 36814411

112. Murthy VL, Naya M, Foster CR et al (2011) Improved cardiac risk assessment with noninvasive measures of coronary flow reserve. Circulation 124:2215–1224

113. Ziadi MC, Dekemp RA, Williams KA et al (2011) Impaired myocardial flow reserve on rubidium-82 positron emission tomography imaging predicts adverse outcomes in patients assessed for myocardial ischemia. J Am Coll Cardiol 58:740–748

114. Murthy VL, Lee BC, Sitek A et al (2014) Comparison and prognostic validation of multiple methods of quantification of myocardial blood flow with 82Rb PET. J Nucl Med 55:1952–1958

115. Taqueti VR, Di Carli MF (2015) Radionuclide myocardial perfusion imaging for the evaluation of patients with known or suspected coronary artery disease in the era of multimodality cardiovascular imaging. Prog Cardiovasc Dis 57:644–653

116. Schinkel AF, Bax JJ, Poldermans D et al (2007) Hibernating myocardium: diagnosis and patient outcomes. CurrProbl Cardiol 32(375–410):106

117. Underwood SR, Bax JJ, vom Dahl J et al (2004) Imaging techniques for the assessment of myocardial hibernation. Report of a Study Group of the European Society of Cardiology. Eur Heart J 25:815–836

118. Schinkel AF, Bax JJ, Delgado V et al (2010) Clinical relevance of hibernating myocardium in ischemic left ventricular dysfunction. Am J Med. 123:978–986

119. Ohira H, Mc Ardle B, Cocker MS et al (2013) Current and future clinical applications of cardiac positron emission tomography. Circ J 77:836–848

120. Ben Bouallègue F, Maïmoun L, Kucharczak F et al (2021) Left ventricle function assessment using gated first-pass 18F-FDG PET: validation against equilibrium radionuclide angiography. J Nucl Cardiol 28:594–603

121. Auer WH, Stern BJ, Baughman RP, Culver DA, Royal W (2017) High-risk sarcoidosis: current concepts and research imperatives. Ann Am Thorac Soc 14:S437–S444

122. Ramirez R, Trivieri M, Fayad ZA, Ahmadi A, Narula J, Argulian E (2019) Advanced imaging in cardiac sarcoidosis. J Nucl Med 60(7):892–898

123. Ramsay SC, Cuscaden C (2020) The current status of quantitative SPECT/CT in the assessment of transthyretin cardiac amyloidosis. J Nucl Cardiol 27(5):1464–1468

124. Okasha O, Kazmirczak F, Chen KHA, Farzaneh-Far A, Shenoy C (2019) Myocardial involvement in patients with histologically diagnosed cardiac sarcoidosis: a systematic review and meta-analysis of gross pathological images from autopsy or cardiac transplantation cases. J Am Heart Assoc 8(10):e011253

125. Youssef G, Leung E, Mylonas I et al (2012) The use of 18F-FDG PET in the diagnosis of cardiac sarcoidosis: a systematic review and metaanalysis including the Ontario experience. J Nucl Med 53:241–248

126. Cegła P, Cieplucha A, Pachowicz M, Chrapko B, Piotrowski T, Lesiak M (2020) Nuclear cardiology: an overview of radioisotope techniques used in the diagnostic workup of cardiovascular disorders. Kardiol Pol 78:520–528

127. Hotta M, Minamimoto R, Awaya T, Hiroe M, Okazaki O, Hiroi Y (2020) Radionuclide imaging of cardiac amyloidosis and sarcoidosis: roles and characteristics of various tracers. Radiographics 40(7):2029–2041

128. Martinez-Naharro A, Baksi AJ, Hawkins PN, Fontana M (2020) Diagnostic imaging of cardiac amyloidosis. Nat Rev Cardiol 17:413–426

129. Fontana M, Ćorović A, Scully P, Moon JC (2019) Myocardial amyloidosis: the exemplar interstitial disease. JACC Cardiovasc Imaging 12(11 Part 2):2345–2356

130. Kyriakou P, Mouselimis D, Tsarouchas A, Rigopoulos A, Bakogiannis C, Noutsias M, Vassilikos V (2018) Diagnosis of cardiac amyloidosis: a systematic review on the role of imaging and biomarkers. BMC Cardiovasc Disord 18(1):1–11

131. Dilsizian V, Freedman NMT, Bacharach SL et al (1992) Regional thallium uptake in irreversible defects: magnitude of change in thallium activity after reinjection distinguishes viable from nonviable myocardium. Circulation 85:627–634

132. Bolli R (1990) Mechanism of myocardial stunning. Circulation 82:723–772

133. Fuster V, Badimon L, Badimon JJ et al (1992) The pathogenesis of coronary artery disease and the acute coronary syndromes. N Engl J Med 326:242–250, 310–318, 127

134. Homans DC, Laxson DD, Sublett E et al (1989) Cumulative deterioration of myocardial function after repeated episodes of exercise-induced ischemia. Am J Physiol 256:H1462–H1471

135. Santos BS, Ferreira MJ (2019) Positron emission tomography in ischemic heart disease. Rev Port Cardiol (Engl Ed) 38(8):599–608

136. Haas F, Haehnel C, Augustin N et al (1997) Prevalence and time course of functional improvement in stunned and hibernating myocardium in patients with CAD and CHF. J Am Coll Cardiol 29:788A

137. Melon PG, DeLandsheere CM, Degueldre C et al (1997) Relation between contractile reserve and positron emission tomographic patterns of perfusion and glucose utilization in chronic ischemic left ventricular dysfunction. J Am Coll Cardiol 30:1651–1659

138. Brunken R, Tillisch J, Schwaiger M et al (1986) Regional perfusion, glucose metabolism, and wall motion in patients with chronic electrocardiographic Q-wave infarctions: evidence for persistence of viable tissue in some infarct regions by positron emission tomography. Circulation 73:951–963

139. Dilsizian V, Bonow RO (1992) Differential uptake and apparent Tl-201 washout after thallium reinjection: options regarding early redistribution imaging before reinjection or late redistribution imaging after reinjection. Circulation 85:1032–1038

140. Dilsizian V, Bonow RO (1993) Current diagnostic techniques of assessing myocardial viability in patients with hibernating and stunned myocardium. Circulation 87:1–20

141. Dilsizian V, Rocco TP, Freedman NMT et al (1990) Enhanced detection of ischemic but viable myocardium by the reinjection of thallium after stress-redistribution imaging. N Engl J Med 323:141–146

142. Perrone-Filardi P, Bacharach SL, Dilsizian V et al (1992) Regional left ventricular wall thickening: relation to regional uptake of F-18-fluorodeoxyglucose and Tl-201 in patients with chronic coronary artery disease and left ventricular dysfunction. Circulation 86:1125–1137

143. Kim YK, Lee DS, Cheon J et al (1999) Myocardial viability assessment by nitroglycerine gated Tc-99m MIBI SPECT: comparison with rest-24-hour redistribution Tl-201 SPECT. J Nucl Med 40:1P

144. Fallavolita JA, Canty JM (1997) F-18 FDG utilization is regionally increased in fasting pigs with hibernating myocardium. J Am Coll Cardiol 29:130A

145. Hansen CL, Corbett JR, Pippin JJ et al (1988) 123-I-phenylpentadecanoic acid and single photon emission computed tomography in identifying LV regional metabolic abnormalities in patients with coronary heart disease: comparison with thallium-201 myocardial tomography. J Am Coll Cardiol 12:78–87

146. Hansen CL, Rastogi A, Sangrigoli R et al (1998) On myocardial perfusion, metabolism, and viability. J NuclCardiol 5:202–204

147. Berman DS, Kiat H, Friedman JD, Wang FP, Van Train K, Metzer L, Maddahi J, Germano G (1993) Separate acquisition rest thallium-201/stress technetium 99m sestamibi dual-isotope myocardial perfusion single-photon emission computed tomography: a clinical validation study. J Am Coll Cardiol 22:1455–1464

148. Guyton AC, Hall JE (1966) Textbook of medical physiology, 9th edn. Saunders, Philadelphia, pp 193–197

149. Suami H, Scaglioni MF (2018) Anatomy of the lymphatic system and the lymphosome concept with reference to lymphedema. In: Seminars in plastic surgery, vol 32. Thieme Medical Publishers, New York, pp 005–011

150. McCance KL (1998) Pathophysiology, biological basis of disease in adults and children. Mosby, St. Louis, pp 968–1023

151. Weissleder R, Thrall JH (1989) The lymphatic system: diagnostic imaging studies. Radiology 172:315–317

152. Ruggiero R, Muz J, Fietsam R Jr (1993) lung transplantation. J Thorac Cardiovasc Surg 106:167–171

153. Uami H, Pan WR, Mann GB, Taylor GI (2008) The lymphatic anatomy of the breast and its implications for sentinel lymph node biopsy: a human cadaver study. Ann Surg Oncol 15:863–871

154. Leak LV (1970) Electron microscopic observations on lymphatic capillaries and the structural components of the connective tissue lymph interface. Microvasc Res 2:361–391

155. Clodius L (1990) Lymphedema. In: McCarthy JG (ed) Plastic surgery. Saunders, Philadelphia, pp 4093–4120

156. Aspelund A, Robciuc MR, Karaman S, Makinen T, Alitalo K (2016) Lymphatic system in cardiovascular medicine. Circ Res 118(3):515–530

157. Zuther JE, Norton S (2013) Lymphedema management. The comprehensive guide for practitioners, 3rd edn. Thieme Medical Publishers, New York/Stuttgart

158. Koolen BB, Valdés ORA, Vogel WV et al (2012) 18F-FDGPET/CT for the assessment of locoregional lymph node involvement and radiotherapy indication in stage II-III breast cancertreated with neo adjuvant chemotherapy. Cancer Res 72:nrP4-02-01

159. Mavi A, Lakhani P, Zhuang H, Gupta NC, Alavi A (2005) Fluorodeoxyglucose-PET in characterizing solitary pulmonary nodules, assessing pleural diseases, and the initial staging, restaging, therapy planning, and monitoring response of lung cancer. Radiol Clin N Am 43(1):1–24

160. Peyton JW, Crosbie J, Bell TK (1981) High colloidal uptake in axillary nodes with metastatic disease. Br J Surg 68:507–509

161. Bergqvist L, Strand SE, Hafstrom L (1984) Lymphoscintigraphy in patients with malignant melanoma: a quantitative and qualitative evaluation of its usefulness. Eur J Nucl Med 9:129–135

162. Baas PC, Schraffordt KH, Hoekstra HJ, Van Bruggen JJ, Van der Weele LT, Oldhoff J (1992) Groin dissection in the treatment of lower-extremity melanoma. Short term and long term morbidity. Arch Surg 127:281–286

163. Morton DL, Wen DR, Wong JH (1992) Technical details of intraoperative lymphatic mapping for early stage melanoma. Arch Surg 127:392–399

164. Alex JC, Weaver DL, Fairbank JT (1993) Gamma-probe-guided lymph node localization in malignant melanoma. Surg Oncol 2:303–308

165. Tojinda N, Clairmon A, Taweewattanasopon N, Boonkhon P, Amornkitticharoen B et al (2017) The heated denatured RBC, the most specific technique for spleen-specific imaging. J Siriraj Radiol 4:19–23

166. Lee GR, Herbert V (1999) Nutritional factors in the production and function of erythrocytes. In: Lee GR et al (eds) Wintrobe's clinical hematology, vol 1, 10th edn. Williams and Wilkins, Baltimore, pp 228–266
167. Das KC, Mohanty D, Garewal G (1989) Nutritional megaloblastosis: from morphology to molecular biology. In: Sapru RP (ed) Medical research monographs. Malhotra Publishing House, New Delhi, pp 1–59
168. Price DC (1996) The hematopoietic system. In: Herbert JC, Eckelman WC, Neumann RD (eds) Nuclear medicine: diagnosis and therapy. Thieme Medical Publishers, New York, pp 764–785
169. Ahuja S, Lewis SM, Szur I (1972) Value of surface counting in predicting response to splenectomy in haemolytic anaemia. J Clin Pathol 25:467
170. Rijke AM, Croft BY, Johnson RA (1990) Lymphoscintigraphy and lymphedema of the lower extremities. J Nucl Med 31:990–998
171. Nawaz MK, Hamad MM, Abdel-Dayem HM (1990) Tc-99m human serum albumin lymphoscintigraphy in lymphedema of the lower extremities. Clin Nucl Med 15:794–799
172. Szuba A, Shin WS, Strauss HW, Rockson S (2003) The third circulation: radionuclide lymphoscintigraphy in the evaluation of lymphedema. J Nucl Med 44(1):43–57
173. Koolen BB, Valdés ORA, Vogel WV et al (2012) 18F-FDG PET/CT for the assessment of locoregional lymph node involvement and radiotherapy indication in stage II-III breast cancer treated with neoadjuvant chemotherapy. Cancer Res 72:nrP4–02–01

10 Digestive System

10.1 Gastrointestinal Tract

The digestive system consists of the gastrointestinal tract, hepatobiliary system (Fig. 10.1), pancreas, and salivary glands. Nuclear medicine is concerned with the evaluation of normal and abnormal functions of the gastrointestinal tract and hepatobiliary system. To date, the role of nuclear medicine in pancreatic disorders is limited to evaluation of its tumors which is dealt with elsewhere in the book.

10.1.1 The Esophagus

10.1.1.1 Anatomical and Physiological Considerations

The human esophagus is a hollow muscular tube that connects the pharynx to the stomach. The upper third consists of striated muscle, the lower third is composed of smooth muscle, and the middle third is a mixture of the two. Functionally, the esophagus has three components: the upper

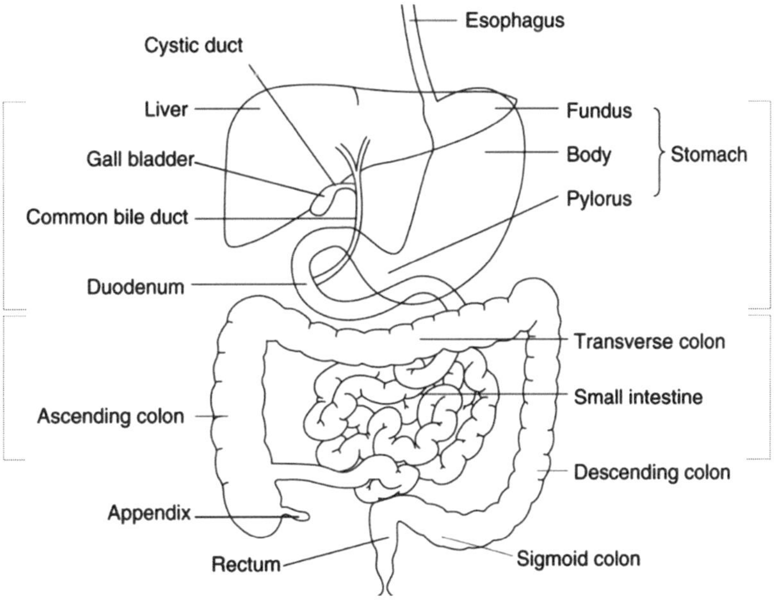

Fig. 10.1 Diagram of the relevant parts of the digestive system

A. H. Elgazzar, *Synopsis of Pathophysiology in Nuclear Medicine*,
https://doi.org/10.1007/978-3-031-20646-7_10

esophageal sphincter (UES), the esophageal body, and the lower esophageal sphincter (LES). These components act to keep the esophagus empty so that swallowed food or liquid is propelled from the pharynx to the stomach and also prevent retrograde movement of gastric or esophageal content.

The upper esophageal sphincter is defined as a high-pressure zone, 2–7 cm long, separating the pharynx from the body of the esophagus. It consists of opening and closing muscles. The esophageal body extends from the UES to the LES and measures 18–24 cm [1]. The lower esophageal sphincter is a high-pressure zone measuring 2–4 cm in length located between the esophageal body and the stomach. At rest, the sphincter is tonically contracted with a normal pressure ranging from 10 to 45 mmHg. On swallowing the LES relaxes and its pressure approaches that of the stomach. The LES remains relaxed until the bolus reaches the end of the esophagus.

Swallowing initiates a progressive series of coordinated propulsive contractions throughout both the striated and the smooth muscle portions of the esophageal body. This form of esophageal motor activity is referred to as primary peristalsis. Intraluminal distention of the esophageal body results in a peristaltic wave at or proximal to the site of distention. This wave is termed secondary peristalsis and serves to clear the esophagus from contents that have not been cleared by primary peristalsis or refluxed gastric contents. Primary and secondary peristaltic waves have similar amplitudes and travel at a velocity of 3–5 cm/s.

Deglutitory inhibition is a unique physiological phenomenon whereby repetitive swallowing inhibits all esophageal body activity while the LES is relaxed. A normal peristaltic contraction will follow the last swallow of such a series and clear the esophagus completely [2].

10.1.2 Esophageal Motility Disorders

Esophageal motility disorders result from sphincter dysfunction or abnormal peristalsis in the body of the esophagus or both. The diagnosis and treatment of motility disorders rest on an understanding of the functional anatomy of the upper esophageal sphincter, esophageal body, and lower esophageal sphincter.

10.1.2.1 Disorders of the UES and Cervical Esophagus

Motor disorders affecting the proximal part of the esophagus result from either neurological abnormalities affecting the extrinsic innervation of the proximal esophagus or skeletal muscle or neuromuscular disorders. These include:

- Neurological diseases.
  - Cerebrovascular accident.
  - Parkinsonism.
  - Amyotrophic lateral sclerosis.
  - Cranial nerve palsy.
- Skeletal muscular disorders.
  - Dermatomyositis.
  - Polymyositis.
  - Muscular dystrophy.
- Cricopharyngeus dysfunction.
- Others.
  - Myasthenia gravis.
  - Amyloidosis.

Because of the difficulty of transferring food bolus from the hypopharynx into the esophageal body across the UES, most patients experience choking or regurgitation of liquids and/or solids. Video fluoroscopy is the best diagnostic modality for diagnosing oropharyngeal dysphagia. Scintigraphy is of limited value.

10.1.2.2 Disorders of Distal Esophagus and LES

Disorders of the distal esophageal body (smooth muscle) and LES can be broadly classified into hypermotility and hypomotility disorders, although overlap is not uncommon.

10.1.2.2.1 Hypermotility Disorders
Hypermotility (spastic) disorders are characterized by high-amplitude, prolonged, or repetitive contractions. They include achalasia and several

Table 10.1 Manometric features of distal esophageal disorders

Disorders	Features
Achalasia	Absent peristalsis in esophageal body
	Incomplete LES relaxation
	Increased LES pressure
Diffuse esophageal spasm	Simultaneous contractions (>10% of wet swallows)
	Intermittent normal peristalsis
	Repetitive contracts
	Prolonged duration of contractions
	High amplitude of contractions
	Incomplete LES relaxation
Nutcracker esophagus	Normal progression of peristalsis
	Mean contractile amplitude 180 mmHg
	Prolonged duration
	Normal LES pressure
Hypertensive LES	Mean LES pressure 45 mmHg
	Normal LES relaxation
	Normal progression of peristalsis

other conditions, particularly the diffuse esophageal spasm (Table 10.1).

Achalasia results from the degeneration of the inhibitory myenteric neurons in the body and the LES region. This leads to a hypertensive LES which relaxes poorly and also causes a peristalsis in the body of the esophagus. Patients usually present with dysphagia to liquids and solids [3, 4].

Several other spastic disorders have been characterized in patients with noncardiac chest pain (Table 10.1). They all share a similar clinical presentation. Diffuse esophageal spasm (DES) is the most severe form. It is less common than achalasia. Some patients with DES progress to achalasia.

10.1.2.2.2 Hypomotility Disorders

A number of systemic conditions are associated with esophageal hypomotility including scleroderma, diabetes mellitus, and amyloidosis. These disorders are characterized by low or absent contractions. The most clinically relevant condition is scleroderma.

Scleroderma (progressive systemic sclerosis) is a multisystem connective tissue disorder that affects the skin and internal organs, especially the vascular system, gastrointestinal tract, lungs, heart, and kidneys. It is more common in women than in men and appears at any age under 50 years. Esophageal involvement occurs in 70–80% of patients. Histopathological findings include smooth muscle atrophy and fibrosis. The end result is impaired muscle contractions in the distal esophagus and incompetence of the LES. Therefore, 50% of patients with scleroderma-associated dysmotility complain of heartburn and/or dysphagia due to gastroesophageal reflux.

10.1.2.2.3 Gastroesophageal Reflux Disease

Gastroesophageal reflux disease (GERD) involves the reflux of chyme from the stomach to the esophagus. The LES may relax spontaneously and transiently 1–2 h after the patient has eaten, allowing gastric contents to regurgitate into the esophagus. The acid is normally neutralized and cleared by peristalsis from the esophagus within 3 min, and the tone of the sphincter is restored. When the reflux does not cause symptoms, it is known as physiological, but in some individuals, it may cause a spectrum of inflammatory responses in the esophagus. GERD is the most prevalent condition originating from the gastrointestinal tract. It is estimated that 20% of the Western adult population suffers from heartburn more than three times a month [5, 6]. It is particularly important in the pediatric age group. GERD is also common among pregnant women, especially during the third trimester. The typical symptom of GERD is heartburn. However, a number of atypical symptoms include noncardiac chest pain, hoarseness, and asthma.

Most children affected with gastroesophageal reflux are between 6 months and 2 years old; they suffer from poor weight gain, vomiting, aspiration, choking, asthmatic episodes, stridor, apnea, and failure to thrive. A small amount of physiological reflux occurs in infants and resolves spontaneously by 8 months of age. Scintigraphy is

Table 10.2 Mechanisms of gastroesophageal reflux disease

Mechanism	Causes
Anti-reflux barrier	Transient LES relaxation
	Incompetent LES
	Slidinghiatushernia
Esophageal clearance	Impaired peristalsis
	Decreased salivary output
Refluxatecomposition	Acid
	Pepsin
	Bile salts
	Pancreatic enzymes
Gastric factors	Delayed gastric emptying
	Acid hypersecretion
	Helicobacter pylori
Defective esophageal mucosal protection	Lack of HCO$_3$ secretion
	Lackofmucussecretion

useful in the diagnosis and is physiological, easily performed, well tolerated by the patient, quantitative, and involves a low radiation dose to the child.

Causes of GERD can be categorized as follows: (a) decreased pressure of LES, (b) transient increase in intra-abdominal pressure, and (c) short intra-abdominal esophageal segment. The mechanisms involved are summarized in Table 10.2. Esophageal body peristalsis plays an important role in clearing refluxed acid in both the upright and the supine positions. Defective primary or secondary peristalsis leads to incomplete clearance of acid. Furthermore, salivary HCO$_3$ usually neutralizes acid that remains in contact with the esophageal mucosa. Thus, impaired salivation may contribute to mucosal injury [7–11].

Delayed gastric emptying is documented in 6–30% of patients with GERD. Theoretically, gastric stasis can contribute to GERD. *Helicobacter pylori* has recently been implicated as having a potential role in the pathogenesis of GERD [12]. *H. pylori* may secrete proinflammatory substances that can damage esophageal mucosa and sensitize vagal afferent nerves or lead to the reduction of LES tone. In contrast, there are data suggesting a protective role for *H. pylori* against GERD [13].

10.2 The Stomach

10.2.1 Anatomical and Physiological Considerations

10.2.1.1 Anatomical Features

The stomach is a storage sac located between the esophagus and duodenum (Fig. 10.1). The proximal stomach consists of the cardia, fundus, and body. The antrum forms the distal stomach and is separated from the duodenum by the pyloric ring. The wall structure of the stomach is similar to that of the rest of the gastrointestinal tract consisting of the mucosa, submucosa, muscularis propria, and serosa. The muscle layer in the antrum is modified to aid the mixing of food. The pyloric ring regulates the emptying of the stomach.

10.2.1.2 Overall Functions

Besides storage, the stomach has a number of exocrine, paracrine, and endocrine functions. The exocrine secretions consist of HCI and pepsin produced by the mucosal parietal cells and chief cells, respectively. These cells are located in the fundus and body of the stomach. Most cells within the lamina propria and submucosa are responsible for the main paracrine function, namely, the release of histamine which in turn stimulates the parietal cells to secrete acid. The antrum secretes the hormone gastrin which enhances gastric emptying and acid secretion. The intrinsic factor (IF) is a glycoprotein secreted by parietal cells. It binds to vitamin B$_{12}$. The IF-B$_{12}$ complex in turn binds to specific receptors on the terminal ileal epithelium. Without IF, B$_{12}$ cannot be absorbed and pernicious anemia develops. Usually, failure to secrete IF results from gastric atrophy which causes the destruction of parietal cells.

10.2.1.3 Gastric Motor Physiology

The motor activity of the stomach serves two main functions: (a) to act as a reservoir for ingested meal and ensure timed delivery of food particles to the duodenum at a rate compatible with optimal digestion and (b) to disperse solids into small particles and to mix them with gastric juice. The functions are accomplished by the coordinated activity of three functionally distinct parts of the stomach: (a) the proximal stomach, including the fundus and proximal body; (b) the distal stomach, including distal body and antrum; and (c) the pylorus, as part of the pyloroduodenal unit.

The proximal stomach has three muscle layers, longitudinal, circular, and oblique. The distal stomach is comprised of two muscle layers: longitudinal and circular. The pyloric sphincter functions, in coordination with the duodenum, as a sieve allowing particles 1 mm or smaller to pass into the duodenum in 2–4-mL aliquots with each gastric peristalsis [3]. Emptying of inert liquids such as 0.9% saline follows first-order kinetics; i.e., the volume of liquid emptied into the duodenum in a given time is a constant fraction of the volume that remains in the stomach (Fig. 10.2) [8, 14]. Emptying of digestible solid particles is characterized by a lag phase and a linear phase

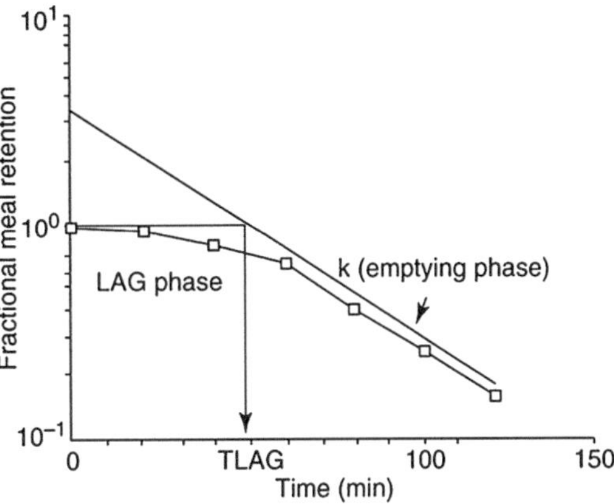

Fig. 10.3 Emptying of digestible solid particles has a lag phase and a linear phase. The curve represents modified power exponential functions (From Siegel et al. [15])

(Fig. 10.3) [15]. However, the components, caloric density, viscosity, osmolarity, and volume of any specific meal will influence gastric emptying rates [16].

10.2.2 Disorders of Gastric Emptying

Conditions that cause abnormal gastric emptying can be divided into two groups: disorders associated with delayed emptying and disorders associated with dumping (Table 10.3). Diabetes is one of the most common causes of delayed gastric emptying in clinical practice. Most afflicted patients have had type I diabetes for more than 10 years, complicated by autonomic and peripheral neuropathy. Delayed emptying of both solids and liquids is attributed to the dysfunction of the proximal and distal stomach, as well as to increased pyloric resistance [17].

Idiopathic gastroparesis is also encountered frequently in patients with bloating, early satiety, and nausea. The exact cause is unclear but it may be related to post-viral gastroenteritis. Delayed gastric emptying is a known and frequent complication of gastric surgery. For instance, vagotomy delays emptying of solids but promotes liquid emptying. Similarly antrectomy can cause rapid emptying of undigested solids and liquids due to the loss of mixing function and loss of pyloric resistance.

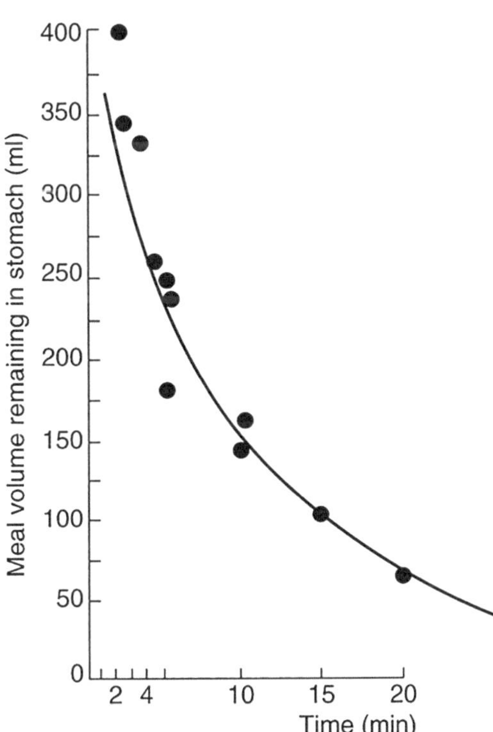

Fig. 10.2 Gastric emptying of 0.9% normal saline follows first-order kinetics (From Brener et al. [14])

Table 10.3 Causes of gastric dysmotility

Condition	Causes
Delayed gastric emptying	Mechanical obstruction
	Gastric outlet obstruction (e.g., tumor and pepticulcer)
	Small intestinal obstruction
	Decreased gastric motility
	Postsurgical gastroparesis (vagotomy, roux-en-Y, fundoplication, etc.)
	Endocrine disorders (DM, hypothyroidism, Addison's disease, hyper- or hypoparathyroidism)
	Drugs (narcotics, anticholinergics, calcium channel blockers)
	Connective tissue diseases (e.g., scleroderma, SLE)
	Muscular disorders (myotonic dystrophy, dermatomyositis)
	Paraneo plastic
	Post-viral
	Neurological disorders (migraine, CVA, Parkinson, dysautonomia)
	Intestinal pseudo-obstruction
	Idiopathic gastroparesis
	Others (anorexia nervosa, uremia, ischemic gastroparesis, pregnancy)
Rapid gastric emptying (dumping)	Duodenal ulcer disease (including ZE syndrome)
	Vagotomy
	Antrectomy
	Idiopathic

10.2.3 Duodenogastric Reflux

Duodenogastric reflux (DGR) has been suggested to occur in normal individuals in both fasting and postprandial periods, although others have suggested that it does not occur physiologically. The amount of refluxed bile in normal subjects is reported to be small and clears rapidly from the stomach. This feature helps separate normal from abnormal subjects in the fasting state.

Pathologically, DGR has been associated with many conditions (Table 10.4), including postgastrectomy/vagotomy, gastric and duodenalulcers, cholecystitis, and gastritis. In some of these conditions, such as duodenal ulcer, duodenal hematoma, and cholecystitis, duodenal irritation is probably the underlying mechanism. Other causes may irritate the duodenal mucosa by the

Table 10.4 Causes of duodenogastric reflux

Causes	
Duodenal ulcer	Gastritis
Acute cholecystitis	Chronic cholecystitis
Enteritis	Pancreatitis
Gastric carcinoma	Surgery
Post-traumatic stress ulceration	Gastric surgery/ vagotomy
Duodenal hematoma	Cholecystectomy
Erosive esophagitis	Gall stone dyspepsia
Physiological/unknown cause	

adjacent pancreatic inflammation. It was also proposed that deficiency of pancreatic secretions can explain DGR since volume, the alkaline pH, and the physiological components of the pancreatic secretions may be important for maintaining the outward flow of gastric contents.

10.3 The Intestines

10.3.1 The Small Intestine

10.3.1.1 Anatomical and Histological Considerations

The small intestine is a hollow muscular cylinder that measures 5–6 min length. It consists of three regions: duodenum, jejunum, and ileum. The intestinal wall is made up of the mucosa, the submucosa, the muscularis, and the serosa. The small intestinal mucosa is fashioned into villi and crypts to increase the surface area and enhance the absorptive function of the small bowel. The mucosa of the villi consists of absorptive columnar epithelial cells (enterocytes) and mucus-secreting goblet cells. Within the crypts the most common cell type is the undifferentiated crypt cell which secretes chloride and water into the lumen. The cryptal so contains pluripotent stem cells. Furthermore, the small bowel harbors the enteroendocrine cells which secrete a number of hormones including secretin, cholecystokinin, gastrin, gastric inhibitory peptide, motilin, glucagon, vasoactive intestinal peptide, somatostatin, and others. These hormones play an important role in gastrointestinal motility. Finally, the intestinal mucosa and laminapropria contain the largest lymphoid organ in man:the gut-associated lymphoid tissue (GALT) [16].

The submucosa consists of connective tissue, lymphocytes, plasma cells, macrophages, mast cells, fibroblasts, eosinophils, nerve fibers, ganglion cells (Meissner's plexus), bloodvessels, and lymphatics.

The muscularis is made of innercircular and outer longitudinal muscle fibers. Between these two layers of smooth muscle lies the myenteric plexus, the network of intramural neurons that is essential for all coordinated and organized motor activity. The extrinsic (autonomic) nerves affect the gastrointestinal motility by means of these enteric nerves.

10.3.1.2 Functional Considerations

Most of the digestion and absorption of nutrients takes place in the small bowel. Moreover, the motor function of the small bowel ensures the mixing of chyme with digestive enzymes and the propulsion of chyme toward the colon. Also, the small bowel plays an important role as a firstline of defense against pathogenic microorganisms and harmful food antigens.

Absorption refers to the process of transporting molecules through the epithelial lining of the gastrointestinal tract into the blood or lymph. Water, electrolytes, monosaccharides, amino acids, small peptides, glycerol, fatty acids, vitamins, and minerals are all absorbed via a number of mechanisms including passive diffusion, facilitated diffusion, active transport, and endocytosis. Although absorption takes place along the entire length of the small intestine, the mucosa incertain regions selectively absorbs specific molecules. For instance, iron is primarily absorbed in the duodenum and proximal jejunum, whereas the terminal ileal mucosa has specific receptors for binding and absorbing vitamin B_{12} and bile salts.

Under physiological conditions the small bowel exhibits two main motor patterns. During the fed state, and as a result of contact with nutrients, a number of neuronal and hormonal signals are elicited including afferent vagal stimulation and the release of cholecystokinin which mediate *segmentation* and *peristalsis*. *Segmentation* is the most frequent movement in the small bowel and is characterized by closely spaced contractions of the circular muscle layer. These contractions divide the small intestine into short neighboring segments. Segmentation helps mix chyme with digestive enzymes. *Peristalsis*, on the other hand, is the progressive contraction of successive sections of circular smooth muscle resulting in the propulsion of chyme toward the colon. Furthermore, during the fed state the small intestine especially the duodenum exerts negative feedback control on gastric emptying via neural and hormonal mechanisms (secretin, cholecystokinin, and gastric inhibitory peptide).

10.3.1.3 Small Intestinal Dysmotility

Motor disorders of the small bowel can lead to symptoms and signs of "functional" as opposed to mechanical small bowel obstruction. Patients frequently complain of abdominal distension, bloating, and abdominal pain, and when small intestinal dysmotility is associated with gastroparesis, nausea and vomiting may be prominent. Small intestinal dysmotility may be acute or chronic. Acute dysmotility is commonly seen following abdominal surgery, severe septicemia, or electrolyte disturbances such as hypokalemia. Chronic dysmotility is termed pseudo-obstruction (Table 10.5).

10.3.1.4 Malabsorption

Malabsorption syndrome is analteration in the ability of the GI tract, usually the small intestine, to absorb one or more nutrients adequately from diet into the bloodstream. These may include fats, proteins, carbohydrates, vitamins, or others. This may result from acquired or congenital defects.

Common causes of malabsorption syndrome include inflammatory bowel disease, tropical sprue, Whipple'sdisease, lactase deficiency, and parasitic diseases. Other causes are past intestinal surgeries, bacterial over growth, gluten enteropathy (non-tropical sprue), AIDS, radiation to the abdomen, diabetes, lymphoma, or motility disor-

Table 10.5 Motor disorders of the small intestine

Cause	Mechanism	Outcome
Acute illness	Altered neuro transmission	Adynamic ileus
Pregnancy	Decreased smooth muscle contraction (progesterone)	Slow transit
Diabetes mellitus	Autonomic dysfunction	Slow or rapid transit
Scleroderma	Smooth muscle fibrosis	Weak contractions
	Neuronal loss in gut wall	Slow transit
Primary pseudo-obstruction	Neuronal loss, plexus degeneration	Weak contractions
		Abnormal MMC
		Slow transit
Myopathies	Myocyte and mitochondrial abnormalities	Weak segmentation and peristalsis

ders. In addition to small bowel disease, malabsorption can occur in those who have had portions of their stomachs removed surgically. The pancreas produces enzymes that help to digest food, so if a condition exists where enzymes are not being produced, it can result in maldigestion or malabsorption. This could include chronic alcoholic pancreatitis, trauma, cystic fibrosis, tumors, or postsurgical states. The diagnosis of malabsorption syndrome and identification of the underlying cause can require extensive laboratory diagnostic testing. Stool collections and cultures are useful as well as certain breath and hormone tests. Scintigraphic imaging and quantitation is also used for some forms.

10.3.1.4.1 Protein-Losing Enteropathy

Protein-losing enteropathy is a condition in which excess protein loss into the gastrointestinal lumen is severe enough to produce hypoproteinemia. It occurs with many of the previously listed conditions causing malabsorption. Furthermore, diseases such as constrictive pericarditis, congestive heart failure, intestinal lymphangiectasia, nephrotic syndrome, and systemic lupusery the matosus may also cause protein loss from the gastrointestinal tract without any observable

mucosal lesions in the bowel. The mechanism of the loss of plasma protein into the gastrointestinal tract in these diseases is not fully understood [18].

10.3.1.4.2 Vitamin B_{12} Malabsorption

Vitamin B_{12} deficiency due to pure dietary inadequacy of this vitamin is very rare and occurs mainly in strict vegetarians. More often gastrointestinal disorders, atrophic gastritis, pernicious anemia, congenital lack or abnormality of gastric IF, and total or partial gastrectomy cause malabsorption and consequent deficiency of this vitamin. Diseases involving the distal ileum such as Crohn's disease, intestinal stagnant loop syndrome, and rarely congenital selective ileal malabsorption with proteinuria (Imerslund-Grasbeck syndrome) may also result in malabsorption of vitamin B_{12}.

10.4   The Colon

10.4.1 Anatomical and Functional Considerations

The colon is a tubular structure that extends from the ileocecal valve to the anal verge (Fig. 10.1). It measures approximately 1–5 m and consists of the cecum, ascending transverse, descending, sigmoid colon, and rectum. Like the small intestine, the colonic wall consists of the mucosal submucosa, muscularis, and serosa. However, the colonic mucosa lacks villi. Also, unlike the small intestine, the external longitudinal muscular layer is gathered into three flat longitudinal ribbons of smooth muscle called teniae coli. The continuous contractions of teniae coli cause sacculations on the wall termed austrations. The primary function of the colon is to absorb water and electrolytes from its contents and to pack feces until defecation. The motility of the colon is geared toward this function. As stated above, throughout the colon, localized segmental contractions take place and result in mixing chyme. In the cecum and ascending colon, retrograde (antipropulsive) contractions also occur.

The net effect of these motility patterns is to slow transit and facilitate the absorption of water and electrolytes. Periodically, massive contractions start in the proximal colon to propel fecal material toward the sigmoid colon where it is stored. One to three times a day, mass contractions sweep the stool toward the rectum. Distension of the rectum by feces initiates the defecation reflex which is mediated by the pelvic nerves and integrated at the level of the sacral spinal cord.

10.4.2 Relevant Colon Diseases

10.4.2.1 Inflammatory Bowel Disease

Inflammatory bowel disease (IBD) refers to two disorders: Crohn's disease (CD) and ulcerative colitis (UC). Both conditions are characterized by chronic relapsing intestinal inflammation. UC affects the colon only, and the inflammation is limited to the mucosa and submucosa in most cases. CD can affect the entire gastrointestinal tract from mouth to anus. The inflammation inCD is granulomatous and transmural. Besides inflammation of the gut, IBD is associated with a number of systemic manifestations includinganterior uveitis, axial, and peripheral arthropathy, primary sclerosing cholangitis, erythema nodosum, and pyoderma gangrenosum.The etiology of IBD is unknown. However, many of the immunological and molecular mechanisms that mediate inflammation have been elucidated in recent years. Genetic predisposition, mucosal immune dysregulation, and environmental agents seem to play a role (Table 10.6). In genetically predisposed individuals, environmental factors can participate in the disease by inducing a broad immunological response characterized by an imbalance between anti-inflammatory mediators. CD consists of segmental involvement by an on specific granulomatous inflammatory process involving all layers of the bowel with skip areas. The disease involves the small bowel in addition to the colon, and rectal sparing is typical. Less commonly it involves the mouth, tongue, esophagus, stomach, and duodenum.

Table 10.6 Pathogenesis of inflammatory bowel disease

Genetic predisposition
 Family clustering
 NOD2 gene variants
 Gene loci on chromosomes 2,3,12

Environmental factors
 Family clustering
 NOD2 gene variants
 Intestinal commensals

Immunological dysregulation
 Pro-inflammatory mediators
 Anti-inflammatory mediators

The primary pathophysiological change of UC is inflammation of the mucosa and the submucosa and formation of crypt abscesses and mucosal ulceration with skip areas. The small intestine is essentially not involved [19, 20].

10.4.2.2 Acute Appendicitis

The appendix is a diverticulum of an average of 10 cm in adults arising from the posteromedial wall of the cecum. This fact accounts for its variable positions (retrocecal, subcecal, retroileal, pre-ileal, or pelvic) and behind much of the diversity in clinical presentations among patients with acute appendicitis.

The pathophysiology of appendicitis begins with obstruction of the narrow appendiceal lumen by causes, including fecaliths, lymphoid hyperplasia (related to viral illnesses such as upper respiratory infections, mononucleosis, or gastroenteritis), gastrointestinal parasites, foreign bodies, and Crohn's disease. Continued secretion of mucus results in elevated intraluminal pressure, leading to tissue ischemia, overgrowth of bacteria, transmural inflammation, appendiceal infarction, and possible perforation. Inflammation may subsequently extend into the parietal peritoneum and adjacent structures causing abdominal abscesses.

Acute appendicitis is the most common reason for emergency abdominal surgery and must be differentiated from other causes of abdominal pain. The overall diagnostic accuracy achieved by medical history, physical examination, and laboratory tests have been approximately 80% as the presentation may be atypical. In atypical cases,ultrasonography and computed tomography (CT) may help lower the rate of unnecessary surgeries. The accuracy rates for ultrasonography range from 71 to 97% and the modality is highly operator dependent and difficult in patients with a large body habitus. The accuracy rate of CT scanning is between 93 and 98%. However, there is controversy regarding the use of contrast media.

The appendix is a diverticulum of an average of 10 cm in adults arising from the posteromedial wall of the cecum. This fact accounts for its variable positions (retrocecal, subcecal, retroileal, pre-ileal, or pelvic) and behind much of the diversity in clinical presentations among patients with acute appendicitis.

The pathophysiology of appendicitis begins with obstruction of the narrow appendiceal lumen by causes, including fecaliths, lymphoid hyperplasia (related to viral illnesses such as upper respiratory infections, mononucleosis, or gastroenteritis), gastrointestinal parasites, foreign bodies, and Crohn's disease. Continued secretion of mucus results in elevated intraluminal pressure, leading to tissue ischemia, overgrowth of bacteria, transmural inflammation, appendiceal infarction, and possible perforation. Inflammation may subsequently extend into the parietal peritoneum and adjacent structures causing abdominal abscesses.

Acute appendicitis is the most common reason for emergency abdominal surgery and must be differentiated from other causes of abdominal pain. The overall diagnostic accuracy achieved by medical history, physical examination, and laboratory tests has been approximately 80% as the presentation may be atypical. In atypical cases, ultrasonography and computed tomography (CT) may help lower the rate of unnecessary surgeries. The accuracy rates for ultrasonography range from 71 to 97% and the modality is highly operator dependent and difficult in patients with a large body habitus. The accuracy rate of CT scanning is between 93 and 98%. However, there is controversy regarding the use of contrast media [21].

10.4.2.3 Colorectal Cancer

The incidence of colorectal cancer is highest in developed countries, such as the United States and Japan, and lowest in developing countries in Africa and Asia. It is the third most common type of cancer in both men and women in the United States. Pathologically most (over 95%) of colorectal cancers are adenocarcinomas. Surgery, chemotherapy, radiation therapy, and immunotherapy are the lines of treatment. Nuclear medicine has an important role in the follow-up to detect recurrence (see Chap. 12). FDG-PET has an important role as it is more sensitive than computed tomography for the detection of metastatic or recurrent colorectal cancer (Fig. 10.4) and may improve clinical management in more than 25% of cases [22]. It is of particular importance to differentiate post-therapy fibrosis and inflammation from a viable tumor in the presacral region.

10.4.2.4 Gastrointestinal Bleeding

The localization of the specific bleeding site in patients presenting with acute GI bleeding remains a serious clinical problem. Acute gastrointestinal bleeding (GIB) can be divided into bleeding in the upper (proximal to the ligament of Treitz) or lower tract. If acute upper GIB is a possibility, lavage with a nasogastric tube should identify acute or subacute bleeding. Endoscopy will localize 80–97% of cases of acute upper bleeding; of this 75% will resolve spontaneously or with conservative medical therapy and 10% will require surgery. Because of the length and tortuosity of the colon and contamination of fecal matter and blood, endoscopy is not that successful in lower GIB cases. Peptic ulcers are the most common cause of upper GIB; other causes include gastritis, esophageal varices, Mallory-Weiss tear, esophagitis with or without hiatal hernia, and carcinoma [23]. The three leading causes of lower GIB are diverticular disease, angiodysplasia, and colorectal cancer. Other causes include inflammatory bowel disease, ischemic colitis, infectious colitis, and anorectal disease

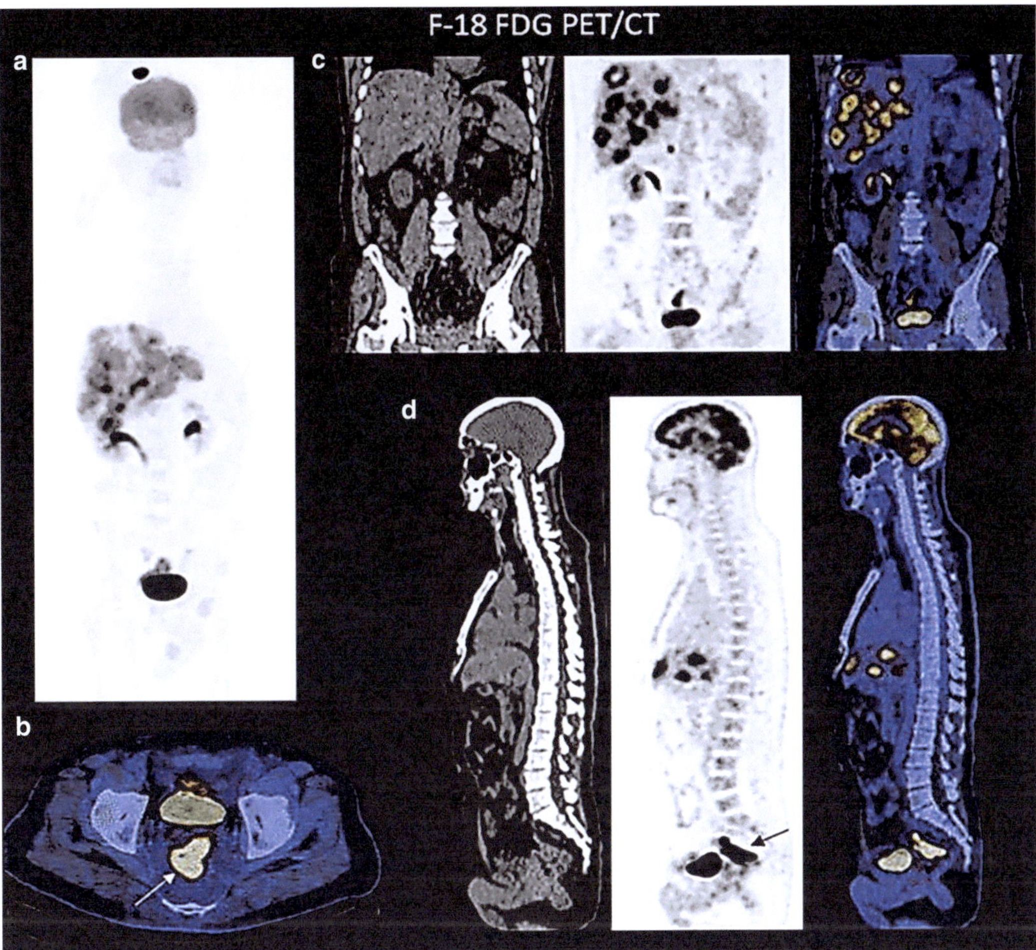

Fig. 10.4 F-18 FDG-PET whole body MIP (**a**), selected transaxial PET/CT fusion image of the lower pelvis (**b**), and selected sagittal (**c**), and coronal (**d**) CT, PET, and PET/CT fusion images (**d**) of a 52-year-old male recently diagnosed with rectal cancer, FDG-PET for initial staging. FDG-PET/CT images demonstrate a hypermetabolic primary rectal tumor (SUVmax, 9.8) (arrows) with multifocal extensive metastatic disease involving both lobes of the liver (SUVmax, 8.6). There are also hypermetabolic lymph nodes in retrocaval, paraortic, and right internal iliac regions, consistent with metastatic disease

(Table 10.7). This bleeding usually resolves spontaneously in 80% of cases and rebleeds in 25%. Angiodysplasias account for 20% of significantly lower GIB and tend to rebleed. Meckel's diverticulum is a vestige of the omphalomesenteric duct that is present in about 2% of the population with two-thirds younger than 2 years. It is an outpouch usually found on the antimesenteric border of the ileum, 50–80 cm proximal to the ileocecal valve. Ectopic gastric mucosa is present in about 30% of cases. Nearly, all diverticula responsible for rectal bleeding contain ectopic gastric mucosa. Bleeding, which is usually massive and painless may result in from ileal mucosal ulceration due to acid secretion. Patients with lower GIB should be stabilized and supported while diagnostic studies are performed. Scintigraphy has emerged as the imaging modality of first choice for localizing bleeding sites in the lower gastrointestinal tract. It is more sensitive to slow or intermittent bleeding, which is a common occurrence.

Table 10.7 Causes of GI bleeding[a]

Upper gastrointestinal bleeding
Esophageal, gastric, and duodenal ulcers
Mallory-Weiss tears
Esophagitis, gastritis, duodenitis, pancreatitis
Neoplasms
Vascular malformations
Varices
Lower gastrointestinal bleeding
Post-polypectomy bleeding
Ischemic colitis
Colorectal polyps/neoplasms
Inflammatory bowel disease
Infectious colitis
Meckel's diverticulum
Neoplasia
NSAID ulcers
Dieulafoy's lesion
Anorectal conditions **such as** rectal varices **and radiation** proctitis

[a][23–26]

10.5 Salivary Gland

10.5.1 Anatomic and Physiologic Considerations

The major salivary glands include the parotid and the submandibular glands. The parotid gland is located behind the mandible and consists of a superficial and a deep part. The main parotid duct (Stensen's duct) runs anteriorly to pierce the buccinator muscle, opening on a papilla on the buccal mucosa opposite the second upper molar tooth. The submandibular gland is smaller than the parotid and lies in the submaxillary triangle just below the mandible. The main duct (Wharton's duct) passes forward and medially to open on a papilla lateral to the frenulum at the base of the tongue. The sublingual glands are situated anteriorly on the floor of the mouth above the mylohyoid muscle, and each gland opens into the oral cavity through several small ducts.

Salivary glands secrete saliva which is a clear, viscous, and watery fluid that contains two major types of protein secretions, a serous secretion containing the digestive enzyme ptyalin and a mucus secretion containing the lubricating aid mucin. Saliva also contains large amounts of potassium and bicarbonate ions and to a lesser extent sodium and chloride ions as well as several antimicrobial constituents, including thiocyanate, lysozyme, immunoglobulins, lactoferrin, and transferrin. Accordingly, saliva provides many several functions including antimicrobial activity, mechanical cleansing action, control of pH, removal of food debris from the oral cavity, lubrication of the oral cavity, remineralization, and maintaining the integrity of the oral mucosa.

10.5.2 Pathophysiology of Relevant Disorders

Nuclear medicine-relevant conditions affecting salivary glands are numerous. These include inflammatory, neoplastic, and mechanical disorders affecting the parenchyma and duct system. Xerostomia is defined as dry mouth resulting from reduced or absent saliva flow. Xerostomia may result from such conditions as mumps, Sjögren's syndrome, sarcoidosis, radiation-induced atrophy, and drug sensitivity.

Inflammation of salivary glands usually presents as diffuse enlargement of the glands, unilateral or bilateral. Bilateral enlargement is caused by inflammation (mumps, Sjögren's syndrome), granulomatous disease (sarcoidosis), or diffuse neoplastic involvement (leukemia and lymphoma). The vast majority of salivary neoplasms occur in the parotid gland. Over two-thirds represent benign mixed or pleomorphic adenomas. Warthin's tumor is another benign tumor that can be bilateral. The more common malignant tumors include mucoepidermoid carcinoma, adenocarcinoma, and squamous cell carcinoma. Plain films are of limited use for evaluating these tumors. Sialography in conjunction with CT is the preferred technique [27]. The CT sialogram demonstrates the location of the tumor within the gland and also defines any involvement of the deep structures of the neck.

The duct system of the parotid and the submandibular glands can be demonstrated by sialography, and the technique is particularly valuable in the diagnosis of diseases that affect the duct system such as calculus, stricture, and sialectasia.

10.5.3 Ascites

Ascites is the accumulation of excess fluid within the peritoneal cavity. It is most frequently encountered in patients with cirrhosis and other forms of severe liver disease, but a number of other disorders may lead to either transudative or exudative ascites. Serous effusion into the peritoneum occurs in cases of general edema of both the cardiac and renal type and is sometimes abundant; some fluid may accumulate also in severe anemias and wasting disease. The most severe ascites, however, results from portal obstruction, the most common cause being cirrhosis of the liver. Hepatic vein occlusion (Budd-Chiari syndrome) is also accompanied by gross ascites.

The pathogenesis of ascites is complex, and multiple factors have been postulated to be involved. In cirrhosis the major vascular obstruction is post-sinusoidal, and the flow of lymph is considerably augmented. The lymphatic vessels, including the thoracic duct, are dilated but nevertheless appear inadequate to deal with the increased volume of lymph. Fluid oozes from the liver surface; this is called the weeping liver [28].

Another factor in the pathogenesis of ascites is hypoalbuminemia, since if this is combined experimentally with portal vein obstruction, ascites develops. It has been postulated that the major factor in the formation of ascites is retention of salt and water by the kidney, followed by an outflow of fluid into the peritoneal cavity. Another factor to consider in the pathogenesis of ascites is the increased capillary pressure in the splanchnic area secondary to portal hypertension. This leads to the formation of transudate.

Surgical management of ascites includes various shunt operations. Most are performed as therapy for esophageal bleeding. Which shunt operation is most effective in relieving ascites has not been established; in fact, ascites is reduced after any type of portosystemic shunt as a consequence of decreased portal flow and decreased intrahepatic congestion. Among the most commonly performed shunts, splenorenal and splenocaval shunts, and their variants have proven effective in relieving ascites. Transjugular intrahepatic portosystemic shunt (TIPS) has been used to reduce portal hypertension in patients with bleeding esophageal varices. TIPS has been shown to relieve intractable ascites as well.

The peritoneovenous shunt is a pressure-activated shunt devised by LeVeen. One line of this shunt lies free in the peritoneal cavity, and the venous opening of the efferent inserts into the SVC near its entrance into the right atrium. Flow into the shunt is maintained if there is a 3–5 cm H_2O pressure gradient between the valve and its venous end. Radionuclide studies using Tc-99m-macroaggregated albumin (MAA) injected intraperitoneally are used to evaluate the patency of the shunts [29].

10.6   Gastrointestinal Scintigraphy

10.6.1 Radionuclide Esophageal Transit Time Study

This study has proven useful and sensitive in detecting esophageal disorders and their involvement in certain systemic disorders.

The patient should fast for 4–6 h. A dose of 250–500 μCi Tc-99m-SC in 10 mL of water is taken through a straw. The multiple-swallow technique is preferred over the single-swallow test because of the considerable intraindividual variations in esophageal emptying among normal subjects and patients. It is preferable to do the imaging with the subject in the supine position to eliminate the effect of gravity; images of 1 s each are acquired to characterize the esophageal transit. Delayed images at 10 min may be helpful in patients with significant stasis of radioactivity in the esophagus. A time–activity curve can be generated; the esophageal transit time is the time interval between the peak activity of the proximal esophageal curve and the peak activity of the distal esophageal curve.

The normal transit time is 15 s, with a distinct peak in each third of the esophagus. A slowing of bolus progression can be noted at the mid-esophagus because of compression by the tracheal bifurcation and aortic arch. Prolonged transit time might be found in several esophageal and systemic disorders such as achalasia, progressive systemic sclerosis, diffuse esophageal spasm, nonspecific motor disorders, nutcracker esophagus, Zenker's diverticulum (an outpouch above the UES that is acquired), esophageal tumors, and esophageal stricture.

10.6.2 Gastroesophageal Reflux Study

The patient should fast for 4 h. The dose is 0.5–1 mCi Tc-99m-SC in 300 mL of acidic orange juice. Imaging is performed with the subject in a supine position at a rate of 1 frame/10 s for 60 min. All frames should be reviewed with contrast enhancement. GER is seen as distinct spikes of activity in the esophagus (Fig. 10.5). The episodes of reflux are graded as high or low level, by duration (less or more than 10 s), and by their temporal relationship to meal ingestion. The salivagram can often reveal aspiration when a GER study is negative.

This scintigraphic study has an 89% correlation with the acid reflux test. The evidence of pulmonary aspiration is valuable in the pediatric age group, though it is seen in up to 25% of cases of aspiration with reflux.

10.6.3 Gastric Emptying Study

The patient should avoid smoking, since it affects emptying, and should fast overnight. The dose is 0.5–1.0 mCi Tc-99 m-SC mixed with egg white or liver pâté as a solid meal. Dynamic images can be taken for 60 min or longer (Figs. 10.6 and 10.7), and if necessary, static delayed images are taken every 15 min until at least 50% of the stomach activity (content) has gone into the bowel. Normally, the stomach should empty 50% of the activity measured at time zero, by 90 min. The lag phase corresponds to maximal filling of the distal stomach when trituration has been completed and the suspended solid particles begin to empty. Lag-phase abnormality may be the earliest finding in diabetic gastroparesis and can be corrected by the drugs used to treat this condition [16].

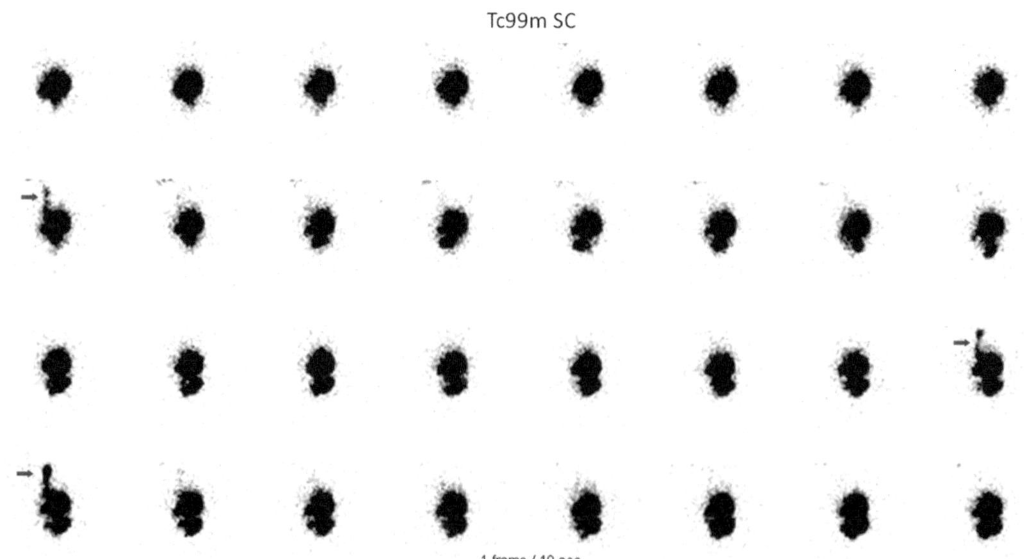

Fig. 10.5 A gastroesophageal reflux study obtained using ⁹⁹ᵐTc-sulfur colloid for a 2-year-old boy demonstrates reflux in three frames (*arrows*)

An ingestible, telemetric device (the wireless motility capsule: WMC) is now commercially available, enabling the measurement of both regional and total GI transit times in a minimally invasive manner without radiationans is an alternative to scintigraphy. The wireless motility capsule measures pH, pressure, and temperature throughout the GI tract, and is used also to calculate gastric emptying [30].

10.6.4 Duodenogastric Reflux Study

The way of detecting duodenogastric reflux is to administer a radiopharmaceutical that can go to the duodenum without passing through the stomach. This can be achieved by using hepatobiliary radiopharmaceuticals in conjunction with stimulation of the gallbladder to empty by a fatty meal. This helps to increase the activity in the duodenum and thus to detect the reflux. The usual protocol is to acquire dynamically for 60 min following i.v. administration of Tc-99 m-IDA derivative (Fig. 10.8). The fatty meal is then ingested by the patient and another dynamic study is obtained for 30 min.

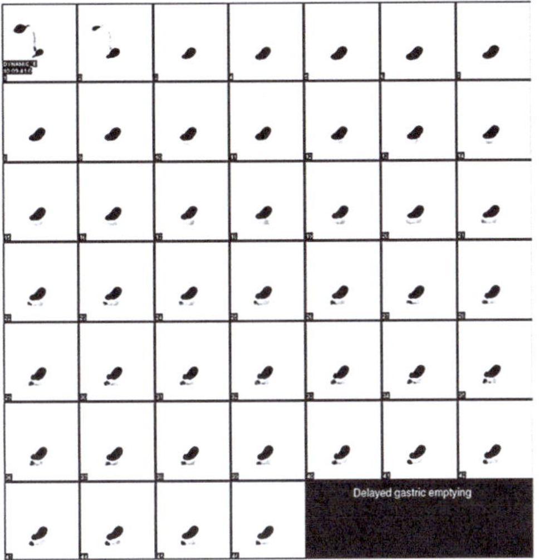

Fig. 10.6 Tc99m sulfur colloid abnormal gastric emptying study. Stomach activity is not adequately decreasing indicating delayed emptying. The half clearance time was more than 160 minutes. Compare with the normal pattern in Fig 10.7

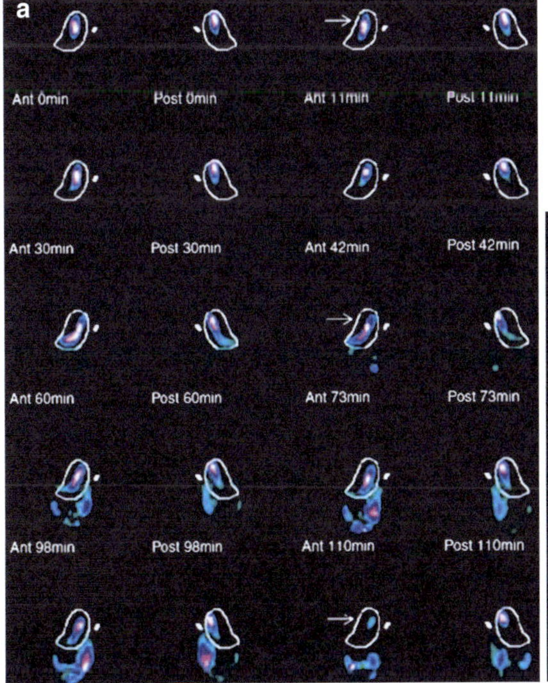

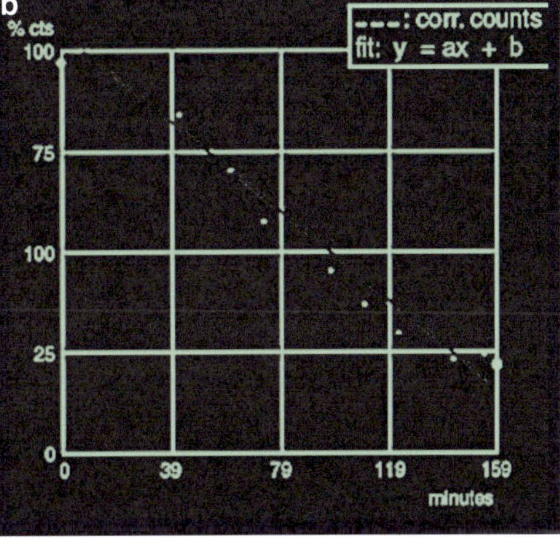

Fig. 10.7 Normal gastric emptying study with progressive clearance of stomach activity as seen visually (**a**) and on time activity curve (**b**)

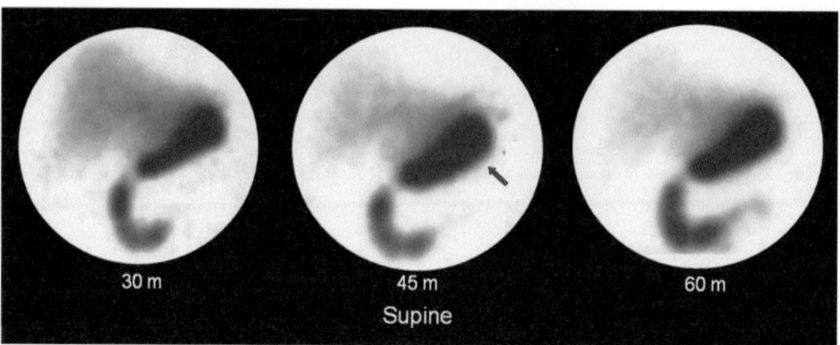

Fig. 10.8 Representative images of a hepatobiliary study of a 32-year-old male patient suspected of having acute cholecystitis. In addition to the nonvisualized gallbladder by 60 min shown in the images presented, significant duodeno-gastric reflux is seen (*arrow*)

10.6.5 Gastrointestinal Bleeding Localization Study

This radionuclide study can detect a bleeding rate as low as 0.1 mL/min. The two common indications for a radionuclide bleeding scan are:

1. Suspected acute ongoing or intermittent lower GIB of unknown localization with nondiagnostic endoscopy.
2. Follow-up of known bleeding to assess treatment effectiveness.

A radionuclide bleeding scan plays only a very small role in the evaluation of upper GIB because of the high accuracy of endoscopy and because of potential interference from radiotracer activity normally excreted by the gastric mucosa. All patients with prior aortic graft surgery and GIB should be considered to have an aortoenteric fistula until proven otherwise.

Two radiopharmaceuticals are available for the study of lower GIB: Tc-99m-labeled RBCs and Tc-99m-sulfur colloid. The technique of Tc-99m-labeled RBCs is preferred (Fig. 10.9). However, for acute or continuous bleeding, a Tc-99 m-SC study may be used, and in this case, images are taken for 30 min, which can detect blood loss of 0.1 mL/min. If this is negative or blood loss is known to be intermittent, a labeled RBC study is used.

10.6.6 Meckel's Diverticulum Study

Scintigraphy is performed using Tc-99m-pertechnetate, since it is taken up by the gastric mucosa contained in Meckel's diverticulum (Fig. 10.10). The radiotracer accumulates in and is excreted from the mucus-secreting cells in the ectopic gastric mucosa regardless of the presence of parietal cells.

The patient should be fasting for 4–6 h to reduce gastric secretion passing through the bowel. With Tc-99m-pertechnetate, Meckel's diverticulum appears at the same time as the stomach and the activity increases in intensity with the stomach; it may change in position during the study and may empty its contents into the bowel. Pharmacological intervention improves the sensitivity of the study. Cimetidine enhances gastric uptake and blocks pertechnetate release from the mucosa. Glucagon is given i.v. 10 min after pertechnetate to inhibit peristalsis and delay emptying of gastric contents into the small bowel.

The sensitivity of Tc-99m-pertechnetate is overall more than 85%, but it drops after adolescence because patients asymptomatic throughout childhood are less likely to have ectopic gastric mucosa. In a recent study on children under 18 years of age, the sensitivity, specificity, PPV, NPV, and accuracy values were 84%, 97%, 90%, 95%, and 94%, respectively [31].

10.6.7 Imaging of Inflammatory Bowel Disease

Scintigraphy with radiolabeled leukocytes (Fig. 10.9) is able to provide a complete survey of the whole intestinal tract, both the small and large bowel, and detects septic complications success-

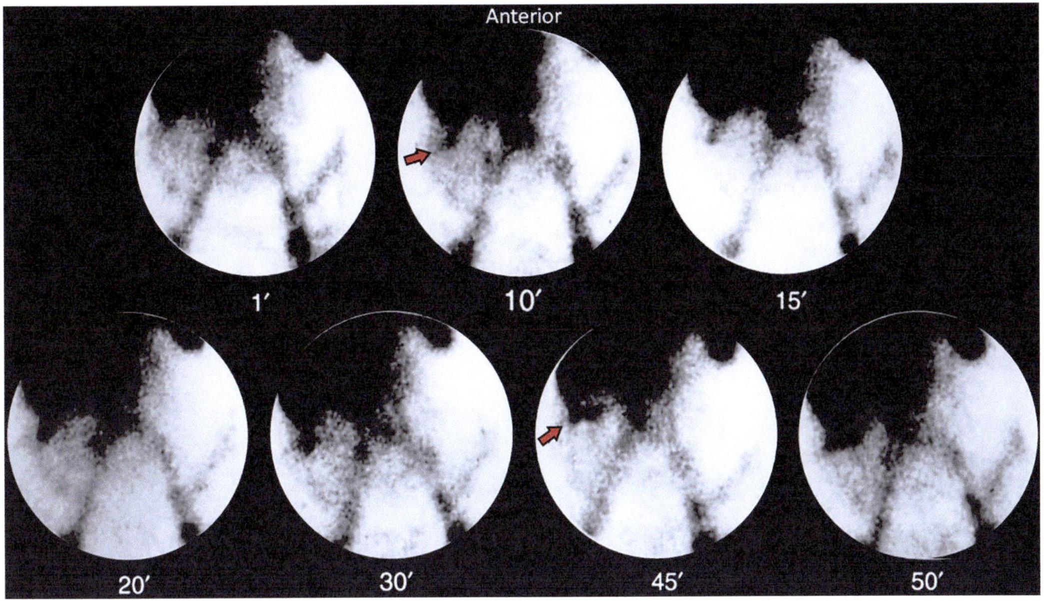

Fig. 10.9 99m-Tc-labeled RBC study for localization of gastrointestinal bleeding showing a focus of extravasated activity in the right hepatic flexure, which progressed later during the study (*arrows*)

fully with negligible risk. Radionuclide procedures are useful in establishing or ruling out IBD in patients with intestinal complaints, in assessing disease severity, and in the evaluation of extraintestinal septic complications [32]. Radiolabeled leukocytes studies offer an accepted radionuclide method for imaging inflammation. Because of the many advantages of technetium-99m (99mTc) over indium-111 (111In), 99mTc-HMPAO-leukocyte scintigraphy is preferred for the investigation of IBD. The 99mTc-HMPAO-leukocyte scintigraphy technique is highly accurate within the first few hours postinjection. It can reliably assess disease activity, but normal scintigraphy does not exclude mild inflammation [33]. Recently, the immunoscintigraphy with 99mTc-antigranulocyte antibodies has been carried out; however, 99mTc-HMPAO is the first-choice agent with SPECT/CT preferred (Fig. 10.11). FDG-PET/CT is very helpful in localization of activity. It is an excellent method for the noninvasive quantification of bowel inflammation and for assessing advancement of the disease [34]. For more details, please refer to Chap. 4.

Scintigraphy is needed in some conditions that cannot be evaluated by morphologic modali-

ties particularly functional conditions such as xerostomia.

Salivary gland scintigraphy is carried out after 5–15 mCi (185–550 MBq) of Tc-99m-pertechnetate is injected into the patient intravenously. Dynamic images are obtained as 1-min frames for 15–20 min. The patient is asked to drink two glasses of water before the study, and a sialagogue (20 mL lemon juice) is given at 10 min to stimulate salivation. The images are obtained for the anterior face and neck in the sitting position, using a low-energy, high-resolution collimator. Extra images for right and left laterals are obtained for 2 min each to localize the activity. Regions of interest (ROI) are drawn and a graph is plotted to assess the function of the salivary glands.

Findings on a normal scan are a stepwise rising curve of activity with an abrupt drop after the sialagogue and a subsequent rise again. In Sjögren's syndrome, there will be a decreased accumulation of radiotracer compared with the thyroid gland and delayed clearance. In Warthin's tumor (adenolymphoma), there is an intense increase in the focal area of activity because it mimics thyroid tissue in pertechnetate uptake [35–37].

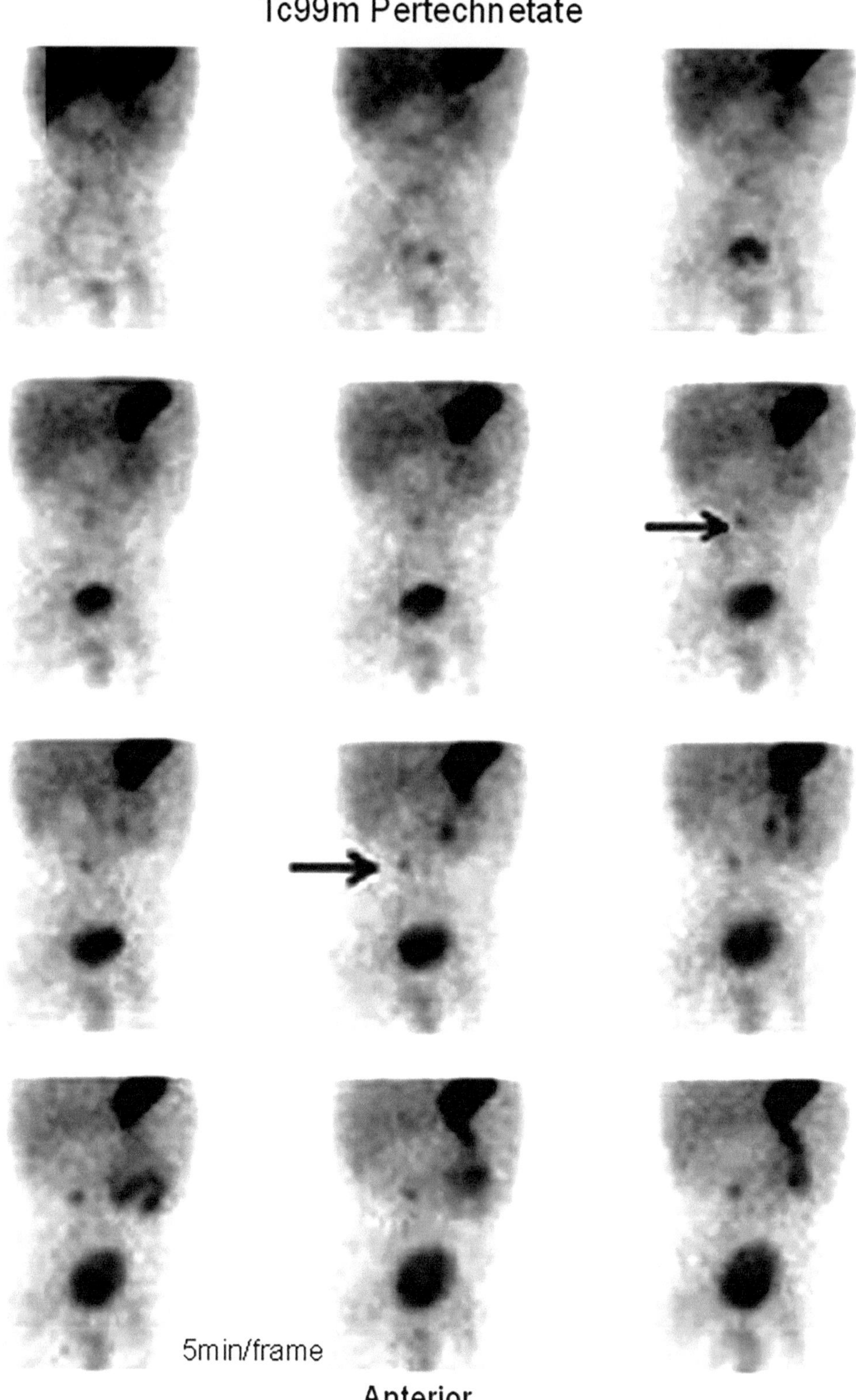

Fig. 10.10 Positive study for Meckel's diverticulum (*arrows*)

Fig. 10.11 In-111 WBC study of a patient with inflammatory bowel disease. On 4-h In-111 WBC images (**a**), there is mild diffuse labeled WBC accumulation in the descending and sigmoid colon (arrow). On 24-h images (**b**), the accumulation in the upper part of the descending colon and splenic flexure are more intense (arrow). SPECT/CT (**c**) more clearly shows the uptake in the colon's splenic flexure (arrow) since there is a superimposition of the spleen and splenic flexure on planar images

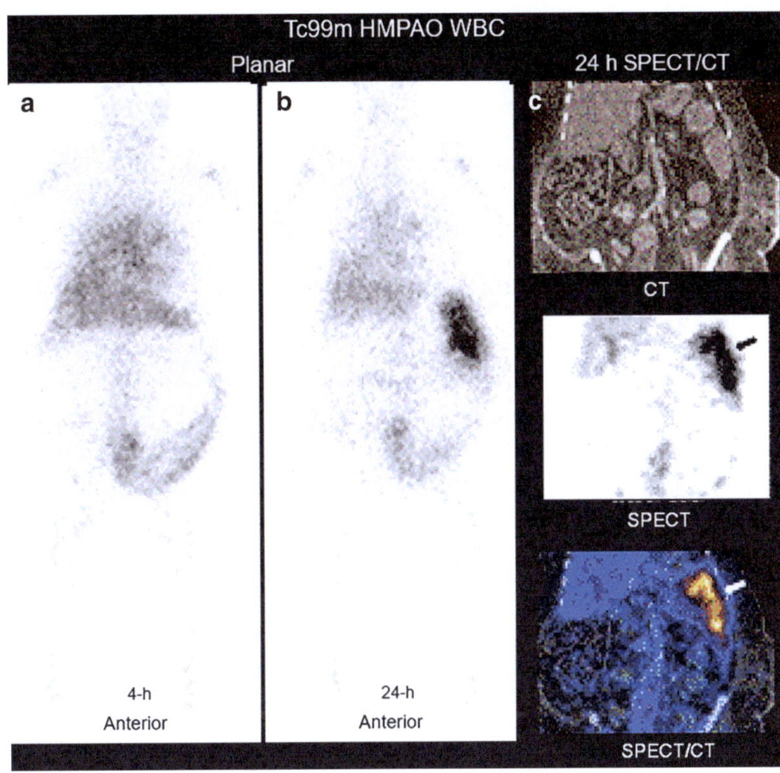

10.6.8 Imaging of Appendicitis

Radioisotope imaging using labeled white blood cells and more recently antigranulocyte antibody technetium (^{99m}Tc) fanolesomab (NeutroSpec) has been used for appendicitis imaging patients with equivocal signs and symptoms of appendicitis. Localized uptake of tracer in the RLQ suggests appendiceal inflammation. Tc-99m-HMPAO-labeled leukocyte showed a sensitivity of 90–98% and specificity of 92–96% [38, 39]. Recent reports suggest a possible role of FDG-PET/CT to diagnose appendicitis [40].

10.6.9 Non-imaging Procedures

10.6.9.1 Carbon-14 Breath Tests

This simple carbon-14 breath test has been utilized increasingly in gastrointestinal practice. The test is based on detection and quantitation of radioactive carbon dioxide originating in the stomach or small intestines and exhaled through the respiratory system after being absorbed into the bloodstream. The test is useful in the diagnosis of several disease processes, particularly *Helicobacter pylori* infections, lactose intolerance, and malabsorption due to bacterial deconjugation of bile acids.

10.6.9.1.1 Helicobacter Pylori Infections

Helicobacter pylori has been known for many years and was previously called *Campylobacter pylori* or *Campylobacter pyloridis*. It is a small, curved, Gram-negative rod found in the stomach and duodenum of many individuals. The prevalence correlates best with socioeconomic status. In the United States, the overall probability of infection was reported as 20–30%. Among African-Americans, the probability is about 50% and approximately 60% of immigrants such as Latinos are affected. The infection approaches 90% in the third-world countries, where it occurs in 10% of children between the age of 2 and 8 years per year and most teens become infected [41].

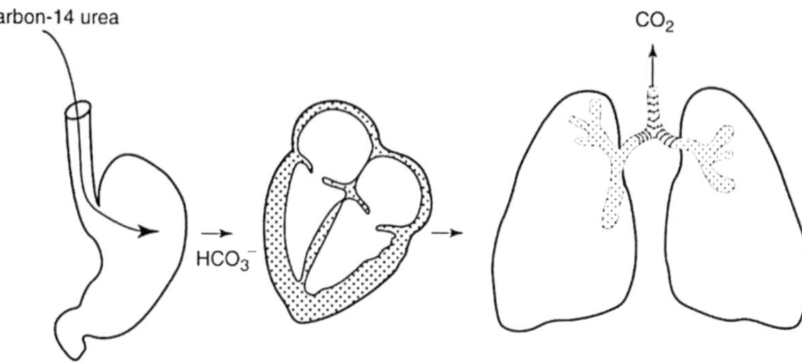

Fig. 10.12 The principle of carbon-14 breath tests

H. pylori infection is known to be associated with several pathological disorders. The organism causes the most common type of nonerosive gastritis, which characteristically involves the antrum and body of the stomach. It is found in almost all patients with duodenal ulcers and approximately 80% of those with gastric ulcer. Other conditions such as gastric ade-nocarcinoma and lymphoma, chronic fatigue syndrome, and acne rosacea are also linked to the organism [41–43]. Recently, it has also been suggested to be involved in the pathogenesis of coronary artery disease.

The diagnosis of *H. pylori* may be obtained by endoscopy specimen, by a blood testidentifying anti-*Helicobacter* infection antibody, or by a carbon-13 or carbon-14 urea breath test. Endoscopy is needed in many cases to detect ulcers and other gross pathological changes. During endoscopy biopsy material is obtained and examined microscopically, in addition to culturing for *H. pylori*. However, endoscopy cannot be used just to find whether *Helicobacter* infection is present and is not justified as a follow-up technique to evaluate the response to therapy. Antibody testing, on the other hand, has the shortcoming of not being suitable for patient follow-ups in antibodies decline slowly after treatment and may remain elevated long after *Helicobacter* has been killed.

H. pylori is able to fight stomach acid containing a large amount of the enzyme urease. Urease converts urea, present in the saliva and gastric juices, into bicarbonate and ammonia, which are strong bases and act as acid-neutralizing agents around the *H. pylori*, protecting it from the stomach acidity. This action of urea hydrolysis is the basis of carbon-14 and carbon-13 urea breath tests.

The test can be performed using a capsule or a liquid containing a minimal amount (2 μ Ci) of carbon-14 urea. The patient swallows a drink or capsule, and 10–20 min later, samples of breath are taken with the patient blowing into a small bottle of liquid. The amount of radioactive carbon dioxide in blood and expired in breath (Fig. 10.12) is detected and quantitated by scintillation counter. In the presence of *H. pylori* infections, the count will be higher than normal. Carbon-14 urea contains a tiny amount of radioactive material, which passes out of the body in a day or so in the urine or breath [42]. The amount of radioactive exposure to the patient from the test is less than the individual normally receives in a half day from nature. It is also equivalent to the radiation dose that an individual absorbs when flying in an airplane for 1 h. Since urea is present in saliva, patients must brush and rinse their teeth before taking the test.

10.6.9.1.2 Lactase Deficiency

Acquired lactase deficiency is a common disorder of carbohydrate absorption. The deficiency of intestinal lactase leads to decreased hydrolysis of ingested lactase in the small intestinal cells as occurs normally. Lactase is one of the most common disaccharides in diet and is a main constituent of milk and other dairy products. The intact lactose is not absorbed and increases the osmotic effect of the small intestinal contents, with subsequent outpouring of liquid into the intestinal lumen. This will result in increased intestinal motility with abdominal cramps, distention, and diarrhea when a patient ingests milk [28].

For lactose intolerance, lactose-1-C-14 together with carrier lactose (50 g) dissolved in 400 mL of water is used. In patients with lactose intolerance, lactase deficiency leads to the inability to split lactose into glucose and galactose and subsequently to CO_2. When carbon-14-labeled lactose-1 is administered to patients with lactase deficiency, there will be decrease dexhalation of labeled carbon dioxide.

10.6.9.1.3 Malabsorption Secondary to Bacterial Overgrowth

Bacterial overgrowth is one of the major reasons for luminal phase malabsorption. Bacterial overgrowth causes deconjugation of bile salts which are absorbed and cycled normally through the enterohepatic circulation but are in effective in micelle formation. Since micelle formation is essential for the normal absorption of free fatty acids and monoglycerides, malabsorption results. Carbon-14-glycine cholate and more recently the carbon-14-xylose breath test are useful in the diagnosis of malabsorption secondary to bacterial overgrowth. Since carbon-14-glycine cholate is a conjugated bile salt, it is absorbed by the ileum and metabolized in the liver. Only a small portion is attached normally by bacteria and causes deconjugation leading to the formation of carbon dioxide that is exhaled. The deconjugation increases within creased bacterial colonization in the intestines, and consequently the amount of labeled carbon dioxide present in the exhaled breath increases [29]. This test is useful in the diagnosis of blind or stagnant loop syndrome and of ileal absorptive function.

10.6.9.2 Schilling's Test

This procedure uses an oral test dose of radiolabeled cyanocobalamin (usually ^{57}Co-B_{12}) with or without added intrinsic factor (IF). The absorption is most frequently measured indirectly by measuring the urinary excretion of the radiolabeled vitamin B_{12}.

10.7 Hepatobiliary System

10.7.1 Anatomical and Physiological Considerations

The liver is the largest organ in the body, weighing between 1200 and 1800 g. The liver lies in the abdominal cavity, where it is split into a large right and a small left lobe by the falciform ligament extending from the anterior abdominal wall. The Couinaud classification divides the liver into eight independent segments numbered 1–8, each of which has its own vascular inflow, outflow, and biliary drainage. The Couinaud segments and their corresponding traditional nomenclature are shown in Fig. 10.13.

Within the lobes and segments are multiple, smaller anatomical units called liver lobules. These lobules are formed of plates of hepatocytes, which are the functional cells of the liver. In addition, the parenchyma of the liver is composed of another type of cells: the reticuloendothelial cells or Kupffer's cells. Almost 90% of the reticuloendothelial cells in the body are found in the liver. The sinusoids are capillaries located between the plates of hepatocytes; they receive a mixture of venous and arterial blood from branches of the portal vein and the hepatic artery, respectively. Blood from the sinusoids drains to central veins that continue to empty into the hepatic vein, which enters the inferior vena cava. Kupffer's cells line the sinusoids and destroy microorganisms.

The liver has digestive, metabolic, hematological, and immunological functions. The hepatocytes synthesize approximately 1 L of bile per day and secrete it into the bile canaliculi, which are small channels between the hepatocytes. The bile canaliculi empty into bile ducts that unite and finally form the right and left hepatic ducts, which join to form the common

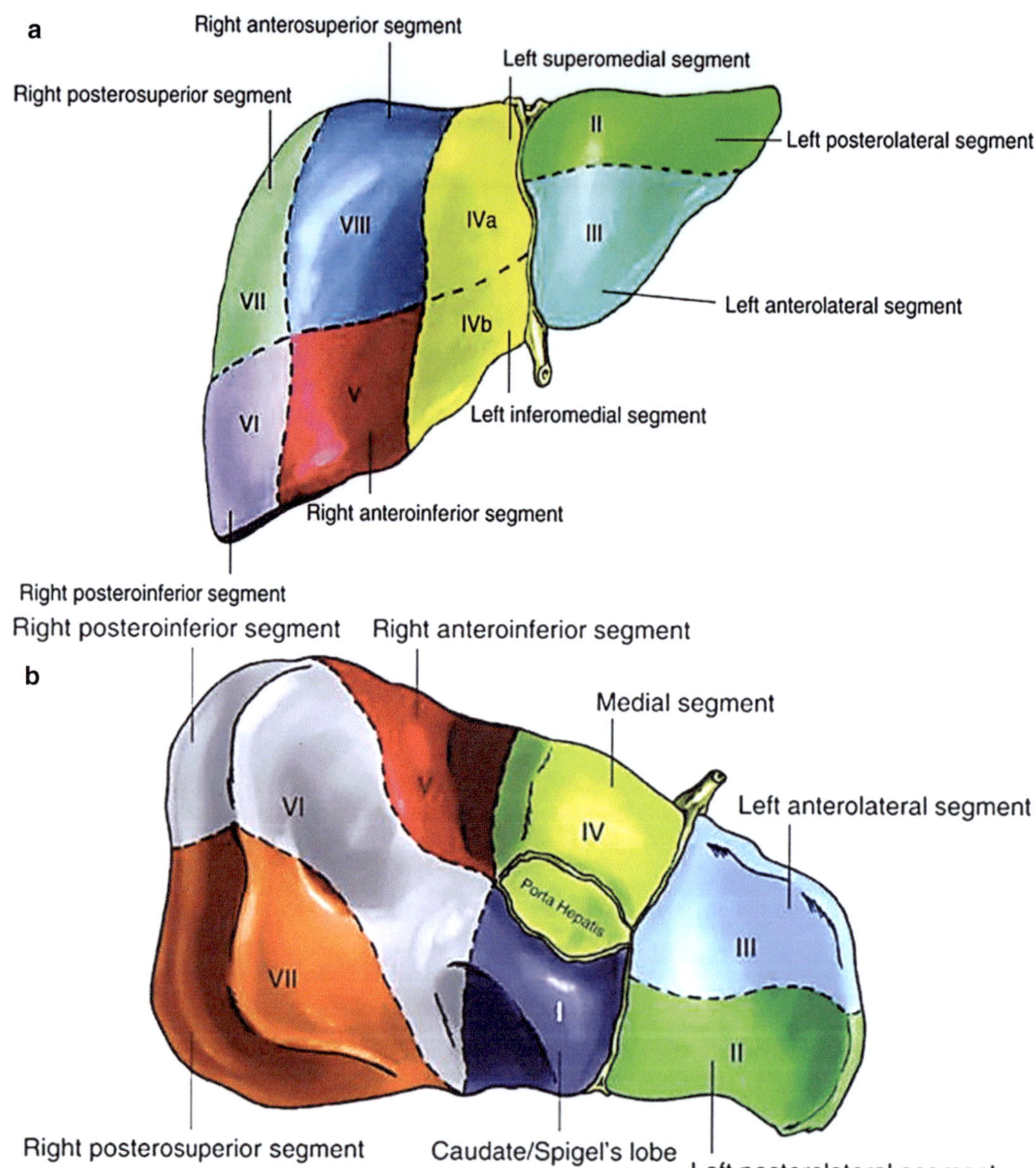

Fig. 10.13 (**a, b**) The Couinaud segments of the liver. (**a**) Anterior surface view; (**b**) visceral surface view. *I*, caudate/Spigel's lobe; *II*, left, posterolateral segment; *III*, left anterolateral segment; *IVa*, left superomedial segment; *IVb*, left inferomedial segment; *V*, right anteroinferior segment; *VI*, right posteroinferior segment; *VII*, right posterosuperior segment; and *VIII*, right anterosuperior segment

hepatic duct. Past the point where the cystic duct begins, the hepatic duct is called the common bile duct, which drains into the duodenum through the major duodenal papilla. Bile is necessary for fat digestion and absorption. Unconjugated bilirubin is converted to water-soluble, conjugated bilirubin by hepatocytes and is secreted with bile. The gallbladder stores bile and ejects it when chyme enters the duodenum and stimulates the secretion of cholecystokinin. The hepatocytes are capable of regeneration. Most regeneration takes place in the left lobe in disease states such as alcoholic damage or chronic hepatitis.

Table 10.8 Radiophramaceuticals for hepatobiliary scintigraphy (Cholescintigraphy)[a]

Radiopharmaceutical	Uptake mechanism	Use
Tc-99 m sulfur colloid	Kupffer cell	Focal nodular hyperplasia, splenosis, liver function
Tc-99 m red blood cells	Blood-pool distribution	Hemangioma, splenosis
Tc-99 m disofenin	Extracted and excreted by the liver similar to bilirubin	Gallbladder and hepatobiliary disorders
Tc-99 m MAA	Blood flow, capillary occlusion	Hepatic arterial perfusion
Tc-99 m mebrofenin	Extracted and excreted by the liver similar to bilirubin	Gallbladder and hepatobiliary disorders
F-18 FDG	Glucose metabolism	Tumor/infection imaging
Gallium-67 citrate	Iron binding	Tumor/infection imaging
Tc-99 m-aglactosyl-neoglycoalbumin (Tc-99 m-NGA) and Tc-99 m-galactosyl human serum albumin (Tc-99 m-GSA)	Binding to the hepatocyte-specific asialoglycoprotein membrane receptors	Assessment of functional liver mass/reserve

[a][44–47]

10.7.2 Hepatobiliary Radiopharmaceuticals

Several radiopharmaceuticals are used for scintigraphic assessment of liver and hepatobiliary disorders (Table 10.8).

Technetium-99m (^{99m}Tc-)-sulfur colloid (SC) is a radiopharmaceutical for liver/spleen imaging. This compound is cleared by cells of the reticuloendothelial system—approximately 85% by Kupffer cells in the liver, 10% by the spleen, and 5% by the bone marrow. Approximately 40–50% of HCCs concentrate hepatobiliary tracers, i.e., ^{99m}Tc-IDA or ^{99m}Tc-PMT. The degree of uptake seems to correlate with tumor differentiation, as well as with survival. ^{99m}Tc-IDA uptake was seen in 70% of well-differentiated tumors, 30% of moderately differentiated tumors, and none in poorly differentiated tumors [48]. The median survival of patients with increased tumor uptake on delayed 99mTc-PMT imaging was found to be significantly longer compared to that of patients with no tumor uptake [49]. Gallium-67, thallium-201, and fluorine-18 fluorodeoxyglucose have been used in patients with HCC in various clinical settings. Wholebody 18F-FDG-PET/CT has proven useful in the early evaluation of residual, intrahepatic recurrent, or extrahepatic metastatic lesions and is able to provide valuable information for the management of HCC recurrence which ultimately helps to establish the best course of treatment and to determine prognosis [44–46].

10.7.3 Evaluation of Liver Diseases

10.7.3.1 Functional Hepatic Mass/Reserve

Assessment of hepatic functional reserve is important prior to major hepatic resection for predicting the outcome of surgery because post-operative liver failure can significantly affect the clinical course. This may require imaging of both the anatomical structure of the liver and the regional functional reserve. Hepatobiliary scintigraphy with technetium-99m (^{99m}Tc) iminodiacetic acid or ^{99m}Tc-galactosyl human serum albumin (GSA) has been used to assess regional hepatic function. Galactosyl human serum albumin (GSA) is a ligand specific to the asialoglycoprotein receptor present exclusively on the plasma membrane of hepatocytes. GSA is bound only by this receptor and then provides valuable information about receptor population density as well as functioning hepatocyte mas [47]. Tc-99m GSA does not compete with bilirubin, which is an additional advantage in the evaluation of hepatic reserve in patients with hyperbilirubinemia.

10.7.3.2 Primary Hepatic Neoplasms and Tumor-like Conditions

10.7.3.2.1 Hepatocellular Carcinoma

While hepatocellular carcinoma (HCC) usually displays marked arterial vascularity on dynamic perfusion imaging, its appearance on static colloid imaging (focally decreased activity) is nonspecific. Sulfur colloid imaging can be used to differentiate regenerating nodules from HCC in a cirrhotic liver. The presence of colloid uptake typically represents regenerating nodules, while decreased uptake is nonspecific but may include HCC [50].

Depending on the degree of differentiation, approximately 40–50% of HCCs concentrate hepatobiliary tracers, i.e., Tc-99m-IDA or Tc-99m-PMT. The degree of uptake seems to correlate with tumor differentiation, as well as with survival [51, 52]. Tc-99m-IDA uptake was seen in 70% of well-differentiated tumors, in 30% of moderately differentiated tumors, and in no poorly differentiated tumors [51]. In another series of 162 patients, the median survival of 82 patients with increased tumor uptake on delayed Tc-99m-PMT imaging was 1013 days, compared with 398.5 days in 80 patients with no tumor uptake [52]. Gallium-67 and thallium-201 were used in the past for evaluation of HCC in various clinical settings. However, the utility of these tracers in HCC appears to have been replaced largely by positron-emitting tracers recently.

10.7.3.2.2 Hepatic Hemangioma

Hemangioma is the most common benign tumor of the liver. Cavernous hemangioma occurs at all ages, but most commonly in adults. Most hemangiomas are of the cavernous type, constituted by dilated non-anastomotic vascular spaces lined by flat endothelial cells and supported by fibrous tissue. Thrombi in different stages of organization are often encountered. Long-standing lesions can show extensive hyalinization or calcification [53].

The sensitivity of planar Tc-99m-RBC imaging is unacceptably low, ranging from 30 to 53% [54–56]. The sensitivity of SPECT RBC imaging is still heavily dependent on the lesion size. Reports published in the 1990s showed an overall sensitivity of 70–80% using single-head SPECT [54–58]. It is remarkable that the specificity and positive predictive value of both planar and SPECT RBC (Fig. 10.14) imaging is essentially 100% [54–57]. A SPECT/CT hybrid system is becoming more widely available, and fusion imaging lowers the false-positive results [59, 60].

10.7.3.3 Focal Nodular Hyperplasia

Focal nodular hyperplasia contains variable quantities of normal hepatic cellular elements, includ-

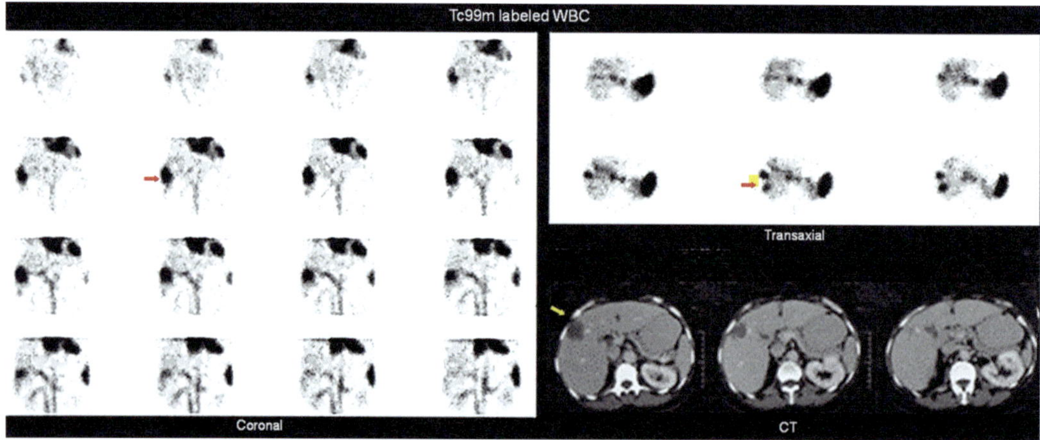

Fig. 10.14 Representative images of a tomographic radionuclide hemangioma study showing a solitary hemangioma corresponding to the finding on CT (*arrow*)

ing Kupffer's cells, hepatocytes, and bile ducts arranged in a characteristic pattern. The characteristic triad suggesting FNH has been described as arterial blood flow, normal colloid uptake, and accumulation of Tc-99m-IDA tracer [61].

Thirty to seventy percent of FNHs have either normal or increased Tc-99m-colloid uptake [62], reflecting the variable quantity of Kupffer's\cells. Decreased Tc-99m-colloid uptake may be seen in approximately one-third of cases [62]. Because of the presence of hepatocytes in FNH, Tc-99m-IDA scintigraphy has also been evaluated for the diagnosis of FNH. Of 25 FNHs in a study, 19 (76%) showed hyperperfusion during the flow phase and 23 (92%) appeared as focal regions of increased uptake during the clearance phase of hepatobiliary imaging. Normal sulfur colloid uptake was seen in 16 (64%) [63]. The detectability of FNH by Tc-99 m-IDA scintigraphy was 92%, greater than that of CT (84%) or MRI (84%).

10.7.3.4 Hepatocellular Adenoma

10.7.3.4.1 Hepatocellular Adenoma
Hepatocellular adenomas typically appear as photopenic defects on Tc-99 m-colloid scintigraphy. In the past, this was attributed to the absence of Kupffer's cells [64]. However, a pathological study demonstrated that all hepatic adenomas studied contained Kupffer's cells [65]. Yet most of these lesions (77%) did not demonstrate Tc-99m-colloid uptake for unknown reasons. The authors found no significant histological difference between those lesions that accumulate colloids and those that do not. They also suggested that adenoma should be added to the differential diagnosis of a hepatic lesion with Tc-99m-colloid uptake because of the presence of uptake in 23% of their cases.

10.7.4 Biliary Tract Diseases

Bile flowing through the common hepatic duct may flow either into the gallbladder or through the common bile duct (CBD) into the duodenum. The quantity of bile flowing in either direction is

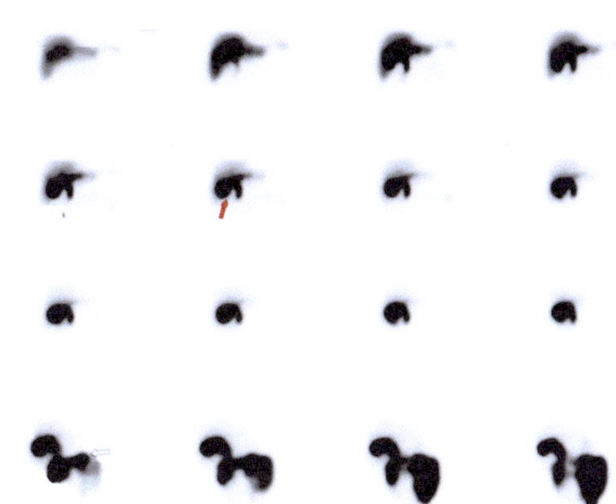

Fig. 10.15 Normal radionuclide hepatobiliary study with prompt visualization of gallbladder (*solid arrow*) and intestinal activity (*open arrow*)

determined to a major degree by the pressure developed by the sphincter of Oddi. In normal individuals, bile flows into the gallbladder when the sphincter of Oddi is contracted. Foods containing lipids and amino acids enter the duodenum and cause the release of endogenous cholecystokinin (CCK) from the duodenum to the upper jejunum, which in turn contracts the gallbladder, dilates the sphincter of Oddi, and increases bile secretion from the hepatocytes. All of these enhance the flow of bile into the duodenum.

On a typical normal cholescintigram performed with Tc-99 m-IDA agents, the CBD and gallbladder are visualized 10–20 min following the intravenous administration of Tc-99 m-IDA (Fig. 10.15). Visualization of the small bowel varies depending on the sphincter tone and the degree of gallbladder filling.

10.8 Acute Cholecystitis

Although it is generally known that acute cholecystitis in 90–95% of cases begins with obstruction of the neck of the gallbladder or the cystic duct by a gallstone, some authors feel that obstruction does not necessarily lead to acute cholecystitis. Nevertheless, obstruction is present in almost all cases of acute cholecystitis. There are other important factors in the pathogenesis of acute cholecystitis, including chemi-

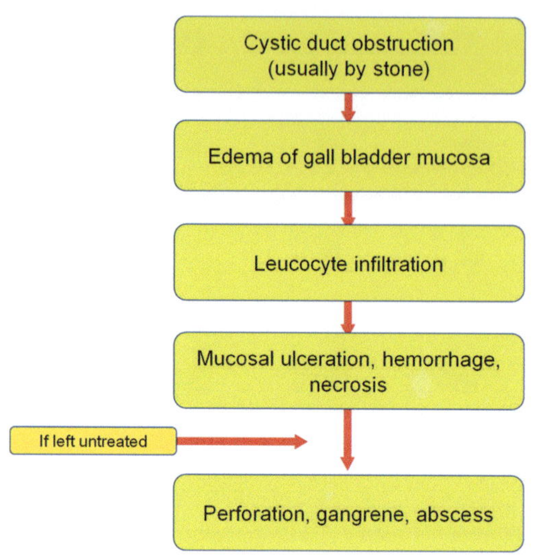

Fig. 10.16 Pathophysiologic features of acute cholecystitis

cal factors such as prostaglandins and bacterial growth. Injury to the gallbladder mucosa by a mechanical or chemical factor stimulates the epithelial cells to secrete fluid. Active fluid secretion in the obstructed gallbladder lumen increases the intraluminal pressure, which may cause impairment of circulation and ischemia of the gallbladder mucosa (Fig. 10.16) and wall. Distention of the gallbladder further enhances formation of prostaglandin, establishing a vicious cycle [66]. Active fluid secretion in the gallbladder wall is markedly reduced by morphine. The acceleration of the process can be reduced by morphine [67].

Approximately 60–70% of patients report prior attacks that resolved spontaneously. The factors regulating the intraluminal pressure may determine the course of an attack of acute cholecystitis. Of the 75% of patients with acute cholecystitis who experience remission of symptoms, approximately one quarter will experience a recurrence of cholecystitis within 1 year, and 60% will have at least one recurrent attack within 6 years [68]. Therefore, the histological pattern of acute cholecystitis is superimposed upon chronic inflammatory changes in at least 90% of cholecystectomy specimens [69].

Acalculous form of acute cholecystitis is less common (less than 10%) in patients with acute cholecystitis [70]. Despite the absence of gallstones, the cystic duct is frequently obstructed by viscous bile, sludge, cellular debris, or edema associated with dehydration [71]. Precipitating factors include severe trauma or burns, the postpartum period following prolonged labor, a major operation, prolonged parenteral hyperalimentation, vasculitis, obstructing tumor of the gallbladder, and parasitic infestation of the gallbladder. It also may be seen with a variety of other systemic diseases (sarcoidosis, cardiovascular disease, tuberculosis, syphilis, actinomycosis, etc.) [68]. Apart from the absence of stones, the pathology of acalculous and calculous cholecystitis is essentially identical [72].

10.8.1 Imaging for Acute Cholecystitis

Acute cholecystitis is the most common indication for cholescintigraphy, which is considered the procedure of choice for its diagnosis [71–75, 78]. Generally, nonvisualization of the gallbladder up to 4 h after radiotracer administration or within 30 min after the administration of morphine sulfate is interpreted as consistent with cystic duct obstruction, provided that there is normal hepatic uptake and excretion. Gallbladder visualization anytime during imaging virtually excludes the presence of acute cholecystitis. The study can be obtained as planar, SPECT, or SPECT/CT. Meta-analysis of 2466 patients showed a sensitivity of 97% and specificity of 90% [73].

Rim sign represents increased IDA activity in the liver parenchyma around the gallbladder fossa (Fig. 10.17). The presence of this sign is frequently associated with acute cholecystitis, which is often complicated, i.e., gangrenous gallbladder [74] and is considered a secondary sign for acute cholecystitis. This pericholecystic activity appears to be caused by increased blood flow to [76] and/or delayed bile excretion from inflamed liver parenchyma adjacent to an inflamed gallbladder [77].

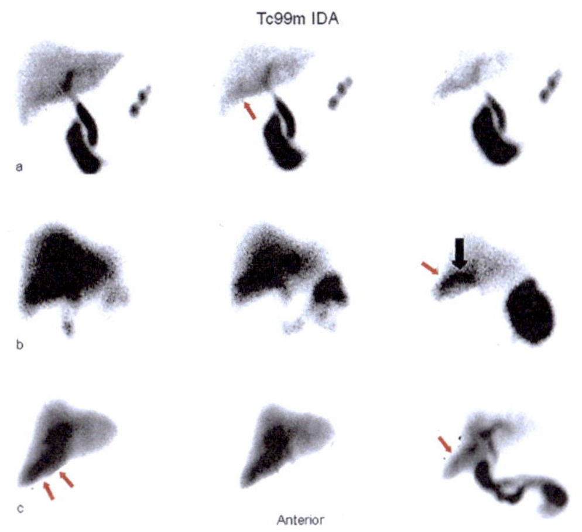

Fig. 10.17 A spectrum of rim signs. (**a**) A mild rim sign is seen in the Tc-99 m-IDA study of patient 1 (*arrow*). The rim sign in (**b**) is quite prominent and clearly seen rim (*arrows*). The rim sign (**c**) is more diffuse and may be confused with the gallbladder. However, this activity is present in the early image (*arrow*) even before the the tracer activity appears in the bile ducts (from Kim [78] with permission)

10.8.2 Chronic Acalculous Biliary Syndromes

This group includes chronic acalculous cholecystitis, cystic duct syndrome, and gallbladder dyskinesis. Approximately 98% of patients with symptomatic gallbladder disease have gallstones. Occasionally, patients have signs and symptoms of gallbladder disease, but no stone can be demonstrated by repeated ultrasound or oral cholecystography [77]. The pathological findings of chronic acalculous cholecystitis are nearly identical to those of chronic calculous cholecystitis, except for the absence of stones [77]. Intermittent acalculous cystic duct obstruction and chronic ischemia with active inflammatory changes have both been postulated as possible pathogenic mechanisms.

Cystic duct syndrome results from a partial acalculous obstruction or narrowing of the cystic duct [75], which may be due to fibrosis, kinking, or adhesion.

Gallbladder dyskinesia histologically shows no abnormal findings. Abnormal and/or inhomo-geneous CCK receptors within the gallbladder, which cause a paradoxical or inhomogeneous response to cholecystokinetic agents, were suggested as a possible mechanism [78].

10.8.2.1 Biliary Sphincter (Sphincter of Oddi) Stenosis/ Obstruction

Biliary Sphincter disorder occurs mostly in patients after cholecystectomy. It is much more common in female patients can be classified into two broad categories: stenosis (by stone or a fixed structural narrowing) and dyskinesia (functional disorder: a primary disorder of tonic/phasic motor activity) [79].

Hepatobiliary imaging with or without pharmacological intervention has also been shown to be useful in patients with SOD, and investigations have focused primarily on patients after cholecystectomy. Although scintigraphic studies on this subject have focused primarily on the differentiation between the presence and absence of SOD, it can be also useful in discriminating between stenosis and functional dyskinesia [80].

10.8.2.2 Interventions in Cholescintigraphy

Several drugs, including cholecystokinin (CCK), morphine, and phenobarbital, have been used to alter biliary kinetics at different levels (i.e., hepatocytes, gallbladder, and/or sphincter of Oddi) in an effort to increase the efficacy of hepatobiliary imaging. Sincalide, a synthetic C-terminal octapeptide of CCK, has been used in the diagnosis of acute cholecystitis in order to empty the gallbladder before cholescintigraphy, so that gallbladder filling can be enhanced during the study if the cystic duct is patent. These agents are also used to evaluate gallbladder ejection fraction (GBEF) and/or sphincter of Oddi response in patients with suspected chronic, acalculous biliary tract diseases to determine who might benefit from cholecystectomy or sphincterotomy.

Table 10.9 Uses of CCK associated with cholescintigraphy

(a)	Administration prioe to cholescitigraphy
	1. Prolonged fasting & total parenetral nutrition
	2. Suspected biliary sphincter (Sphincter of Oddi) dysfunction
(b)	Admistration after 60 min study
	1. Chronic acalculous cholecystitis
	2. Differentiate common bile duct obstruction from functional etiology
	3. Exclude acalculous form of acute cholecystitis when gall bladder is visualized

10.8.2.3 Cholecysystokinin (CCK) Administration

CCK is a polypeptide hormone normally released from mucosal cells of the proximal small bowel in response to fat and protein ingested. CCK is bound to receptors in the gallbladder and sphincter of Oddi resulting in gallbladder wall contraction and sphincter of Oddi relaxation. CCK can be used in several situations as one of the interventions with cholescintigraphy. It may administered before cholescintigraphy or after the 60-min study ends (Table 10.9).

10.8.3 CCK Pre-Cholescintigraphy Administration for the Diagnosis of Acute Cholecystitis

Administration of CCK prior to injection of Tc-99 m-IDA will induce gallbladder emptying with a reduction of intraluminal pressure. It was introduced as a means of reducing potential false-positive results for acute cholecystitis and shortening the total imaging time [81]. The rationale of this approach is that gallbladder emptying before initiating the study is generally followed by more reliable gallbladder filling during the cholescintigraphy. Although sincalide pretreatment of all patients may not be necessary, it is often used in conditions such as alcoholism and total parenteral nutrition and during a prolonged fasting state, because functional resistance to tracer inflow may result from distention of the gallbladder with viscous contents. Fasting for 24 h or longer is a routine indication for the pre-administration of sincalide in many laboratories.

10.8.4 CCK Pre-Cholescintigraphy Administration for Suspected Biliary Sphincter (Sphincter of Oddi) Dysfunction

CCK is infused at a dose of 0.02 μg/kg over 3–10 min, 15 min prior to injection of IDA derivative and then the study is carried out for the initial standard of 60 min [44]. If the condition is not post-cholecystectomy, a longer infusion for 45–60 min is carried out after the initial cholescintigraphy study, and GBEF is determined if it is useful in predicting the outcome of sphincterotomy.

10.8.4.1 CCK Post-Cholescintigraphy Administration for Acalculous Biliary Syndromes

Determination of GBEF after CCK administration is important for confirmation of this group of disorders and also in predicting the outcome of surgery. The technique for administration of CCK is of the utmost importance. Comparison of various sincalide doses for a 3-min infusion technique demonstrated that 10 ng/kg (the rate of 3.3 ng/kg/min) produces maximal gallbladder emptying [44]. With further increase of the dose rate, i.e., 20 ng/kg/3 min, the GBEF actually decreases. The normal GBEF value using 10 ng/kg/3 min was established as greater than 35%. Falsely reduced GB emptying associated with a 3-min infusion of 20 ng/kg of sincalide is illustrated well in Fig. 10.18 [82]. However, Ziessman et al. showed that even the infusion at a so-called physiological rate (10 ng/kg infused over 3 min) produces an excessively variable GBEF response to establish a clinically useful and reproducible normal range compared with the same dose infused over a longer period, i.e., 10 ng/kg infused for 60 min [83].

10.8.4.2 Morphine Augmentation

The administration of morphine sulfate (morphine) results in contraction of the sphincter of Oddi. This, in turn, causes an increase in the intraductal pressure and forces the bile to flow into the gallbladder if the cystic duct is patent [84–86]. A widely used protocol as an alternative to delayed imaging involves the administration of 0.04 mg/kg morphine intravenously over 3 min at 1 h after the injection of

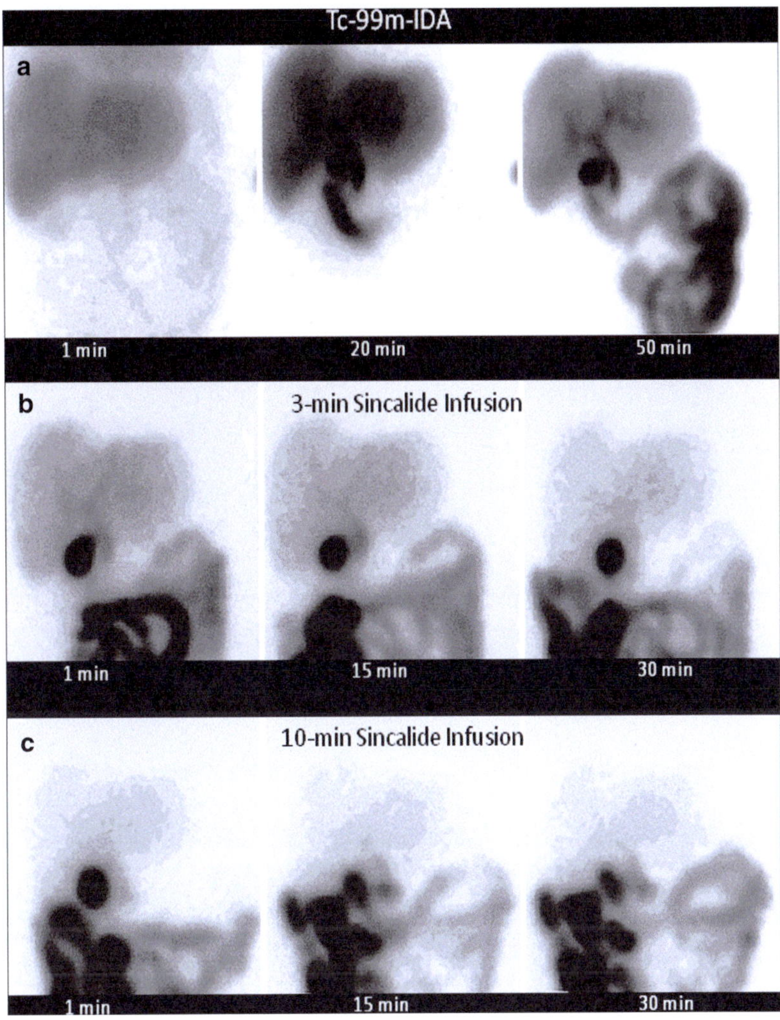

Fig. 10.18 A hepatobiliary scan using Tc-99m-IDA was performed in a patient with suspected chronic acalculous biliary disease. The scan shows prompt visualization of the GB and small bowel (**a**). Following a 3-min infusion of 20 ng/kg sincalide, the GB is poorly contracted, with an EF of approximately 10% (**b**). Immediately after this, a 10-min infusion of the same dose produced a GBEF of 80% (**c**)

a radiotracer, provided that activity is seen in the bowel. After morphine administration, imaging is continued for an additional 30 min (Fig. 10.19).

10.8.5 Hyperbilirubinemia

Cholescintigraphy is often performed to differentiate surgical jaundice (CBD obstruction and biliary atresia) from medical jaundice (intrahepatic cholestasis and/or hepatocellular disease) in both adults and neonates. Alternatively, CBD obstruction or intrahepatic cholestasis is occasionally detected incidentally on cholescintigraphy performed in patients who present with abdominal pain.

10.8.6 Common Bile Duct Obstruction

Cholescintigraphy is useful for the diagnosis of biliary obstruction in patients with normal ultrasonography and who are not clearly jaundiced and only mild liver dysfunction as if serum bilirubin levels are high, bilirubin occupies the available receptors and blocks the IDA uptake since both have the same mechanism for uptake by hepatocytes. Prompt hepatic uptake of IDA that persists for 2–4 h (sometimes even up to 24 h) without evidence of biliary excretion is the obstructive pattern that has been commonly described [87, 88].

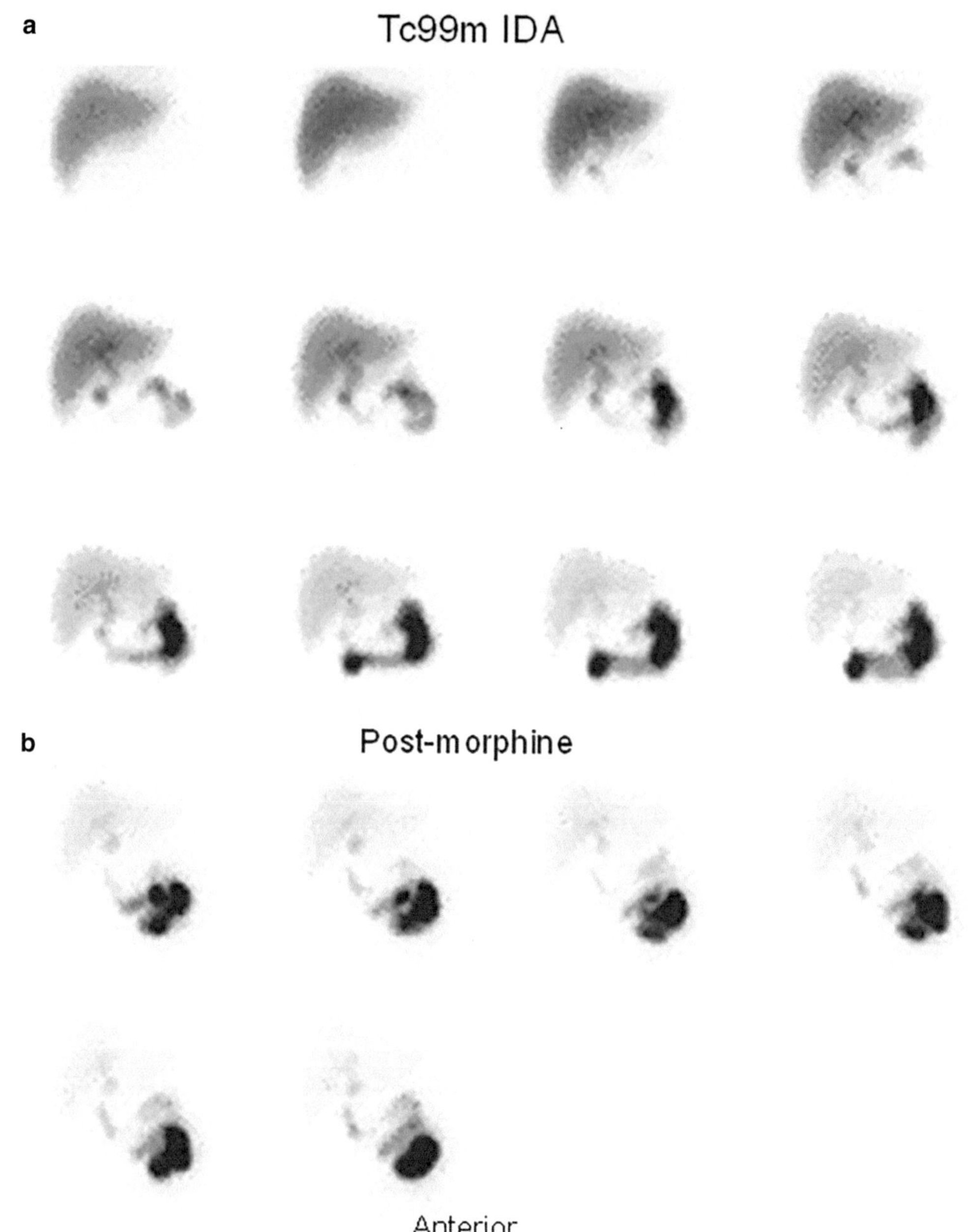

Fig. 10.19 Hepatobiliary study showing nonvisualization of gallbladder during the routine study (**a**) and after low-dose morphine injection (**b**) in a patient suspected of having acute cholecystitis. The CBD and small bowel are promptly visualized but the gallbladder is not visualized for up to 60 min. Following morphine administration, the gallbladder did not show filling. The finding indicates obstruction of the cystic duct which indicates acute cholecystitis in the clinical setting of this patient

10.8.7 Neonatal Hyperbilirubinemia

Persistent jaundice is considered to be pathological beyond 3 weeks of age in full-term babies and 4 weeks in preterm babies. Cholestasis with conjugated hyperbilirubinemia can be due to a wide variety of abnormalities including extrahepatic biliary tree abnormalities (i.e., extrahepatic biliary atresia (EHBA) and choledochal cyst) or intrahepatic diseases (i.e., interlobular bile duct paucity or neonatal hepatitis syndrome).

If there is no excretion in an infant less than 2 months of age (Fig. 10.20) and the initial uptake suggests liver dysfunction, and then neonatal hepatitis syndrome should be suspected. Cholescintigraphy is most useful in excluding the diagnosis of biliary atresia with a sensitivity and negative predictive value of virtually 100% when intestinal and/or extrahepatic biliary activity is seen

(Fig. 10.21). Patients are typically premedicated with phenobarbital, 5 mg/kg daily in two divided doses given for 5 days. Ursodeoxycholic acid, an additional choleretic agent, may also be given at a dose of 20 mg/kg daily in two divided doses in order to optimize bile flow prior to the study.

Phenobarbital stimulates the hepatic transport system for organic anions. This is primarily achieved by induction of hepatic microsomal enzymes, thereby increasing bilirubin conjugation and excretion situations.

10.8.8 Evaluation of Complications after Hepatobiliary Surgery

The increase in the number of laparoscopic cholecystectomies and liver transplantations leads to increased utilization of cholescintigraphy for the

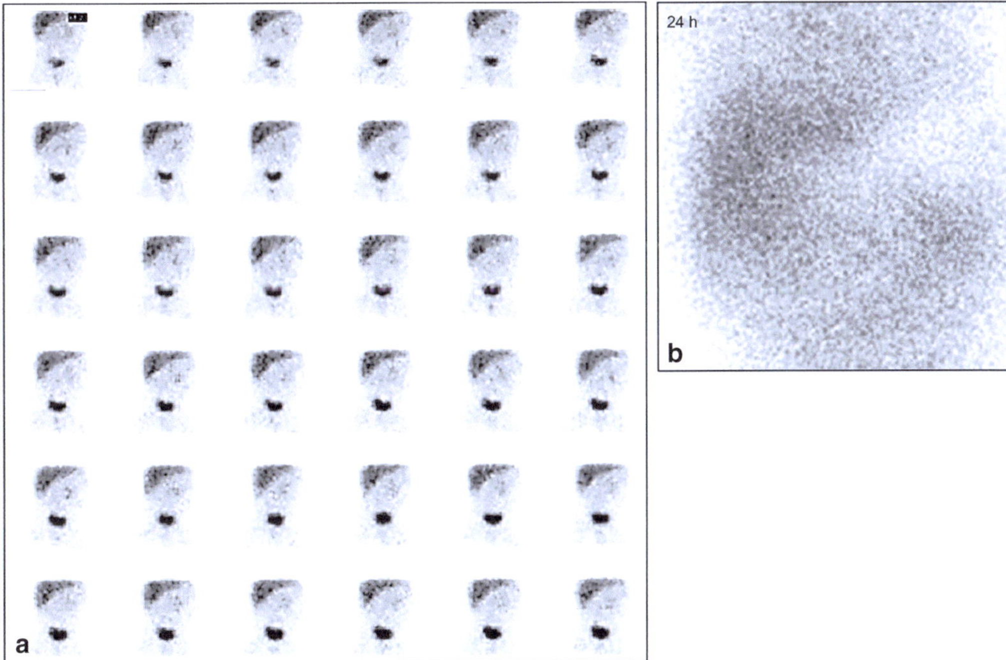

Fig. 10.20 Hepatobiliary study in a neonate carried out for 60-min (**a**) and delayed 24-h image (**b**) illustrating no secretion of activity in the intestine as well as non-visualization of the gallbladder. Biliary atresia in such case cannot be excluded and since the function of the liver in adequate it is more likely than neonatal hepatitis

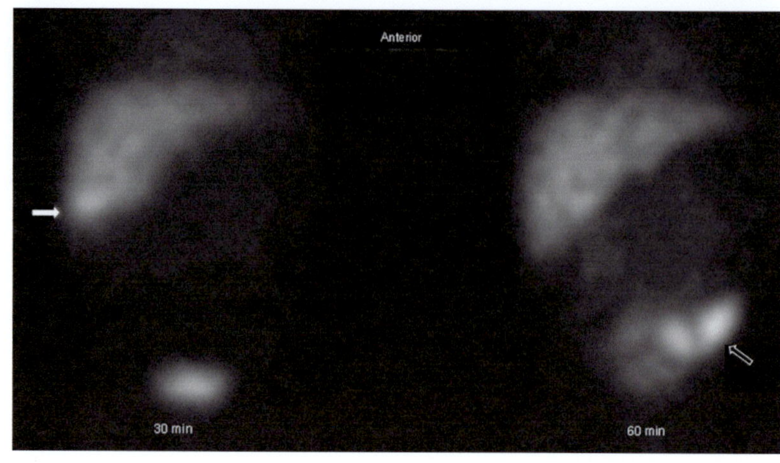

Fig. 10.21 ^{99m}Tc-Mebophenin study of a 1-month-old baby boy with neonatal jaundice. The gallbladder (*solid arrow*)is visualized by 30 min and the intestinal activity (*open arrow*) by 60 min excluding biliary atresia

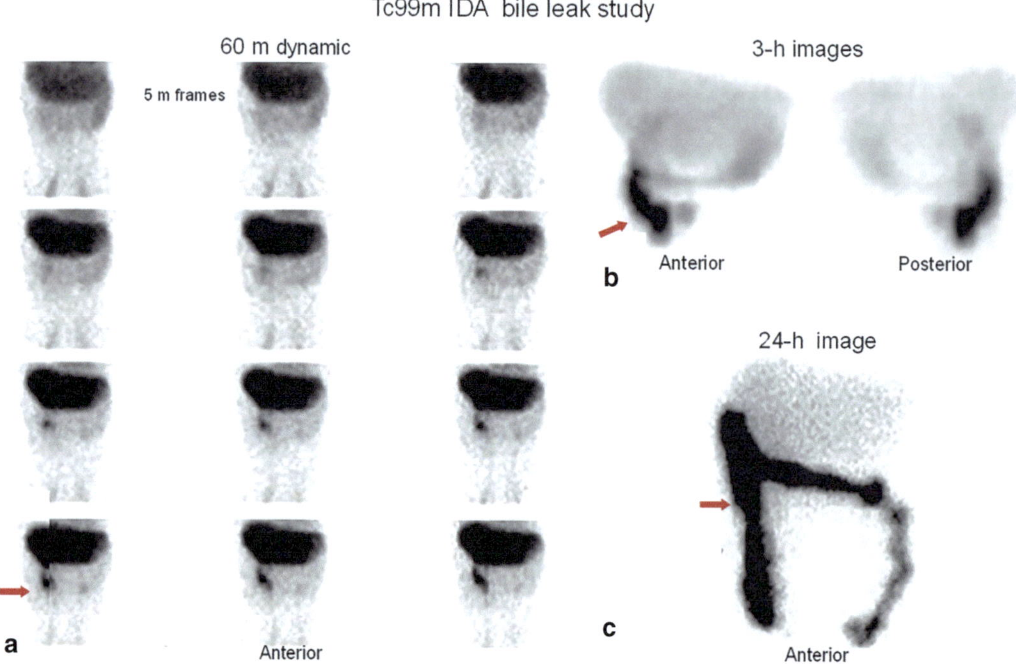

Fig. 10.22 Bile leak study of a patient who underwent liver transplantation 20 days earlier

evaluation of postoperative complications [89]. Bile duct complications include bile leaks (Fig. 10.22), common bile/hepatic duct injuries or strictures, retained biliary calculi, and obstruction. When ultrasonography or CT shows a fluid collection, cholescintigraphy can be helpful not only in confirming but also in excluding biloma. The addition of SPECT/CT imaging can help in localization and improve the accuracy of the study.

References

1. Kuo B, Urma D (2006) Esophagus-anatomy and development. GI Motility online. https://doi.org/10.1038/gimo6
2. Mittal RK (2011) Upper esophageal sphincter. In: Mittal RK (ed) Motor function of the pharynx, esophagus and its sphincters. Morgan and Claypool life sciences, San Rafael, California. Available from: http://www.ncbi.nih.gov/nooks/NBK54282

3. Wong RKH, Waysonovitch CL (1995) Achalasia. In: Castell DO (ed) The esophagus, 3rd edn. Little Brown, Boston, pp 219–245

4. Oude Nijhuis RAB, Zaninotto G, Roman S, Boeckxstaens GE, Fockens P, Langendam MW, Bredenoord AJ (2020) European guidelines on achalasia: united European gastroenterology and European Society of Neurogastroenterology and Motility recommendations. United European Gastroenterol J 8(1):13–33

5. Sama SK, Daniel EE, Waterfall WE (1977) Myogenic and neural control systems for esophageal motility. Gastroenereology 73:1345–1352

6. Howard PJ, Heading RC (1992) Epidemiology of gastro-esophageal reflux disease. World J Surg 16:288–293

7. Sidhu AS, Triadafilopoulos G (2008) Neuroregulation of lower esophageal sphincter function as treatment for gastro-esophageal reflux disease. World J Gastroenterol 14:985–990

8. Lacy BE, Weiser K (2008) Esophageal disorders: medical therapy. J Clin Gastroenterol 42:652–658

9. Penaginie R, Schoeman MN, Dent J, Tipnett MD, Holloway RH (1996) Motor events underlying gastroesophageal reflux in ambulant patient with reflux esophagitis. Neurogastroenterol Motil 8:131–141

10. Kahrilas PJ, Manka M, Shi G, Joehl RJ (2000) Increased frequency of transient lower esophageal sphincter relaxation induced by gastric distention in reflux patients with hiatal hernia. Gastroenterology 118:688–695

11. Galmiche JP, Janssens J (1995) The pathophysiology of gastroesophageal reflux disease: an overview. Scand J Gastroenterol Suppl 211:7–18

12. Labenz J, Malfertheiner P (1997) Helicobacter pylori in gastroesophageal reflux disease: causal agent, independent or protective factor? Gut 41.277–280

13. Fallone CA, Barkun AN, Friedman G, Mayrand S, Loo V, Beech R, Best L, Joseph L (2000) Is helicobacter pylori eradication associated with GERD? Am J Gastroenterol 95:914–920

14. Brener W, Hendrix TR, McHugh PR (1983) Regulation of the gastric emptying of glucose. Gastroenterology 85:76–82

15. Siegel JA, Urbain JL, Adler LP, Charkes ND, Maurer AH, Krevsky B, Knight LC, Fisher RS, Malmud LS (1988) Biphasic nature of gastric emptying. Gut 29:85–89

16. Minami H, McCallum RW (1984) The physiology and pathophysiology of gastric emptying in humans. Gastroenterology 86:1592–1600

17. Loo FD, Palmer DW, Soergel KH, Kalbfleisch JH, Wood CM (1984) Gastric emptying in patients with diabetes mellitus. Gastroenterology 86:485–494

18. Greenberger NJ, Isselbacher KJ (1998) Disorders of absorption. In: Fauci AS, Braunwald E, Isselbacher KJ, Fauci AS, Braunwald E, Isselbacher KJ, Martin JB (eds) Harrison's principles of internal medicine, 14th edn. McGraw-Hill, New York, pp 1616–1633

19. Hatoum OA, Binion DG (2005) The vasculature and infammatory bowel disease: contribution to pathogenesis and clinical pathology. Infamm Bowel Dis 11:304–313

20. Rogler G, Biedermann L, Scharl M (2018) New insights into the pathophysiology of infammatory bowel disease: microbiota, epigenetics and common signalling pathways. Swiss Med Wkly 148:w14599

21. Old JL, Dusing RW, Yap W, Dirks J (2005) Imaging for suspected appendicitis. Am Fam Physician 71:71–78

22. Whiteford MH, Whiteford HM, Yee LF, Ogunbiyi OA, Dehdashti F, Siegel BA, Birnbaum EH, Fleshman JW, Kodner IJ, Read TE (2000) Usefulness of FDG-PET scan in the assessment of suspected metastatic or recurrent adenocarcinoma of the colon and rectum. Dis Colon Rectum 43:759–767

23. Aabakken L (2005) Non variceal upper gastrointestinal bleeding. Endoscopy 37:195–200

24. Carney BW, Khatri G, Shenoy-Bhangle AS (2019) The role of imaging in gastrointestinal bleed. Cardiovasc Diagn Ther 9(Suppl 1):S88

25. Strate LL, Gralnek IM (2016) Management of patients with acute lower gastrointestinal bleeding. Am J Gastroenterol 111(4):459

26. Zurkiya O, Walker TG (2015) Angiographic evaluation and management of nonvariceal gastrointestinal hemorrhage. Am J Roentgenol 205(4):753–763

27. Stone DN, Mancuso AA, Rice D, Hanafee WN (1981) Parotid CT sialography. Radiology 138:393–397

28. Arroyo V, Bernadi M, Epstein M (1998) Pathophysiology of ascites and functional renal failure in cirrhosis. J Hepatol 6:239

29. Singh A (1996) Peritoneovenous shunts: patency studies. In: Henkin RE, Bles MA, Dillehay GL, Halama JR, Karesh SM, Wagner PH, Zimmer AM (eds) Textbook of nuclear medicine. Mosby, New York, pp 1041–1052

30. Wang YT, Mohammed SD, Farmer AD, Wang D, Zarate N, Hobson AR, Scott SM (2015) Regional gastrointestinal transit and pH studied in 215 healthy volunteers using the wireless motility capsule: influence of age, gender, study country and testing protocol. Aliment Pharmacol Ther 42(6):761–772

31. Nogueira HJV (2020) Detection of ectopic gastric mucosa using scintigraphy in pediatric patients

32. Gyorke T, Duffek L, Bratfai K et al (2000) The role of nuclear medicine in inflammatory bowel disease. A review with experiences of a specific bowel activity using immunoscintigraphy with ^{99m}Tc anti-granulocyte antibodies. Eur J Radiol 3:183–192

33. Lantto E (1994) Investigation of suspected intra-abdominal sepsis: the contribution of nuclear medicine. Scand J Gastroenterol Suppl 203:11–14

34. Perlman SB, Hall BS, Reichelderfer M (2013) PET/CT imaging of inflammatory bowel disease. Semin Nucl Med 43:420–426

35. Saha GB (2009) Fundamentals of nuclear pharmacy, 6th edn. Springer, New York

36. Sarkady E, Sapi Z, Toth V, Kiss S (1999) Warthin-like tumor of the thyroid: a case report. Pathol Oncol Res 5:315–317

37. Loutfi I, Nair MK, Ebrahim AK (2003) Salivary gland scintigraphy: the use of semi quantitative analysis for uptake and clearance. J Nucl Med Technol 31(2):81–85

38. Katabathina VS, Zafar AM, Suri R (2015) Clinical presentation, imaging, and management of acute cholecystitis. Tech Vasc Interv Radiol 18:256–265

39. Kipper SL (1999) The role of radiolabeled leukocyte imaging in the management of patients with acute appendicitis. Q J Nucl Med 43:83–92

40. Bourgeois S, Van Den Berghe I, Frank De Geeter MD (2016) 18 incidental finding of silent appendicitis on F-FDG PET/CT in a patient with small cell lung adenocarcinoma. Hell J Nucl Med 19:164–166

41. Graham DY, Malaty HM, Evans DG et al (1991) Epidemiology of Helicobacter pylori in asymptomatic population in the United States. Gastroenterology 100:1495–1501

42. Parsonnet J, Friedman GD, Vandersteen DP et al (1991) Helicobacter pylori infection and the risk of gastric carcinoma. N Engl J Med 325:1127–1131

43. O'Connor A (2021) The urea breath test for the noninvasive detection of helicobacter pylori. In: Helicobacter pylori. Humana, New York, pp 15–20

44. Tulchinsky M, Ciak BW, Debelke D, Hilsom A, Holes-Lewis KA et al (2010) SNM practice guidelines for hepatobiliary scintigraphy 4.0. J Nucl Med Technol 38:210–218

45. Lambie H, Cook AM, Scarsbrook AF, Lodge JPA, Robinson PJ, Chowdhury FU (2011) Tc^{99m}-hepatobiliary iminodiacetic acid (HIDA) scintigraphy in clinical practice. Clin Radiol 66:1094–1105

46. Rassam F, Olthof PB, Richardson H, van Gulik TM, Bennink RJ (2019) Practical guidelines for the use of technetium-99m mebrofenin hepatobiliary scintigraphy in the quantitative assessment of liver function. Nucl Med Commun 40(4):297–307

47. Imura S, Shimada M, Utsunomiya T (2015) Estimation of hepatic functional reserve. Hepatol Res 45:10–19

48. Yumoto Y, Yagi T, Sato S, Nouso K, Kobayashi Y, Ohmoto M, Yumoto E, Nagaya I, Nakatsukasa H (2010) Preoperative estimation of remnant hepatic function using fusion images obtained by ^{99m}Tc-labelled galactosyl-human serum albumin liver scintigraphy and computed tomography. Br J Surg 97(6):934–944

49. Mitsumori A, Nagaya I, Kimoto S, Akaki S, Togami I, Takeda Y, Joja I, Hiraki Y (1998) Preoperative evaluation of hepatic functional reserve following hepatectomy by technetium-99m galactosyl human serum albumin liver scintigraphy and computed tomography. Eur J Nucl Med 25:1377–1382

50. Fujimoto H, Uchiyama G, Araki T et al (1991) Exophytic regenerating nodule of the liver: misleading appearance on iodized-oil CT. J Comput Assist Tomogr 15:495–497

51. Calvet X, Pons F, Bruix J et al (1988) Technetium-99m DISIDA hepatobiliary agent in diagnosis of hepatocellular carcinoma: relationship between detectability and tumor differentiation. J Nucl Med 29:1916–1920

52. Hasegawa Y, Nakano S, Hiyama T et al (1991) Relationship of uptake of technetium-99m(Sn)-N-pyridoxyl-5-methyltryptophan by hepatocellular carcinoma to prognosis. J Nucl Med 32:228–235

53. Lin J, Westerhoff M (2021) Vascular neoplasms of the liver. Clin Liver Dis (Hoboken) 17:261–266

54. Ziessman HA, Silverman PM, Patterson J et al (1991) Improved detection of small cavernous hemangiomas of the liver with high-resolution three-headed SPECT. J Nucl Med 32:2086–2091

55. Langsteger W, Lind P, Eber B et al (1989) Diagnosis of hepatic hemangioma with ^{99m}Tc-labeled red cells: single photon emission computed tomography (SPECT) versus planar imaging. Liver 9:288–293

56. Krause T, Hauenstein K, Studier-Fischer B et al (1993) Improved evaluation of technetium-99m-red blood cell SPECT in hemangioma of the liver. J Nucl Med 34:375–380

57. Birnbaum BA, Weinreb JC, Megibow AJ et al (1990) Definitive diagnosis of hepatic hemangiomas: MR imaging versus Tc-99m-labeled red blood cell SPECT. Radiology 176:95–101

58. Jhuang J-Y, Lin L-W, Hsieh M-S (2011) Adult capillary hemangioma of the liver: case report and literature review. Kaohsiung J Med Sci 27:344–347

59. Zheng JG, Yao ZM, Shu CY, Zhang Y, Zhang X (2005) Role of SPECT/CT in diagnosis of hepatic hemangiomas. World J Gastroenterol 11:5336–5341

60. Schillaci O, Danieli R, Manni C, Capoccetti F, Simonetti G (2004) Technetium-99m-labelled red blood cell imaging in the diagnosis of hepatic haemangiomas: the role of SPECT/CT with a hybrid camera. Eur J Nucl Med Mol Imaging 31:1011–1015

61. Tanasescu D, Brachman M, Rigby J et al (1984) Scintigraphic triad in focal nodular hyperplasia. Am J Gastroenterol 79:61–64

62. Welch TJ, Sheedy PF Jr, Johnson CM et al (1985) Focal nodular hyperplasia and hepatic adenoma: comparison of angiography, CT, US, and scintigraphy. Radiology 156:593–595

63. Kotzerke J, Schwarzrock R, Krischek O et al (1989) Technetium-99m DISIDA hepatobiliary agent in diagnosis of hepatocellular carcinoma, adenoma, and focal nodular hyperplasia (letter). J Nucl Med 30:1278–1280

64. Salvo AF, Schiller A, Athanasoulis C et al (1977) Hepatoadenoma and focal nodular hyperplasia; pitfalls in radiocolloid imaging. Radiology 125:451–455

65. Lubbers PR, Ros PR, Goodman ZD et al (1987) Accumulation of technetium-99m sulfur colloid by hepatocellular adenoma: scintigraphic-pathologic correlation. AJR Am J Roentgenol 148:1105–1108

66. Jivegard L, Thornell E, Svanvik J (1987) Pathophysiology of acute obstructive cholecystitis: implications for nonoperative management. Br J Surg 74:1084–1086

67. Jivegard L, Thornell E, Bjorck S, Svanvik J (1985) The effects of morphine and enkephaline on gallbladder function in experimental cholecystitis. Inhibition of inflammatory gallbladder secretion. Scand J Gastroenterol 20:1049–1056

68. Greenberger NJ, Isselbacher KJ (1991) Diseases of the gallbladder and bile ducts. In: Wilson JD, Braunwald E, Isselbacher KJ et al (eds) Harrison's principles of internal medicine, 12th edn. McGraw-Hill, New York, pp 1358–1368

69. Freitas JE (1994) Cholescintigraphy. In: Murray IPC, Ell PJ (eds) Nuclear medicine in clinical diagnosis and treatment. Churchill Livingstone, London, pp 77–86

70. Ziessman HA (2014) Hepatobiliary scintigraphy in 2014. J Nucl Med Technol 42:249–259

71. Ziessman HA (2010) Nuclear medicine hepatobiliary imaging. Clin Gastroenterol Hepatol 8:111–116

72. Kumar V, Abbas A, Aster JC (2014) Robbins and Cotzan, pathologic basis of disease, 9th edn. Saunders, Philadelphia

73. Shea JA, Berlin JA, Escarce JJ et al (1994) Revised estimates of diagnostic test sensitivity and specificity in suspected biliary tract disease. Arch Intern Med 154:2573–2581

74. Ziessman HA (2003) Acute cholecystitis, biliary obstruction and biliary leakage. Semin Nucl Med 38:279–296

75. Kiewiet JJ, Leeuwenburgh MM, Bipat S, Bossuyt PM, Stoker J, Boermeester MA (2012) A systematic review and metaanalysis of diagnostic performance of imaging in acute cholecystitis. Radiology 264:708–720

76. Colletti PM, Cirimelli KM, Radin DR et al (1989) Radionuclide angiography in suspected acute cholecystitis: further observations. Clin Nucl Med 14:867–873

77. Nahrwold DL (1991) Chronic cholecystitis and cholelithiasis. In: Sabiston DC (ed) Textbook of surgery, 14th edn. Saunders, Philadelphia, pp 1057–1063

78. Kim CK (1998) Scintigraphic evaluation of the liver and biliary tract. In: Gazelle SG, Saini S, Mueller PR (eds) Hepatobiliary and pancreatic radiology: imaging and interventions. Thieme, New York, pp 108–153

79. Bolen G, Javitt NB (1982) Biliary dyskinesia: mechanisms and management. Hosp Pract 17:115–130

80. Misra DC Jr, Blossom GB, Fink-Bennett D et al (1991) Results of surgical therapy for biliary dyskinesia. Arch Surg 126:957–960

81. Fink-Bennett D (1991) Augmented cholescintigraphy: its roles in detecting acute and chronic disorders of the hepatobiliary tree. Semin Nucl Med 21:128–139

82. Zech ER, Simmons LB, Kendrick RR et al (1991) Cholecystokinin enhanced hepatobiliary scanning with ejection fraction calculation as an indicator of disease of the gallbladder. Surg Gynecol Obstet 17:21–24

83. Ziessman HA, Fahey FH, Hixson DJ (1992) Calculation of a gallbladder ejection fraction: advantage of continuous sincalide infusion over the three-minute infusion method. J Nucl Med 33:537–541

84. Torsoli A, Corazziari E, Habib FI, Cicala M (1990) Pressure relationships within the human bile tract. Normal and abnormal physiology. Scand J Gastroenterol Suppl 175:52–57

85. Murphy P, Solomon J, Roseman DL (1980) Narcotic anesthetic drugs: their effect on biliary dynamics. Arch Surg 115:710–711

86. Dedrick DF, Tanner WW, Bushkin FL (1980) Common bile duct pressure during enflurane anesthesia: effects of morphine and subsequent naloxone. Arch Surg 115:820–821

87. Zeman RK, Lee C, Jaffe MH et al (1984) Hepatobiliary scintigraphy and sonography in early biliary obstruction. Radiology 153:793–798

88. Miller DR, Egbert RM, Braunstein P (1984) Comparison of ultrasound and hepatobiliary imaging in the early detection of acute total common bile duct obstruction. Arch Surg 119:1233–1237

89. Rayter Z, Tonge C, Bennett C et al (1991) Ultrasound and HIDA: scanning in evaluating bile leaks after cholecystectomy. Nucl Med Commun 12:197–202

11.1 Anatomic and Physiologic Considerations

11.1.1 Anatomy

The central nervous system consists of the brain and the spinal cord. The major anatomic divisions of the brain are the cerebrum and the cerebellum, together weighing about 1400 g in the adult. Brain cells are classified as glia or neurons. About 10,000 different types of neurons totaling approximately 100 billion neurons comprise the human brain. The cerebral cortex consists of two hemispheres connected by a large mass of white matter called the corpus callosum. The surface layer of each hemisphere is folded into gyri comprising the gray matter. The brain is divided into functional areas called the frontal lobe (anterior to the central sulcus) and the parietal lobe (posterior to this sulcus). The occipital lobe lies below the parieto-occipital sulcus, and the temporal lobe is situated below the lateral sulcus (Figs. 11.1 and 11.2).

Knowledge of cross-sectional anatomy of the brain (Figs. 11.3, 11.4, and 11.5) is a prerequisite for proper interpretation of brain imaging since

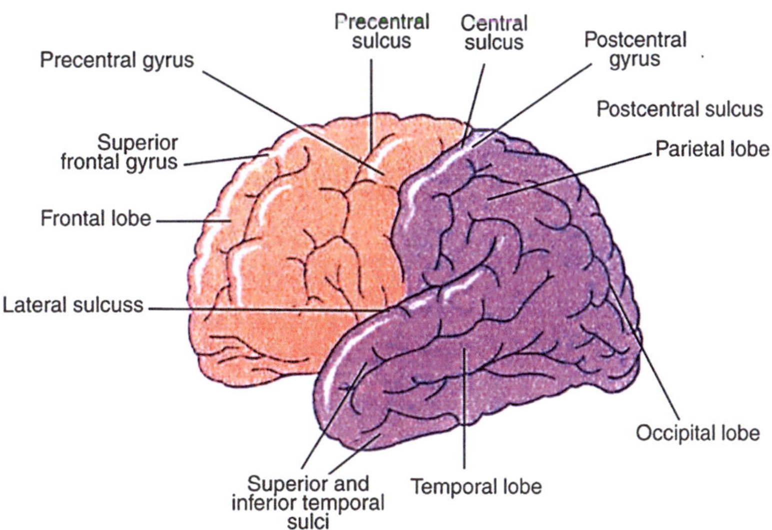

Fig. 11.1 Diagram of the lateral surface of the brain illustrating its main anatomical features

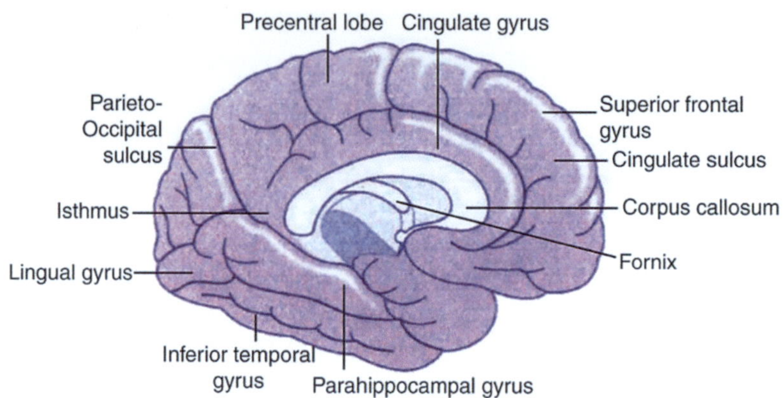

Fig. 11.2 Diagram of the brain illustrating the main internal structures

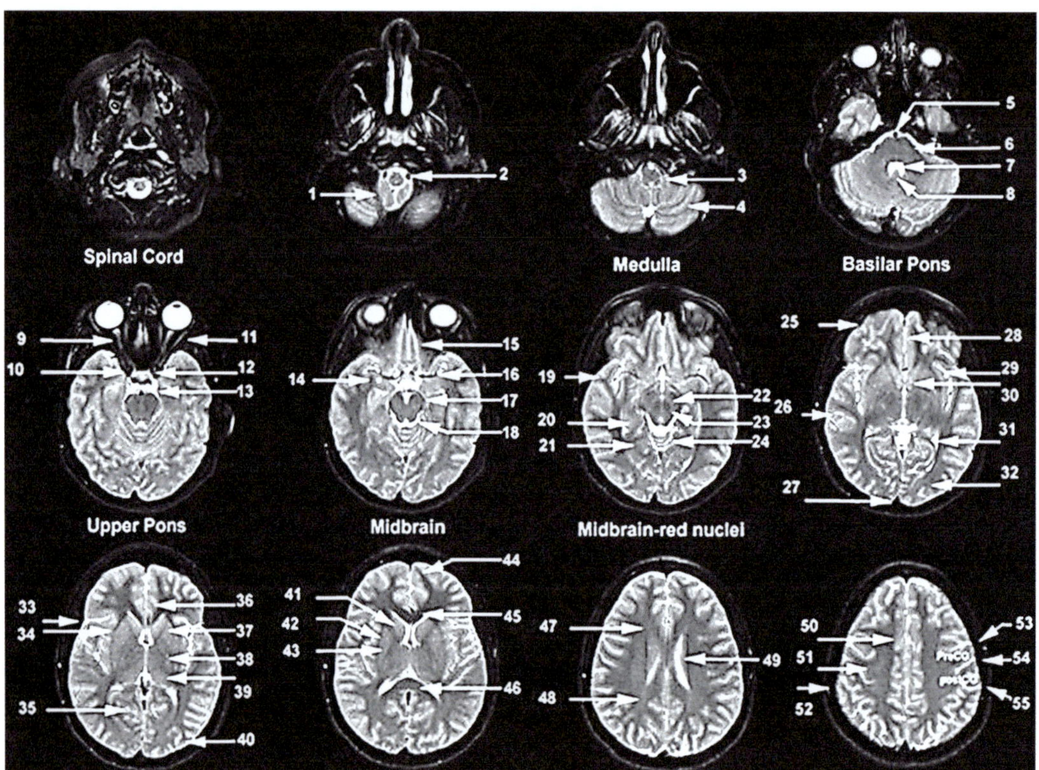

Fig. 11.3 Axial T2-weighted MR images. (*1*) Cerebellar tonsil, (*2*) vertebral artery, (*3*) medulla, (*4*) cerebellar hemisphere, (*5*) basilar artery, (*6*) pons, (*7*) fourth ventricle, (*8*) uvula, (*9*) optic nerve, (*10*) internal carotid artery siphon, (*11*) lateral rectus muscle, (*12*) pituitary gland, (*13*) ambient cistern, (*14*) amygdala, (*15*) gyrus rectus, (*16*) middle cerebral artery, (*17*) posterior cerebral artery, (*18*) mesencephalic cistern, (*19*) temporal pole, (*20*) hippocampus, (*21*) parahippocampal gyrus, (*22*) substantia nigra, (*23*) red nucleus, (*24*) cerebellar vermis, (*25*) frontal lobe, (*26*) temporal lobe, (*27*) superior sagittal sinus, (*28*) gyrus rectus, (*29*) insular cortex, (*30*) anterior commissure, (*31*) posterior horn lateral ventricle, (*32*) occipital lobe, (*33*) Sylvian fissure, (*34*) external capsule, (*35*) calcarine sulcus, (*36*) cingulate gyrus, (*37*) anterior limb of the internal capsule, (*38*) posterior limb of the internal capsule, (*39*) thalamus, (*40*) occipital lobe, (*41*) head of the caudate nucleus, (*42*) putamen, (*43*) globus pallidus, (*44*) frontal pole, (*45*) genu of the corpus callosum, (*46*) splenium of the corpus callosum, (*47*) forceps minor, (*48*) forceps major, (*49*) caudate nucleus, (*50*) cingulate gyrus, (*51*) centrum semiovale, (*52*) calvarial marrow, (*53*) precentral sulcus, (*54*) central sulcus, (*55*) postcentral sulcus. PreCG, precentral gyrus; PostCG, postcentral gyrus

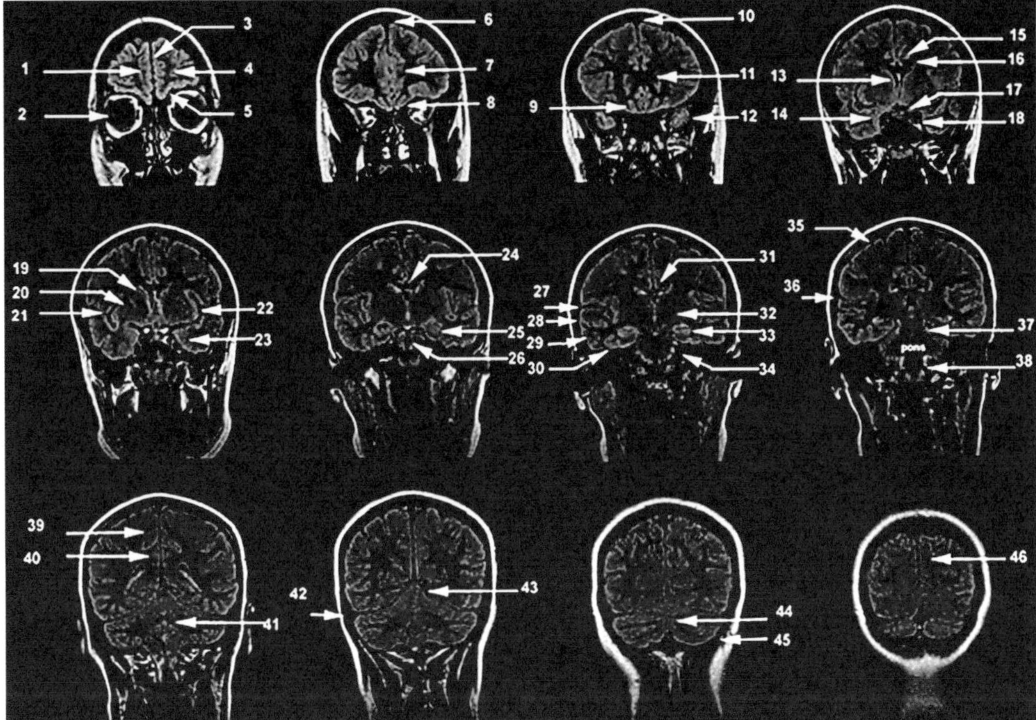

Fig. 11.4 Coronal FLAIR MR images. (*1*) Superior frontal gyrus, (*2*) orbit, (*3*) interhemispheric fissure, (*4*) frontal pole, (*5*) orbital gyrus, (*6*) superior sagittal sinus, (*7*) cingulate gyrus, (*8, 9*) gyrus rectus, (*10*) superior sagittal sinus, (*11*) genu of the corpus callosum, (*12*) temporal pole, (*13*) anterior horn lateral ventricle, (*14*) mesial temporal lobe, (*15*) cingulate gyrus, (*16*) corpus callosum, (*17*) optic nerve, (*18*) cavernous sinus, (*19*) head of the caudate nucleus, (*20*) lenticular nucleus, (*21*) Sylvian fissure, (*22*) insular cortex, (*23*) amygdala, (*24*) corpus cal- losum, (*25*) hippocampus, (*26*) basilar artery, (*27*) Sylvian fissure, (*28*) superior temporal gyrus, (*29*) middle temporal gyrus, (*30*) inferior temporal gyrus, (*31*) cingulate gyrus, (*32*) thalamus, (*33*) parahippocampal gyrus, (*34*) vestibulocochlear nerve, (*35*) central sulcus, (*36*) Sylvian fissure, (*37*) mesencephalon, (*38*) medulla, (*39*) paracentral lobule, (*40*) cingulate gyrus, (*41*) fourth ventricle, (*42*) transverse sinus, (*43*) tentorium, (*44*) cerebellar vermis, (*45*) cerebellar hemisphere, (*46*) cuneus

tomographic imaging is the rule in current functional neuroimaging. The interpretation of brain SPECT and PET studies depends on a background of neuroanatomy which with current techniques allows co-registration of MRI and CT with the functional SPECT and PET images (Figs. 11.3, 11.4, and 11.5).

11.1.2 Physiology

11.1.2.1   Perfusion

Blood flow utilization by neurons is primarily related to synaptic activity at the neuron cell body; thus, gray matter requires about four times as much blood flow as white matter. In the normal brain, the overall determinant of regional cerebral blood flow (rCBF) is dependent on vascular integrity, cerebral anatomy, and cerebral function. Since diseases of the brain can disrupt one or more of these functions, for accurate diagnosis it is important to integrate these three physiological functions with the pattern of rCBF change from normal to arrive at an accurate diagnosis of disease. Perfusion changes noted with SPECT radiotracers are appreciated due to the differences in the cortical gray to white matter perfusion related to the large amount of neurons in the cortex. Coupling of perfusion and metabolism provides functional information regarding

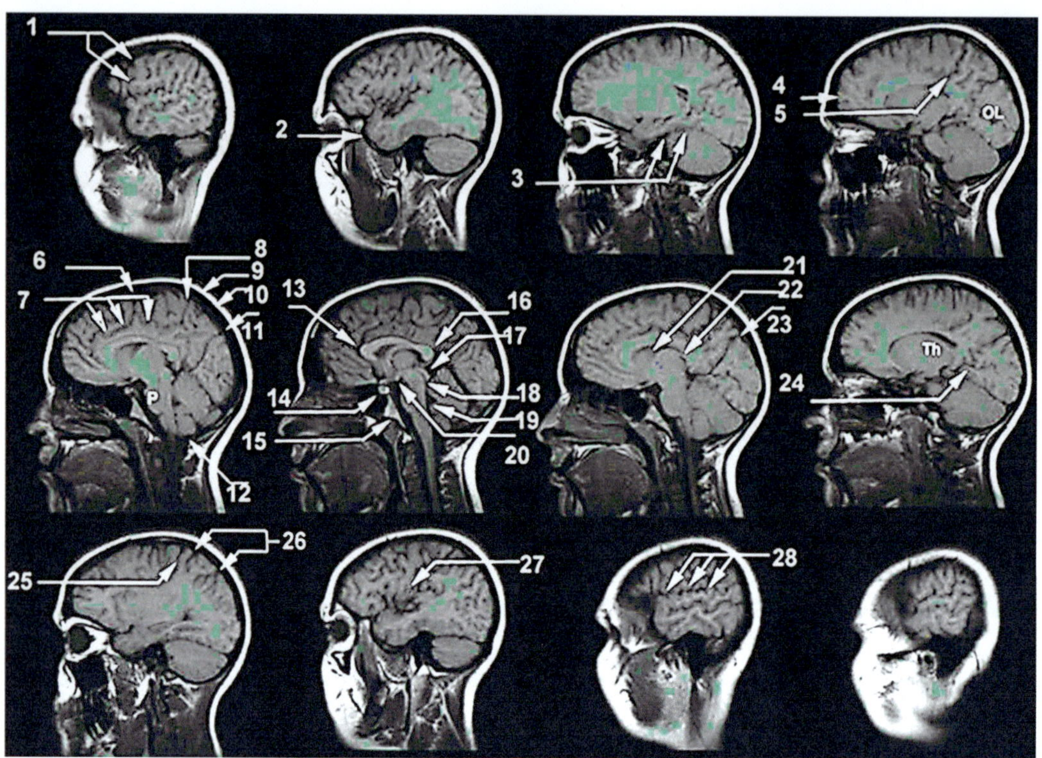

Fig. 11.5 Sagittal T1-weighted MR images. (*1*) Central sulcus, (*2*) temporal pole, (*3*) parahippocampal gyrus, (*4*) frontal pole, (*5*) ascending branch of cingulate sulcus, (*6*) paracentral sulcus, (*7*) cingulate sulcus, (*8*) ascending branch of cingulate sulcus, (*9*) scalp, (*10*) calvarium, (*11*) superior sagittal sinus, (*12*) cerebellar tonsil, (*13*) genu of the corpus callosum, (*14*) pituitary gland, (*15*) clivus, (*16*) splenium of the corpus callosum, (*17*) tectal plate, (*18*) aqueduct of the third ventricle, (*19*) fourth ventricle, (*20*) mammillary body, (*21*) head of the caudate nucleus, (*22*) thalamus, (*23*) parieto-occipital sulcus, (*24*) calcarine sulcus, (*25*) central sulcus, (*26*) postcentral sulcus, (*27*) insular cortex, (*28*) Sylvian fissure. *OL* occipital lobe, *P* pons, *Th* thalamus

the state of the patient during tracer injection with 99mTc-HMPAO and 99mTc-ethyl cysteinate dimer (ECD).

11.1.2.2 Metabolism

In the brain, glucose metabolism provides approximately 95% of adenosine triphosphate (ATP) required for brain function. Under normal physiological conditions, glucose metabolism is tightly connected to neuronal activity. ^{18}F-FDG is an analog of glucose and is taken up by living cells via the normal glucose pathway. ^{18}F-FDG is suitable for imaging regional cerebral glucose consumption with PET since it accumulates in neuronal tissue depending on facilitated transport of glucose and hexokinase-mediated phosphory-

lation. The rationale behind its use as a tracer for cancer diagnosis depends on an increased glycolytic activity in neoplastic cells. The cell alterations related to neoplastic transformation are associated with functional impairments that are discernible before structural alterations occur. Therefore, changes in neuronal activity induced by disease are reflected in an alteration of glucose metabolism.

^{18}F-FDG PET is currently the most accurate in vivo method for the investigation of regional human brain metabolism in health and disease states when conventional morphologic diagnostic modalities (i.e., CT, MRI) do not yet detect any evident for lesions.

11.1.2.3 Cerebrospinal Fluid (CSF)

CSF is a clear fluid similar to blood plasma. The intracranial and spinal cord structures float in CSF and are protected from jolts and blows. Principally, the choroid plexus in the lateral, third, and fourth ventricles produces the major portion of CSF. Normally, between 125 and 150 mL of CSF is circulating within the ventricles and subarachnoid space at any given time. Approximately 600 mL of CSF is produced daily. The CSF normally drains from the lateral ventricles sequentially through the interventricular foramen of Monro, the third ventricle, and the cerebral aqueduct of Sylvius into the fourth ventricle and then leaves the ventricular system through the median foramen of Magendie and two lateral foramina of Luschka. Here, the CSF enters the subarachnoid space. Along the base of the brain, this space extends into a number of lakes called cisterns. The CSF is absorbed through the pacchionian granulations of the pia-arachnoid villi into the superior sagittal sinus.

11.2 Pathophysiology of Relevant Diseases

11.2.1 Cerebrovascular Disease

Cerebrovascular disease, also referred to as stroke, includes all disorders in which an area of the brain is temporarily or permanently affected by lack of blood flow or bleeding. Cerebrovascular diseases include stroke; carotid, vertebral, and intracranial stenoses; aneurysms; and vascular malformations.

The cause may be a blockage of the blood vessel, referred to as "ischemic stroke," or due to a blood vessel which has burst, referred to as "hemorrhagic stroke." Ischemic disease may cause stroke due to plaque rupture or pieces of plaque which have blocked a narrowed artery or when the person's carotid artery has become completely blocked by plaque buildup. In hemorrhagic form, when a person's blood vessel that supplies blood to their brain bursts, it prevents normal blood flow to their brain and permits blood to leak into an area of their brain, destroying tissue.

11.2.2 Dementia

Approximately 3 to 4% of the adult population in the USA demonstrates significant cognitive impairment. In general, the causes of dementia include primary neurodegenerative disorders with the most prevalent being Alzheimer's disease, followed by frontotemporal dementia, Lewy body dementias, Parkinsonian dementia, progressive supranuclear palsy, Pick's disease, cortical basilar degeneration, Huntington's disease, and Wilson's disease [1]. Vascular dementias are categorized as multi-infarct, Binswanger's, and cerebral autosomal dominant arteriopathy with subcortical infarctions and leukoencephalopathy. Inflammatory etiologies include multiple sclerosis and vasculitis. Infectious etiologies include syphilis, human immunodeficiency virus, Lyme disease, and other viral disease and fungal diseases. Cancers are a rare cause of dementia which can be attributed to metastatic disease to the brain. Other causes and physical abnormalities include trauma and hydrocephalus.

It has been documented that approximately 80% of all dementias are attributable to Alzheimer's disease or Lewy body dementia. Vascular dementia comprises approximately 18% of the dementias, with the other dementias less common [2].

11.2.2.1 Alzheimer's Disease (AD)

AD is the most common cause of dementia in the elderly. AD is rarely familial. The sporadic form occurs usually after 65 years of age and accounts for most cases; it most likely results from a combination of genetic and environmental influences.

The only confirmed risk factors for sporadic AD are age and the presence of the E4 allele of *APOE* (apolipoprotein E). The brain of a patient with AD of ten shows marked atrophy, with widened sulci and shrinkage of the gyri. In the great majority of cases, every part of the cerebral cortex is involved; however, the occipital pole is often relatively spared. The cortical ribbon may be thinned and ventricular dilatation apparent, especially in the temporal horn, due to atrophy of the amygdala and hippocampus.

Microscopically, there is a significant loss of neurons, in addition to shrinkage of large cortical neurons. The neuropathological hallmarks of AD include extracellular amyloid plaques and intracellular neurofibrillary tangles. The plaques are spherical structures consisting of a central core of fibrous protein known as amyloid that is surrounded by degenerating or dystrophic nerve endings. Neurofibrillary tangles are found inside neurons and are composed of paired helical filaments of hyperphosphorylated microtubule-associated tau protein. The intracellular deposition may cause disruption of normal cytoskeletal architecture with subsequent neuronal cell death. Neuritic plaques and neurofibrillary tangles are not distributed evenly across the brain in AD but are concentrated in vulnerable neural systems.

11.2.2.2 Other Causes of Dementia

Pick's disease is a rapidly progressing frontal lobe type dementia. Primary progressive aphasia (PPA) is an uncommon type of degenerative dementia characterized by gradual impairment of language function that remains neuropsychologically focal for several years with sparing of the memory domain [3]. Compared with other neurodegenerative disorders that initially affect cognition followed by language impairment, many patients with PPA retain their cognitive functions allowing them to continue with their activities of daily living [3]. "Word-finding" or "naming" difficulty (dystonia) is the most common and earliest clinical presentation of PPA [4].

11.2.3 Epilepsy

Regional cerebral perfusion evaluation in patients with epilepsy has proven to be of significant clinical value for identification of the epileptogenic focus location. The underlying pathophysiology concerning the advantages of using regional cerebral perfusion tracers in epilepsy is based on the clinical observation of an increase in cortical blood flow in the area of seizure discharge on surgery. Therefore, the most valuable use of ^{99m}Tc-HMPAO evaluation of the epilepsy patient is to localize the epileptogenic focus during the ictal state.

11.2.4 Brain Tumors

Brain tumors may be primary or metastatic. Primary tumors are classified by the type of tissue in which they arise. Gliomas come from glial cells such as astrocytes, oligodendrocytes, and ependymal cells. The gliomas, accordingly, include three types: astrocytic tumors (astrocytomas) may grow anywhere in the brain or spinal cord. In adults, astrocytomas most often arise in the cerebrum. In children, they occur in the brainstem, the cerebrum, and the cerebellum. A grade III astrocytoma is sometimes called anaplastic astrocytoma. A grade IV astrocytoma is usually called glioblastoma multiforme (the most aggressive type of all primary brain tumors).

Oligodendroglial tumors (oligodendrogliomas) arise in the cells that produce myelin which is the fatty covering that protects nerves. The tumors usually arise in the cerebrum. They grow slowly and usually do not spread into surrounding brain tissue. Ependymomas usually develop in the lining of the ventricles. They may also occur in the spinal cord. Some primary brain tumors are made up of both astrocytic and oligodendrocytic tumors. These are called mixed gliomas.

Meningiomas arise from the meninges, they are usually benign. Because these tumors grow very slowly, the brain may be able to adjust to their presence; meningiomas may grow quite large before they cause symptoms. Schwannomas are benign tumors that grow from Schwann cells, which produce the myelin that protects peripheral nerves. Acoustic neuromas are a type of schwannoma, they occur mainly in adults. These tumors affect women twice as often as men. Other rare tumors are craniopharyngiomas, pituitary tumors, primary CNS lymphoma, pineal gland tumors, and primary germ cell tumors of the brain. Most primary brain tumors do not metastasize, but if they do metastasize, intracranial spread generally precedes distant spread.

Metastatic brain tumors are five times more common than primary brain tumors. The most common types of cancer that cause metastatic brain tumors are lung cancer, breast cancer, melanoma, colon cancer, renal cell carcinoma, and thyroid cancer. Metastatic brain tumors from non-CNS primary tumors may be the first sign of malignancy. Nonetheless, the signs and symptoms of brain metastases simulate those of primary brain tumors.

Brain tumors, primary or metastatic, produce neurological manifestations by several mechanisms. Tumors can invade and infiltrate normal parenchymal tissue, disrupting normal function. Since brain is contained in the limited volume of the cranial vault, growth of intracranial tumors with accompanying edema may cause increased intracranial pressure. Tumors may generate new blood vessels (angiogenesis), disrupting the normal blood–brain barrier and promoting edema. Small, critically located tumors may damage specific neural pathways traversing the brain. Tumors located adjacent to the third and fourth ventricles may impede the flow of cerebrospinal fluid causing obstructive hydrocephalus.

The cumulative effects of tumor invasion, edema, and hydrocephalus may elevate the intracranial pressure which impairs cerebral perfusion. Compartmental rise of intracranial pressure may lead to shifting or herniation of tissue under the falx cerebri, through the tentorium cerebelli, or through the foramen magnum. Leptomeningeal infiltration may present with dysfunction of multiple cranial nerves.

11.2.5 Hydrocephalus

The term hydrocephalus generally refers to those conditions that produce an imbalance between the rate of production and absorption of the cerebrospinal fluid, leading to dilatation of the ventricular system. Hydrocephalus normally occurs as a result of obstruction to the flow and absorption of CSF, although there are rare cases of choroid plexus papillomas causing hydrocephalus by overproduction of CSF.

Hydrocephalus is traditionally classified as communicating and noncommunicating, based on whether ventricular obstruction is present. In the former, the ventricular system continues to communicate with the subarachnoid spaces outside the brain through the fourth ventricular foramina of Luschka and Magendie. Noncommunicating hydrocephalus correspondingly refers to the presence of occlusion within the ventricular system. Hydrocephalus may be either congenital or acquired. Arnold-Chiari malformation, Dandy-Walker malformations, and aqueductal stenosis/atresia are common causes of the congenital variety. In the acquired type, many pathological conditions, including inflammatory, infectious, traumatic, and neoplastic disorders, can cause hydrocephalus [5, 6].

Noncommunicating hydrocephalus can be the result of intraventricular mass, aqueductal obstruction, or fourth ventricular obstruction. Communicating hydrocephalus, however, results from meningitis, meningeal carcinomatosis, or cerebral dural sinus thrombosis, otitis idiopathic in elderly patients. Normal-pressure hydrocephalus (NPH) is a communicating hydrocephalus of particular interest to nuclear medicine professional since radionuclide cisternography is useful in its diagnosis and management.

In NPH, the usual flow of CSF is impaired somewhere in the intracranial subarachnoid space, resulting in a reversal of CSF flow and dilatation of the lateral ventricles. There is free communication between the ventricular system and the subarachnoid pathways and no elevation of CSF pressure. Clinically, the entity occurs in patients 50–70 years of age and is characterized by dementia, gait disturbances, and fecal and urinary incontinence. Most commonly, this condition results from subarachnoid hemorrhage or meningoencephalitis.

11.2.6 Cerebrospinal Fluid Leakage

Leaking of CSF may be etiologically classified into:

1. Traumatic: occurring in about 30% of basilar skull fractures. Two percent of all head injuries develop a CSF fistula. This leak is usually unilateral, scanty, and seen within 48 h after trauma and resolves in 1 week.
2. Nontraumatic: taking place in tumors (pituitary, brain, and skull), skull infections, and congenital defects (encephalocele). This leak is profuse and may persist for years. Infection complicates the untreated leak in 25–50% of cases.

CSF rhinorrhea may occur anywhere from the frontal sinus to the temporal bone. The cribriform plate is the most susceptible to fracture and rhinorrhea. Otorrhea is much less common [7, 8].

11.2.7 Brain Death

Death is an irreversible, biological event that consists of permanent cessation of the critical functions of the organism as a whole. It implies permanent absence of cerebral and brain stem functions. Brain death then qualifies as death (as brain is essential for integrating critical functions of the body). The equivalence of brain death with death is largely but not universally accepted.

The concept of irreversible coma or brain death was first described in 1959, predating widespread organ donation. The fundamental definition of brain death has substantively remained constant over time and across countries (although specific details of diagnostic criteria differ). Many conditions are known to cause brain death (Table 11.1).

Table 11.1 Causes of brain death

Trauma and subarachnoid hemorrhage: Most common
Intracerebral hemorrhage
Hypoxic ischemic encephalopathy
Ischemic stroke
Any condition causing permanent widespread brain injury

11.3 Scintigraphic Evaluation of CNS Diseases

11.3.1 Radiopharmaceuticals

In addition to ^{111}In-DTPA and ^{99m}Tc-DTPA used for CSF imaging (radionuclide cisternography), there are three main classes of radiopharmaceuticals available for functional brain imaging in nuclear medicine.

1. Regional cerebral blood flow agents.

   SPECT radiopharmaceuticals used for measuring regional cerebral blood flow (rCBF) are lipophilic agents which are transported from the arterial vascular compartment to the normal brain tissue compartment by diffusion and are distributed proportionally to regional tissue blood flow. After this first phase of transport, the tracers are essentially irreversibly trapped in the tissue compartment. The two major blood flow agents used in brain SPECT imaging are technetium-99 m hexamethyl propylene amine oxime (^{99m}Tc-HMPAO) and technetium-99 methyl cysteinate dimer (^{99m}Tc-ECD) [9–11]. Xenon-133 (^{133}Xe) is unique since it is freely diffusible and not trapped in the tissues. Inhaled or i.v. injection of ^{133}Xe dissolved in saline can more accurately and quantitatively provide measurements of blood flow by determination of the clearance rate of this tracer from the cerebral compartment, after a brief uptake period [12]. The major PET radiopharmaceutical used to measure cerebral perfusion is ^{15}OH$_2$O [5].
2. Regional cerebral metabolism agents.

   These radiopharmaceuticals are transported to the brain tissues by regional cerebral blood flow, but subsequent regional cerebral distribution reflects the utilization rate of the tracer in a cerebral metabolic pathway. Currently, there are no SPECT tracers that specifically measure normal cerebral metabolism. However, in brain tumor imaging, where the blood–brain barrier is broken, ionic tracers such as thallium-201 [13] or other SPECT tracers such as ^{99m}Tc-methoxyisobutylisonitrile (^{99m}Tc-MIBI) [14] can be used to detect new, recurrent, or residual viable tumor. The PET radiopharmaceutical predominantly used is fluorine-182-fluoro-2-deoxy-D-glucose ($^{18F\text{-}FDG}$) [15]. [^{18}F]-fluoro-3'-deoxy-3'-L-FLUOROTHYMIDINE (FLT) is a newer tracer used to indicate tumor proliferation to more specifically identify new, recurrent, or residual viable brain tumor.

3. Central nervous system receptor-binding agents.

This class of radiotracers important in brain imaging is central nervous system receptor-binding agents, which measure neuronal receptor density and binding affinity [16]. InSPECT, a dopamine transporter receptor-binding agent which has been well characterized is ^{123}I-i of lupane. This benzamide compound has been used to image the dopaminergic (D2) transporter system in the corpus striatum [10].

Table 11.2 Summarizes the radiopharmaceuticals used for Imaging CNS conditions.

Table 11.2 Radiopharmaceuticals for CNS imaging

In-111-DTPA
Tc99m DTPA
Tc99m-Hexamethylpropyleneamine oxime (99mTc-HMPAO)
Tc99m-ethyl cysteinate dimer (99mTc-ECD)
^{133}Xe for quantitative regional cerebral blood flow
O-15-water for quantitative regional cerebral perfusion measured by PET
Thallium-201
Tc99m-Hexakis-2-methoxy-2-isobutyl isonitrile (99mTc-Sestamibi)
F-18-Fluoro-2-deoxy-D-glucose (F-18-FDG)
L-methyl-C-11 methionine (C-11-MET)
O-(2-F-18 fluoroethyl)-L-tyrosine (F-18-FET)
3, 4-Dihydroxy-6-$^{18F\text{-fluoro-I}}$-phenylalanine (^{18}F-FDOPA)
F-18-Fluoromisonidazole (F-18-FMISO)
3'-deoxy-3'-F-18-fluorothymidine (18F-FLT)
Ga-68 DOTATATE

11.3.2 Scintigraphic Imaging Techniques

SPECT (Fig. 11.6) and PET (Fig. 11.7) imaging are both used for brain imaging. ^{18}F-FDGPET studies should be performed during "a resting state" (e.g., eyes open, ears unoccluded in a dark room with minimal ambient noise). Procedures to minimize head movement during scan acquisition should be implemented using well-tolerated head immobilization procedures. The use of medications and the behavioral state of patients at the time of the scan also should be carefully taken into account since they may produce changes in cerebral metabolism that could alter ^{18}F-FDG tracer distribution.

The normal brain has high ^{18}F-FDG uptake (Fig. 11.7), and therefore administration of approximately 10 mCi ^{18}F-FDG i.v. is sufficient. The PET scanner should be of the latest generation, full ring and multislice to cover the entire brain. The 3D acquisition mode should be used to accommodate lower dosimetry and to improve the count statistics of the data. Measured attenuation correction should be employed. The image should be reconstructed with the standard clinical reconstruction including all necessary corrections (such as for random, scatter, and attenuation). Quality control with calibration phantoms should be performed in order to assure qualitative accuracy (e.g., using the Hoffman brain phantom) and quantitative accuracy (e.g., using a uniform cylinder phantom) and should be run periodically to assess scanner stability [17].

For CSF imaging a radionuclide (usually^{111}In-DTPA) is injected into the CSF system, usually via the lumbar subarachnoid space. For NPH, skull imaging is performed up to 72 h following injection of the radiopharmaceutical in the anterior, posterior, lateral, and vertical projections. For CSF leak, images are also obtained for the same duration and projections, depending on the suspected site of leakage [6, 7].

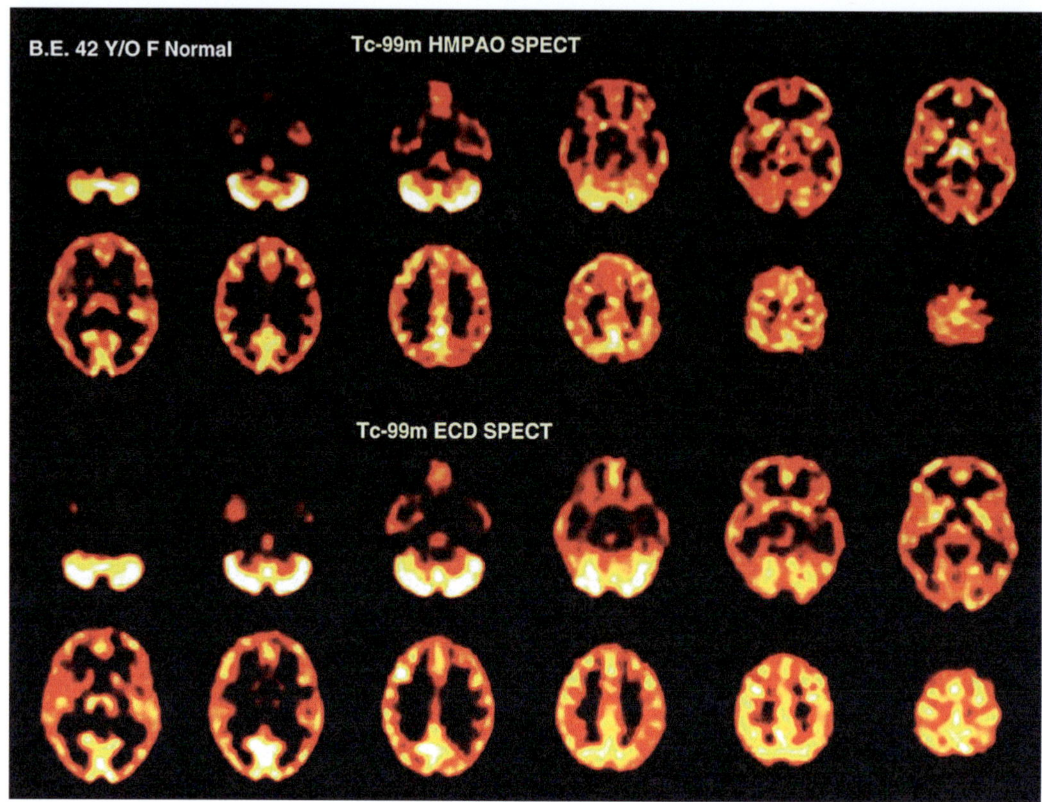

Fig. 11.6 Images of a ^{99m}Tc-HMPAO brain SPECT scan (**a**) compared with a ^{99m}Tc-ECD brain SPECT scan (**b**) for a 42-year-old normal female. There is high uptake of tracer in the cerebellum (*top row*), the thalamus and basal ganglia (second row from *top*), and the primary visual cortex. There is high uptake in all cortical structures compared to white matter. The ^{99m}Tc-HMPAO brain SPECT scan shows increased tracer uptake in the thalami but less uptake in the parietal and occipital regions, as compared to the ^{99m}Tc-ECD brain SPECT scan

11.3.3 Major Clinical Applications of Scintigraphy

11.3.3.1 Cerebrovascular Disease

Diamox-enhanced SPECT is useful in assessment of vascular reserve and is of value in identification of patients at risk for stroke [18]. Diamox SPECT scans may provide objective evidence for the selection of patients with a high-grade asymptomatic carotid stenosis who will benefit from carotid endarterectomy (Fig. 11.8).

The standard vasoreactive stress protocol is to first perform a resting state ^{99m}Tc-HMPAO brain SPECT scan to assess the blood flow to the vascular territories of the brain. In many cases in patients with TIA, the blood flow is often symmetric or may show small regions of cortical hypoperfusion due to small embolic infarctions. The vasoreactive challenge SPECT is best to perform the rest-vasoreactive comparative test on two separate days using the same dose. After the intravenous administration of one gram of Diamox and waiting 15 min, there is an increase in CO_2 in the brain which causes dilatation of the vasculature. There is an increase in the blood flow to normal brain of about 30%, and areas of hemodynamic constraint can be identified since CVD patients may be at the limit of their vasoreactive reserve before Diamox and, therefore, will illustrate no increase in perfusion as compared to normal vascular territories of the brain which can accommodate a 30% increase in blood flow [1, 18].

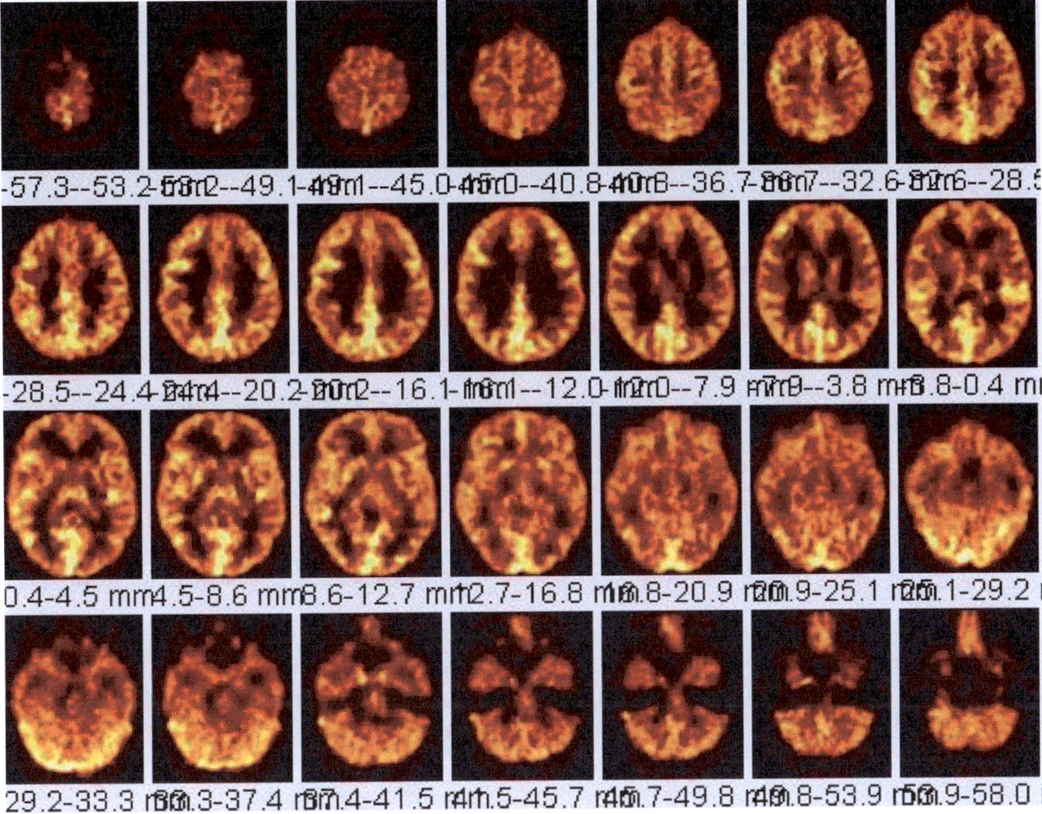

Fig. 11.7 Normal PET in a 36-year-old normal female volunteer underwent fully dynamic ^{18}F-FDG PET at rest

11.3.3.2 Alzheimer's Disease

The rationale for imaging as a diagnostic tool for Alzheimer's disease is based on the condition's associated reduction in metabolic brain activity. This can be visualized on both ^{18}F-FDG brain PET and ^{99m}Tc-HMPAO or ^{99m}Tc-ECD brain SPECT. There is a reduction of brain glucose metabolism identified on PET due to reduced neuronal metabolism and synaptic activity. A reduction in brain perfusion on regional cerebral perfusion SPECT is identified as a decrease in blood flow and reduction in neuronal and synaptic activity (proportional to the blood flow) in areas of reduced metabolism caused by amyloid deposition, a finding characteristic of Alzheimer's disease. The characteristic findings on ^{18}F-FDG brain PET and regional cerebral perfusion SPECT are as follows: (1) often bilateral involvement with asymmetry of reduction in the posterior temporoparietal cortical areas, (2) reduction of metabolism and blood flow to the posterior cingulate gyrus, and (3) less common primary visual cortex involvement (which is more common in Lewy body dementia).

11.3.3.2.1 SPECT Imaging

Alzheimer's disease is characterized by low global blood flow with accentuation of the diminution in the posterior temporoparietal lobes, relative sparing of the thalamus and corpus striatum as well as the sensorimotor cortex, and late involvement of the frontal lobes (Fig. 11.9). In the differential diagnosis of both Alzheimer's disease and vascular dementia, the cerebellum is often useful as a structure for semiquantitative normalization of blood flow since it is relatively uninvolved in most cases of progressive cerebral cognitive decline.

It is important to distinguish, on a rCBF brain SPECT scan, the differences between a progres-

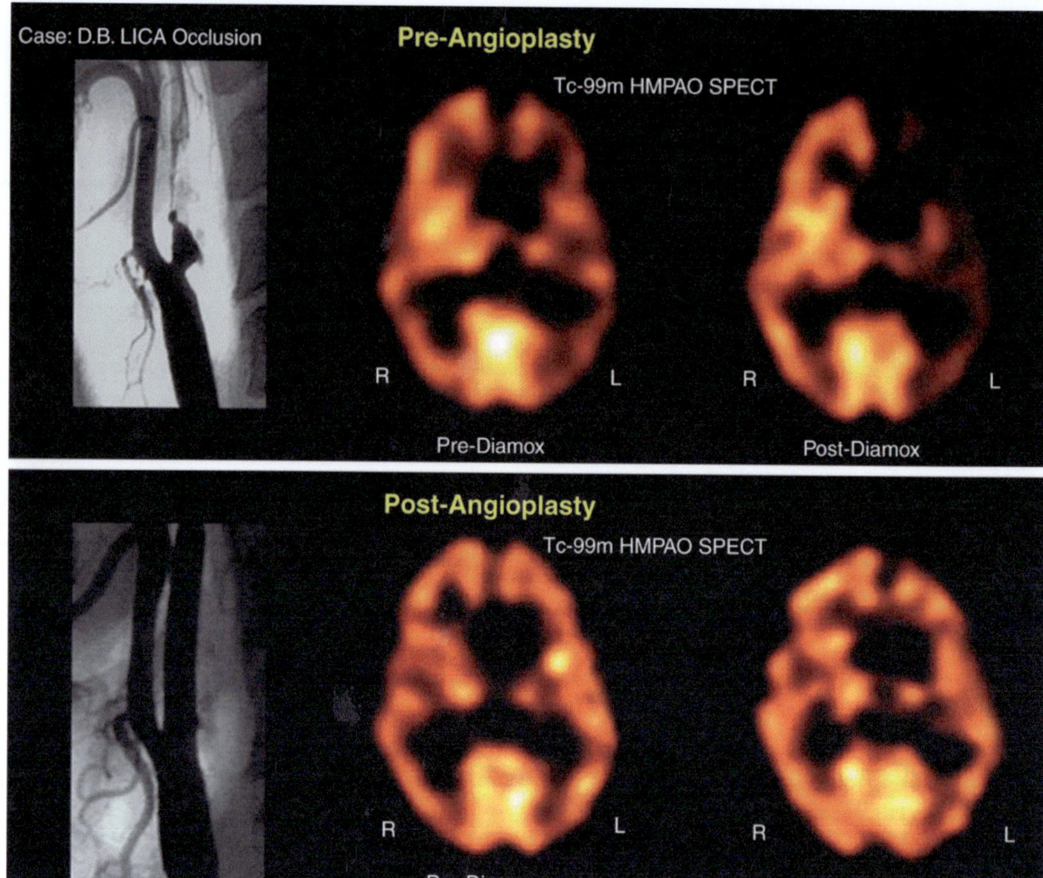

Fig. 11.8 Angiogram showing complete left ICA occlusion in a patient with transient ischemic symptoms (**a**). The resting scan (**b**) shows slight reduction of blood flow to the left ICA distribution. The post-Diamox scan (**c**) shows significant relative reduction of rCBF to the left ICA territory as compared to the remainder of the brain. The *bottom row of images* shows the results after angioplasty. The angiogram (**d**) now shows a patent left internal carotid artery. The resting ⁹⁹ᵐTc-HMPAO brain SPECT scan (**e**) shows a more symmetric perfusion of tracer distribution at rest. More importantly, after Diamox, there is no relative reduction in the left hemisphere as compared to the right hemisphere (**f**)

sive degenerative dementia such as Alzheimer's disease and a vascular dementia, usually from hemodynamic compromise or embolic vascular disease at the internal carotid artery level or higher. The importance of this differentiation now extends beyond the theoretical issue of clinical diagnosis and prognosis, since currently therapeutic protocols have now been established for these two causes of memory impairment [19].

11.3.3.2.2   ¹⁸F-FDGPET Imaging

Accurate and early diagnosis of Alzheimer's disease (AD) is vital to ensure patients receive the proper treatment, research is targeted correctly, and prevention and cures are found. However, it can be difficult to distinguish between AD and other forms of dementia, or even from other reversible disorders such as severe depression.

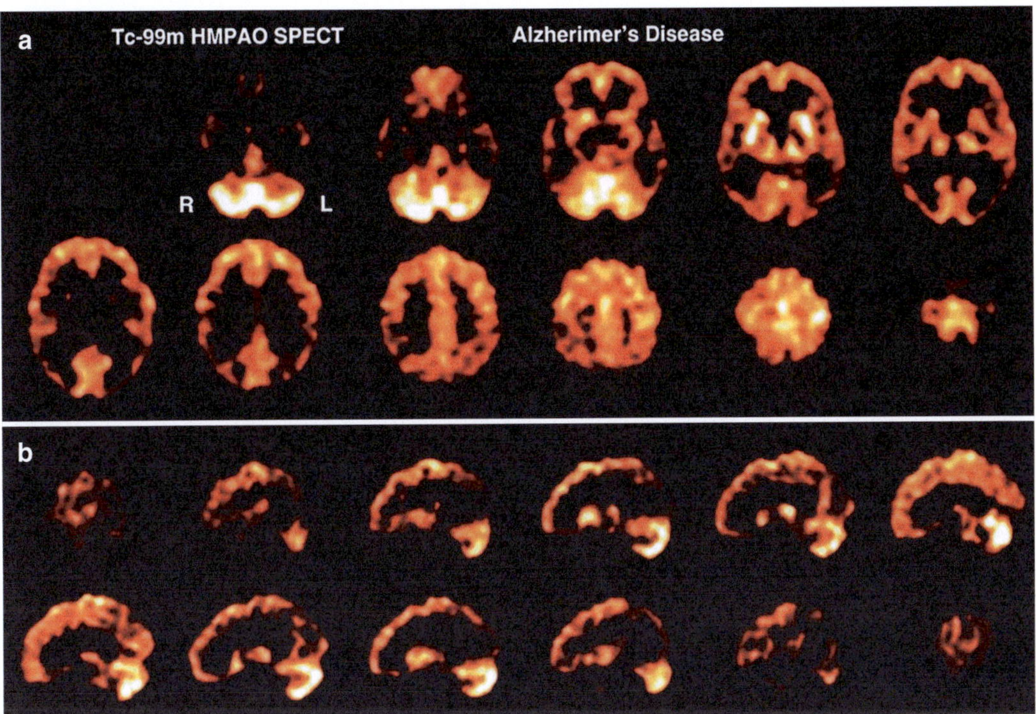

Fig. 11.9 ^{99m}Tc-HMPAO brain SPECT scan of a 67-year-old female with Alzheimer's disease. Transverse sections (**a**) and sagittal sections (**b**) show global decrease in blood flow to essentially all cortical structures (relative to the cerebellum) with accentuation of the decrease in the posterior temporal parietal region. There is relatively spared uptake in the cerebellum, caudate head, lentiform, and thalamus

The Center for Medicare and Medicaid Services (CMS) decided that an ^{18}F-FDG brain PET scan (Fig. 11.10) is reasonable and necessary in patients with a recently established diagnosis of dementia with documented cognitive decline for at least 6 months who have met the criteria for both Alzheimer's disease and frontotemporal dementia and who have been evaluated for specific alternate neurodegenerative diseases or causative factors for which the cause of clinical symptoms remains uncertain.

11.3.3.3 Vascular Dementia

Patients with vascular dementia may show relatively normal perfusions in areas not involved with vascular disease. These patients may benefit from a revascularization procedure before any further dementia or frank infarction occurs. A common form of vascular dementia is produced by small embolic events, and, therefore, small punctate cortical ribbon breaks may be observed in these patients. In addition, there tends to be more involvement of the frontal lobes as compared to the posterior regions of the brain. Finally, the subcortical structures or internal capsule region may demonstrate asymmetry in blood flow due to the presence of small embolic events in these locations. Figure 11.11 illustrates a case of vascular dementia.

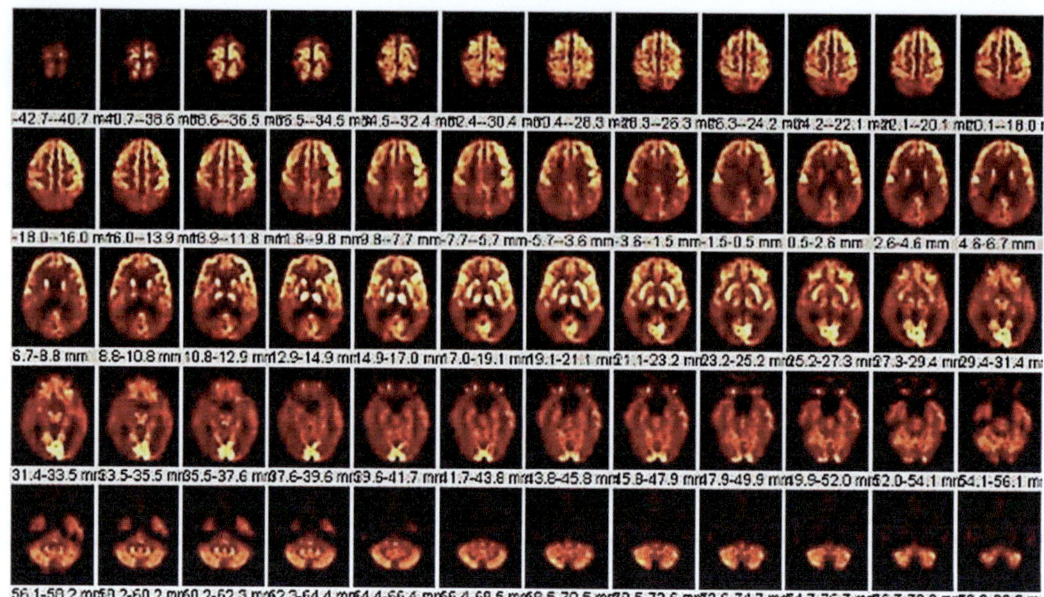

Fig. 11.10 ^{18}F-FDG brain PET scan in transverse section illustrating significant reduction in regional glucose metabolism in the posterior temporoparietal lobes bilaterally. The patient is a 52-year-old male with symptoms of cognitive impairment and memory loss for 2 years. The patient satisfied the ADRDA criteria for probable Alzheimer's disease with a Folstein Mini Mental Status measuring 16 out of 30. In addition to significant reduction of ^{18}F-FDG uptake involving the temporoparietal lobes bilaterally, there is also significant reduction in the posterior cingulate gyrus region. There is relative sparing in the sensorimotor cortical area and basal ganglia region

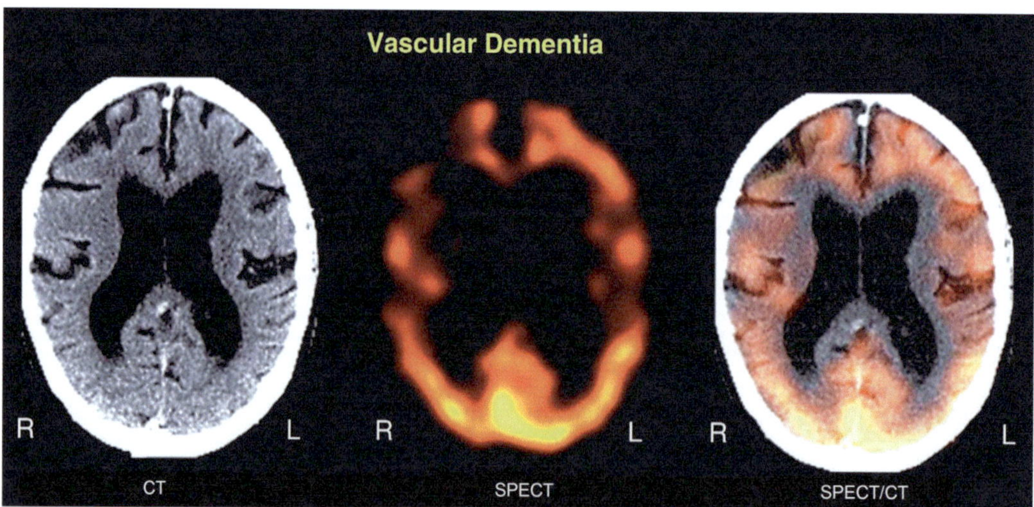

Fig. 11.11 Sixty-two-year-old male with bilateral MCA chronic ischemia and transient ischemic attacks. The image shows a CT scan of the patient (*left*), a corresponding section from the ^{99m}Tc-HMPAO brain SPECT scan (*middle*), and the CT SPECT fusion image (*right*). The CT scan shows atrophy with areas of tissue loss characteristic of small embolic infarctions. The ^{99m}Tc-HMPAO brain SPECT scan through the same level shows the regular uptake in the cortical structures with diminutions at the 2 o'clock and 4 o'clock as well as the 8 o' clock and 11 o'clock positions, which is characteristic of embolic disease. There is no reduction of rCBF to the posterior portion of the brain as noted in the case of Alzheimer's disease (Fig. 11.9)

11.3.3.4   Epilepsy: Epileptogenic Focus Localization Imaging

11.3.3.4.1   Ictal ⁹⁹ᵐTc-HMPAO or ⁹⁹ᵐTc-ECDSPECT

In order to perform these studies, ⁹⁹ᵐTc-HMPAO must be readily available at the patient's bedside allowing for rapid injection by a trained technologist or other personnel immediately available at the time of seizure onset. The ictal injection should be performed in a rapid bolus fashion such that the entire tracer is injected before the seizure abates. The patient is then stabilized and transferred to the SPECT scanner within several hours to receive a brain SPECT scan which will indicate the regional cerebral perfusion at the time of ictus. This method is feasible since ⁹⁹ᵐTc-HMPAO is irreversibly trapped in the epileptogenic hyperemic region at the time of seizure and during the period between injection and scan there is essentially no redistribution. The subsequent scan (albeit several hours after the injection) still shows hyperemia in the region of the epileptogenic focus. Several articles [20–23] characterize the brain propagation patterns of the epileptogenic electrocortical discharge and resultant rCBF hyperemia to allow for more accurate localization of the epileptogenic focus (Figs. 11.12) in cases where two or more cortical areas are seen to be hyperemic on the brain SPECT scan. A very common pattern of propagation of activity observed in frontal lobe seizures is ipsilateral basal ganglia activation and contralateral cerebellar activation. Automated Injector was introduced to monitor epilepsy [24].

11.3.3.4.2   ¹⁸F-FDG Brain PET Assessment in the Interictal State

It has been shown that ictal SPECT in patients with extra-temporal lobe epilepsy has superior localization capability as compared to interictal ¹⁸F-FDGPET. Conversely, if ictal SPECT is not available, identification of the epileptogenic focus during the interictal state using ⁹⁹ᵐTc-HMPAO is less sensitive compared to interictal ¹⁸F-FDGPET. In cases of suspected temporal lobe epilepsy, the preferred diagnostic method is to perform interictal ¹⁸F-FDGPET in addition to ictal and interictal SPECT.

11.3.3.5   Psychiatry and Learning Disabilities

Studies have shown a relationship between rCBF and negative depressive symptoms [25]. The diagnostic application of rCBF SPECT brain scanning in psychiatry is limited (on an individual patient basis).

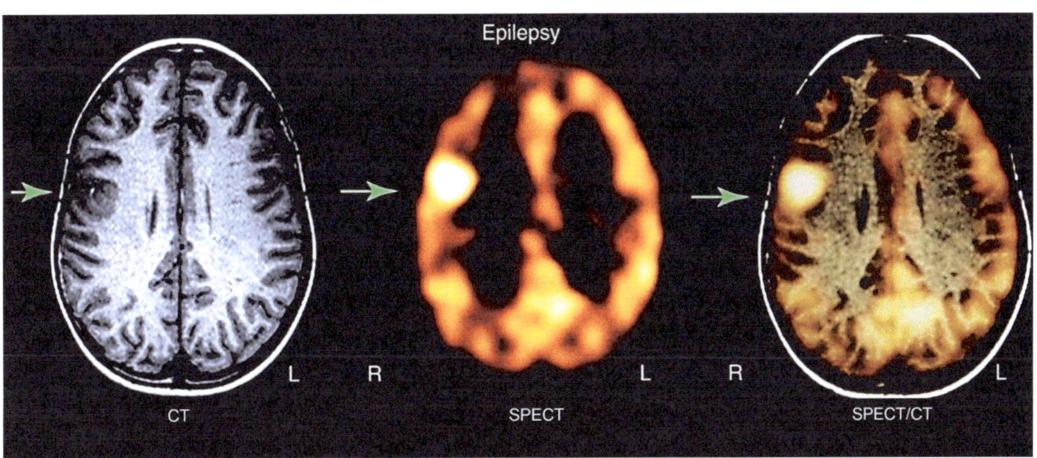

Fig. 11.12 Frontal lobe epilepsy in a 9-year-old right-handed boy. The MRI (*left*) is normal. The ⁹⁹ᵐTc-HMPAO brain SPECT scan (*middle*) reflects the regional cerebral perfusion at the time the tracer was injected during the epileptogenic seizure. ASPECTMRI fusion image (*right*) clearly identifies the location of the focus on the MRI scan

11.3.3.6   Brain Death

Diagnosis of brain death is clinical with tests available for confirmation and documentation. These confirmatory tests include:

1. EEG with no physiological brain activity.
2. Absent cerebral circulation on angiography or scintigraphy (the principal legal sign in the USA and many European countries).
3. Confirmatory imaging for brain death:
   (a) Cerebral angiography.
       Lack of intracranial perfusion other than filling of the superior sagittal sinus is strongly confirmatory of brain death on a selective 4-vessel angiogram with iodinated contrast medium.
   (b) Radionuclide scanning.
       No tracer uptake in the brain parenchyma indicates brain death (Fig. 11.13). This study is increasingly used as an alternative to cerebral angiography. Imaging uses a radioactively labeled substance that readily crosses the blood–brain barrier such as ^{99m}Tc-HMPAO.

11.3.3.7   Brain Tumors

Identification of viable tumor after brain tumor therapy is a significant clinical problem since distinction between necrosis and residual or recurrent viable tumor cannot be accurately evaluated by either computed tomography or magnetic resonance imaging [26–28]. Functional imaging can distinguish cerebral necrosis from viable brain tumor and determine viability grade [29–31]. This can be determined by ^{201}Tl, ^{99m}Tc-sestamibi, or ^{18}F-FDGPET imaging.

The main utility of thallium in brain SPECT imaging is in the visualization of primary and metastatic CNS tumor. Blood–brain barrier (BBB) breakdown in any lesion of the brain allows the passage and localization of thallium-201. After intravenous administration, the first 5 min of ^{201}Tl uptake depends on rCBF, rCBV, and BBB breakdown. Subsequently the uptake depends on active transport by the tumor cell [32], tumor grade [33], and activity of the Na$^+$/K$^+$ ATPase pump. Thallium-201 is therefore an extremely sensitive but sometimes nonspecific indicator of residual recurrent viable tumor since there is nonspecific uptake in regions of blood–brain barrier breakdown not due to tumor.

Early response to treatment can theoretically be determined by comparing ^{99m}Tc-MIBI or ^{201}Tl uptake before and after a course of radiation or chemotherapy. Decline in the $^{99m\text{Tc-MIBI}}$ or ^{201}Tl uptake ratio may indicate lethal injury or decreased viability of neoplastic cells and effective response to treatment.

Each of the tracers shows increased uptake in recurrent viable tumor. It has been postulated that

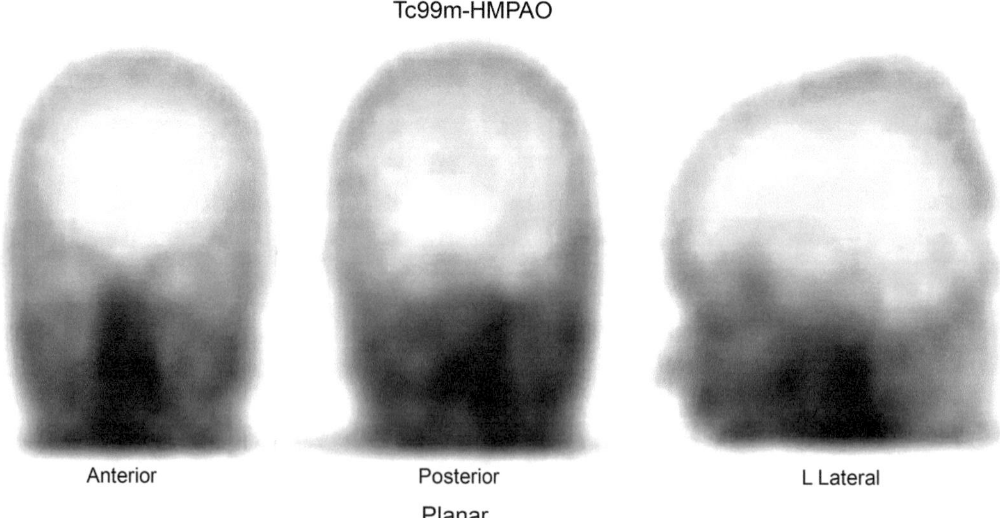

Fig. 11.13 Brain death: No intracranial activity is seen on planar ^{99m}Tc HMPAO study compared to Fig. 11.14 which shows normal findings

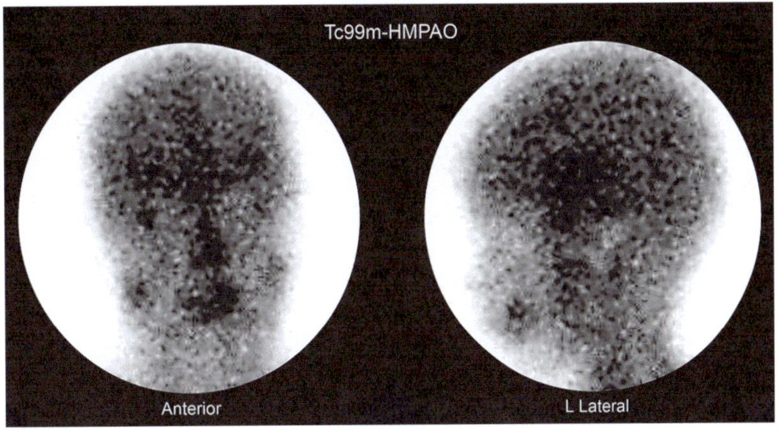

Fig. 11.14 Cerebral perfusion imaging of a 16-month-old boy after near-drowning incident. After injection 6 mCi of ^{99m}Tc-HMPAO IV study was obtained. The static images demonstrate radiotracer activity in the brain. These findings are not suggestive of brain death

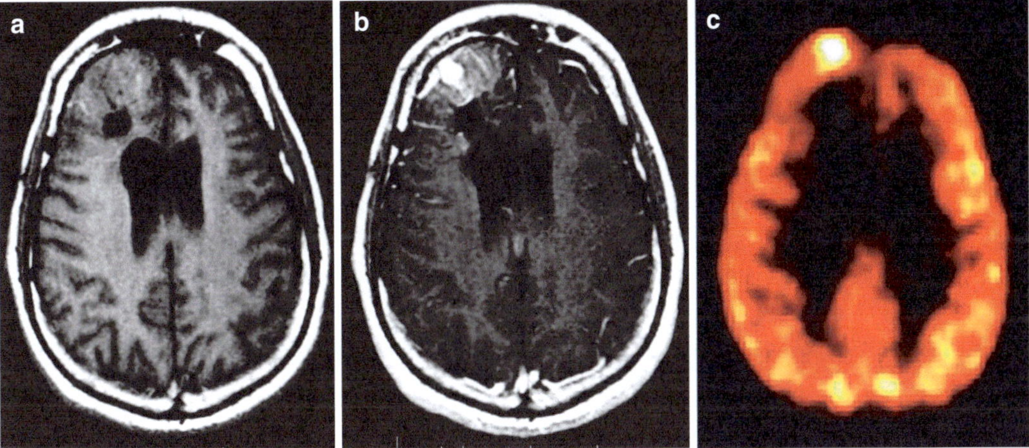

Fig. 11.15 Non-contrast MRI scan (**a**) with abnormality involving the right frontal lobe. Contrast MRI scan (**b**) shows enhancement in the right frontal lobe. Pet (**c**) shows a focal area of increased ^{18}F-FDG uptake involving the right frontal lobe consistent with high-grade transformation and recurrence of tumor in the right frontal lobe 8 years after initial diagnosis, therapy, and complete remission

thallium-201 is taken up by the sodium-potassium ATPase activity and reflects global cellular energetics. Conversely, the uptake of ^{99m}Tc-MIBI is related to mitochondrial energetics, and high uptake of ^{99m}Tc-MIBI possibly indicates a poor prognosis since the tumor continues to have a high glycolytic rate, glucose utilization, and good repair mechanisms. The reduction of MIBI immediately after chemotherapy indicates that there is DNA damage (both to the nucleus and the mitochondrial DNA) with impairment of the TCA cycle and involved glycolytic enzymes. This compromises the production of ATP and cripples the cellular reparative mechanisms such that the tumor is less able to recover from chemotherapy damage and, therefore, the patient has a better prognosis. It is suggested that the use of MIBI before and after

chemotherapy treatment may be used as an indicator for the efficacy of a specific type of chemotherapy, possibly after one dose. This would permit several trials to be performed to determine the most efficacious chemotherapy before complete treatment is instituted allowing the patient to remain relatively refractory from the hematological and other side effects of the chemo therapy.

^{18}F-FDG is a less sensitive but more specific tracer for the detection of recurrent or residual viable tumor (Fig. 11.15) as compared to thallium-201 which is a more sensitive but less specific tracer due to nonspecific BBB breakdown accumulation. The lack of sensitivity of ^{18}F-FDG is due to the fact that it is taken up by the normal brain. The lack of specificity of thallium-201 is due to the fact that it accumulates at the site of blood–brain barrier breakdown prior to its uptake through the Na⁺/K⁺ ATPase pump. However, early and delayed uptake ratio significantly improves specificity.

Recently somatostatin imaging agents such as gallium 68 dotatate (^{68}Ga-DOTATATE) PET have allowed for high sensitivity as well as improved image resolution for detection of neuroendocrine tumors. Over the past few years, its role in tumor detection has also been extended to meningiomas [34].

11.3.3.8 Parkinsonism

Parkinsonism is a chronic and progressive movement disorder that belongs to a group of conditions called motor system disorders, which are the result of the loss of dopamine-producing brain cells. It presents with bradykinesia, rigidity, tremor at rest, and postural instability. Similar set of symptoms occur in other conditions such as multiple system atrophy, progressive supranuclear palsy, corticobasal degeneration, drug-induced Parkinsonism, vascular Parkinsonism, and psychogenic Parkinsonism. 50,000–60,000 new cases of PD are diagnosed each year, adding to the one million people who currently have PD. Anatomical imaging is of little help when determining the integrity of the dopaminergic system. Ioflupane, N-u-fluoropropyl-2a-carbomethoxy-3a-(4-iodophenyl) nor tropane, also called FP-CIT or Ioflupane, labeled with ^{123}I (^{123}I-Ioflupane) and is commercially known as DaTSCAN is useful in the differential diagnosis of tremor. This compound is a cocaine analog substance and in the USA is classified as a Schedule II controlled substance. It can demonstrate the location and concentration of DaTs in the synapses. It can be used in differentiating patients with essential tremors from those with presynaptic Parkinsonian syndromes (Figs. 11.16a, b). 3–5 mCi is administered by slow intravenous injection (over ~20s) followed by a saline flush. SPECT is then obtained 3–6 h after injection. DaTSPECT with ^{123}I-ioflupane is a radionuclide imaging study that evaluates the integrity of nigrostriatal dopaminergic synapses by visualizing the presynaptic DaTs [35–37].

11.3.3.9 Radionuclide Cisternography

When hydrocephalus is suspected, the goal of imaging evaluation in general is to identify any abnormality of the ventricular or the subarachnoid space morphology and, if other unexplained ventriculomegaly is present, to demonstrate the site and nature of any impediment to the flow of

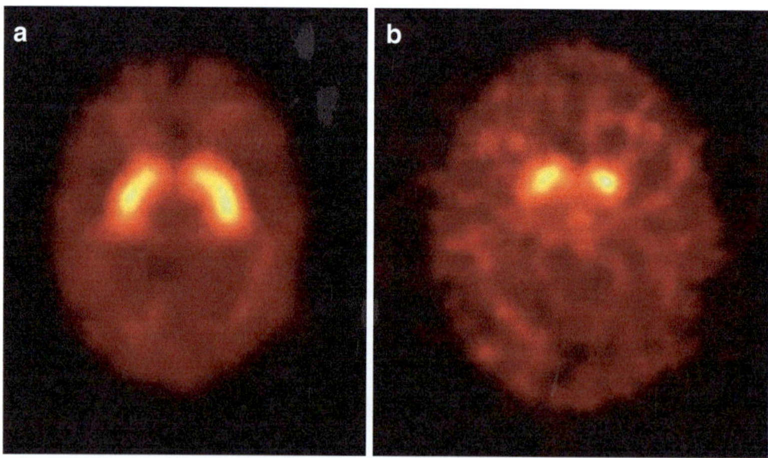

Fig. 11.16 Delayed images of ^{123}I-β-CIT (DaT SCAN). Images were obtained 4 h after the intravenous injection of 5 mCi of ^{123}I-β-CIT in two patients. The normal pattern (a) is seen in the left-hand side (a) with almost complete clearance of the tracer from all cortical and white matter regions of the brain except for the corpus striatum, which appears as "bright" comma-shaped objects in the center of the brain. There is symmetry comparing the left corpus striatum to the right corpus striatum. The specificity of binding is due to the specific prevalence of dopamine uptake in these brain structures. (**b**) The *image on the right* shows significant reduction of uptake, which is asymmetric. This is indicative of the loss of the dopaminergic input from the substantia nigra, which is the etiology of Parkinson's disease

CSF. MRI is generally the best imaging method for achieving this goal. It also visualizes CSF movement and evaluates ventricles and sulci. On T_2-weighted images, the low signal intensity of CSF flowing in the cerebral aqueduct stands out in contrast to the high signal intensity of the adjacent tectum of the mesencephalon, a useful sign of aqueductal patency [5]. In children with patent anterior fontanels, the ventricular size can be assessed by ultrasound. When NPH is suspected, scintigraphy becomes the procedure of choice, since other morphological modalities are not specific. The procedure has proven to be the most specific in differentiating patients with normal-pressure hydrocephalus (NPH) from those with other forms of degenerative brain disorder who would clearly not benefit from surgical treatment (Fig. 11.17) by ventricular shunting.

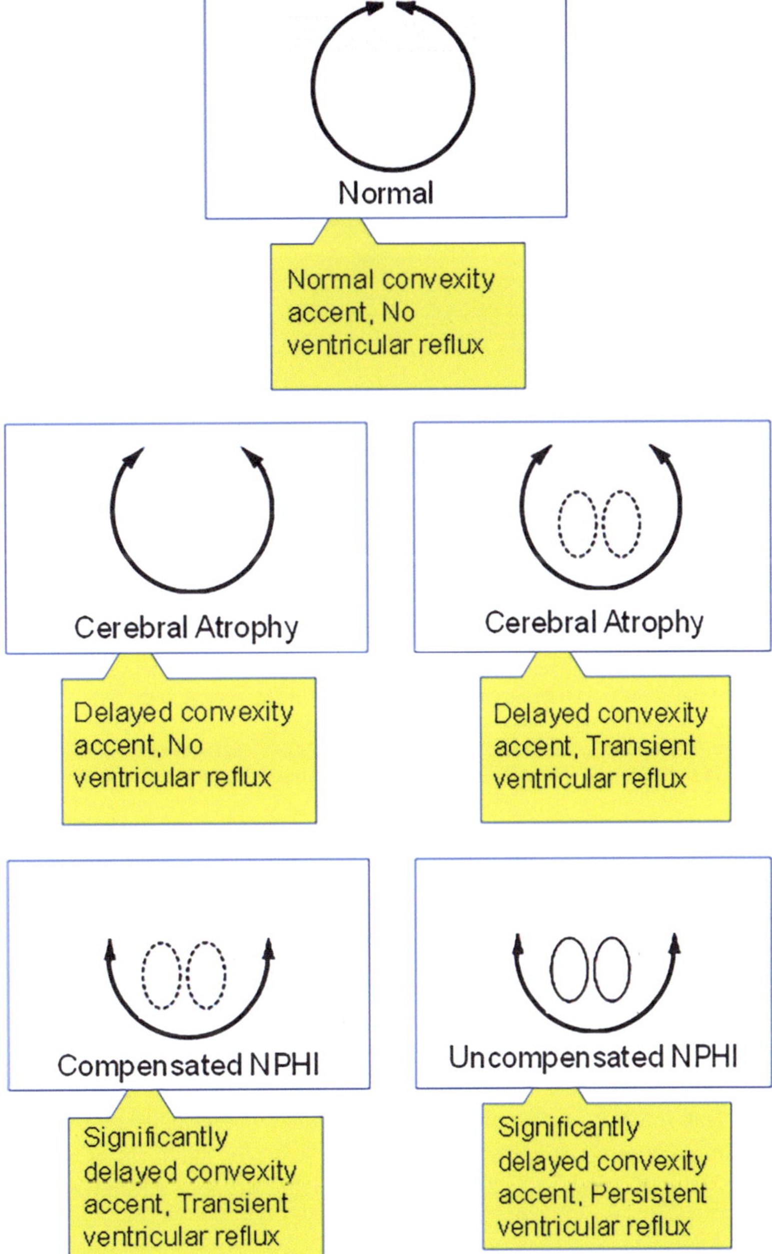

Fig. 11.17 Diagram illustrating different patterns seen on ^{111}In-DTPA cisternography. He pattern of uncompensated normal-pressure hydrocephalus is the pattern that indicates benefit from shunting surgery

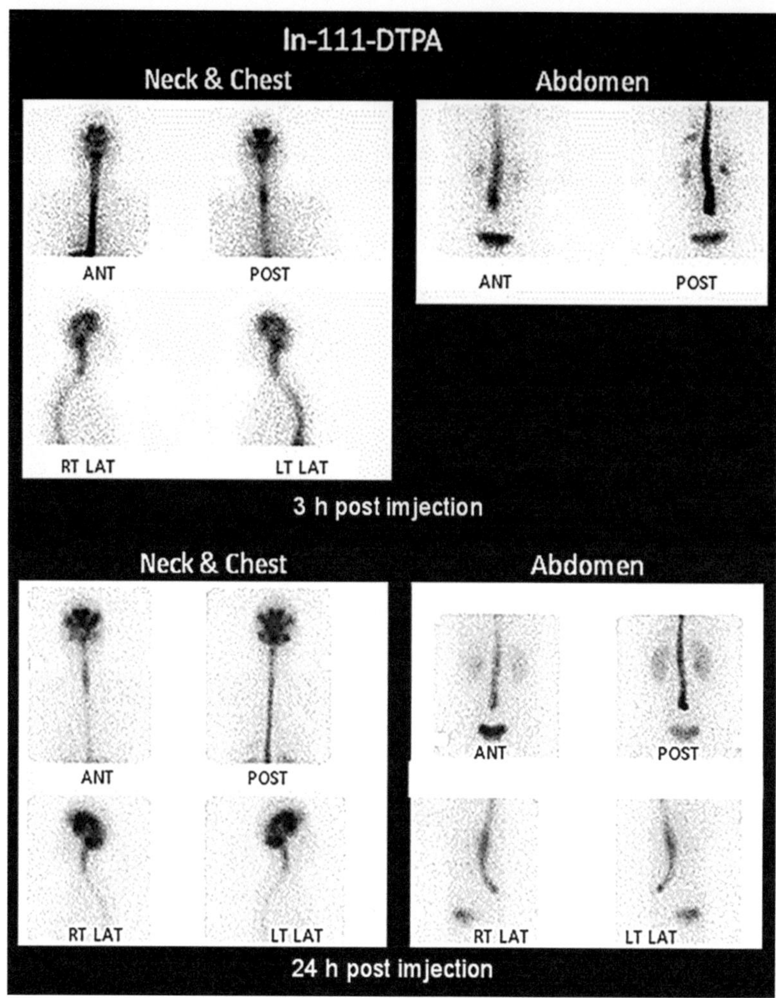

Fig. 11.18 Normal-pressure hydrocephalus (NPH): A 70-year-old female with headaches presents for evaluation of hydrocephalus. After injection of 1.0 mCi ^{111}In-DTPA into the subarachnoid space, planar images of the head and abdomen were obtained at 3 (*top 2 rows*) and 24 h (*bottom 2 rows*). Early (3 h postinjection) images show radiopharmaceutical accumulation in the ventricular system, as well as in the lumbar and basilar cistern portions of the subarachnoid space, with no tracer seen to ascend over the convexities. Repeat imaging was performed at approximately 24 h after injection, and there is again seen the tracer accumulation in the ventricles, with accumulation in the basilar cisterns, but no radiotracer is seen sent over convexities. Findings of persistent tracer in the lateral ventricles with no ascend over the convexities are consistent with normal-pressure hydrocephalus

A radionuclide (usually ^{111}In-DTPA) is injected into the CSF system, usually via the lumbar subarachnoid space. For NPH, skull imaging is performed up to 72 h following injection of the radiopharmaceutical in the anterior, posterior, lateral, and vertical projections. For CSF leak images are also obtained for the same duration and projections, depending on the suspected site of leakage [6, 7]. Normally activity ascends over cerebral convexities by 24 h with no ventricular reflux.

There are characteristic findings in NPH (Fig. 11.18). Imaging performed as early as 2–4 h postinjection shows radioactivity in the lateral ventricles which persists for 24–48 h, indicating ventricular reflux [6]. There is delayed clearance of the tracer as evidenced by minimal visualization of the convexities as late as 24–48 h.

Radionuclide studies have proven to be a sensitive and accurate method of detecting CSF leaks [7, 8]. The site is most likely to be identified during heavy leakage. Imaging in the appropriate projections is important; posterior imaging is used for otorrhea, whereas lateral and anterior imaging is used for rhinorrhea. Alternatively, radioactive counts may be obtained from an absorbent material placed in the orifice in question to determine whether CSF is indeed leaking.

Radionuclide CSF studies are also used in the evaluation of patency of ventriculoperitoneal (VP) shunts. Figure 11.19 shows patient with history of hydrocephalus, and VP shunt presents for evaluation of VP shunt patency. Radiotracer activity is seen only within the ventricular system, and none is seen within the VP shunt tubing. There was radiotracer activity in the peritoneal cavity, to suggest a patent shunt.

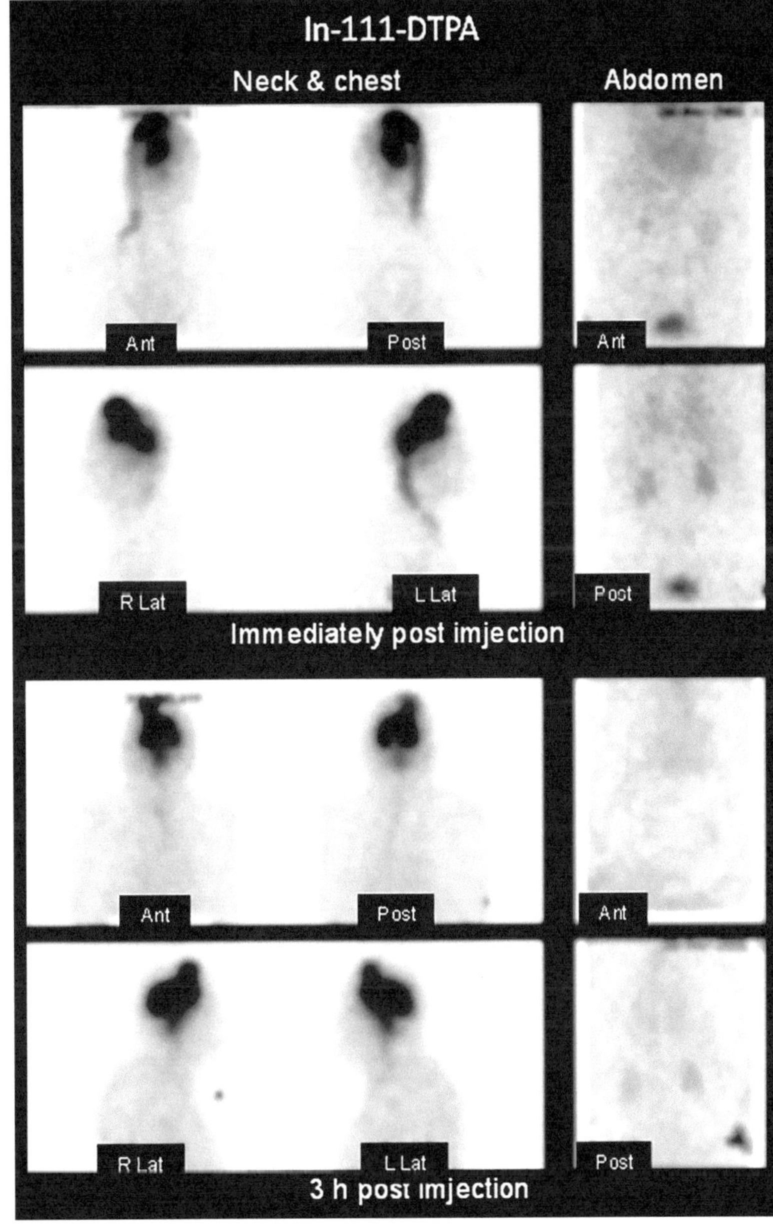

Fig. 11.19 VP shunt study: A 35-year-old male patient with history of hydrocephalus and VP shunt presents for evaluation of VP shunt patency. Following administration of 1.0 mCi ^{111}In-DTPA intrathecally, scintigraphic images were obtained of the head, chest, and abdomen in the anterior and lateral projections immediately and 3 h after radiotracer injection. Radiotracer activity is seen only within the ventricular system, and none is seen within the VP shunt tubing. There was no spillage seen into the peritoneal cavity. Findings consistent with obstructed VP shunt

References

1. Ropper AH, Brown RJ (eds) (2005) Adams and Victor's principles of neurology. McGraw-Hill, New York

2. von Strauss E, Viitanen M, De Ronchi D, Winblad B, Fratiglioni L (1999) Aging and the occurrence of dementia: findings from a population-based cohort with a large sample of nonagenarians. Arch Neuro 156:587–592

3. Mesulam MM, Johnson N, Grujic Z, Weintraub S (1997) Apolipoprotein genotypes in primary progressive aphasia. Neurology 49:51–55

4. Westbury C, Dan B (1997) Primary progressive aphasia: a review of 112 cases. Brain Lang 60:381–406

5. Brodley WG, Kortman KE, Burgoyne B (1986) Flowing cerebrospinal fluid in normal and hydrocephalic states. Appearance on MRI Imaging Radiology 159:611

6. Shih WJ, Ryo UY (1988) Radionuclide brain imaging. In: Yeh SD, Chen DC (eds) Nuclear medicine update. Chinese American Society of Nuclear Medicine. The Society of Nuclear Medicine, ROC, Taipei, pp 246–271

7. Kawaguchi S, Lio M, Murata Het al (1986) Comparative study of NPH by RN cisternography and CT scan in aged. J Nucl Med 27:84

8. Silberstein EB (1983) Brain scintigraphy in the diagnosis of the sequelae of head trauma. Semin Nucl Med 13:153

9. Saha GB, MacIntyre WJ, Go RT (1994) Radiopharmaceuticals for brain imaging. Semin Nucl Med 24:324–349

10. Lassen NA, Blasberg RG (1988) Technetium-99m-d,l-HM-PAO, the development of a new class of 99mTc-labeled tracers: an overview. J Cereb Blood Flow Metab 8:S1–S51

11. Walovitch RC, Hill TC, Garrity ST, Cheesman EH, Burgess BA et al (1989) Characterization of technetium-99m-L, L-ECD for brain perfusion imaging, part 1: pharmacology of technetium-99mECD in nonhuman primates. J Nucl Med 30:1892–1901

12. Lassen NA (1985) Cerebral blood flow tomography with xenon-133. Semin Nucl Med 15:347–356

13. Mountz JM, Raymond PA, McKeever PE, Modell JG, Hood TW et al (1989) Specific localization of thallium-201 in recurrent high grade astrocytoma by microautoradiography. Cancer Res 49:4053–4056

14. O'Tuama LA, Treves ST, Larar JN (1993) Thallium-201 versus technetium-99m-MIBISPECT in evaluation of childhood brain tumors: a within-subject comparison. J Nucl Med 34:1045–1051

15. Conti PS (1995) Introduction to imaging brain tumor metabolism with positron emission tomography (PET). Cancer Investig 13:244–259

16. Meegalla S, Plossl K, Kung MP, Chumpradit S, Stevenson DA et al (1996) Tc-99m-labeled tropanes as dopamine transporter imaging agents. Bioconjug Chem 7:421–429

17. Bartenstein P, Asenbaum S, Catafau A, Halldin C, Pilowski L et al (2002) European Association of Nuclear Medicine procedure guidelines for brain imaging using F-18FDG. Eur J Nucl Med Mol Imaging 29:BP43–BP48

18. Cikrit DF, Dalsing MC, Harting PS, Burt RW, Lalka SG et al (1997) Cerebral vascular reactivity assessed with acetazolamide single photon emission computer tomography scans before and after carotid endarterectomy. Am J Surg 174:193–197

19. Cummings JL (2004) Alzheimer's disease. N Engl J Med 351:56–67

20. Kuzniecky R, Mountz JM, Thomas F (1993) Ictal^{99m}Tc-HM-PAO brain single photon emission computed tomography in electroencephalographic non-localizable partial seizures. J Neuroimaging 3:100–102

21. Laich E, Kuzniecky R, Mountz JM, Liu HG, Gilliam F et al (1997) Supplementary sensorimotor are a epilepsy: identification of the epileptogenic zone and propagation pathways using ictal SPECT. Brain 120:855–864

22. Knowlton RC, Lawn ND, Mountz JM, Buddhiwardhan O, Miller S et al (2004) Ictal single-photon emission computed tomography imaging in extratemporal lobe epilepsy using statistical parametric mapping. J Neuroimaging 14:324–330

23. Knowlton RC, Lawn ND, Mountz JM, Kuzniecky RI (2004) Ictal SPECT analysis in epilepsy: subtraction and statistical parametric mapping techniques. Neurology 63:10–15

24. Kim S et al (2013) Clinical value of the first dedicated, commercially available automatic injector for ictal brain SPECT in Presurgical evaluation of pediatric epilepsy: comparison with manual injection. J Nucl Med 54(5):732–738

25. Galynker II, Cai J, Ongseng F, Finestone H, Dutta E, Serseni D (1998) Hypofrontality and negative symptoms in major depressive disorder. J Nucl Med 39:608–612

26. Wilms G, Marchall G, Demaerel PH (1991) Gadolinium enhanced MRI of intracranial lesions. A review of indications and results. Clin Imaging 15:153

27. Valk PE, Dillon WP (1991) Diagnostic imaging of central nervous system radiation injury. In: Gutin PH, Leibel SA, Sheline GE (eds) Radiation injury to the central nervous system. Raven Press, New York, pp 211–237

28. Mountz JM, Deutsch G, Kuzniecky R, Rosenfeld SS (1994) Brain SPECT: 1994 update. In: Freeman LM (ed) Nuclear medicine annual. Raven Press, New York, pp 1–54

29. Schwartz RB, Holman BL, Polk JF et al (1998) Dual-isotope single-photon emission computerized tomography scanning in patients with glioblastoma multiforme: association with patient survival and histopathological characteristics of tumor after high-dose radiotherapy. J Neurosurg 89:60

30. Kaplan WD, Takvorian T, Morris JH et al (1987) Thallium-201 brain imaging: a comparative study with pathologic correlation. J Nucl Med 28:47
31. Black KL, Hawkins RA, Kim KT et al (1989) Use of thallium-201 SPECT to quantitate malignancy grade of gliomas. J Neurosurg 71:342
32. Lastoria S, Castelli L, Vergara E et al (1990) Human gliomas radioimmunoimaging with I-131BC-2 murine IgG: preliminary report. J Nucl Med Allied Sci 34:173
33. Ueda T, Kaji Y, Wakisaka S et al (1993) Time sequential single photon emission computed tomography studies in brain tumour using 201Tl. Eur J Nucl Med 20:138
34. Dressen MS et al (2019) Complementary Molecular and Metabolic Characterization of Meningiomas with DOTATATE and FDG-PET: Advancing Treatment Planning and Prognostication. Clin Nucl Med 44(1):e26–e27
35. Cummings JL, Henchcliffe C, Schaier S et al (2011) The role of dopaminergic imaging in patients with symptoms of dopaminergic system neurodegeneration. J Brain 134:3146–3166
36. Djang DSW, Janssen MJR, Bohnen N (2012) SNM practice guidelines for dopamine transporter imaging with I-123I of Lupane SPECT. J Nucl Med 53:154–163
37. Gerasimou G, Costa DC, Papanastasiou E, Bostanjiopoulou S, Arnaoutoglou M et al (2012) SPECT study with I-123-I of Lupane (DaTSCAN) in patients with essential tremor. Is there any correlation with Parkinson's disease? Ann Nucl Med 26:337–344

12.1 Principles of Tumor Pathology and Biology

12.1.1 Tumor Pathology

The classification and typing of tumors depend mainly on the histopathological diagnosis, which is made on the basis of gross and microscopic examination of tissues. Tumor classification is based on histogenesis, degree of cellular differentiation (i.e., well or poorly differentiated), and biological behavior (benign vs. malignant). All tumors, whether benign or malignant, have two components: (1) proliferating neoplastic cells and (2) supportive stroma, which is host derived and made up of connective tissue andblood vessels. While the neoplastic cells determine the nature of the tumors, tumor growth and evolution depend on the stroma [1]. In the past, the general concept was that neoplasms of certain phenotypes arise from their normal cell counterpart. However, evidence that accumulated over the years has proven the inaccuracy of this histogenetic assumption. It is now believed that most tumors arise from immature cells that can transform and acquire phenotypic features similar to those of one or more normal cell types. For example, rhabdomyosarcomas are tumors that show rhabdomyoblastic differentiation rather than tumors that arise from striated muscle cells [2]. In some instances, the immature cells can undergo divergent differentiation into two cell types, as in the case of mixed tumors of the salivary gland (Fig. 12.1), or they have the capacity to differentiate into any adult cell type, as in teratoma.

12.1.1.1 Tumor Biologic Behavior

The categorization of tumors into benign and malignant is an oversimplification of the wide behavioral range of neoplasms. There are tumors that exhibit intermediate behavior. This has led to the introduction of a third category designated as "borderline or undetermined," which represents low-grade malignant tumors that can mostly be managed by conservative therapeutic approach.

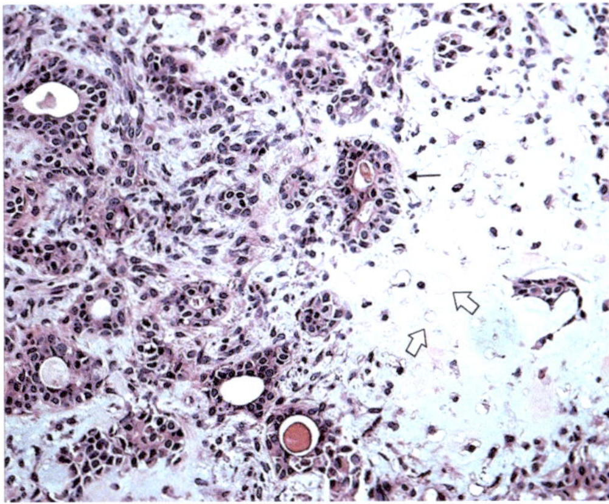

Fig. 12.1 Benign mixed tumor of salivary gland (pleomorphic adenoma). The tumor consists of an epithelial component "glands" (*arrow*) and a mesenchymal component "cartilage" (*open arrows*)

A. H. Elgazzar, *Synopsis of Pathophysiology in Nuclear Medicine*,
https://doi.org/10.1007/978-3-031-20646-7_12

The best examples are borderline tumors of the ovary and uterine smooth muscle of low malignant potential. Currently, the malignant category is restricted to tumors that have metastatic properties.

12.1.1.1.1 Benign Tumors

A tumor is considered benign when its gross and microscopic characteristics are relatively innocent, implying that it will remain localized and cannot spread to other sites. A benign tumor is generally composed of well-differentiated cells that resemble their normal counterpart. In general, the addition of the suffix -oma to the cell of origin describes benign tumors; for example, adenoma indicates a benign tumor of epithelial cell origin. Tumors that arise from mesenchymal tissues are designated according to their putative cell of origin (e.g., fibroma, chondroma, lipoma, and leiomyoma). Benign tumors can also be classified on the basis of their macroscopic pattern; for example, papillomas are benign epithelial tumors with certain growth characteristics, such as exophytic or finger-like projections.

12.1.1.1.2 Malignant Tumors

The classification of malignant tumors essentially follows that of benign tumors, with some exceptions. Malignant neoplasms arising from epithelial cells are termed carcinomas. Carcinomas are further classified on the basis of the type of epithelium, for example, glandular as adenocarcinoma (Fig. 12.2), squamous as squamous cell carcinoma (Fig. 12.3), and transitional as transitional cell carcinoma. Malignant epithelial tumors that have not extended through the underlying basement membrane are described as in situ carcinoma. Malignant tumors arising from mesenchymal tissue are broadly designated as sarcomas (Fig. 12.4). These are further subclassified on a histogenetic basis according to the normal tissue they resemble or its embryonal counterparts, for example, fibrosarcoma, chon-

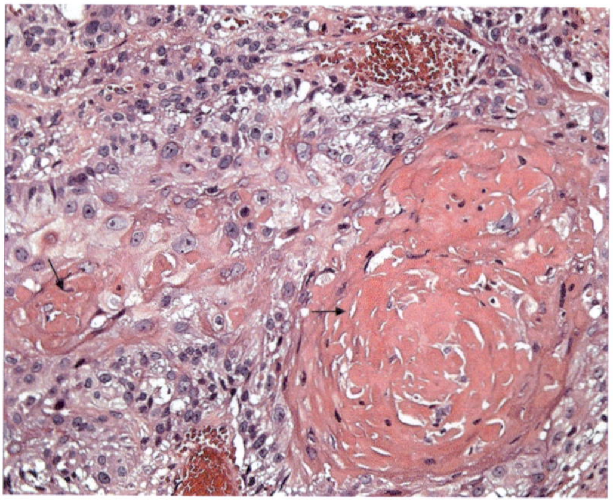

Fig. 12.3 Squamous cell carcinoma. The tumor consists of well-differentiated squamous cells forming keratin pearls (*arrows*)

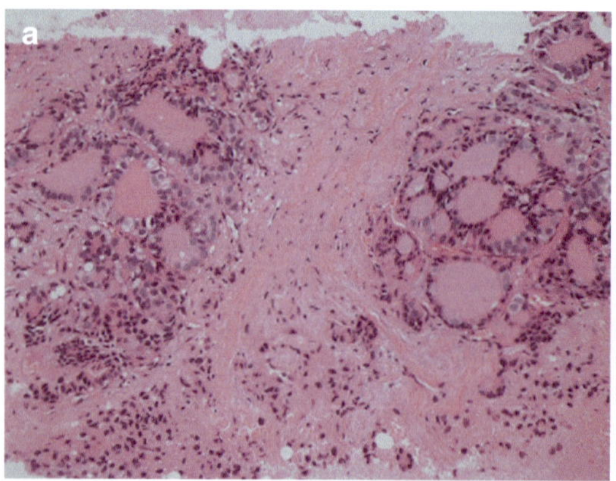

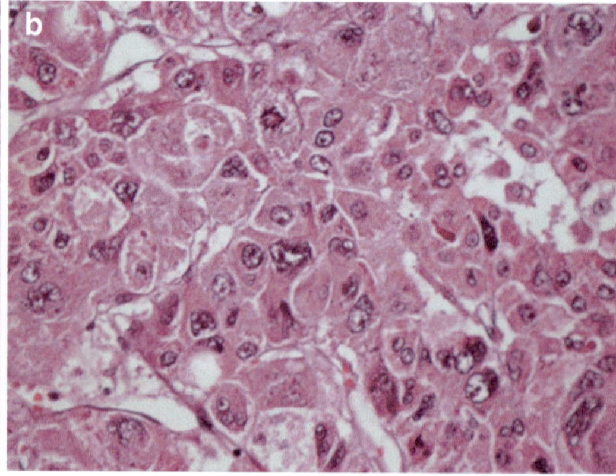

Fig. 12.2 Adenocarcinoma. (**a**) Example of adenocarcinoma in a case of metastatic thyroid cancer in the liver (H&E × 20) illustrating the glandular architecture. (**b**) A high power field of another adenocarcinoma (hepatocellular carcinoma) illustrating the typical cellular features of malignancy. Note the variation in cell size, abnormal chromatin pattern, prominent nucleoli, and abnormal mitosis (H&E × 40)

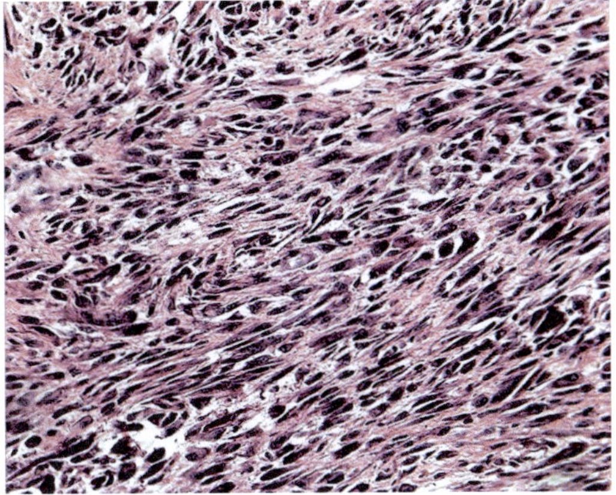

Fig. 12.4 Soft tissue sarcoma consisting of pleomorphic spindle cells, illustrating the features of malignancy as variable cell size and shapes and increased nuclear/cytoplasmic ratio

drosarcoma, leiomyosarcoma, and rhabdomyosarcoma. There are tumors that do not follow any classifi cation scheme, and they have been identified by trivial names, such as seminoma and melanoma. Other tumors carry eponyms, such as Hodgkin's disease and Ewing's sarcoma. Tumors within a single organ or single type of epithelium are further subclassified into different types; each has its own characteristics, prognosis, and response to therapy. Malignant tumors that extend into surrounding tissue without respecting normal tissue boundaries are capable of invading lymphatics and blood vessels and can be transported to distant sites. Several salient abnormalities are helpful to the pathologist in making the morphological diagnosis of such tumors, and they are expressed in two ways: First, there are abnormalities that affect individual cells in the form of cytological features and increased mitotic activity. Cytological features of malignancy include cell enlargement, increased ratio of nuclear to cytoplasmic area, pleomorphism (variation in size and shape), clumping of nuclear chromatin, and big nucleoli (Fig. 10.2b). Second, there are abnormalities that affect intercellular relationship, i.e., altered orientation of neoplastic cells and stroma leading to disorganization [3].

12.1.1.2   Tumor Grading

Grading is a scheme that attempts to determine the degree of malignancy and is based on the evaluation of certain parameters that vary according to the system used. These broadly include degree of tumor cellularity, resemblance of tumor cells to their normal forbears morphologically and functionally, cellular pleomorphism or anaplasia, mitotic activity (number and abnormality), and necrosis [4]. Tumors may be graded on four-tier, three-tier, or two-tier scales, depending on the tumor type. In general, a three-grade system has proven to be the most reproducible: well, moderately, and poorly or undifferentiated, or grades I, II, and III, where grade 1 is well differentiated (low grade); grade 2, moderately differentiated (intermediate grade); and grade 3, poorly differentiated (high grade).

12.1.1.3   Tumor Staging

Staging of cancer depends on the size of the primary neoplasm, its extent to regional lymph nodes, and the presence or absence of metastasis. Cancer care is a cooperative, multidisciplinary endeavor; therefore, all disciplines involved in cancer care are to work well together, they must be able to communicate with precision. The TNM system has been developed by the American Joint Committee on Cancer (AJCC), and European Union International Contre le Cancer (UICC) commissions on cancer to allow systematic categorization and description of cancer patients. In this fashion, disease progression patterns, natural history, and treatment outcome can be more reliably documented when applied to the individual patient. The objectives of a staging system can be briefly summarized as follows: (a) to aid the clinician in planning treatment, (b) to give some indication of prognosis, (c) to assist in the evaluation of end results, (d) to facilitate the exchange of information between treatment centers, and (e) to assist in the continuing investigation of cancer. The TNM system meets these requirements. It is an expression of the anatomical extent of disease and is based on the assessment of three components:

T The extent of primary tumor.
N The absence or presence and extent of regional lymph node metastases.
M The absence or presence of distant metastases.

TNM clinical–diagnostic staging allows for pretreatment characterization via clinical examination and specific diagnostic studies. TNM surgical-evaluative staging is applied following a major surgical exploration or biopsy. TNM postsurgical treatment-pathological staging characterizes the extent of the cancer following thorough examination of the resected surgical specimen. TNM retreatment staging is applied in instances where the initial therapy has failed and additional treatment decisions are being considered. TNM autopsy staging is the final staging, done after the postmortem study.

12.1.1.4 Tumor Growth Rate

Generally, most benign neoplasms grow slowly, and most malignant neoplasms grow much faster. However, there are many exceptions since some benign neoplasms grow more rapidly than some cancers. For example, uterine leiomyomas (benign smooth muscle tumors) may increase rapidly in size during pregnancy (hormonal effect). The rate of growth of malignant tumors correlates in general with their level of differentiation. Rapidly growing malignant neoplasm often contains central areas of ischemic necrosis because the tumor blood supply, derived from the host, fails to keep pace with the oxygen needs of the expanding mass of cells [1].

12.2 Tumor Biology

Developing cancer cells must acquire a variety of characteristics not generally found in nontransformed cells. The cancer cell represents the culmination of a complex process of developing capacity for largely unregulated growth. The main characteristics that differentiate the cancer cell from the precancerous or noncancerous cell are capabilities of self-sufficiency in growth signals, insensitivity to antigrowth signals, evasion of apoptosis, limitless replicative potential, sustained angiogenesis, and a potential for tissue invasion and metastasis. In addition, the enabling characteristic of genetic instability was noted as a driving force for acquiring these cell characteristics.

12.2.1 Cell Growth and Cell Cycle

Normal cell proliferation (also known as cell growth or cell division) is essential for tissue homeostasis in the adult body. When stimulated to divide, a normal cell progresses through a tightly regulated process known as the cell cycle. The cell cycle is a complex circuit composed of positive and negative protein regulators, the role of which is to duplicate DNA specifically during S phase and to segregate it evenly into two identical progeny during M phase (see Fig. 2.3 Chap. 2). When a cell leaves the dormant state of G0 and enters a metabolically active phase during G1, the destiny of the cell cycle pivots in the equilibrium as the decision to undergo division must be made at the restriction point [5]. Because G1 is such an essential phase of the cell cycle, it is not astonishing that many oncogenic perturbations have been found as targeted amplifications or mutations of G1-specific protein regulators.

12.2.2 Tumor Neovascularization (Angiogenesis)

Cell survival and proliferation are dependent on an adequate supply of oxygen and nutrients and the removal of toxic metabolites. Tumor cells still require nutrients and oxygen in order to grow. Since oxygen can diffuse radially from capillaries for only 150–200 μm, the growth of tumor masses greater than 1 mm in diameter depends on the formation of new blood vessels, also known as tumor neovascularization or angiogenesis. Neovascularization is a feature of neoplasia. Neovascularization supplies nutrients and oxygen and is required not only for continued tumor growth but also for metastasis [1].

Tumor-associated angiogenic factors may be produced by tumor cells or may be derived from inflammatory cells (e.g., macrophages) that infiltrate tumors. The two most important tumor associated angiogenic factors are vascular endothelial growth factor (VEGF) and basic fibroblast growth factor. The tumor cells not only produce angiogenic factors but also induce antiangiogenesis molecules. The molecular basis of the angiogenesis is not entirely clear but may involve increased production of angiogenic factors or loss of angiogenesis inhibitors. Hypoxia within the growing tumor favors angiogenesis by release of hypoxia-inducible factor-1 (HIF-1) [1]. HIF-1 controls transcription of VEGF. The wildtype TP53 gene seems to inhibit angiogenesis by inducing the synthesis of the antiangiogenic molecule thrombospondin-1. With mutational inactivation of both TP53 alleles (a common event in many cancers), the levels of thrombospondin-1 drop precipitously, tilting the balance in favor of angiogenic factors. Because of the important role of angiogenesis in tumor growth, extensive publications concentrated on antiangiogenesis therapy and the results are very promising.

12.2.3 Distinguishing Features of Tumor Cells

Cancer is a genetic disease resulting from multiple, sequential genetic changes affecting oncogenes, tumor suppressor genes, and modifiers [6]. Because of this multistep process, most human malignancies show various degrees of genetic heterogeneity even if they originate from single cells. The multistep progression model determines that cells pass through a number of distinctive intermediate stages of evolution from normalcy to full malignancy [7]. The evolved tumor cells vary significantly from their normal counterparts. Tumor cells have distinguishing morphological and structural features that are different from those of the cells of origin. Moreover, the abnormal cells show altered interaction with neighboring cells.

12.2.3.1 Loss of Contact Inhibition of Growth

Normal cells have an ordered growth pattern and a predicted relationship with their neighboring cells, and that growth pattern is predominantly two-dimensional. Further normal cell division is inhibited by contacts made with other cells; this is the phenomenon of contact inhibition [8]. In contrast, tumor cells exhibit loss of contact inhibition and continue to display a disordered growth pattern.

12.2.3.2 Growth Regulatory Pattern

Another feature that distinguishes normal growth from malignant proliferation is the reduced dependence of the latter on the presence of the known stimulatory and inhibitory growth factors. The diversion from the control of the growth regulatory factors can be explained, in part, by the discovery of biochemical changes within cancer cells resulting from some genetic alterations. Thus, when normal cells are grown in culture, they continue to divide for a limited number of generations and then experience a senescent crisis, in which most cells stop dividing and die and no cells survive to establish permanent cell lines. Conversely, human tumor cells usually have an unlimited potential for growth and are thus immortalized [9]. This distinctive growth factor independence or autonomy has been attributed to several mechanisms including ability of tumor cells to secrete mitogenic growth factors that have a growth stimulatory ability on the same cell that has released them [10].

12.2.3.3 Ability to Escape Immune Surveillance Pathways (Immune Evasion)

Another characteristic feature of human malignancy is its ability to escape the human immune surveillance pathways. It is known that human tumor cells express on their surfaces novel antigens that are not present on the surfaces of their transformed progenitors. One type of novel antigen may be common to many different types of malignancy and may be recognized by the natural killer lymphocytes even without specific prior immunization [5]. In other instances, novel antigens specific to a particular type of tumor may be displayed. According to one theory of tumorigenesis, all individuals develop abundant transformed cells over the course of their lives, but most of these cells are recognized and destroyed by one or another module of the host's immune mechanisms. Support for this theory stems from the observation of the substantial increase in the incidence of malignancy in patients with acquired immune deficiency syndrome, in patients with organ transplants receiving intensive immunosuppressive agents, and in patients with other immune deficiency disorders. It has been proven that tumor cells may escape the host immune system by downregulating the expression of HLA antigens, which normally assist lymphocyte recognition of the target cells.

12.2.3.4 Metabolic Alterations

Tumor cells exhibit a vast array of metabolic differences distinguishing them from their untransformed counterparts. This is illustrated primarily in simplified metabolic activities and by an increased synthesis of material necessary for cell division. Some of the most striking metabolic alterations include the utilization of anaerobic pathways and the increased utilization of glucose transport [11].

12.2.4 Invasion and Metastasis

Malignant neoplasms disseminate by one of the three pathways: (1) seeding within body cavities—an example of this is carcinoma of the colon that may penetrate the wall of the gut and reimplant at other sites in the peritoneal cavity, (2) lymphatic spread which is the preferred way of spread by carcinomas in general, or (3) hematogenous spread which is favored by sarcomas.

The ability of a tumor to metastasize is a multifaceted phenomenon which requires several prerequisites [12]: (a) invasion by tumor cells through adjacent structures, (b) entrance of tumor cells into blood or lymphatic vessels, (c) survival of tumor cells within the circulation and avoidance of the immune system, and (d) implantation in a foreign tissue with establishment of a new tumor locus. Most carcinomas arise in epithelial cell layers with an underlying basement membrane. Invasive tumors frequently secrete enzymes, including collagenases, heparanase, and stromelysin, that are capable of degrading this type of physical barrier [13]. Once a tumor has eroded through the wall of a blood or lymphatic vessel, individual tumor cells may detach and circulate through the body as an embolus. Encasing these cells in clots of fibrin or in aggregates of platelets may protect them from destruction by the immune system. The presence of tumor cells in the circulation does not necessarily lead to metastases. However, these circulating cells have to "home" preferentially to a specific target organ. This pattern has been described as the "seeds" and "soil" model and has been demonstrated experimentally and observed consistently in oncological practice. It is not clear how these patterns of metastases arise, but some evidence suggests that tumor cells can respond to specific chemotactic signals. Moreover, specific receptors have recently been identified on the surfaces of metastasizing tumor cells that cause them to adhere to complementary structures displayed by endothelial cells in certain organs [14].

12.2.5 Carcinogenesis

Carcinogenesis or oncogenesis is a process by which normal cells are transformed into cancer cells. It is well known that agents that induced damage to the DNA (mutagens) have potential carcinogenic effects. The progenitor tumor cells that sustain genetic alterations are said to undergo somatic mutations that promote the multistep process of neoplastic development.

12.2.5.1 Genetic Mutations and Cellular Oncogenes

Enormous scientific evidence has accumulated over more than half a century to indicate that neoplastic transformation occurs as a direct consequence of alterations to the cell genome. Four basic approaches have been used to identify genes involved in cancer: (a) the study of cancer-causing viruses, (b) bioassays for cancer genes in tissue culture systems, (c) localization of genes at sites of chromosomal alteration in tumor specimens, and (d) isolation of genes for cancer predisposing familial syndromes. It is well known that agents that induce damage to the DNA (mutagens) have potential carcinogenic effects. The DNA found in the nucleus of every living cell encodes the heritable or genetic information necessary to direct the development of that organism from a single fertilized cell to the mature organism. Therefore, the progenitor tumor cells that sustain genetic alterations are said to undergo somatic mutations that promote the multistep process of neoplastic development. From many studies, it became very clear that some of the information encoding cancerous behavior of the donor cells could be passed to the recipient cells via DNA molecules. It was not until the early 1980s that, with the advent of gene cloning, it was possible to isolate these cellular oncogenes (Table 12.1). Activation of cellular oncogenes is a

Table 12.1 Cellular oncogenes implicated in human cancer

Category	Proto-oncogene	Mode of activation	Associated human tumor
Growth factors			
PDGF-βchain	*SIS*	Overexpression	Astrocytoma
			Osteosarcoma
Fibroblast growth factors	*HST-1*	Overexpression	Stomach cancer
	INT-2	Amplification	Bladder cancer
			Breast cancer
			Melanoma
TGFa	*TGFa*	Overexpression	Astrocytomas
			Hepatocellular carcinomas
HGF	*HGF*	Overexpression	Thyroid cancer
Growth factor receptors			
EGF receptor family	*ERB-B1(ECFR)*	Overexpression	Squamous cell carcinomas of lung, gliomas
	ERB-B2		Breast and ovarian cancers
CSF-1 receptor	*FMS*	Point mutation	Leukemia
Receptor for neurotrophic factors	*RET*	Point mutation	Multiple endocrine neoplasia 2A and B, familial medullary thyroid carcinomas
PDGF receptor	*PDGF-R*	Overexpression	Gliomas
Proteins involved in signal transduction			
GTP binding	*K-RAS*	Point mutation	Colon, lung, and pancreatic tumors
	H-RAS	Point mutation	Bladder and kidney tumors
	N-RAS	Point mutation	Melanomas
Non-receptor tyrosine kinase	*ABL*	Translocation	Chronic myeloid leukemia
WNT signal transduction	*β-Catenin*	Point mutation	Hepatoblastomas, hepatocellular carcinoma
		Overexpression	
Nuclear regulatory proteins			
Transcriptional activators	*C-MYC*	Translocation	Burkitt's lymphoma
Cell cycle regulators			
Cyclins	*CYCLIND*	Translocation	Mantle cell lymphoma
		Amplification	Breast and esophageal cancers
	CYCLINE	Overexpression	Breast cancer
Cyclin-dependent kinase	*CDK4*	Amplification or point mutation	Glioblastoma, melanoma

complex process that involves a variety of somatic mutational mechanisms. The c-myc oncogene develops its malignant properties through mechanisms that affect the level of expression of its encoded proteins without any associated alteration in its protein structure. Recently, the prognostic significance of c-myc in lymphoma has also been described [15]. Conversely, a quantitative change in the structure of the encoded proteins may be responsible for oncogene activation. In chronic myelogenous leukemia, for example, the abl gene undergoes fusion with a fully unrelated gene, bcr. The bcr-abl hybrid protein encoded by these fused genes differs substantially in structure and function from the normal abl proto-oncogene protein [16].

It was clear, however, that single oncogenes were not capable of inducing transformation of fully normal cells into totally malignant cells. Instead, the action of a single oncogene usually induces only partial progression to malignancy. Fortunately, this has served as a protective mechanism to prevent the development of cancers in response to single oncogenes that arise through isolated genetic mishaps. Therefore, it appears that each step through which cells pass in the progression from normalcy to malignancy (multistep carcinogenesis) is characterized by a distinct genetic change, often one that creates an oncogene. However, the precise number of the distinct steps for most human tumors is poorly understood. Nonlethal genetic damage may be acquired by the action of environmental agents, such as chemicals, radiation, or viruses, or it may be inherited in the germ line. The current hypothesis implies that cancer formed as a result of clonal expansion of a single progenitor cell that has incurred the genetic damage (i.e., tumors are monoclonal). This theory has been supported by many studies that revealed clonality in neoplasm that have been assessed readily in women who are heterozygous for polymorphic X-linked markers, such as the enzyme glucose-6-phosphate dehydrogenase or X-linked restriction fragment length polymorphisms or in clonality assessed in lymphoid neoplasm. Mutant alleles of proto-oncogenes are called oncogenes [17, 18]. Three classes of normal regulatory genes—growth-promoting proto-oncogenes; growth-inhibiting cancer suppressor genes (antioncogenes); and genes that regulate programmed cell death, or apoptosis—are the principal targets of genetic damage [1]. They are considered dominant because they transform cells despite the presence of their normal counterpart. In addition to the three classes of genes mentioned earlier, a fourth category of genes, those that regulate repair of damaged DNA, is pertinent in carcinogenesis.

12.2.5.2 Growth-Promoting Proto-Oncogenes

Genes that promote autonomous cell growth in cancer cells are called oncogenes. They are derived by mutations in proto-oncogenes and are characterized by the ability to promote cell growth in the absence of normal growth-promoting signals. Their products, called oncoproteins, resemble the normal products of proto-oncogenes except that oncoproteins are devoid of important regulatory elements, and their production in the transformed cells does not depend on growth factors or other external signals. All normal cells require stimulation by growth factors to undergo proliferation. Many cancer cells acquire growth self-sufficiency, however, by acquiring the ability to synthesize the same growth factors to which they are responsive. Such is the case with platelet-derived growth factor (PDGF) and transforming growth factor α (TGF-α). Many glioblastomas secrete PDGF, and sarcomas make TGF-α.

12.2.5.3 Growth Factor Receptors

There are several oncogenes that encode growth factor. Those oncogenes represent either mutation or overexpression of normal forms of growth factor receptors. Mutant receptor proteins can send continuous mitogenic signals to cells, even in the absence of the growth factor in the environment [1]. Overexpression can render cancer cells hyperresponsive to normal levels of the growth factor, a level that would not normally trigger proliferation. Among the examples of overexpression is the receptor called HER2 (ERBB2), which is present in 30% of breast cancers and present in variable percentages in other human cancer. Breast cancers which are positive for Her2 are more sensitive to the mitogenic effects of small amounts of growth factors, and a high level of HER2 protein in breast cancer is associated with poor prognosis. The clinical significance of HER2 in breast cancers is clearly evident in the treatment of breast cancer with anti-HER2 antibodies which block the extracellular domain of this receptor [19, 20].

12.2.5.4 Signal-Transducing Proteins

Mutations in genes that encode various components of the signaling pathways are a common process in cancer. These signaling molecules couple growth factor receptors to their nuclear targets. The most important members in this category are RAS and ABL. Approximately 30% of all human tumors contain mutated versions of the RAS gene. In some tumors, such as colon and pancreatic cancers, the incidence of RAS mutations is even higher [1]. The activated RAS in turn activates downstream regulators of proliferation, including the RAFMAP kinase mitogenic cascade, which flood the nucleus with signals for cell proliferation. In chronic myeloid leukemia and certain acute leukemias, this activity is unleashed because the ABL gene is translocated from its normal abode on chromosome 9 to chromosome 22, where it fuses with part of the breakpoint cluster region (BCR) gene. The BCR-ABL hybrid gene has potent tyrosine kinase activity, and it activates several pathways, including the RAS-RAF cascade just described. The crucial role of BCR-ABL in transformation has been confirmed by the dramatic clinical response of patients with chronic myeloid leukemia after therapy with an inhibitor of ABL kinase called STI 571 (Gleevec); this is another example of rational drug design emerging from an understanding of the molecular basis of cancer.

12.2.5.5 Nuclear Transcription Factors

Growth autonomy in neoplasm may occur as a consequence of mutations affecting genes that regulate transcription of DNA such as MYC oncogene that has been localized to the nucleus. The MYC proto-oncogene is expressed in virtually all cells, and the MYC protein is induced rapidly when quiescent cells receive a signal to divide. The MYC protein binds to the DNA, causing transcriptional activation of several growth related genes, including cyclin-dependent kinases (CDKs), whose product drives cells into the cell cycle. In normal cells, MYC levels decline to near basal level when the cell cycle begins. In contrast, oncogenic versions of the MYC gene are associated with persistent expression or overexpression, contributing to sustained proliferation. The classic example is the dysregulation of the MYC gene resulting from a t(8; 14) translocation that occurs in Burkitt's lymphoma [1].

12.2.5.6 Tumor Suppressor Genes and Tumor Progression

While oncogenes play a critical role in tumorigenesis, another group of genes known as tumor suppressors appears to be equally significant. These tumor suppressor genes, as the name implies, function in the normal cells to restrict cellular proliferation. However, tumor suppressor genes are involved in tumorigenesis when they suffer genetic inactivation or loss-of-function mutations, affecting the two redundant copies of these genes and resulting in the elimination of that important barrier to cell growth. The loss of wild-type tumor suppressor genes such as Rb and p53 is associated with a wide variety of human tumors. Many proto-oncogenes transform in model systems in which the wildtype gene is overexpressed or expressed in the wrong cell type; similarly, overexpression or inappropriate expression of some proto-oncogenes, such as c-myc, is thought to be tumorigenic in some human tissues. The most commonly mutated tumor suppressor gene in human cancer is p53, with at least 50% of tumors having abnormal p53 genes [21]. The gene participates in a cell cycle checkpoint signal transduction pathway that causes either a G1 arrest or apoptotic cell death following DNA damage. Loss of p53 function during tumorigenesis can thus result in both inappropriate progressions through the cell cycle after DNA damage and survival of a cell that might otherwise have been destined to die.

Another newly discovered tumor suppressor gene is the p16. Since its discovery as a CDKI (cyclin-dependent kinase inhibitor) in 1993, the tumor suppressor p16 has gained widespread importance in tumor biology [22]. The frequent mutations and deletions of p16 in human cancer cell lines first suggested an important role for p16 in carcinogenesis. APC is another tumor suppressor gene [23] and its loss is common in colon cancer. APC is a cytoplasmic protein whose function in normal cells is to bind another protein called β-catenin and bring about its degradation. β-Catenin is a transcriptional factor, and, if APC function is defective by mutation, accumulated level of β-catenin occurs in the cells, driving cell proliferation. Individuals born with one mutant allele develop hundreds to thousands of adenomatous polyps in the colon during their teens or 20s. If the cells develop a second mutation of the normal inherited gene on the other allele, it leads to development of carcinoma of the colon.

12.2.6 Apoptosis

Each day, approximately 50–70 billion cells die in the average adult because of programmed cell death. The morphological self destruction cells go through when experiencing programmed cell death has been termed apoptosis and is executed by a family of intracellular proteases, called caspases [24]. These physiological deaths culminate in fragmentation of cells into membrane-encased bodies, which are cleared through phagocytosis by neighboring cells without inciting inflammatory reactions or tissue scarring. Defects in the processes controlling apoptosis can extend cell life span, contributing to neoplastic cell expansion independent of cell division [25].

12.2.7 Hereditary Cancer

The evidence now indicates that for many types of cancer, including the most common forms, there exist not only environmental influences but also hereditary predispositions. Our list of genes whose mutations can account for hereditary cancer is increasing. Hereditary forms of cancer can be divided into three categories:

12.2.7.1 Inherited Cancer Syndromes

Inherited cancer syndromes include several well-defined cancers in which inheritance of a single mutant gene greatly increases the risk of a person developing a tumor. The predisposition to these tumors shows an autosomal dominant pattern of inheritance. Childhood retinoblastoma is the most striking example of this category. Familial adenomatous polyposis is the other classic example. For most the development of the clinical features is age dependent, and that development may be early in life, as with hereditary retinoblastoma, or relatively later in life as with colorectal carcinoma.

12.2.7.2 Familial Cancers

Almost all the common types of cancers that occur sporadically have been reported to occur in familial forms. Examples include carcinomas of the colon and breast. Inherited susceptibility to breast cancer has been an area of intensive investigation for the past 10 years. Early work focused on identifying modes of transmission, which culminated in the identification of chromosome 17q12–21 as the first human genomic region that harbored an autosomal dominant susceptibility gene for breast cancer (BRCA1) in 1990. BRCA1 was subsequently identified, followed shortly by the identification of BRCA2 [26]. Research has elucidated much about the mutation spectrum and mutation frequency of these genes in specific populations in the past 3 years and is beginning to identify potential functions. Whereas progress in this area has been rapid and much is now known about inherited susceptibility to breast cancer, much more needs to be done to make these discoveries useful in the diagnosis, treatment, and ultimately prevention of breast cancer.

12.2.7.3 Autosomal Recessive Syndromes of Defective DNA Repair

One of the best-studied examples is xeroderma pigmentosum, in which DNA repair is defective. It is a rare autosomal recessive disease character-

Table 12.2 Biological characteristics of cancer cells

Self-sufficiency in growth signals
Loss of sensitivity to antigrowth signals
Evasion of apoptosis
Evasion of immune surveillance
Loss of capacity for senescence
Loss of contact inhibition
Sustained angiogenesis
Immortality
Genetic instability
Ability to invade neighboring tissues
Ability to form metastases at distant sites

ized by deficiency of endonuclease, the enzyme partly responsible for repair of DNA damage. Children with this disorder develop multiple squamous cell carcinomas [18].

In summary, the molecular pathogenesis of cancer is a complex process requiring the disruption of a number of regulatory pathways. There are a vast number of molecules and genes in a cell that can regulate cell growth. Defects in any of these that shift the balance toward uncontrolled growth, invasiveness, and decreased cell death and other characteristics of cancer cells (Table 12.2) lead to cancer. Recent progress during the last 20 years in understanding these pathways has been tremendous and may explain not only the molecular paradigms for the development of cancer phenotypes, but also finally being brought to force as new cancer therapeutics. Molecular-targeted agents have already made dramatic differences in the treatment of cancers that were previously considered untreatable. The next decade will continue to see explosive growth in novel cancer diagnosis particularly molecular and in therapeutics targeting the different pathways that define a cancer cell.

12.3 Tumor Imaging with Pathophysiological Correlation

Understanding tumor biology is crucial for the use of radionuclide agents for tumor imaging and therapy. For example, the features of proliferation, apoptosis, necrosis, angiogenesis, and cell receptors lead to the discovery of newer radiopharmaceuticals and direct the use of various radiopharmaceuticals for imaging and treatment of tumors based on the biological features. The use of positron-emitting radionuclide imaging has revolutionized the imaging of physiologically and pathologically important molecules. It provides data at both a molecular and metabolic level needed for the evaluation and treatment for effective patient management. It has a major role in cancer detection and more importantly in staging and follow-up of many tumors. In the view of lack of PET, particularly in developing countries, utilizing non-PET radiotracers in managing tumors and in particular in monitoring therapeutic effects of chemoradiotherapy is feasible. Accordingly a brief discussion of such radiopharmaceuticals and their applications is included in this chapter.

12.3.1 Basis of Uptake of Tumor Radiopharmaceuticals

Several radionuclides are useful in imaging tumors. There are similarities and differences in the mechanisms of uptake of the radiopharmaceuticals currently used for tumor imaging (Table 12.3). The choice of radiopharmaceutical depends on the tumor location, the pathology, and the availability of the radiopharmaceutical and the equipment used. The following is a brief on conventional and PET radiopharmaceuticals including agents in the pipeline (Fig. 12.5).

12.3.1.1 Conventional Radiopharmaceuticals

There are numerous radiopharmaceuticals that are used for the differentiation of benign from malignant lesions including gallium-67 citrate, thallium-201 chloride, and ^{99m}Tc-sestamibi. However, with the advent of ^{18}F-FDG as well as computed tomography (CT) and magnetic resonance imaging (MRI), many of the others are not routinely used. The most notable of which is gallium-67 (^{67}Ga) citrate. It was used as a tumor imaging agent initially for Hodgkin's lymphoma. Approximately 90% of Hodgkin's lymphomas

Table 12.3 Tumor imaging radiopharmaceuticals

Radiotracer	Basis of uptake
99mTc-hexakis-methoxy-isobutyl-isonitrile(MIBI)/99mTc-tetrofosmin	Passive diffusion and mitochondrial retention
123I-orI-131-metaiodobenzylguanidine(MIBG)	Active uptake via the epinephrine transporter to enter neuroendocrine cells and store in the neurosecretory granules
201Tl	Sodium pump, ATPase activity
111In-/99mTc-pentetreotide	Detects overexpression of somatostatin receptors in neuroendocrine tumors
111In-capromabpendetide	A monoclonal antibody which recognizes a transmembrane glycoprotein expressed by poorly differentiated and metastatic prostatic carcinoma
67Ga-citrate	Forms a complex with transferrin or lactoferrin for which receptors are overexpressed by tumor cell membrane
18F-fluorodeoxyglucose (FDG)	Increased glucose metabolism
11C-carbon-thymidine	DNA uptake to reflect DNA replication/cellular proliferation
18F-fluorothymidine (FLT)	
11C-carbon-methionine (MET)	Protein synthesis, amino acid transport
18F-fluoroethyltyrosine (FET)	
18F-fluoro-methyl-tyrosine(FMT)	
18F-fluoro-dihydroxyphenylalanine (F-DOPA)	
18F-fluoro-acetate	Membrane lipid synthesis
11C-carbon-choline	
18F-fluoro-choline (FCH)	
18F-fluoromisonidazole (FMISO)	Incorporation into cell constituents under hypoxic conditions
64Cu-copper-ATSM	
18F-fluoro-annexinV	Binding to phosphatidyl serine which comes out of cells due to apoptosis
18F-fluoro-galacto-RDG	Targeting integrin overexpressed on tumor derived endothelial cells
18F-fluoro-deoxyarabinofuranosylnucleosides (FEAU,FIAU,FMAU)	Reporter genes
18F-fluoro-estradiol(FES)	Receptor binding (estrogen)
Ga-68-gallium-DOTATOC/DOTANOC	Receptor binding (somatostatin)

are gallium avid pretreatment [27]. It was later found that 67Ga was also useful in other types of malignancies such as non-Hodgkin's lymphoma, melanoma, hepatocellular carcinoma, and lung cancers among others. 67Ga is trapped on the transferrin or lactoferrin receptors and then passes through the cytoplasm intracellularly [28–30]. Therefore, when transferrin-binding sites in the plasma are saturated by iron, gallium stays in free form in plasma; it will not bind to the transferrin and will not pass across the cell membrane. As a result in these conditions of transferrin saturation, 67Ga citrate uptake will be less sensitive for detection of inflammatory and malignant disease. Background activity will be high and the quality of the scan will be poor. When indicated, these

patients were given a dose of 10 mCi (370 MBq) for adults or 75–100 uCi/kg for pediatric patients. Whole body images with or without SPECT were performed initially at 48–72 h and at 5–10 days as needed [31]. 67Ga citrate is still used in centers where PET service is not available, in spite of its poor physical characteristics, relatively poor sensitivity, and lack of specificity. This is due primarily to its lower cost and long half-life of 3 days, which makes it suitable for worldwide delivery. Those centers that have access to 18F-FDG PET/CT imaging do not recommend 67Ga citrate studies for tumor imaging but are still used for chronic infection localization.

Although predominantly a myocardial perfusion agent, thallium-201 chloride (201Tl) has been

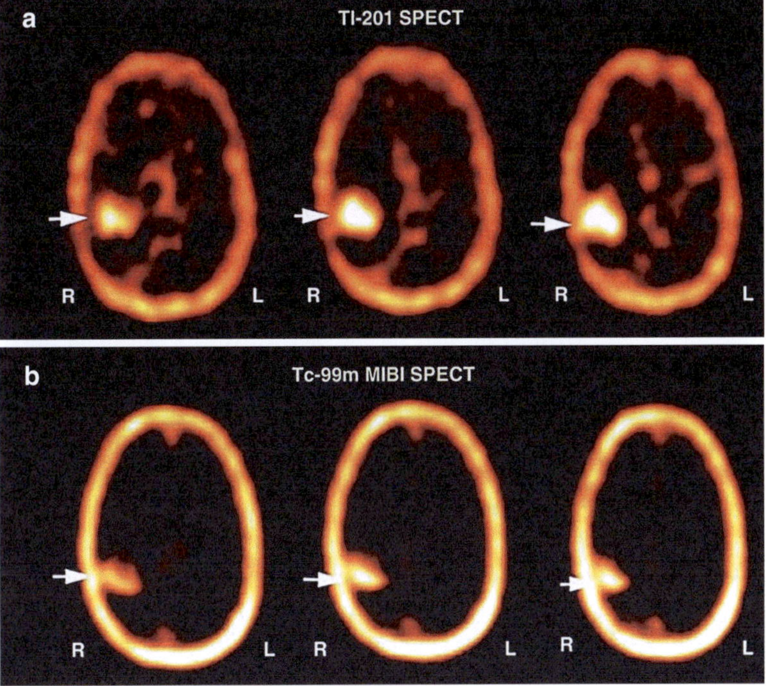

Fig. 12.5 ^{201}Tl (**a**) and ^{99m}TcMIBI (**b**) SPECT scans of a 45-year-old female with high grade brain tumor in the right temporal lobe who had chemotherapy then recurrence. Each tracer shows increased uptake in recurrent viable tumor (*arrows*)

used to image viable benign and malignant tumors throughout the body. It was found that ^{201}Tl was also useful in malignancies including lung, breast, thyroid, glioblastomas, and some sarcomas. However, the use of ^{201}Tl below the diaphragm is limited due to the normal uptake in the liver, spleen, kidneys, and intestines. Chemotherapy and radiation therapy do not alter the uptake of thallium as they do with gallium. ^{201}Tl chloride has a mechanism of uptake in the cell related to the sodium pump, ATPase activity, angiogenesis, and ill-formed and well-formed new blood vessels [32–34]. The typical administered dose is 3–4 mCi (111–148 MBq). Imaging can be performed as early as 10 min postinjection since it localizes in active neoplasms such as lymphoma. Delayed imaging at 3 h can provide enhanced target-to-background ratios [35].

Technetium-99 m sestamibi (^{99m}Tc) has also been found useful for a number of tumors including breast, thyroid, and CNS neoplasms. ^{99m}Tc-sestamibi uptake is related to the electrical gradient difference across the cell membrane and mitochondrial uptake. Retention of this radiopharmaceutical inside the cell, however, is thought to be inversely proportional to the multidrug resistance of its glycoprotein content and its activation in the cell [36–38]. The typical administered dose is 20–30 mCi (740–1110 MBq). Imaging can be performed at 10–20 min postinjection and as far as 2 h delayed imaging since there is little washout from malignant lesions [39, 40].

Indium-111 pentetreotide (OctreoScan) is a somatostatin analog which has been found to be useful for evaluation of neuroendocrine tumors, particularly in carcinoid tumors and gastrinomas. It has also been used to assess patients with lymphomas and granulomatous diseases [41]. Somatostatin is a 14-amino acid peptide that inhibits the release of pituitary hormones as well as the release of certain intestinal and pancreatic peptides such as insulin, glucagon, gastrin, VIP, gastric inhibitory polypeptide, secretin, motilin, and cholecystokinin. Since there is a large quantity of somatostatin receptors in neuroendocrine tumors, radiolabeled analogs are useful for imaging. The typical administered dose of In-111 pentreotide is 3.0–6.0 mCi (111–222 MBq). Imaging can be performed at 4 and 24 h with an option of

48 h imaging to confirm equivocal findings. SPECT imaging is helpful and increases the sensitivity of the examination. The normal distribution includes the blood pool, thyroid, kidneys, bladder, liver, gallbladder, spleen, and bowel.

Metaiodobenzylguanidine (MIBG) can be labeled as either Iodine-123 or Iodine-131. MIBG is a guanethidine analog and resembles norepinephrine making it useful for the detection and evaluation of pheochromocytomas and neuroblastomas [42]. MIBG can also be utilized to evaluate other tumors with a lower affinity such as carcinoid tumors, paragangliomas, and medullary thyroid carcinoma. The ability of MIBG to detect extra-adrenal tumors is integral to the proper staging. The typical administered dose of MIBG for adults is 500 uCi (18.5 MBq) for I-131 or 10–30 mCi (370–1110 MBq) for I-123. Imaging with I-131 MIBG is performed 1 and 2 days after injection and can be repeated at day 3. Imaging with I-123 MIBG is performed between 20 and 24 h with optional delayed images at up to 48 h. When evaluating for pheochromocytomas, the sensitivity and specificity of I-123 MIBG are 88 and 84%, respectively [43]. When evaluating for neuroblastomas, the sensitivity and specificity of I-123 MIBG are 90 and 94%, respectively [44].

12.3.1.2 PET Radiopharmaceuticals

12.3.1.2.1 Glucose Metabolism Agents

Fluorine-18-2-deoxy-D-glucose (^{18}F-FDG) diagnoses, stages, and restages many cancers with an accuracy ranging from 80 to 90%. PET/CT has become a standard procedure in the management of many cancer patients [45]. ^{18}F-FDG uptake in the cell is related to several glucose transporters in the cell membrane which allow active ^{18}F-FDG passage across the membrane to the cytoplasm and trapping without further metabolism. One of the biochemical characteristics of malignant cells is an enhanced rate of glucose metabolism due to increased number of these cell surface glucose transporter proteins (such as Glut-1 and Glut-3) and increased intracellular enzyme levels of hexokinase and phosphofructokinase which promote glycolysis [46, 47]. FDG is phosphorylated to FDG-6-phosphate which, unlike glucose-6-phosphate, cannot be metabolized further and remains trapped in the cell. Imaging needs to be performed in the fasting state in order to minimize competitive inhibition of FDG uptake by glucose [48]. It is recommended that patients fast for a minimum of 4 h prior to FDG administration. Patients should also be well hydrated for the exam and avoid any type of exercise or strenuous work at least 24 h before scanning [49]. A serum glucose level should be obtained prior to FDG administration since image quality is significantly influenced by plasma glucose levels. A commonly used glucose cutoff level is 200 mg/dl. An elevated level will cause an increase in soft tissue uptake and lead to decreased accumulation in tumors. In addition, diabetic patients will have to adjust insulin requirements and are best imaged early in the morning prior to the first meal and insulin (or other hypoglycemia medications). Insulin will also affect image quality by increasing accumulation in skeletal muscles which will in turn decrease accumulation in tumors [50]. FDG PET imaging is performed approximately 60 min following the intravenous administration of 10–20 mCi of FDG (0.14–0.21 mCi/kg of body weight) [49]. For pediatric patients, a dose of 0.15–0.30 mCi/kg is recommended with a minimum dose of 1 mCi [51]. The most common PET acquisition is from the base of the skull to the mid thighs, but some institutions have also recommended imaging from the top of the skull to the feet in all patients as unsuspected malignancies can be found outside the typical field of view in up to 4% of patients. In the following cases images should be obtained from top of the head to toes: melanoma and other skin malignancies, paraneoplastic syndromes, primary unknown tumors, multiple myeloma, neuroblastoma, and extremity tumors [52].

12.3.1.2.2 Bone Seeking Agent

F-fluoride is a sensitive agent for detecting altered osteogenic activity with a mechanism of uptake

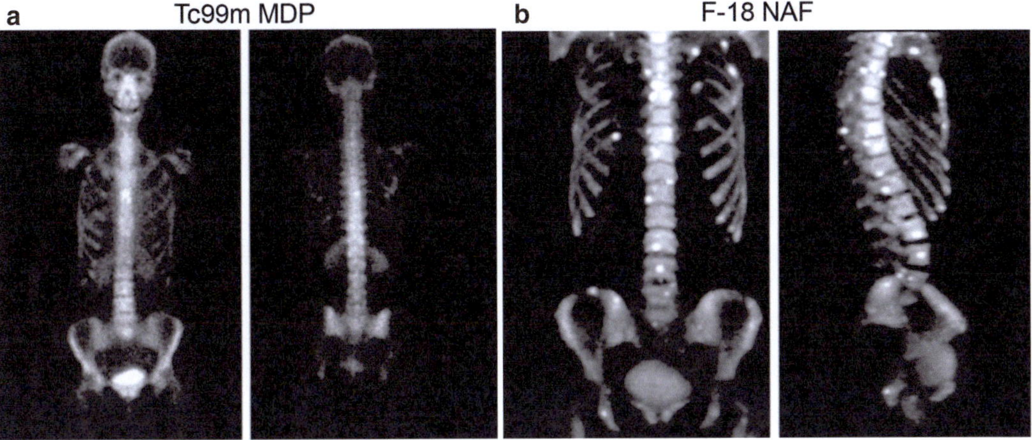

Fig. 12.6 Bone scan (**a**) showing metastases at the manubrium sterni and the thoracic spine. F-18–PET scan (maximum-pixel-intensity projection) showing more lesions indicating disseminated metastatic bone disease (**b**)

similar to that of ^{99m}Tc-MDP (Fig. 12.6). The radiotracer accumulates in the vicinity of metastatic lesions in bone like MDP. However, 18F-fluoride has the advantage of faster blood clearance and higher bone uptake. Deposition of the radiotracer in bone is secondary to the blood flow to the bone as well as the efficiency of the bone to extract the fluorine ions from the blood which are not bound to serum proteins [53]. Given these characteristics, studies have shown that this is more accurate and sensitive for detection of bone metastasis when compared to the current gold standard bone scan as well as MRI [54]. However, one of the drawbacks to this modality is the lack of physiologic information in regard to the soft tissues. At times, both ^{18}F-FDG and 18F-fluoride studies are needed on a given patient. This is typically done as two separate studies on different days which are both inconvenient for the patient and increases radiation exposure from the CT component of both studies. Some have suggested that both ^{18}F-FDG and 18F-fluoride can be combined in a single PET/CT scan by administering the two radiopharmaceuticals simultaneously or in sequence. Preliminary studies have shown this to increase the sensitivity for detecting bone lesions compared with ^{18}F-FDG which only scans with the benefit of additional soft tissue evaluation [55].

12.3.1.2.3   Proliferation Agents

Currently, only ^{18}F-FDG is widely accepted and used in clinical practice for proliferation imaging. ^{18}F-fluorodeoxythymidine (^{18}F-FLT) is an amino acid agent labeled with ^{18}F that can be used to measure tumor cell proliferation [56–58]. The agent is transported into the cell by the same nucleoside carrier as thymidine [59]. The agent is then phosphorylated within the cell by thymidine kinase-1 (TK_1) which is upregulated in rapidly dividing tumor cells (thymidine kinase activity is a marker of cellular proliferation) [56, 60]. Because ^{18}F-fluorodeoxythymidine is resistant to catabolism by thymidine phosphorylase, there is prolonged intracellular retention of the agent [50]. Based on ^{18}F-FLT uptake, an overall reduction in the proliferative activity of gross tumor volumes was observed across the duration of treatment. This information may be useful to monitor changes in cellular proliferation occurring during treatment, to provide valuable prognostic information, and to adapt treatment based on individual biologic response [61].

Other agents of cell growth and proliferation imaging are based on utilization of the uptake of the molecules that are needed for synthetic pathways, including labeled amino acids for measuring transport and protein synthesis and nucleosides for DNA synthesis. Example of such agent to track cancer cell proliferation is C-11 thymidine, which is taken up into DNA but not by RNA to map proliferation and has been used mainly for brain tumors [62]. ^{11}C-methionine is another example, which seeks amino acid transport. A higher correlation with proliferation of lung tumors was seen for C11-4DST than for (18)F-FDG [63]. C-11-labeled agents however have very short half-life. For this reason, F-18-radiolabeled tracers are preferred. This radiotracer was also used to evaluate the response to radiation therapy in patients with lung cancer (NSCLC).

^{11}C-choline (^{11}C-CHOL) is an agent that is incorporated into tumor cells by conversion into ^{11}C-phosphorlycholine which is trapped inside the cell. This is followed by synthesis of ^{11}C-phosphatidylcholine which constitutes a main component of cell membranes. Because tumor cells duplicate very quickly, the biosynthesis of cell membranes is also very fast, and there is increased uptake of choline and upregulation of the enzyme choline kinase [64]. Essentially, the uptake of ^{11}C-CHOL in tumors represents the rate of tumor cell proliferation [65]. ^{11}C-CHOL is very rapidly cleared from the blood, and optimal tumor-to-background contrast is reached within 5 min [64, 66].

12.3.1.2.4 Hypoxia Agents

It has been established that hypoxic tumor cells are more resistant than aerobic cells to ionizing radiation and chemotherapy. Hypoxic cells are more resistant to radiation therapy and therefore require additional radiation to achieve adequate cell killing, which might exceed the tolerance of the surrounding normal tissues, called the tumor bed [67, 68].

Accordingly, tumor hypoxia is an important factor in relapse-free survival. The potential importance of tumor hypoxia as a cause of treatment failure in patients treated with radiation has been recognized for a long time. Methods have been developed to add compounds to act as hypoxic cytotoxin to potentiate the effect of radiation. Accordingly, evaluation of tumor hypoxia can help in patient's management. PET/CT imaging using F-18-misonidazole (FMISO) is used in evaluating hypoxia and in evaluating prognosis in patients receiving radiation therapy and certain chemotherapy [69, 70].

^{18}F-fluoromisonidazole (^{18}F-FMISO) acts as a bioreceptor molecule and is incorporated into cell constituents under hypoxic conditions [67]. Unfortunately, there is slow cellular uptake and slow washout from non-hypoxic tissues. ^{62}Cu-ATSM is another tumor hypoxia agent, which accumulates in hypoxic tissues where it is reduced, trapped, and has the advantage of rapid clearance from non-hypoxic tissue [67, 68].

12.3.1.2.5 Receptor Imaging Agents

The increased expression of various types of receptors on the cell surface is a unique biomarker for specific types of cancers. For example, somatostatin receptor is a unique characteristic of neuroendocrine tumors. 68-Ga-DOTATATE and the newly approved 64-Cu-DOTATATE are radiolabeled somatostatin analogs for the diagnosis and pretreatment evaluation of neuroendocrine tumors with PET. There are five types of somatostatin receptors characterized (sst1 to sst5), but sst2 is the predominant one in neuroendocrine tumors [71]. Studies have demonstrated that the sensitivity of these agents was up to 96% with a specificity of up to 100% in the diagnosis of neuroendocrine tumors on PET. In addition, this was found to be superior than conventional somatostatin receptor scintigraphy and diagnostic CT in diagnosis, staging, and restaging [72–74].

The advent of 64-Cu-DOTATATE allows for a lower radiation-dose option with superior lesion detection rates compared to 68-Ga [75]. In addition, these radiotracers are linked to a therapy arm with Lutetium-177 for the treatment of neuroendocrine tumors. Further discussion on theranostics will be reviewed in another chapter.

Estrogen receptors (ER) are a unique biomarker of breast cancers and can be evaluated using the radiolabeled estrogen analog 18F-estradiol. The advantage of this type of imaging is the ability to assess the estrogen receptor status of tumor lesions throughout the body. The mainstay for treatment of this type of tumor is endocrine therapy, however, resistance can occur with progression. Imaging with 18F-estradiol can help clinicians predict response to therapy and select optimal treatment in the future while sparing patients from unnecessary chemotherapy. For the detection of ER+ breast cancer, 18F-estradiol imaging has a sensitivity of 84% and specificity of 98% [76].

Human epidermal growth factor receptor 2 (HER2 or erb2) is a member of the ERbBs or type 1 receptor kinase family involved in cell development, proliferation, and differentiation. Tumors that overexpress HER2 show high rate of proliferation and are associated with more aggressive disease, poor prognosis, and shorter overall survival. Approximately 20% of invasive ductal breast cancers are classified as HER2 positive. Zr-89 Trastuzumab is a radiolabeled monoclonal antibody which targets HER2. HER2 PET helps noninvasively assess HER2 expression in tumors and identify patients who may benefit from HER2-targeted therapy, to monitor the change in HER2 status during therapy, and selecting cases for targeted radionuclide therapy [77]. Prostate-specific-membrane antigen (PSMA) is a cell surface glycoprotein overexpressed on prostate cancer cells. Its expression is 100-1000 fold higher in prostate cancer than in other tissues and the levels increase with higher tumor stage and grade (Gleason score). 68Ga-PSMA and 18F-PSMA are analogs for the diagnosis and pretreatment of prostate cancer with PET. It has been established that PSMA PET-CT imaging has superior diagnostic accuracy than conventional imaging with CT or MRI in men with high-risk prostate cancer. 18F-PSMA has several advantages over 68-Ga such as a longer half-life (110 min vs. 68 min), can be produced in larger quantities due to the cyclotron production vs. generator-produced, and greater spatial resolution due to the lower positron energy. As in neuroendocrine tumors, imaging with PSMA tracers is linked to the therapy arm with Lutetium-177 for the treatment of prostate cancer [78, 79].

12.3.1.2.6 Tumor Stroma Agents

We are now coming to the age where we have the potential to image and treat a wide variety of malignancies using a single target. Imaging and therapy for neuroendocrine tumors and prostate cancer discussed in this chapter are dependent on unique biomarkers (DOTATATE and PSMA). The introduction of fibroblast activation protein (FAP), however, has the potential of transforming our treatment strategy. FAP is a serine proteinase which is expressed on the cell surface of activated fibroblasts during wound healing, fibrotic processes, and the stroma of many malignancies. Normal fibroblasts can be differentiated from the cancer-associated fibroblasts by the expression of FAP. In cancer associated-fibroblasts, FAP promotes tumor growth and progression while being overexpressed in various types of malignancies. Approximately 90% of a tumor's mass can be attributed to these cancer-associated fibroblasts [80, 81].

Accordingly, FAP is a potential target for theranostics with a wide variety of applications. Studies have already been performed with promising results using FAP inhibitors (FAPIs). A recent study evaluating 68Ga-FAPI PET/CT in 28 different kinds of cancer demonstrated high uptake in many prevalent cancers including breast, esophageal, lung, pancreatic, head and neck, and colorectal [82]. In addition, the therapeutic application of 90Y-FAPI has been performed on a patient with advanced breast cancer with equally encouraging results [83]. Alpha emitters have also been shown in mice to be an effective treatment in pancreatic cancer. Multiple additional studies are being performed to evaluate FAP as a viable target for theranostics but it could bring us a step closer to the development of a universal cancer therapy.

12.3.1.2.7 Angiogenesis Imaging Agents

Tumor growth depends on the balance between proangiogenic and antiangiogenic molecules. Inhibition of angiogenesis is a current target to develop new anticancer medication against solid tumors. Recent advances enabled tumor angiogenesis imaging, and the targets include vascular endothelial growth factor (VEGF) and vascular endothelial growth factor receptor, integrin $\alpha_v\beta_3$, matrix metalloproteinase, endoglin (CD105), and E-selectin. Tumor angiogenesis imaging will help in further understanding the mechanisms of tumor angiogenesis and evaluating the efficacy of novel antiangiogenic therapies. Molecular imaging has enormous potential in improving the efficiency of the drug development process, including the specific area of anti-angiogenic drugs. Radiolabeled VEGF isoforms were tested for imaging angiogenesis using SPECT and PET. A few radiolabeled anti-VEGF antibodies have been also reported for PET imaging [84]. The alpha (v) beta3 integrin is an important cell adhesion receptor involved in tumor-induced angiogenesis and tumor metastases. The RGD-containing glycopeptide cyclo(-Arg-Gly-Asp-D-Phe-Lys (sugar amino acid) with 4-nitrophenyl2-^{18}F0fluoropropionate has been studied in vitro as well as in tumor mouse models [85]. These studies suggested that this^{18}F-labeled compound is suitable for noninvasive PET imaging of angiogenesis status of a tumor and subsequent monitoring of treatment response, especially when the primary target of the therapy was angiogenesis.

12.3.1.2.8 Apoptosis Detection Agents

All chemotherapeutic agents and radiation therapies induce programmed cell death (apoptosis). Detection of apoptosis by noninvasive imaging is another interesting area. Annexin V, an endogenous protein labeled with technetium-99 m, has led the way to detect apoptosis [86]. The mechanism of ^{99m}Tc-annexin uptake is through its binding with phosphatidylserine, which is normally present in the inner aspect of a normal cell membrane that becomes externalized during the process of apoptosis. Labeling annexin V with ^{18}F has been reported. The capability of PET to provide better quantification may further increase the utility of this method in the near future and may provide greater insight into the therapeutic response in patients with cancer [86].

12.3.1.2.9 Labeled Reporter Gene

Reporter gene labeling is a common concept in cell tracking. Most commonly used genes are coding regions for alkaline phosphatase, firefly luciferase, and chloramphenicol acetyltransferase. The corresponding gene product (a protein) can metabolize a substrate into a detectable product (a color, fluorescence, or chemical). Hence, the reporter gene label enables cell detection by an assay. The disadvantage of these tracking methods is the requirement of a biopsy or even animal sacrifice for the performance of cell tracking. Several methods have been developed to track transplanted cells/stem cells in vivo. Advances in molecular genetics made it possible to introduce gene therapy as a treatment option in the near future in conjunction with other treatment modalities in cancer patients. The success of gene therapy depends on several steps like delivery of the gene to the targeted tumor cells, then the gene needs to be incorporated into the native gene of the tumor cells, and afterward the delivered gene should get translated into a final product. The difficulties faced during gene therapy are the (1) variability of uptake of the gene of interest by the targeted cells, (2) uncertainty of incorporation of this gene to the native gene, and (3) variable expression of this gene after incorporation. A noninvasive imaging modality to identify and quantify the extent of success of these steps of gene therapy is essential to implement gene therapy in clinical practice for cancer patients. Currently, PET gene therapy imaging studies with radiolabeled probes use HSV1-tk as the reporter gene [87], and several other PET tracers, which are analogs of uracil and thymidine, are being developed.

12.3.2   Scintigraphic Imaging and its Clinical Uses

Nuclear medicine has a major and increasing role in the management of malignant tumors. With the developments toward molecular imaging and the advancement of equipment used for imaging particularly after combining the nuclear medicine instruments with morphological modalities, it has even become a more integral part of management protocols. This role includes detection of malignant tumors, staging and restaging of the disease, early detection of recurrence, evaluation of the response to therapy, and prediction of the prognosis.

Radionuclide diagnosis and therapy for tumors depend on the characteristics of tumors which include:

- Increased vascularization.
- Increased blood flow.
- Newly proliferated capillaries with more permeable walls.
- Increased metabolic activity of cells.
- Increased energy demand.
- High density of some common or specific antigens.
- Several specific receptors.

Understanding the cell biology of tumors and their features including the angiogenesis, cell proliferation, necrosis, apoptosis, and specific cell receptors has led and will lead to the development of new imaging methods to evaluate various aspects of the tumor to help improve the diagnostic and therapeutic capabilities. Furthermore, this understanding has led to the development of newer methods to treat tumors as well as the development of newer drugs.

The pathophysiological characteristics of tumors are utilized in several scintigraphic clinical applications effectively including diagnosis, staging, and evaluation of the response to therapy, selection of drug therapy, and prediction of prognosis.

12.3.2.1   Tumor Detection

Early diagnosis provides the best chance for cure. Histopathology is the gold standard to differentiate benign and malignant lesions. Therefore, if a tumor is superficial or accessible for any form of biopsy, it should be the next investigation of choice if not contraindicated. Various imaging modalities play a role in the diagnosis of tumors which are not accessible easily for biopsy or when needle biopsy is associated with serious consequences. The goal of an imaging modality is to identify a pathological process correctly noninvasively at the earliest so that curative treatment (most often surgery) can be offered. Molecular derangement occurs at the very beginning of the disease process, and the final result of anatomically detectable abnormalities occurs much later [88]. Accordingly, functional imaging is suited for earlier detection of the malignant process. CT, the most frequently used imaging modality, relies on the differentiation between benign and malignant lesions on the basis of certain criteria involving the size of the lesion and the interval increase in size over a short period of time detected by repeated imaging, the regular irregular margins of the lesion, the presence of capsular demarcation, the heterogeneity, and the presence of microcalcification. Similar criteria are used in mammography for breast cancer screening. All these parameters are nonspecific and too many patients are therefore sent for unnecessary biopsy [48]. Conversely, functional imaging is unique in that it can provide unperturbed physiological information. It usually uses a molecular probe for imaging. The probe could be already existing in the tumor, like MR spectroscopy, to detect concentration of ATP/ADP, thereby measuring tumor energy metabolism in tissue by imaging the 31 P of ATP/ADP [89]. The probe can be introduced from outside like 18 F-FDG for PET scanning to measure the glucose metabolism in tissue. In this case, the administered quantity is so small (<10 µg) that while portraying the pathway of interest, it leaves that pathway completely intact [88]. Nuclear medicine radiopharmaceuticals used for the differentiation of benign from malignant lesions include gallium-67 citrate, thallium-201 chloride, 99 m Tc-sestamibi, and fluorine-18 fluorodeoxyglucose (FDG). These radiopharmaceuticals have been used for the diagnosis of tumors and in differentiating benign from malignant disease. Although differentiating benign from malignant lesions is achieved in many locations with high degree of accuracy, it has not achieved a level to replace histological examination since the sensitivity and specificity are not 100%. Small cancer lesions can be missed, and false positives occur due to uptake of some radiotracers by pathologies other than cancer such as inflammation. Dual acquisition using early and delayed imaging with quantitation using thallium-201, 99 m Tc-MIBI, and FDG PET as well as the use of image fusion or combined modality as PET/CT helps decrease the false-positive results. FDG PET is valuable in the early detection of tumor (Fig. 12.7, 12.8, and 12.9) and can help in its diagnosis [90]. The indeterminate lung nodule is an important example illustrating this. It is estimated that solitary pulmonary nodules are detected in 52 per 100,000 people in the USA. Thirty percent of these will be considered benign based on an initial examination for history of risk factors and standard radiographs. The remaining 70% are considered indeterminate, requiring the examination—often by CT. Of the cases sent to CT, 78% are diagnosed indeterminate or malignant, and 75% will be referred to surgery, resulting in approximately 68,000 thoracotomies annually. Twenty percent of these thoracotomies will yield a benign diagnosis. Based on published data, PET would reduce the number of unnecessary thoracotomies, resulting in only a 6% yield of benign diagnosis for resected solitary pulmonary nodules [91–94]. A lesion that present high SUV values on PET study should be considered malignant until proven otherwise. A lesion that is PET negative has a low probability of being a malignancy (under 5% [88]). However, one must consider all characteristics of a lesion prior to discounting its

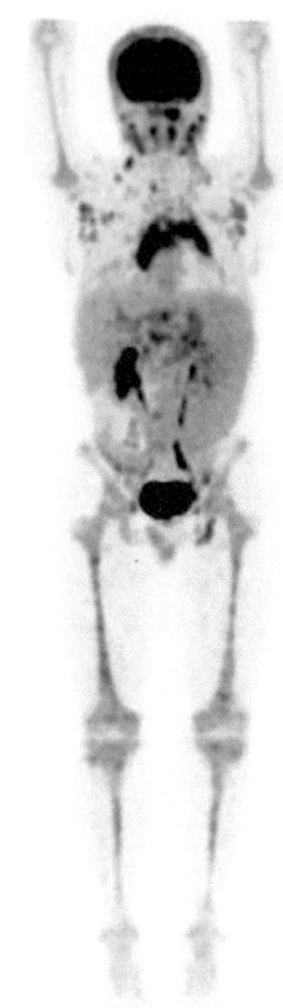

Fig. 12.7 FDG PET/CT. Patient is a 19-year-old male presenting with acute lymphoblastic lymphoma for initial staging. Extensive FDGavid lymphadenopathy is seen including the head and neck, chest, abdomen, and pelvis with associated massive splenomegaly. There is also FDG avidity within the enlarged thymus and diffuse bone marrow activity. Increased FDG activity throughout the stomach with associated wall thickening, equivocal for malignancy F-18 FDG 10 Nuclear Oncology

malignant potential. Follow-up exams with CT should be performed on PET-negative nodules to ensure stability [95]. If the lesion grows, further evaluation with tissue diagnosis should be obtained. Patients who have a negative FDG PET exam but are subsequently shown to have lung cancer may have an overall better survival compared to patients with positive FDG exams [89]. However, SUV criteria to diagnose malignancy should be used very cautiously, as there are several factors mentioned earlier that can influence the value of SUV.

Fig. 12.8 FDG-18 whole body MIP (**a**); selected transaxial CT, PET, and PET/CT fusion image of the abdomen (**b**) of a 54-year-old male with incidentally discovered enlarged mediastinal lymph nodes on a CT angiography of the neck/done for a bleeding cavernoma of the brain. FDG PET/CT images show a large FDG avid right renal cell carcinoma with widespread metastasis to the lungs, mediastinal lymph nodes, left adrenal gland, and multiple bones

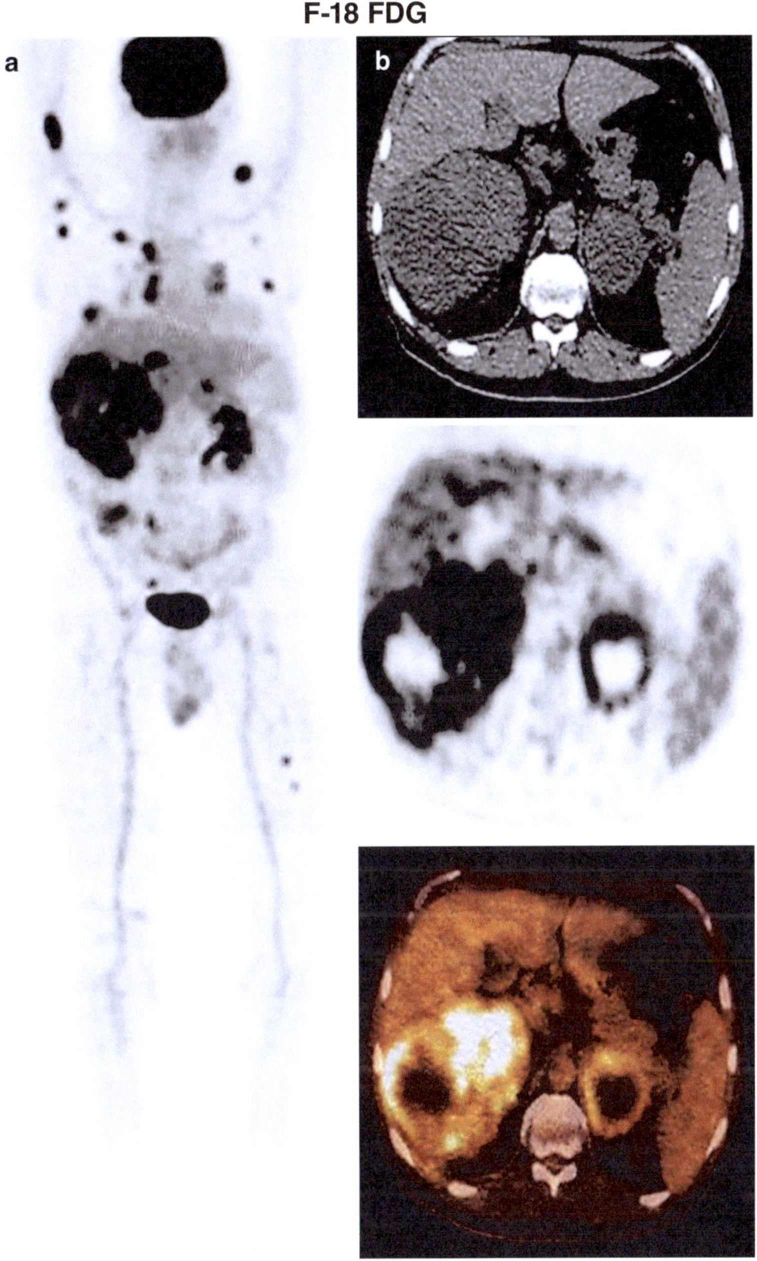

If PET is not available, other options are as follows: for lung cancer, thallium should be utilized when the lesion is larger than 2 cm in size, and for breast cancer, brain tumors, and bone and soft tissue tumors, thallium-201 or 99 m Tcsestamibi should be utilized.

F-18 FDG

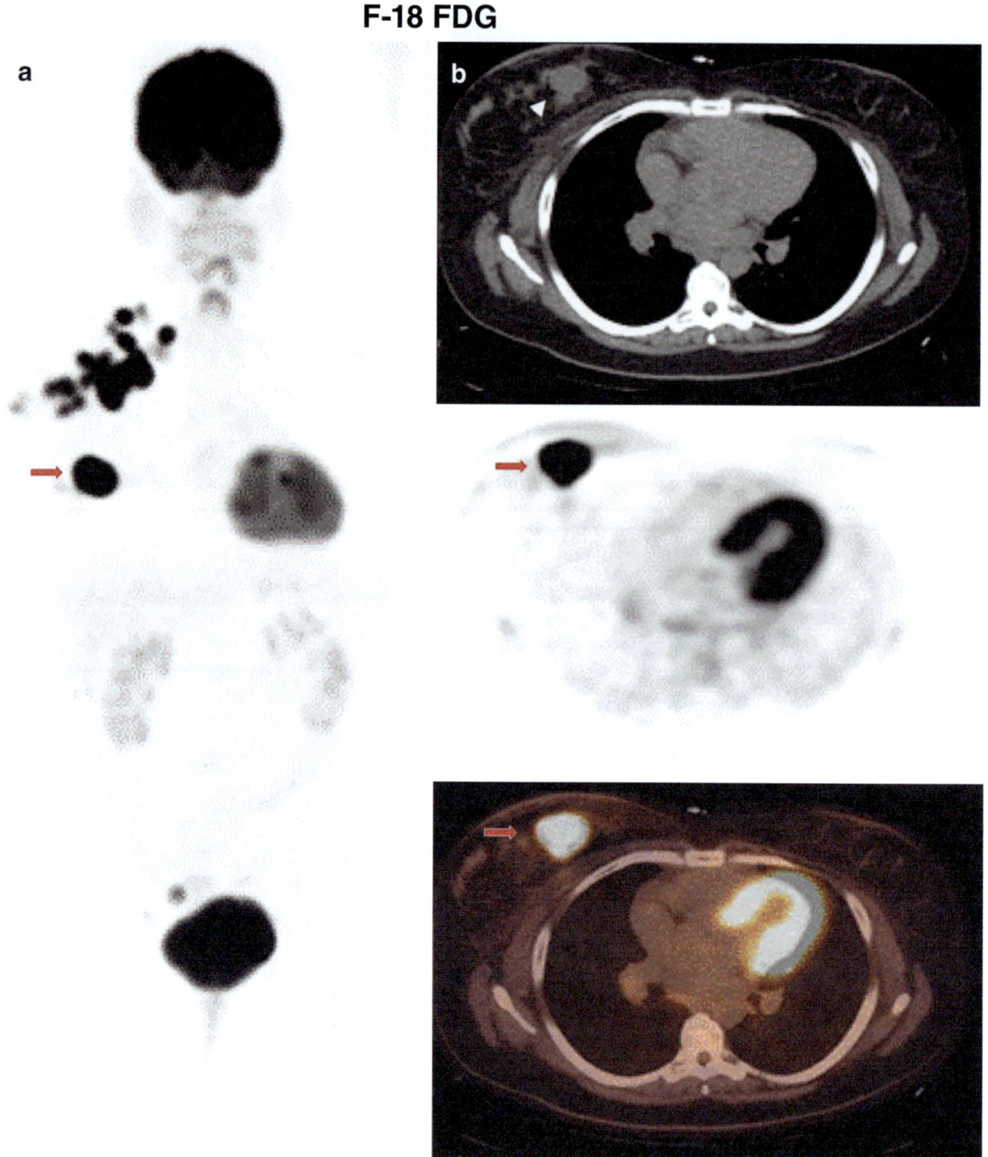

Fig. 12.9 A 34-year-old female presenting with a right breast mass. FDG PET/CT images show an intensely hypermetabolic right breast mass (*arrow*) with multiple hypermetabolic right axillary lymph nodes onwhole body MIP (**a**). Representative transaxial cut (**b**) shows again the primary breast tumor ON PET and Fused PET/CT images (*arrows*) corresponding to CT finding (*arrowhead*) Biopsy revealed right breast invasive ductal carcinoma with metastatic right axially lymph nodes

12.3.2.2 Staging and Restaging

Nuclear medicine has a more important role in staging malignant tumors compared to tumor diagnosis (Figs. 12.10, 12.11, 12.12, 12.13, and 12.14). Accurate staging of malignant lesions at the time of initial presentation is of utmost importance to provide appropriate management for a particular patient (Figs. 10.6 and 10.7). Overstaging can inappropriately deprive a patient from receiving curative treatment. Conversely, understaging can subject a patient to undergo a futile but drastic treatment that can even increase the morbidity and mortality (e.g., pneumonectomy in case of stage III or IV lung cancer) without any increase in the chance of cure. Staging has been mostly performed according to the find-

Fig. 12.10 An FDC
study of a patient with
known colon cancer as
part of the work up for
staging. The study
shows metastases to the
liver and abdominal
lymph nodes (*arrows*)

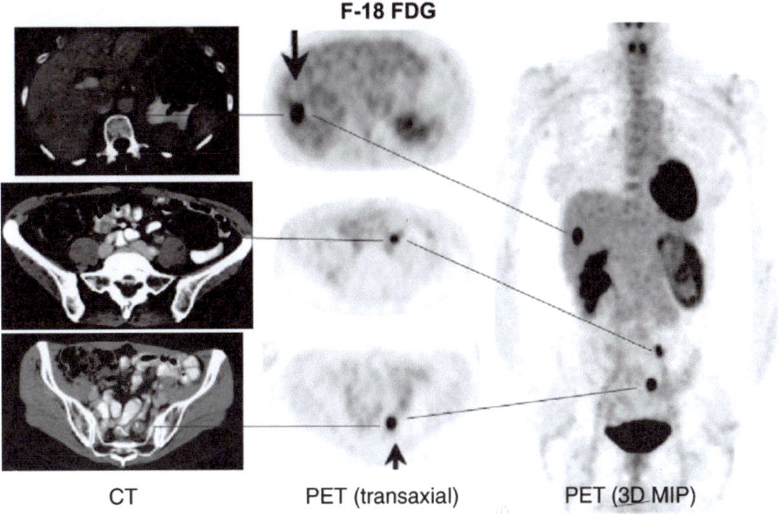

Fig. 12.11 ^{18}F-FDG study for staging of a patient
recently diagnosed with non-small cell right lung
cancer. CT showed increased sizes of lymph nodes
ipsi- and contra-laterally. The question was whether
the patient had stage N2 or N3 to determine
resectability. The FDG study shows only ipsilateral
lymph node metastasis (*arrow*), indicating minimal
N2, M0 stage (Courtesy of Professor Osama Sabri,
Leipzig)

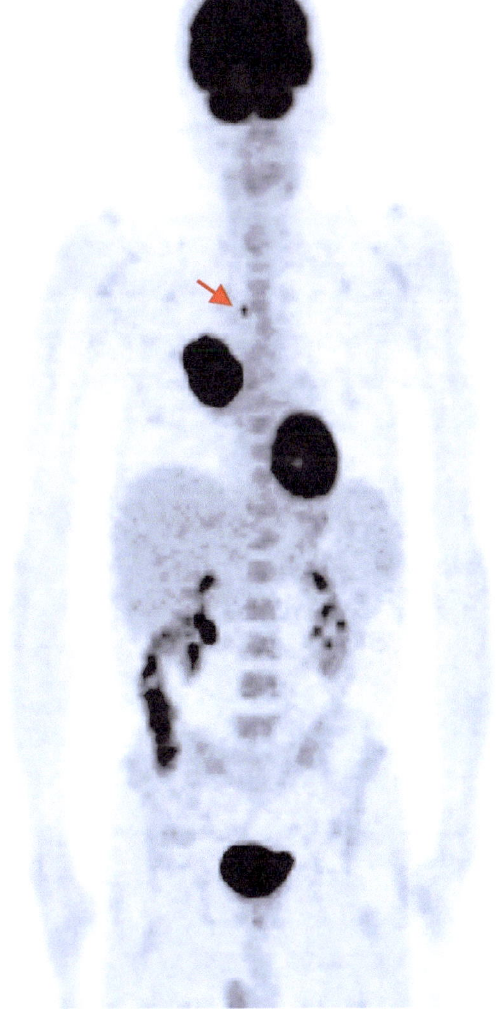

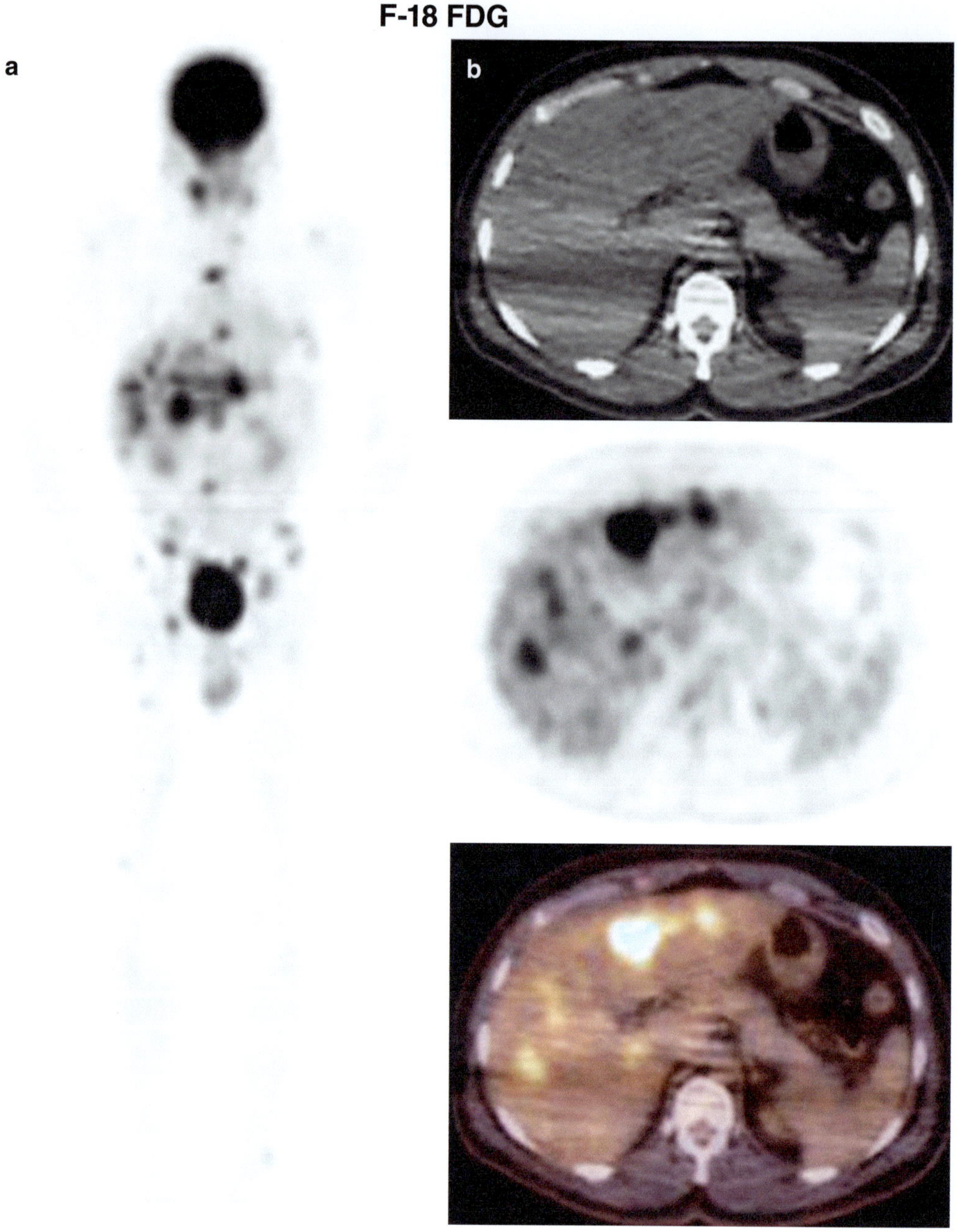

F-18 FDG

Fig. 12.12 F-18 FDG whole body MIP (**a**); selected transaxial CT, PET, and PET/CT fusion image of the abdomen (**b**) images of a 33-year-old male with nasal melanoma, showing widespread metastatic disease involving the lungs, liver, cervical lymph nodes, abdominal cavity, musculoskeletal system, left thyroid gland, and skin

F-18 FDG

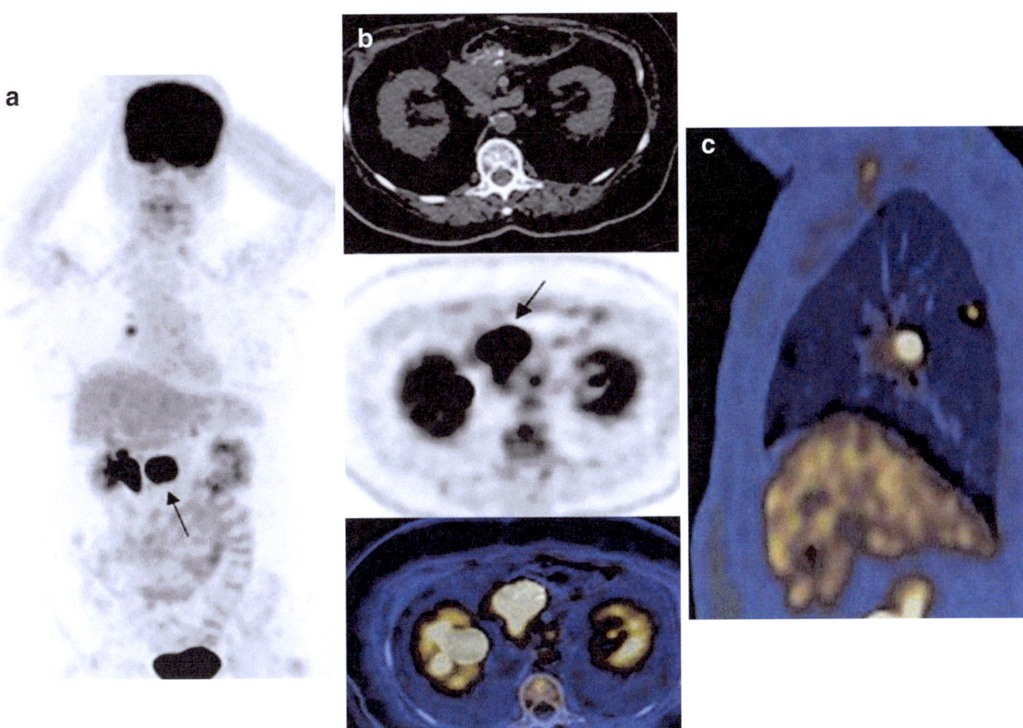

Fig. 12.13 F-18 FDG whole body MIP (**a**); selected transaxial CT, PET, and PET/CT fusion image of the abdomen (**b**), and selected sagittal and transaxial PET/CT fusion images of the chest and upper abdomen (**c**) *for a 51*-year-old female with history of adenocarcinoma of the hepatic flexure of the colon and metastases to mesenteric nodes and omentum, operated in 2015. Now with possible recurrence and referred for restaging. There is a large hypermetabolic mass in the region of the surgical clips/anastomosis in the mid-abdomen (arrows) (SUVmax, 19.7), consistent with recurrent tumor. There are also hypermetabolic lymph nodes in the right hilum and left diaphragmatic region as well as hypermetabolic right posterior lung nodules which are suspicious for metastatic disease

ings of noninvasive imaging modalities such as CT or MRI, in addition to other guided invasive procedures for the purpose of biopsy [96]. CT criteria for staging lymph node involvement depend mostly on the size of the lymph nodes. If they are more than 1 cm in the mediastinum, for example, the lymph nodes are considered to be positive for malignant involvement [97]. However, microscopic involvement of these lymph nodes is not related to their size. Metastatic malignant cells can involve small lymph nodes. Large lymph nodes can be due to inflammatory response without metastatic involvement. For the same reasons that have been mentioned with regard to primary lesions, the accuracy of the staging depends on the resolution of the systems, the location of the lymph nodes, and the intensity of uptake of the radiopharmaceutical in the adja-

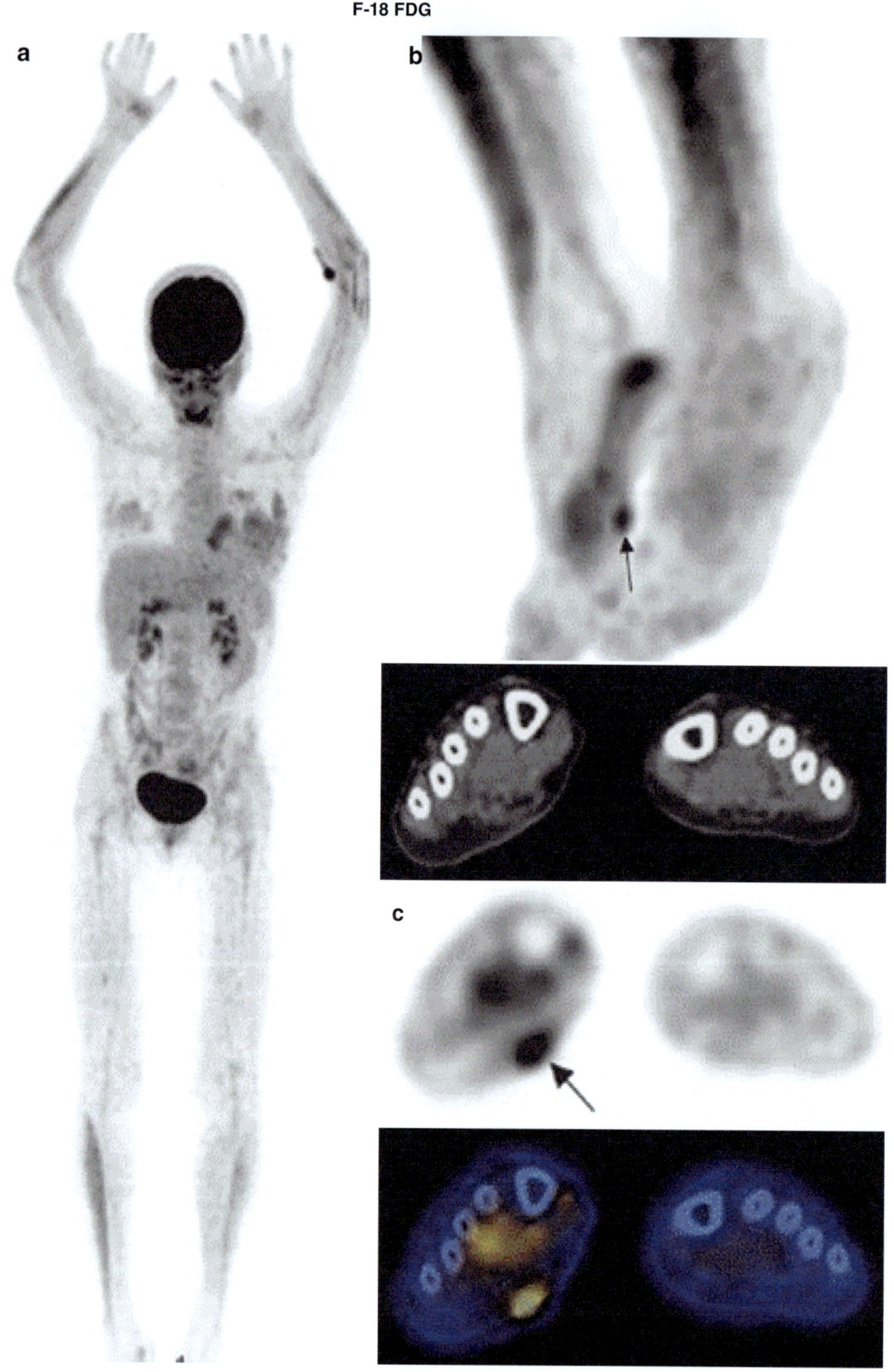

Fig. 12.14 F-18 FDG PET whole body MIP (**a**), MIP image of the feet (**b**), and selected transaxial CT, PET, and PET/CT fusion images of the feet (**c**) of a thirty-year-old female with biopsy (incisional)-proven malignant melanoma in the sole of the right foot. Focal hypermetabolic activity with some thickening of the skin in the mid-sole of the right foot is seen, consistent with the biopsy-proven tumor (arrows) (SUVmax of 2.3). Diffuse activity adjacent and posterior to this lesion is muscular. On whole body images, there is no evidence of metastatic disease. Increased activity in the breasts, more on the left, is due to lactation

cent regions. Nuclear medicine procedures, especially 18 F-FDG PET, have a higher degree of accuracy compared with X-ray CT or MRI, with the advantage of functionally verifying and determining whether the draining lymph nodes are involved in metastatic invasion. For example, the accuracy of X-ray CT in staging mediastinal disease in lung cancer is approximately 70%; MRI is slightly higher at around 80%, while 18 F-FDG accuracy is better than 90% [98–101].

Proper staging commonly requires surgical, pathological, and microscopic verification. Even with nuclear medicine procedures, however, certain invasive procedures cannot be avoided. For example, in patients with primary pulmonary nodules, if the CT scan does not show evidence of enlargement of mediastinum nodes and the 18 F-FDG PET study shows that there is unilateral or bilateral mediastinal lymph node increased uptake, this will be considered as metastatic nodal involvement until surgeons have to weigh the results of these studies in order to decide whether to completely avoid invasive staging procedures and be satisfied with the results of the PET studies or perform guided biopsy.

The same problem holds for the staging of axillary nodal involvement, which is one of the most important factors for the staging and prognosis of breast cancer as the sensitivity of any nuclear medicine procedure, including 18 F-FDG PET studies, is no more than 90% [102, 103]. Although sentinel node imaging does not image the cancer, it can identify the lymph node/nodes where the primary tumor drains. Sentinel lymph node localization by either the radionuclide or the blue dye technique is the most acceptable alternative to total axillary node dissection [104].

12.3.2.3 Prediction of Prognosis

Once the staging of cancer is established, the management of that particular patient is mainly based on the stage and associated clinical factors (comorbid conditions). However, for most of stage III and IV solid tumors, the response rate to the first-line chemotherapy treatment is approximately 30–40% with few exceptions such as the cases of lymphoma and testicular tumor.

Therefore, a significant number of patients will not respond to the first-line chemotherapy and will require more aggressive second-line treatment, which is usually associated with more bone marrow toxicity. In the case of patients who had already received the first-line treatment with associated toxicities leading to decreasing bone marrow reserve, oncologist has to wait till the patient's bone marrow reserve comes back to near normal level so that the patient can tolerate the second-line treatment. It is possible that during this waiting period tumor burden increases further and potentially decreases the chance for response to the second-line treatment. It is well known that chemotherapeutic agents (e.g., alkylating agents) as well as radiotherapy can cause late complications like solid tumors, leukemias, non-Hodgkin's lymphomas, cardiac diseases, pulmonary fibrosis, gonadal problems, and thyroid disorders (thyroiditis, thyroid nodules, hypo- and hyperthyroidism) [105]. These effects are dose dependent. Therefore, they are more likely to occur but also more likely to occur earlier in patients who received first-line treatment followed by second-line treatment compared to the patients who received the second-line treatment at the beginning and did not require any other treatment. Early detection of nonresponders to first-line treatment and starting more aggressive treatment protocol not only increase the likelihood of complete response to the treatment but also at the same time potentially decrease the incidence of long term complications associated with tumoricidal treatments. This is very important particularly when more and more new treatment regimens are invented to increase the long-term disease-free survival. Recently, there is not only increase in the cure rate for some cancers as lymphoma and testicular tumors, but also these cured patients are living long (more than 10–15 years) and they can experience long-term toxicities related to the treatment. Correlation studies with histology showed that high mitotic counts tend to be associated with higher glycolytic rates, and higher glycolytic rates tend to have poor prognosis. Higher glycolytic rate, determined by FDG uptake, was shown to be associated with high-grade tumors and poor prognosis [106]. Study in head and neck cancer patients showed that SUV higher than 10 is associated with poorer prognosis [107]. It was found that a low pre-therapy FDG uptake (metabolic rate of glucose [MRgl] < 20 mmol/min/100 g tissue) predicated complete local response [108]. Conversely, increase in SUV correlated with increase in tumor proliferative potential (MIB-1 and PCNA), cellularity, and overall advanced stage as well as shorter survival compared to low SUV group [109–112]. Kunkel et al. [70] found that an SUV of less than 4 predicted 80% survival at 3 years after treatment, and the similar number for SUV >4 was only 43% in patients with head and neck cancer. Although endocrine therapy is an effective method to treat estrogen receptor (ER)-positive breast cancer, approximately 30–40% of all hormone receptor-positive tumors display de novo resistance. 18 F-FMISO PET/CT can be used to predict primary endocrine resistance in ER-positive breast cancer [113, 114].

12.3.2.4 Prediction of Drug Resistance

Drug resistance is a major problem in the treatment of cancer [115]. Resistance to treatment with anticancer drugs results from a variety of factors including individual differences in patients and somatic cell genetic variations in tumors even those from the same tissue of origin. Multidrug resistance is the principal mechanism by which many cancers develop resistance to chemotherapy and is a major factor in the failure of many forms of chemotherapy. It affects a variety of solid and blood cancers. Tumors usually consist of mixed populations of malignant cells, some of which are drug sensitive and others are drug resistant. Chemotherapy kills drug-sensitive cells but leaves behind a higher proportion of drug resistant cells. As the tumor begins to grow again, chemotherapy may fail because the remaining tumor cells are now resistant. Resistance to therapy has been correlated to the presence of at least two molecular "pumps" in tumor cell membranes that actively expel chemotherapy drugs from the interior. This allows tumor cells to avoid the toxic effects of the drug or molecular processes within the nucleus or the cytoplasm and eject anticancer drugs from

cells. The two pumps commonly found to cause chemoresistance in cancer are P-glycoprotein and multidrug resistance-associated protein (MRP). Knowledge about the mechanisms of cancer drug resistance will help design strategies to circumvent resistance and develop drugs that are less susceptible to known resistance mechanisms which will be important in improving drug delivery and distribution in patients [7, 115]. These glycoproteins are responsible for the outward cellular transport of a variety of chemotherapeutic agents (such as daunorubicin, vincristine, and adriamycin). In men there are two closely related genes—MDR1 and MDR3. They have similar structures. MDR1 has been labeled P-glycoprotein (PGP), or p170, because of its molecular weight of 170 kD. It consists of 12 transmembrane domains and two binding sites for ATP, which provides the necessary energy for drug transport [4]. The PGP appears to function as an efflux pump that removes a variety of toxins from the cell, not confined only to chemotherapy. Drug resistance leads to defective drug transport into the cells, enhanced drug elimination from the cells, decreased metabolic activation of drugs, increased drug inactivation, altered target proteins with reduced affinity for cytotoxic agents, and overproduction of specific target proteins. A noninvasive imaging may have a potential role in the selection of patients in whom the modulation of Pgp may be beneficial before and after chemotherapy. As well, this imaging could be helpful to evaluate the efficacy of the Pgp modulation therapy. 99 m Tc-sestamibi is a substrate for the P-glycoprotein pump, and a correlation exists between the efflux rate of 99 m Tc-sestamibi and the expression of P-glycoprotein in breast cancer. By performing early and delayed 99 m Tc-sestamibi imaging of patients with breast cancer, the washout rate of sestamibi can be determined. Lack of significant tracer washout indicates a low risk for chemoresistance [116]. Conversely, a high washout rate was associated with a high probability of chemoresistance (sensitivity 100%, specificity 80%, and positive predictive value 83%) [117]. In these patients, the use of chemorevertant or chemomodulator agents could be justified [117].

The multidrug-resistant energy-dependent P-glycoprotein pump system (MDR-Pgp) may play a role in the resistance of lung cancer to certain chemotherapeutic agents. Determination of MDR-Pgp at time of diagnosis may provide information regarding which treatment protocol would be best for each individual patient. P-glycoprotein recognizes certain chemotherapy agents as substrates (such as paclitaxel, a taxane agent) and is involved with their transport out of the cell. P-glycoprotein also works to prevent intracellular accumulation of some lipophilic cationic radiopharmaceuticals such as Tc-tetrofosmin. Cancers with low uptake of Tc-tetrofosmin likely have overexpression of MDR-Pgp and are more likely to be associated with a poor response to certain chemotherapy agents [118].

12.3.2.5 Evaluation of Therapy and Detecting Recurrence

Patients can respond differently to the same treatment protocol, and accordingly individualization of therapy should be more appropriate. Tumor volume changes observed during follow-up morphological studies in principle can be used for evaluation of response to antitumor therapy. However, it is not early enough before the patient develops considerable toxicity and side effects from the prescribed chemotherapy since it takes considerable time to see the size changes.

After initial treatment, early discrimination of tumor recurrence from post-treatment changes is a clinical problem. There are problems in developing methods that are sensitive to early changes during the course of treatment and for the discrimination of tumor tissue from surrounding normal tissue, fibrous tissue, and necrotic tissue in the posttherapy period. Adding to the problem is that tumors have heterogeneous pathology that is not always clearly distinct from those of normal tissue and the induction of complex deformations in the surrounding tissues after treatment. There is a whole list of functional imaging modalities currently available for clinical and research purposes which include optical imaging, different types of MR imaging (diffusion-weighted imaging, tensor imaging, MR spectroscopy, etc.), and also several radionuclide imaging techniques. MR spectroscopy provides biochemical information on steady-state processes, and the information from MR spectroscopy has not replaced the kinetic and metabolic information from nuclear medicine techniques.

The role of imaging viable tumors is increasing because of the problems encountered by MRI and CT, especially after surgical, radiation, or chemotherapy treatment in differentiating post-therapy changes from residual viable tumor tissue, local recurrence, or necrosis [119]. As a result different radiopharmaceuticals play an important role in different malignancies for evaluation of treatment response and for detection of recurrence. Radiopharmaceutical agents like gallium (in lymphoma) and FDG (in lymphoma, head and neck cancer, breast cancer, and others) show good results in predicting the response to a treatment regimen as early as after 1–3 cycles of chemotherapy [4] (Figs. 12.15, 12.16, 12.17, 12.18, and 12.19).

Quantification of radiopharmaceutical uptake in tumors is an important factor for evaluating treatment response and for other purposes as well. In nuclear medicine intensity of radiopharmaceutical uptake relative to the normal tissue has been used to differentiate benign from malignant lesions. This has been calculated using different approaches, such as tumor-to-background ratio and standard uptake value. Comparison between early and delayed tumor-to-background ratio of 201 Tl chloride has been proposed in order to differentiate false-positive 201 Tl chloride uptake due to inflammatory lesions or postoperative changes from true-positive uptake due to the malignant lesion [120, 121]. It is presumed that with delayed images there will be lower background activity and, accordingly, the 201 Tl chloride uptake ratio in malignant lesions increases in the delayed images compared with the early images. Conversely, with benign lesions lesion-to-background ratio in the delayed images is lower due to washout of 201 Tl chloride activity from the benign cells and extravascular and intravascular components of the lesion. It is also believed that malignant cells retain 201 Tl chloride longer, with less washout. They might even continue to accumulate 201 Tl chloride in the

Gallium-67

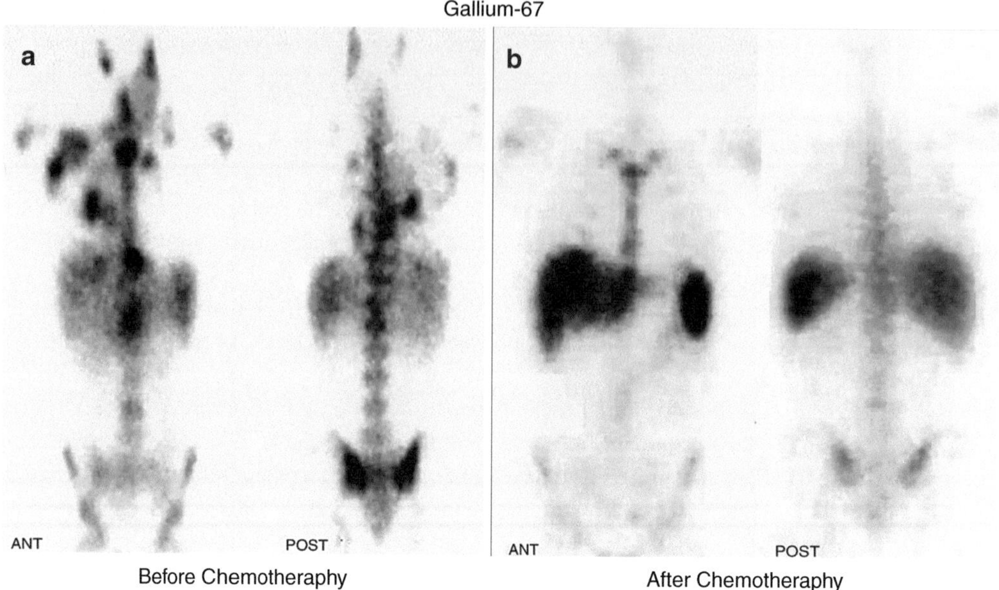

Fig. 12.15 ^{67}Ga initial (**a**) and post-therapy (**b**) studies of a patient with non-Hodgkin's lymphoma showing excellent response to chemotherapy since the pre-therapy significant uptake has disappeared on the follow-up study

Tallium-201

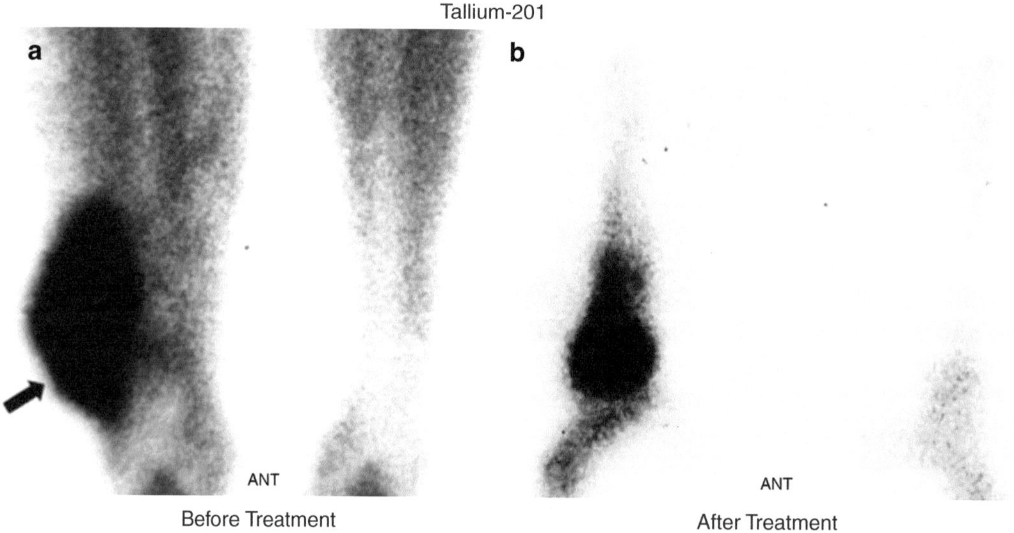

Fig. 12.16 ^{201}Tl study of a patient with Ewing's sarcoma of the right distal tibia. (**a**) Prechemotherapy study with significant radiotracer accumulation (*arrow*). Follow-up (**b**) post-therapy study shows significantly decreasing uptake at the site of the tumor reflecting the response to therapy

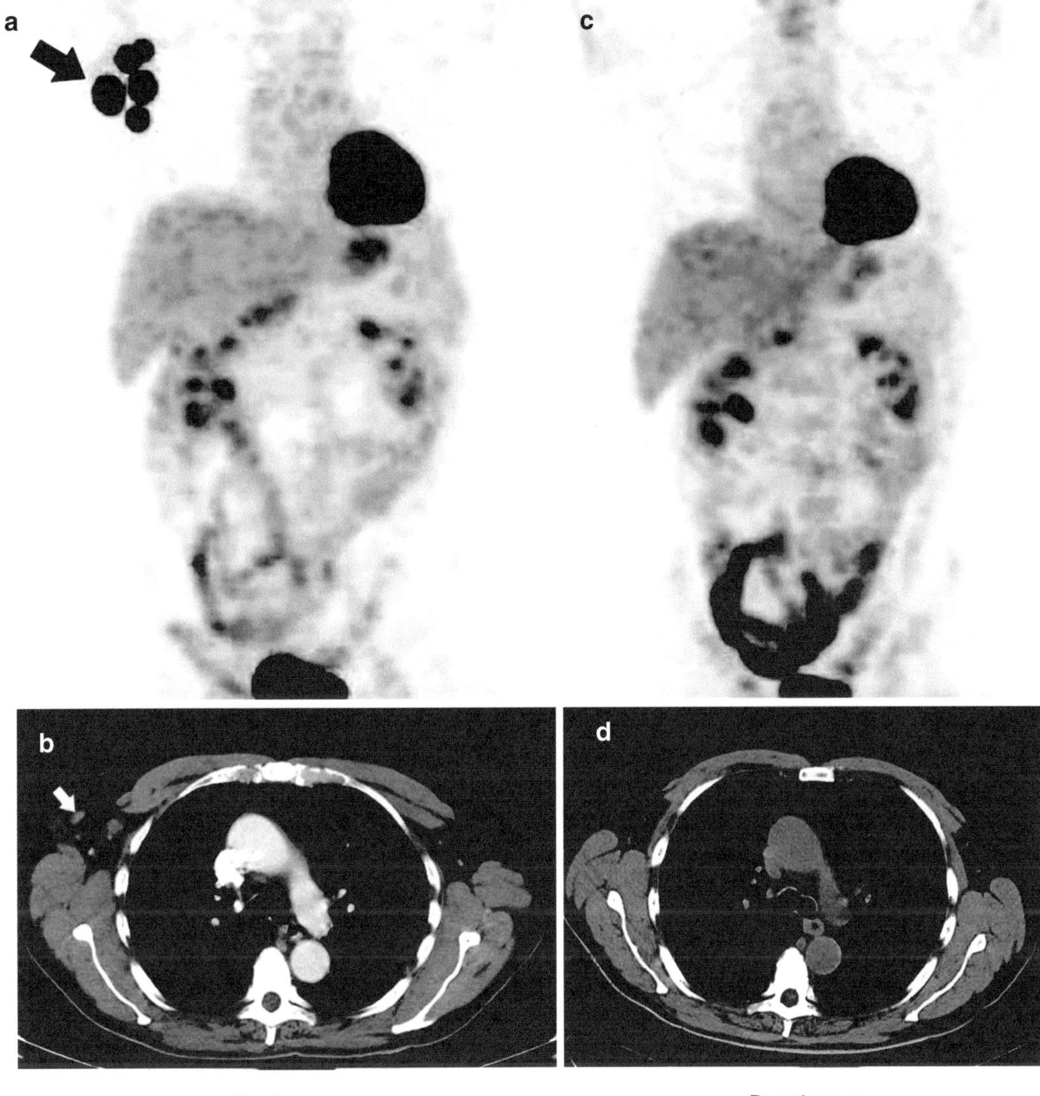

Pre-therapy   Post-therapy

Fig. 12.17 FDG-PET/CTstudy for non-Hodgkin's lymphoma. The pre-therapy images (**a**, **b**) show multiple lymph nodes with intense FDG uptake (*arrow*). On post-therapy images (**c**, **d**) the FDG uptake is no longer seen (**c**) and significant decrease in size of lymph nodes with some disappeared on CT (**d**)

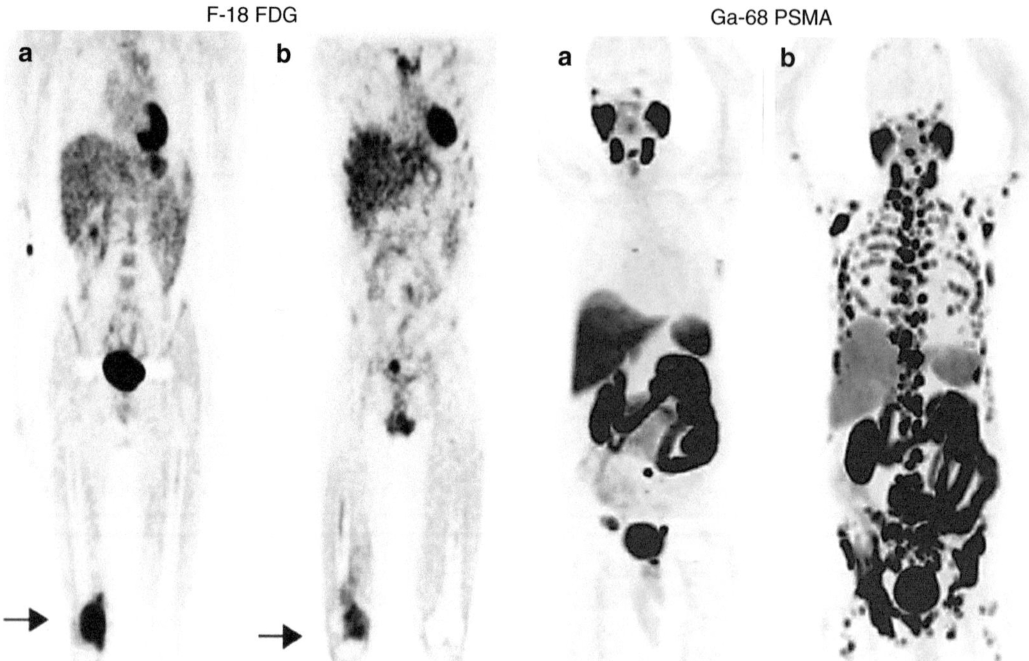

Fig. 12.18 A case with osteogenic sarcoma of the right distal femur. FDG PET to assess response to chemotherapy. On pretherapy FDG PET study (**a**), there is a large markedly hypermetabolic tumor in the right distal femur with SUV max of 9.6 (arrow). Post-chemotherapy FDG PET study to assess response to chemotherapy (**b**) shows significant decrease in metabolic activity of the tumor (SUVmax, 4.2) (arrow) and reduction in tumor size, indicating good response to treatment with some residual disease

Fig. 12.19 Ga-68 PSMA ligand PET MIP images in 2015 (**a**) and 2017 (**b**) for a 69-year-old patient with history of prostate cancer diagnosed in 2014. Patient is on hormone therapy. PSA is raised from 10 to 90 in 2017. PSMA ligand image in 2015 shows primary tumor in the prostate gland as well as lymph node metastases in the pelvis and metastatic uptake in several bones. Ga-68 PSMA ligand image in 2017 demonstrates extensive bone metastases in the axial and peripheral skeleton as well as lymph node metastases in the pelvis and focal uptake in the primary tumor

delayed images, leading to a higher tumor-to-background ratio. Calculations have been made by subtracting the delayed from early ratios in order to calculate the washout index. If the product of this subtraction is positive, it means washout of thallium from the lesion, indicating its possible benign nature, while if the result of the subtraction is negative, it indicates buildup of thallium concentration with time and the possible malignant nature of the lesion. The reverse has also been proposed, i.e., subtracting the early from the delayed ratio to calculate the washout or buildup ratios.

Attempts are being made with 18 F-FDG comparing early (1 h following injections) SUV and lesion-to-background ratios with the same SUV or ratios calculated from the delayed images (2–3 h following injection) to improve the ability to differentiate malignancy from other tissues. It is important to realize that there are many reservations to applying these principles in the initial diagnosis for the purpose of differentiation between benign and malignant disease and for follow-up purposes. The factors affecting SUV values (Table 12.4) are as fol-

Table 12.4 Factors affecting SUV calculation

1. Plasma glucose level
2. Time between injection and imaging
3. Change in body weight
4. Patient motion
5. Partial volume effects in small lesions
6. Image reconstruction method
7. Region of interest
8. Method of attenuation correction

lows: (a) high plasma glucose level at the time of injection (diabetes, steroid used during chemotherapy, etc.) can falsely decrease the SUV; (b) time between injection and imaging can influence the SUV (it is assumed that after 45 min the tumor uptake curve reaches a plateau, but it may not be always true, so comparison of pre-therapy SUV with post-therapy SUV requires attention for this time and preferably should not be more than 5 min of difference); (c) significant change in body weight is not unlikely after chemoradiotherapy, so attention should be paid for adjustment of SUV so that pre- and posttreatment SUVs are comparable (as fat has very low FDG uptake, SUV corrected to either lean body mass or surface area is preferable); and (d) other factors that can affect the SUV include (i) patient motion (due to lesion blurring also during breathing in along lesion particularly located at the anterior and lower lung fields), (ii) partial volume effects in lesions smaller than two and a half times the scanner resolution at full width half-maximum, appropriate recovery coefficients, which represent the ratio of apparent to true isotope concentration in the structure of interest, can be used to correct for partial volume effects. SUVs are obtained by placing a region of interest on the PET images, (iii) image reconstruction (SUV measurements from filtered back projection (FBP) images underestimate the true activ-

ity concentration by about 20%—this is much greater than iterative reconstruction (IR) images which underestimate activity concentration by about 5% [122]), (iv) the size of the region of interest affects the radioactivity measurements: the larger the region of interest, the lower the mean SUV. In the clinical setting, the maximum SUV within the region of interest, which represents the highest radioactivity concentration in one voxel within the tumor, is most frequently being used.

12.3.2.6 Radiotherapy (RT) Planning

Planning Radiotherapy is used for curative intent in the tumors of the following organs: head and neck, female genital organs, lymphomas, breast, primary brain tumors, prostate, unresectable sarcomas, and skin cancer. However, despite the development of RT, the most common site of recurrence for solid tumors is the local recurrence. This fact led to the concept of using fused metabolic and anatomical image to define target volume for RT. This image not only will allow inclusion of the metabolically active tumor and spare the normal structure from radiation, but also it will allow to provide an extra boost of radiation to the part of the tumor with very high metabolic activity or hypoxic (seen by metabolic imaging with misonidazole PET). Studies showed that FDG PET can be useful for radiotherapy planning (Fig. 12.20). The advantages of PET/CT during RT planning are (1) the ability to detect systemic metastases thereby helping to avoid unnecessary/aggressive RT, (2) the ability to delineate metabolically active tissue not picked up on CT thereby modifying the planned target volume and reducing the risk of geographical misses, (3) the ability to accurately target delineation in RT which helps protect vital normal structures, and (4) the ability to decrease interobserver variability in drawing target volumes for RT.

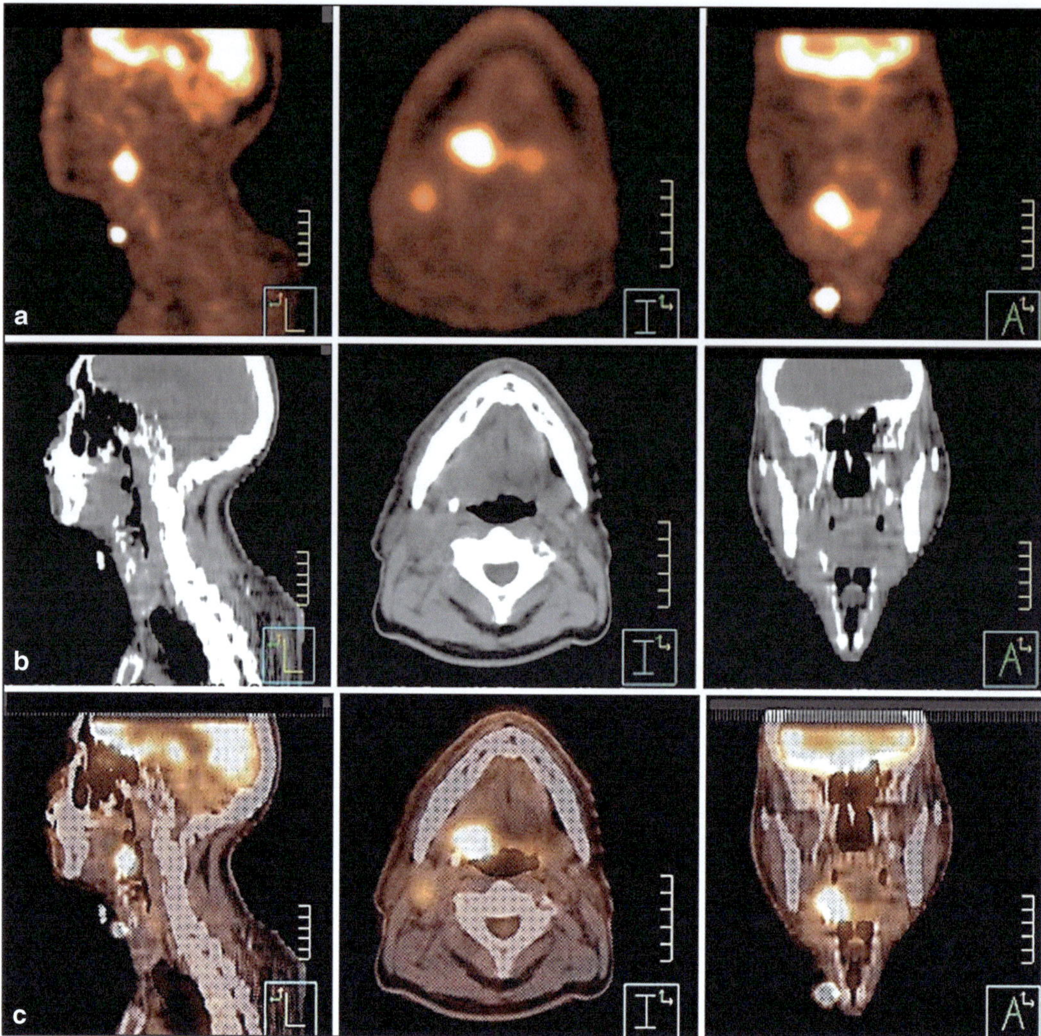

Fig. 12.20 Example of RT planning PET/CT scan [PET (**a**), CT (**b**) and fused PET/CT (**c**) images] for a head and neck cancer patient. The hot circular activity in front of the patient's neck below the chin outside on the skin is a dual PET and CT marker. This is a sodium-22 coin (a positron emitter). Therefore, seen in both PET (as hot) and CT (as metallic density in the middle panel) images. The fused images were used in this patient to draw the gross tumor volume which included both the tumor at the right base of the tongue and a right-sided cervical lymph node as seen in the lower panel trans-axial images

References

1. Kumar V, Abbas A, Aster JC (2020) Robbins and Cotzan, pathologic basis of disease, 10th edn. Saunders, Philadelphia
2. Devita VT, Hellman S, Rosenberg SA (2011) Cancer: principles and practice of oncology, 9th edn. Lippincott, Philadelphia
3. Holland JF, Bast RC, Morton DL, Frei EIII, Kufe DW, Weichselbaum RR (2009) Cancer medicine, 6th edn. Williamsand Wilkins, Baltimore
4. Collan Y (1989) General principles of grading lesions in diagnostic histopathology. Pathol Res Pract 185:539–543
5. Herberman RB, Ortaldo JR (1981) Natural killer cells as an initial defense against pathogens. Science 2:24–30
6. Heichman KA, Roberts JM (1994) Rules to replicate by. Cell 79:557–562
7. Foulds L (1969) Neoplastic development, vol 2. Academic, London
8. Abercrombie M, Heaysman JE (1954) Observations on the social behaviour of cells in tissue culture.

II. Monolayering of fibroblasts. Exp Cell Res 6:293–306

9. Todaro GJ, Green H (1963) Quantitative studies of the growth of mouse embryo cells in culture and their development into established lines. J Cell Biol 17:299–313

10. Sporn MB, Todaro GJ (1980) Autocrine secretion and malignant transformation of cells. N Engl J Med 303:878–880

11. Warburg OH (1930) The metabolism of tumors: investigations from the Kaiser Wilhelm Institute for biology constable. Constable, London

12. Yokota J (2000) Tumor progression and metastasis. Carcinogenesis 3:497–503

13. Recklies AD, Tiltman KJ, Stoker TA, Poole AR (1980) Secretion of proteinases from malignant and nonmalignant human breast tissue. Cancer Res 40:550–556

14. Gunthert U, Hofmann M, Rudy W, Reber S, Zoller M, Haussmann I, Matzku S, Wenzel A, Ponta H, Herrlich P (1991) A new variant of glycoprotein CD44 confers metastatic potential to rat carcinoma cells. Cell 65:13–24

15. Knutsen T (1998) Cytogenetic changes in the progression of lymphoma. Leuk Lymphoma 31:1–19

16. Faderl S, Talpaz M, Estrov Z, Kantarjian HM (1999) Chronic myelogenous leukemia: biology and therapy. Ann Intern Med 131:207–219

17. Underwood JCE (2000) General and systemic pathology, 3rd edn. Churchill Livingstone, London

18. Stevens ALJ (2000) Pathology, 2nd edn. Mosby, London

19. Eisenhauer EA (2001) From the moleculetothe-clinic–inhibiting HER2 to treat breast cancer. N Engl J Med 344:841–842

20. Harari D, Yarden Y (2001) Molecular mechanisms underlying ErbB2/HER2 action in breast cancer. Oncogene 19:6102–6114

21. Kirsch DG, Kastan MB (1998) Tumor-suppressor p53: implications for tumor development and prognosis. J Clin Oncol 16:3158–3168

22. Liggett WH Jr, Sidransky D (1998) Role of the p16 tumor suppressor gene in cancer. J Clin Oncol 16:1197–1206

23. Fearnhead NS, Britton MP, Bodmer WF (2001) The ABC of APC. Hum Mol Genet 10:721–733

24. Reed JC (1999) Dysregulation of apoptosis in cancer. J Clin Oncol 17:2941–2953

25. Eichhorst ST, Krammer PH (2001) Derangement of apoptosis in cancer. Lancet 4:345–346

26. Blackwood MA, Weber BL (1998) BRCA1 and BRCA2: from molecular genetics to clinical medicine. J Clin Oncol 16:1969–1977

27. Israel O, Mekel M, Bar-Shalom R et al (2002) Bone lymphoma: 67Ga scintigraphy and CT for prediction of outcome after treatment. J Nucl Med 43:1295–1303

28. International Survey of PET/CT Operations and Oncology Imaging (2010) Academy of molecular imaging. Accessed 19 Sept 2012. http://www.ami-maging.org/index.php?option=com_content&task=view&id=181

29. Larson SM, Rasey JS, Allen DR, Nelson NJ (1979) A transferrin-mediated uptake of gallium-67 by EMT-6 sarcoma. I. Studies in tissue culture. J Nucl Med 20:837–842

30. Berry JP, Escaig F, Poupon MF, Galle P (1983) Localization of gallium in tumor cells. Electron microscopy, electron probe microanalysis and analytical ion microscopy. Int J Nucl Med Biol 10:199–204

31. Ziessman H, O'Malley J, Thrall J (2006) Nuclear medicine: the requisites in radiology. Mosby, Philadelphia, Print

32. Gehring PJ, Hammond PB (1967) The interrelationship between thallium-201 chloride and potassium in animals. J Pharmacol Exp Ther 155:187–201

33. Britten JS, Blank M (1968) Thallium-201 chloride-201 chloride activation of the (Na + K +) activated ATPase of rabbit kidney. Biochim Biophys Acta 159:160–166

34. Sessler MJ, Geck P, Maul FD, Hor G, Munz DL (1986) New aspects of cellular thallium-201 chloride-201 chloride uptake: Tl+-Na+-2Cl-cotransport is the central mechanism of ion uptake. Nucl Med 23:24–27

35. Abdel-Dayem HM et al (1994) Role of Tl-201 chloride and Tc-99m-sestamibi in tumor imaging. Nucl Med Annual:181–234

36. Piwnica-Worms D, Holman BL (1990) Noncardiac applications of hexakis-(alkylisonitrile) technetium-99m complexes. J Nucl Med 31:1166–1167

37. Piwnica-Worms D, Chiu ML, Budding M, Kronauge JF, Kramer RA, Croop JM (1993) Functional imaging of multidrug-resistant P-glycoprotein with an organotechnetium complex. Cancer Res 53:977–984

38. Ballinger JR, Sheldon KM, Boxen I, Erlichman C, Ling V (1995) Differences between accumulation of 99mTc-MIBI and 201Tl-thallous chloride in tumour cells: role of P-glycoprotein. Q J Nucl Med 39:122–128

39. Henze M, Mohammed A, Schlemmer HP et al (2004) PET and SPECT for detection of tumor progression in irradiated low-grade astrocytoma: a receiver-operating-characteristics analysis. J Nucl Med 45:579–586

40. Taillefer R (1999) The role of 99mTc-sestamibi and other conventional radiopharmaceuticals in breast cancer diagnosis. Semin Nucl Med 29:16–40

41. Kwekkeboom D, Krenning EP, de Jong M (2000) Peptide receptor imaging and therapy. J Nucl Med 41(10):1704–1713

42. Freitas JE (1995) Adrenal cortical and medullary imaging. Semin Nucl Med 25:235–250

43. Wiseman GA, Pacak K, O'Dorisio MS et al (2009) Usefulness of 123I-MIBG scintigraphy in the evaluation of patients with known or suspected primary or metastatic pheochromocytoma or paraganglioma: results from a prospective multicenter trial. J Nucl Med 50:1448–1454

44. Shulkin BL, Shapiro B (1998) Current concepts on the diagnostic use of MIBG in children. J Nucl Med 39:679–688

45. Czernin J, Phelps ME (2002) Positron emission tomography scanning: current and future applications. Annu Rev Med 53:89–112

46. Delbeke D (1999) Oncological applications of FDG PET imaging: brain tumors, colorectal cancer, lymphoma and melanoma. J Nucl Med 40:591–603

47. Ak I, Stokkel MP, Pauwels EK (2000) Positron emission tomography with 2-[18F]fluoro-2-deoxy-D-glucose in oncology. Part II. The clinical value in detecting and staging primary tumours. J Cancer Res Clin Oncol 126:560–574

48. Lowe VJ, Naunheim KS (1998) Current role of positron emission tomography in thoracic oncology. Thorax 53:703–712

49. Shankar LK, Hoffman JM, Bacharach S et al (2006) Consensus recommendations for the use of ^{18}F-FDG PET as an indicator of therapeutic response in patients in national cancer institute trials. J Nucl Med 47:1059–1066

50. Coleman RE (1999) PET in lung cancer. J Nucl Med 40:814–820

51. Jadvar H, Alavi A, Mavi A et al (2005) PET in pediatric diseases. Radiol Clin N Am 43:135–152

52. Osman MM, Chaar BT, Muzaffar R et al (2010) $^{18F\text{-}FDG}$ PET/CT of patients with cancer: comparison of whole-body and limited whole-body technique. AJR Am J Roentgenol 195:1397–1403

53. Sodium Fluoride F18 injection investigator's brochure. http://imaging.cancer.gov/images/documents/Generic-NaF_IB_Edition1_10-2009.pdf

54. Even-Sapir E, Metser U, Flusser G et al (2004) Assessment of malignant skeletal disease: initial experience with 18F-fluoride PET/CT and comparison between ^{18}Ffluoride PET and 18F-fluoride PET/CT. J Nucl Med 45:272–278

55. Lin FI, Rao JE, Mittra ES et al (2012) Prospective comparison of combined ^{18}F-FDG and 18F-NaF PET/CT vs. ^{18}F-FDG PET/CT imaging for detection of malignancy. Eur J Nucl Med Mol Imaging 39:262–270

56. Rasey JS, Grierson JR, Wiens LW, Kolb PD, Schwartz JL (2002) Validation of FLT uptake as a measure of thymidine kinase-1 activity in A549 carcinoma cells. J Nucl Med 43:1210–1217

57. Buck AK, Halter G, Schirrmeister H, Kotzerke J, Wurziger I et al (2003) Imaging proliferation in lung tumors with PET: $^{18F\text{-}FLT}$ versus ^{18}F-FDG. J Nucl Med 44:1426–1431

58. Been LB, Suurmeijer AJ, Cobben DC, Jager PL, Hoekstra HJ, Elsinga PH (2004) [18F]FLT-PET in oncology: current status and opportunities. Eur J Nucl Med Mol Imaging 31(12):1659–1672. https://doi.org/10.1007/s00259-004-1687-6

59. Van Waarde A, Cobben DC, Suurmeijer AJ, Maas B, Vaalburg W et al (2004) Selectivity of ^{18}F-FLT and ^{18}F-FDG for differentiating tumor from inflammation in a rodent model. J Nucl Med 45:695–700

60. Cobben DC, Jager PL, Elsinga PH, Maas B, Suurmeijer AJ et al (2003) 3′-(18)F-fluoro-3′-deoxy-L-thymidine: a new tracer for staging metastatic melanoma? J Nucl Med 44:1927–1932

61. Everitt S, Hicks RJ, Ball D, Kron T, Schneider-Kolsky M et al (2009) Imaging cellular proliferation during chemo-radiotherapy: a pilot study of serial ^{18}F-FLT positron emission tomography/computed tomography imaging for non–small-cell lung cancer. Int J Radiat Oncol Biol Phys 75:1098–1104

62. Yomo S, Oguchi K (2017) Prospective study of ^{11}C–methionine PET for distinguishing between recurrent brain metastases and radiation necrosis: limitations of diagnostic accuracy and long-term results of salvage treatment. BMC Cancer 17:713

63. Minamimoto R, Toyohara J, Seike A, Ito H, Endo H et al (2012) 4′-[methyl-11C]-thiothymidine PET/CT for proliferation imaging in non-small cell lung cancer. J Nucl Med 53:199

64. Pieterman RM, Que TH, Elsinga PH, Pruim J, van Putten JW et al (2002) Comparison of (11)C-choline and (18)F-FDG PET in primary diagnosis and staging of patients with thoracic cancer. J Nucl Med 43:167–172

65. Hara T, Inagaki K, Kosaka N, Morita T (2000) Sensitive detection of mediastinal lymph node metastasis of lung cancer with 11C-choline PET

66. Torizuka T, Kanno T, Futatsubashi M, Okada H, Yoshikawa E et al (2003) Imaging gynecologic tumors: comparison of ^{11}C-choline PET with ^{18}F-FDG PET. J Nucl Med 44:1051–1056

67. Kostakoglu L, Goldsmith SJ (2004) PET in the assessment of therapy response in patients with carcinoma of the head and neck and of the esophagus. J Nucl Med 45:56–68

68. Bradley JD, Perez CA, Dehdashti F, Siegel BA (2004) Implementing biologic target volumes in radiation treatment planning for non-small cell lung cancer. J Nucl Med 45(Suppl 1):96S–101S

69. Huang T, Civelek A, Zheng H et al (2013) F-18 misonidazole PET imaging of hypoxia in micrometastases and macroscopic xenografts of human non-small cell lung cancer: a correlation with autoradiography and histopathological findings. Am J Nucl Med Mol Biol 3:142–153

70. Richin D, Hicks RJ, Fisher R et al (2006) Prognostic significance of F-18 misonidazole positron emission tomography-detected tumor hypoxia in patients with advanced head and neck cancer randomly assigned chemo-radiation with or without tirapazamine: a substudy of Tasman radiation oncology group 98.2. J Clin Oncol 24:2098–2104

71. Poeppel TD, Binse I, Petersenn S et al (2011) 68Ga-DOTATOC versus 68Ga-DOTATATE PET/CT in functional imaging of neuroendocrine tumors. J Nucl Med 52:1864–1870

72. Yang J, Kan Y, Ge BH et al (2013) Diagnostic role of Gallium-68 DOTATOC and Gallium-68 DOTATATEPET in patients with neuroendocrine tumors: a meta-analysis. Acta Radiol 55:389–398

73. Sandström M, Velikyan I, Garske-Román U et al (2013) Comparative biodistribution and radiation dosimetry of 68Ga-DOTATOC and 68Ga-DOTATATE in patients with neuroendocrine tumors. J Nucl Med 54:1755–1759

74. Gabriel M, Decristoforo C, Kendler D et al (2007) 68Ga-DOTA-Tyr3-octreotide PET in neuroendocrine tumors: comparison with somatostatin receptor scintigraphy and CT. J Nucl Med 48:508–518

75. Delpassand ES, Ranganathan D, Wagh N, Shafie A, Gaber A et al (2020) 64Cu-DOTATATE PET/CT for imaging patients with known or suspected somatostatin receptor–positive neuroendocrine tumors: results of the first U.S. prospective, reader-masked clinical trial. J Nucl Med 61:890–896

76. Fowler AM, Linden HM (2017) Functional estrogen receptor imaging before Neoadjuvant therapy for primary breast cancer. J Nucl Med 58:560–562

77. Bensch F, Brouwers AH, Lub-de Hooge MN et al (2018). 89Zr-trastuzumab PET supports clinical decision making in breast cancer patients, when HER2 status cannot be determined by standard work up) Eur J Nucl Med Mol Imaging 45:2300–2306

78. Lenzo NP, Meyrick D, Turner JH (2018) Review of Gallium-68 PSMA PET/CT imaging in the Management of Prostate Cancer. Diagnostics (Basel) 8(1):16

79. Hofman MS, Lawrentschuk N, Francis RJ et al (2020) Prostate-specific membrane antigen PET-CT in patients with high-risk prostate cancer before curative-intent surgery or radiotherapy (proPSMA): a prospective, randomised, multicentre study. Lancet 395:1208–1216

80. Langbein T, Weber WA, Eiber M (2019) Future of Theranostics: an outlook on precision oncology in nuclear medicine. J Nucl Med 60:13S–19S

81. Kratochwil C, Flechsig P, Lindner T et al (2019) 68Ga-FAPI PET/CT: tracer uptake in 28 different kinds of cancer. J Nucl Med 60:801–805

82. Lindner T, Loktev A, Altmann A et al (2018) Development of Quinoline-based Theranostic ligands for the targeting of fibroblast activation protein. J Nucl Med 59:1415–1422

83. Yilmaz S, Ozhan M, Sager S et al (2011) Metformin-induced intense bowel uptake observed on restaging FDG PET/CT study in a patient with gastric lymphoma. Mol Imaging Radionucl Ther 20:114–116

84. Cai W, Rao J, Gambhir SS, Chen X (2006) How molecular imaging is speeding up antiangiogenic drug development. Mol Cancer Ther 5:2624–2633

85. Haubner R, Wester HJ, Burkhart F, Senekowitsch-Schmidtke R, Weber W, Goodman SL, Kessler H, Schwaiger M (2001) Glycosylated RGD-containing peptides: tracer for tumor targeting and angiogenesis imaging with improved biokinetics. J Nucl Med 42:326–336

86. Blankenberg FG, Strauss HW (2001) Will imaging of apoptosis play a role in clinical care? A tale of mice and men. Apoptosis 6:117–123

87. Herschman HR (2004) PET reporter genes for noninvasive imaging of gene therapy, cell tracking and transgenic analysis. Crit Rev Oncol Hematol 51:191–204

88. Weissleder R, Mahmood U (2001) Molecular imaging. Radiology 219:316–333

89. Marom EM, Sarvis S, Herndon JE 2nd, Patz EF Jr et al (2002) T1 lung cancers: sensitivity of diagnosis with fluorodeoxyglucose PET. Radiology 223:453–459

90. Schoder H, Larson SM, Yeung HW (2004) PET/CT inoncology: integration into clinical management of lymphoma, melanoma, and gastrointestinal malignancies. J Nucl Med 45:72S–81S

91. Bury T, Corhay JL, Duysinx B, Daenen F, Ghaye B, Barthelemy N, Rigo P, Bartsch P (1999) Value of FDG-PET in detecting residual or recurrent nonsmall cell lung cancer. Eur Respir J 14:1376–1380

92. Magnani P, Carretta A, Rizzo G, Fazio F, Vanzulli A, Lucignani G, Zannini P, Messa C, Landoni C, Gilardi MC, Del Maschio A (1999) FDG/PET and spiral CT image fusion for mediastinal lymph node assessment of non-small cell lung cancer patients. J Cardiovasc Surg 40:741–748

93. Marom EM, McAdams HP, Erasmus JJ, Goodman PC, Culhane DK, Coleman RE, Herndon JE, Patz EF Jr (1999) Staging non-small cell lung cancer with whole-body PET. Radiology 212:803–809

94. Gambhir SS, Czernin J, Schwimmer J, Silverman DH, Coleman RE, Phelps ME (2001) A tabulated summary of the FDGPET literature. J Nucl Med 42:1S–93S

95. Patz EF (2000) Evaluation of focal pulmonary abnormalities with FDGPET. Radiographics 20:1182–1185

96. Young H, Baum R, Cremerius U, Herholz K, Hoekstra O, Lammertsma AA, Pruim J et al (1999) Measurement of clinical and subclinical tumour response using [18F]-fluorodeoxyglucose and positron emission tomography: review and 1999 EORTC recommendations. European Organization for Research and Treatment of cancer (EORTC) PET study group. Eur J Cancer 35:1773–1782

97. Rosen EL, Turkington TG, Soo MS, Baker JA, Coleman RE (2005) Detection of primary breast carcinoma with a dedicated, large field of view FDGPET mammography device: initial experience. Radiology 234:527–534

98. Hanson JA, Armstrong P (1997) Staging intrathoracic non-small-cell lung cancer. Eur Radio 17:161–172

99. Moog F, Bangerter M, Diederichs CG, Guhlmann A, Merkle E, Frickhofen N, Reske SN (1998) Extranodal malignant lymphoma: detection with FDGPET versus CT. Radiology 206:475–481

100. Steinert HC, Hauser M, Allemann F, Engel H, Berthold T, von Schulthess GK, Weder W (1997) Non-small cell lung cancer: nodal staging with FDGPET versus CT with correlative lymph node mapping and sampling. Radiology 202:441–446

101. Bury T, Dowlati A, Paulus P, Corhay JL, Hustinx R, Ghaye B, Metal R (1997) Whole-body 18FDG positron emission tomography in the staging of non-small lung cancer. Eur Respir J 10:2529–2534

102. Kubota K, Matsuzawa T, Amemiya A, Kondo M, Fujiwara T, Watanuki S, Metal I (1989) Imaging of breast cancer with (18F)fluorodeoxyglucose and positron emission tomography. J Comput Assist Tomogr 13:1097–1098

103. Tse NY, Hoh CK, Hawkins RA, Zinner MJ, Dahlbom M, Choi Y, Maddahi J (1992) The application of positron emission tomographic imaging with fluorodeoxyglucose for the evaluation of breast disease. Ann Surg 216:27–34

104. Vidal-Sicart S, Olmos RV (2012) Sentinel node mapping for breast cancer: current situation. J Oncol 2012:361341. https://doi.org/10.1155/2012/361341

105. Barnwell JM, Arredondo MA, Kollmorgen D, Gibbs JF, Lamonica D, Carson W, Zhang P et al (1998) Sentinel node biopsy in breast cancer. Ann Surg Onco l5:126–130

106. Kogel KE, Sweetenham JW (2003) Current therapies in Hodgkin's disease. Eur J Nucl Med Mol Imaging 30(Suppl1):S19–S27

107. Okada J, Oonishi H, Yoshikawa K, Itami J, Uno K, Imaseki K, Arimizu N (1994) FDG-PET for predicting the prognosis of malignant lymphoma. Ann Nucl Med 8:187–191

108. Kunkel M, Forster GJ, Reichert TE, Jeong JH, Benz P, Bartenstein P, Wagner W et al (2003) Detection of recurrent oral squamous cell carcinoma by[18F]-2-fluorodeoxyglucose-positron emission tomography: implications for prognosis and patient management. Cancer 98:2257–2265

109. Halfpenny W, Hain SF, Biassoni L, Maisey MN, Sherman JA, McGurk M (2002) FDG-PET. A possible prognostic factor in head and neck cancer. Br J Cancer 86:512–516

110. Brun E, Ohlsson T, Erlandsson K, Kjellen E, Sandell A, Tennvall J, Wennerberg J et al (1997) Early prediction of treatment outcome in head and neck cancer with 2-18FDGPET. Acta Oncol 36:741–747

111. Kitagawa Y, Sano K, Nishizawa S, Nakamura M, Ogasawara T, Sadato N, Yonekura Y (2003) FDG-PET for prediction of tumour aggressiveness and response to intra-arterial chemotherapy and radiotherapy in head and neck cancer. Eur J Nucl Med Mol Imaging 30:63–71

112. Minn H, Lapela M, Klemi PJ, Grenman R, Leskinen S, Lindholm P, Bergman J et al (1997) Prediction of survival with fluorine-18-fluoro-deoxyglucose and PET in head and neck cancer. J Nucl Med 38:1907–1911

113. Cheng J et al (2013) 18F-fluoromisonidazole PET/CT: a potential tool for predicting primary endocrine therapy resistance in breast cancer. J Nucl Med 54:333–340

114. Groheux D, Giacchetti S, Moretti J-L, Porcher R, Espié M et al (2011) Correlation of high 18F-FDG uptake to clinical, pathological and biological prognostic factors in breast cancer. Eur J Nucl Med Mol Imaging 38:426–435

115. Ullah MF (2008) Cancer multidrug resistance (MDR): a major impediment to effective chemotherapy. Asian Pac J Cancer Prev 9:1–6

116. Kostakoglu L, Goldsmith SJ (2003) 18F-FDGPET evaluation of the response to therapy for lymphoma and for breast, lung, and colorectal carcinoma. J Nucl Med 44:224–239

117. Luker GD, Luker KE, Sharma V et al (1999) Assessment of multidrug resistance. Nuclearoncology. Springer, Berlin/Heidelberg/NewYork, pp 371–382

118. Kao CH, Hsieh JF, Tsai SC, Ho YJ, Changlai SP, Lee JK (2001) Paclitaxel-based chemotherapy for non-small cell lung cancer: predicting the response with 99mTc-tetrofosmin chest imaging. J Nucl Med 42:17–20

119. Wallner KE, Galieich JH, Malkin MG, Arbit E, Krol G, Rosenblum MK (1989) Inability of computed tomography appearance of recurrent malignant astrocytoma to predict survival following reoperation. J Clin Oncol 7:1492–1496

120. Abdel-Dayem HM, Scott AM, Macapinlac HA, El-Gazzar AH, Larson SM (1994) Role of thallim-201 chloride in tumor imaging. In: Freeman LM (ed) Nuclear medicine annual. Raven, NewYork, pp 181–234

121. Ganz WI, Nguyen TW, Benedetto MP, Friden A, Topchik S, Serafini A, Sfakianakis G (1993) Use of early, late and SPECT thallium-201 chloride-201 chloride imaging in evaluating activity of soft tissue and bone tumors (abstract). J Nucl Med 34:32P

122. Jana S, Mahadeo S, Heller S, Isasi CR, Blaufox MD (2005) Influence of PET scanners, lesion size, and attenuation correction methods on SUV in FDG-PET imaging (abstract). J Nucl Med 46:328

Basis of Therapeutic Nuclear Medicine

13.1 Radionuclide Therapy

Therapeutic applications of nuclear medicine are expanding (Table 13.1). Until 5–10 years ago, the use of radioisotopes in therapy was limited predominantly to treatment of hyperthyroidism and thyroid cancer with I-131, polycythemia rubra vera with P-32, bone metastases (palliative) with strontium-89 (Sr-89), rhenium-186 (Re-186), samarium-153 (Sm-153), tin-117 m (Sn-117), liver tumor, and metastases with Y-90 microspheres and neuroblastoma, pheochromocytoma and paraganglioma with I-131 MIBG. In recent years, Lu-177 and Y-90 labeled somatostatin analogs for the treatment of neuroendocrine tumors (NETs), Lu-177 labeled PSMA ligands and Ra-223 dichloride for metastatic prostate cancer have been increasingly used.

It is not the objective of this chapter to discuss different protocols and experiences in the treatment of various conditions using radioisotopes. Rather, the objective is to explore some of the pathological features of the disease processes being treated, and the underlying theory behind the action of the radioisotopes that induce therapeutic effects.

Generally, treatment options for cancer may be local (surgery or external beam radiation) or systemic. The role of nuclear medicine focuses on a targeted systemic approach, whether dealing with a primary tumor or with its metastatic foci.

Table 13.1 Therapeutic applications of nuclear medicine

Oncologic
1. Lymphomas and leukemias
2. Polycythemia rubra vera
3. Solid tumors (thyroid carcinoma, neuroblastoma, ovarian, prostate, breast, osteogenic sarcoma, others)
4. Treatment of metastasis-induced bone pain
Non-oncologic
1. Benign thyroid disease particularly hyperthyroidism
2. Radionuclide synovectomy
3. Bone marrow ablation
4. Intravascular radionuclide therapy for prevention of restenosis

13.2 Treatment of Hyperthyroidism

For more than 60 years, iodine-131 has been used to treat most cases of Graves' disease and hyperfunctioning nodules. It has become the modality of choice in treating Graves' disease, with the result that surgeons are becoming less and less experienced in thyroidectomy since the number of operations has decreased significantly. In a recent Canadian survey study, endocrinologists were found to be the most common to prescribe I-131 for

A. H. Elgazzar, *Synopsis of Pathophysiology in Nuclear Medicine*,
https://doi.org/10.1007/978-3-031-20646-7_13

malignant, while nuclear medicine physicians were the most in prescribing it for benign disease [1].

The normal thyroid gland varies in shape between individuals, and the average weight is approximately 20 g. The gland utilizes iodine for the synthesis of thyroid hormones (see Chap. 6). The cells of the gland do not differentiate between stable iodine and radioactive iodine. Accordingly, if radioactive iodine is administered, it is trapped and then organified by thyroid follicular cells exactly like nonradioactive iodine.

13.2.1 Pathophysiology

After oral administration, I-131 iodide is absorbed rapidly from the upper gastrointestinal tract, 90% within 60 min. After entering the bloodstream, the iodide is distributed in the extrathyroid compartment similar to the stable iodide and leaves this compartment to be taken up by the thyroid and by renal excretion. Approximately 20% of the administered activity is taken up normally by the thyroid gland. A small amount of I-131 is also found in the salivary glands, gastric mucosa, choroid plexus, breast milk, and placenta. Up to 75% is excreted by the kidney and 10% by fecal excretion. Approximately 40% of the administered activity has an effective half-life of 0.43 days while 60% has an effective half-life of 7.6 days.

Graves' disease is the most common form of hyperthyroidism, comprising approximately 56% of all cases. It is also the major immunologically mediated form. It occurs most commonly in young women and is characterized by symptoms of hyperthyroidism with or without ophthalmopathy and dermopathy. Rarely, lymphadenopathy and splenomegaly may be present. The thyroid gland is usually diffusely enlarged but sometimes normal in size. The condition is an autoimmune process with autoantibodies directed against the TSH receptors on thyroid follicular cells which may be stimulatory and/or destructive [2]. Thyroid stimulatory antibodies include long-acting thyroid stimulator (LATS). This antibody is detected in most patients with Graves' disease and behaves like TSH, stimulating the production of thyroid hormones and consequently trapping and organifying radioiodine. The other stimulatory antibody is the LATS protector, the antibody that prevents

degradation of LATS; accordingly, it helps to stimulate thyroid cells indirectly. The disease is associated with other autoimmune disorders such as pernicious anemia and myasthenia gravis.

Graves' disease is also known to be associated in Caucasians with HLA B8, DR2, and DR3 and with an inability to secrete certain glycoproteins coded for on chromosomes 6 and 19. A 50% concordance rate is seen among monozygous twins while 5% concordance is noted in dizygous twins. These facts suggest a genetic susceptibility to the disease. The observation that *Yersinia enterocolitica* and *Escherichia coli* and other Gram-negative organisms contain TSH binding sites raised the possibility that the initiating event in the pathogenesis of the disease may be infectious in genetically susceptible individuals.

Histologically, there is hyperplasia of the thyroid epithelium, sometimes with papillary unfolding. Lymphocytic infiltration is present, usually less than in other forms of autoimmune diseases such as postpartum thyroiditis. Little colloid storage is also seen. With time, the untreated gland will show progressive fibrosis and the end stage will lead to hypothyroidism, which may be considered part of the natural history of the disease [3, 4].

Thyroid scintigraphy shows uniform uptake throughout the gland or, less commonly, varying degrees of nonuniform uptake. This nonuniformity is related predominantly to different stages of involution of the disease with variable amounts of fibrosis based on the duration of the disease or the presence of nodules (Fig. 13.1). The presence of a TSH-dependent functioning nodule in a diffusely toxic gland has been referred to as Marine–Lenhart's syndrome (Fig. 13.1). Since the function of such nodule is much less than the surrounding hyperfunctioning tissue, it appears scintigraphically cold.

Ophthalmopathy occurs in approximately 50% of patients with Graves' disease [5]. Infiltration of extraocular muscles by an inflammatory reaction consisting predominantly of lymphocytes is the main pathological feature of ophthalmopathy. These lymphocytes are believed to be sensitized to antigens common to the orbital muscles and thyroid gland. Similar inflammatory infiltrates may also be present in the dermis, causing dermopathy or pretibial myxedema which may be present in up to 10% of patients with unclear etiology.

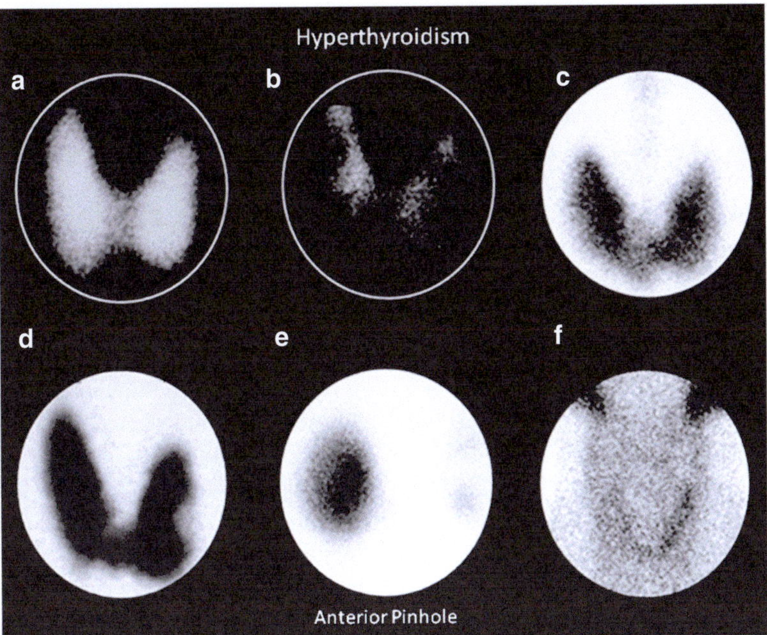

Fig. 13.1 Examples of thyroid scans of patients with hyperthyroidism illustrating patterns that affect the treatment strategy using iodine-131. (**a**) Illustrates pattern of uniform uptake in a patient with Graves' disease. Note that scans of patients during recovery phase of thyroiditis may simulate Graves' disease scintigraphically and show high uptake. Example (**b**) shows a diffusely toxic gland with mild nonuniformity. Example (**c**) shows a diffusely toxic gland with significant nonuniformity and multiple cold nodules. Example (**d**) shows a scan of a patient with Graves' disease and a colloid nodule illustrating another pattern of "Marine–Lenhart" syndrome which is more resistant to iodine-131 therapy. Compare this pattern to that of multiple toxic nodules (Fig. 6.2, Chap. 6). This pattern also needs to increase activity per gram of tissue for successful treatment. Example (**e**) is for autonomous single toxic adenoma which is treated by relatively high activity. Example (**f**) is of a patient with subacute thyroiditis. Scan shows decreased and nonuniform uptake. ONN recovery the scan may resemble and may be mistaken for Graves' disease if the patient is referred first during this phase and history and lab results are important for differentiation

Single thyroid nodules can, via an autonomous function, secrete sufficient thyroid hormone to cause hyperthyroidism. These nodules are usually greater than 3 cm in diameter in order to be capable of producing this level of function [6]. Hyperfunction may also arise in a gland containing multiple nodules [7]. In this case, the secretion of thyroid hormones can be either from hyperfunctioning nodules that are assumed to be autonomous or from the internodule parenchyma, which may be an expression of Graves' disease in an otherwise nodular goiter. The nodules in the latter situation may be cold or a mixture of cold and hot, hypertrophic nodules. The term Plummer's disease, or toxic nodular goiter, has been used to designate hyperthyroidism in glands with both single and multiple toxic nodules. The term nodular toxic goiter may be reserved for a toxic gland that contains nodules that are not hyperactive. The presence of cancer in toxic nodular goiter is extremely rare and varies from 0.1 to 0.9%. The toxic nodular goiter may have a cold nodule representing a TSH-dependent adenoma. Scintigraphic imaging cannot exclude malignancy in the cold nodule that is not TSH dependent.

The therapeutic effects of I-131 sodium iodide are due to the emission of ionizing radiation from the decaying radionuclide. In benign conditions such as Graves' disease, division of some metabolically active cells is prevented by the effect of this ionizing radiation. Cell death is another mechanism activated when the cells are exposed to high levels of radiation, particularly when high doses are given to patients with toxic adenoma, where the suppressed normal thyroid tissue is essentially spared with the delivery of a very high concentration to the cells of the toxic nodule. Cell death is followed by replacement with connective tissue, which may lead to hypothyroidism, depending on the number of cells destroyed and replaced by fibrous nonfunctioning tissue. Since 90% of the radiation effects of I-131 are due to beta radiation, which has a short range in tissue of 0.5 mm, the extrathyroid radiation and consequently the side effects are minimal. It has been estimated that 15% of patients treated with I-131 may show worsening ophthalmopathy [8, 9]. Since posttreatment hypothyroidism has been associated with exacerbation of ophthalmopathy, lower-dose radioactive iodine or starting replacement hormones early (2 weeks) after therapy along with the use of prednisone 40–80 mg per day tapered over 3 months may prevent severe eye disease in up to two-thirds of patients [10, 11]. It is interesting that cigarette smoking has been also implicated as a risk factor for progression of Graves' ophthalmopathy [9].

13.2.2 Factors Affecting the Dose of I-131 Used for Therapy of Hyperthyroidism

Several factors affect the therapeutic dose to be administered to patients suffering from hyperthyroidism. These include some parameters related to the patient, such as age, sex, medical history, and duration of treatment with antithyroid medications and factors related to the gland itself, particularly its size, the level of radioiodine uptake, scintigraphic findings of uniform or nonuniform uptake, and whether nodules are present. Additionally, the dose is dependent on how the therapist defines the goals of therapy. If the control of thyrotoxicosis is the most important consideration, the total dose or the dose per gram of estimated thyroid tissue weight will be higher than when the therapist is trying to avoid or delay hypothyroidism [12]. Using empirical low-dose iodine therapy to avoid hypothyroidism has been shown to result in persisting hyperthyroidism in up to 54% of patients [13]. Additionally, it has been found that the rate of hypothyroidism is not different among those treated with low- and high-dose radioiodine [14].

13.3 Treatment of Differentiated Thyroid Cancer

Radioactive iodine is the mainstay of therapy for residual, recurrent, and metastatic thyroid cancer that takes up iodine and cannot be resected, for presumed disease (adjuvant therapy), and ablation of residual thyroid tissue. Radioactive iodine adjuvant therapy is routinely recommended after total thyroidectomy for American Thyroid Association (ATA) high-risk differentiated thyroid cancer patients [15]. Per ATA, radioactive iodine remnant ablation is not routinely recommended after lobectomy or total thyroidectomy for patients with unifocal papillary microcarcinoma, in the absence of other adverse features [15]. The tissue of normal thyroid and its tumors expresses a variety of oncogenes, growth factors, and growth factor receptors. There is increased expression of some oncogenes, namely, c-myc/c-fos, and c-ras, in some epithelial and medullary thyroid carcinomas.

C-myc mRNA and c-fos mRNA are found in high levels in papillary carcinomas compared with the surrounding normal thyroid tissue. Patients with an unfavorable prognosis were twice as likely to overexpress c-myc as patients with a good prognosis [16].

Ras oncogenes were found in 80% of follicular and 20% of papillary carcinomas. This high prevalence of transforming ras oncogenes in follicular carcinomas may explain its aggressive behavior in comparison to papillary carcinoma and may suggest a role of this oncogene in the metastatic phenotype of this cancer [17]. Recently, a tissue-specific oncogene associated with papillary carcinoma has been identified.

Excessive growth factor and increased expression of oncogenes encoding growth factors or growth factor expression, such as the oncogene of c-ras B were identified in papillary carcinoma, adenomas, and anaplastic carcinoma.

Besides the importance of growth factors in the development of thyroid carcinoma, links have also been found to certain risk factors. The most important of these is radiation exposure. Exposure to radiation following the explosion of the atomic bombs in Japan, as well as after head and neck radiation, resulted in a 30-fold increase in the incidence of thyroid cancer [18].

About 90% or more of thyroid carcinomas are well differentiated, of the papillary, papillofollicular, follicular, and Hürthle-cell types, which take up iodine and accordingly can be successfully treated with I-131. The therapeutic effects on differentiated thyroid cancer, where larger doses of radioactive iodide are administered, are based on destruction of cells of the residual thyroid tissue and the functioning carcinoma cells by the high dose of administered radionuclide. The mortality of patients treated with subtotal thyroidectomy and limited I-131 therapy was found to be three to four times higher than that of patients treated with total thyroidectomy and I-131 therapy to ablate known foci of radioiodine uptake [19] (Fig. 13.2). Because of the larger dose of radionuclide and the lower uptake by the tissue in the case of thyroid cancer, more side effects can be seen, particularly transient sialadenitis, than in the treatment of hyperthyroidism. This, however, does not justify using limited therapy such as 30 mCi. A recent study con-

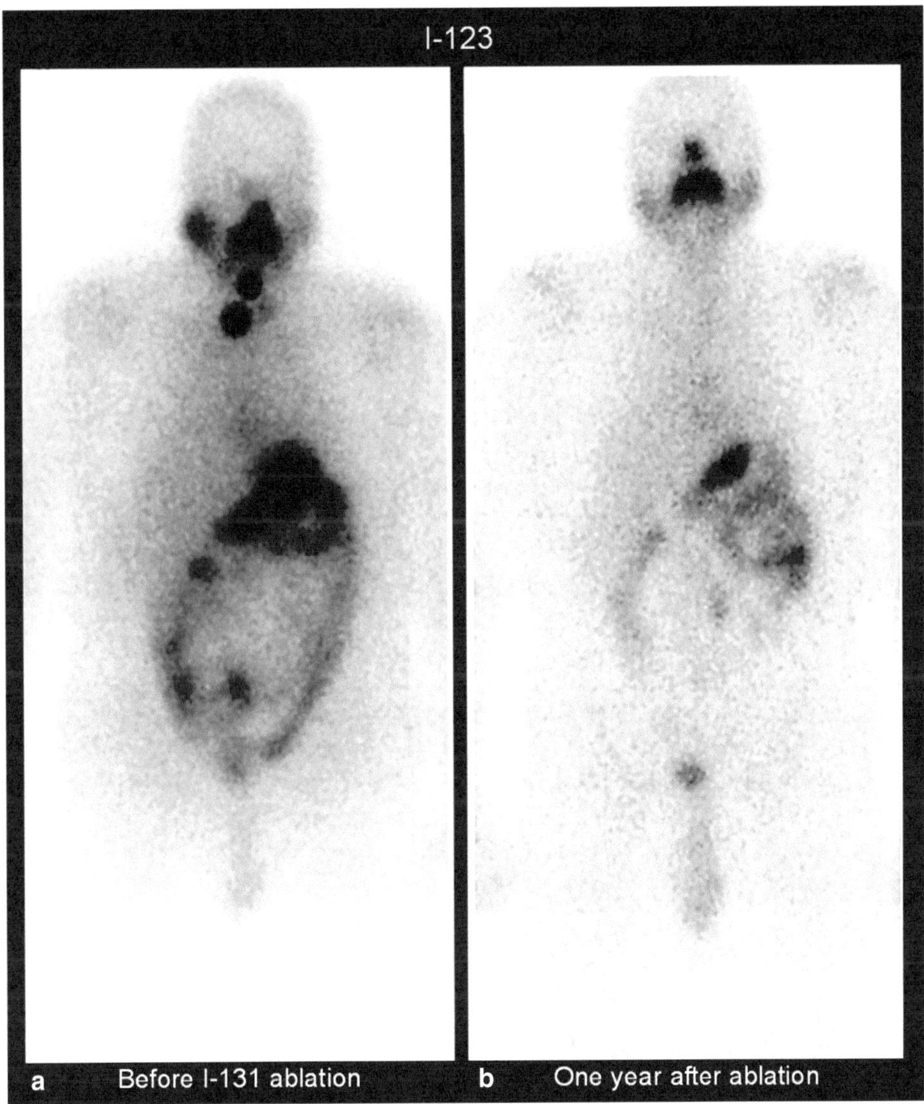

Fig. 13.2 ^{123}I whole-body scan (**a**) for a patient with papillary thyroid carcinoma treated with total thyroidectomy. The scan shows neck activity (*arrows*). Follow-up scan (**b**) one year after I-131 ablation shows complete resolution. Follow-up I-123 whole-body scan in a patient with papillary thyroid carcinoma treated with total thyroidectomy and I–131 ablation showing resolution of the neck activity 1 year after I-131 postoperative ablation

firmed the high rate of efficiency of the high ablative dose of 100 mCi of I-131, particularly in patients with less than 2% neck uptake values [20]. This study confirmed also that success rate is dependent on the pre-therapy neck uptake. The success rate was 94% when pre-ablation uptake was less than 2, 80% with uptake between 2 and 5, and 60% when the uptake value was more than 5% [20].

Thyroglobulin and calcitonin are the major tumor markers for thyroid cancer of the follicular epithelium and parafollicular C cells, respectively. These markers are unique, in the sense that they are not only specific for tumor tissue but are also specific components of normal thyroid tissue. Thyroglobulin is an iodinated glycoprotein essential for the synthesis and storage of thyroid hormones. Since thyroglobulin is produced exclusively by thyroid tissue, only very small amounts can be found in the blood after thyroidectomy and ablative radioiodine therapy. Accordingly, any post-therapeutic elevation of its levels indicates either remnant thyroid tissue, requiring further ablative treatment, or the presence of metastases or local recurrence. Other tumor markers used for many other tumors, such as carcinoembryonic antigen (CEA) and tissue polypeptide antigen (TPA), are not specific for thyroid cancer. TPA, which is a cytokeratin-related nonspecific proliferation marker, has a sensitivity of 40–60% for thyroid cancer. However, it has a good correlation with tumor progression or therapeutic response, with a high positive predictive value of 90%. Evaluation of ablative therapy and follow-up of patients post-ablation to monitor disease recurrence has further improved and facilitated by the availability of recombinant human thyrotropin as well as the use of F-18 FDG positron emission tomography. The value of recombinant human thyrotropin (rhTSH) rests on providing the opportunity to obtain diagnostic whole-body I-131 scan under adequate TSH elevation as well as representative thyroglobulin levels while the patients receiving their thyroid hormone [21]. FDG-PET is useful in evaluating patients in instances where radioiodine imaging fails to identify known or suspected recurrent or metastatic disease [22]. Additionally,

the use of Tl-201 and Tc-99 m MIBI particularly when FDG-PET is not available is of value for this purpose [23].

There are many purposes to ablate postoperative normal residual thyroid tissue with I-131. Residual thyroid tissue, if large, can cause start artifact and obscure the surrounding nodal uptake on radioiodine images. It can also take up most of the activity and leave a small amount of activity for metastatic foci. It can mimic local/regional diseases. It can harbor micrometstases. Residual thyroid tissue will also continue producing Tg and make Tg measurements unreliable. The usual amount of I-131 activity for ablation of the thyroid remnant is 1.11–3.7 GBq (30–100 mCi), which depends on the radioactive iodine uptake measurement and amount of residual thyroid tissue.

13.4 Treatment of Pain Secondary to Skeletal Metastases

Approximately 75% of patients with advanced cancer have pain, with a high percentage due to skeletal metastases. Bone metastases cause intractable pain, which affects the quality of life for the patient, especially if it is associated with immobility, anorexia, and anxiety, with the consequent long-term use of narcotic analgesics. The mechanism of bone pain may not be clear in many of these patients and could be due to cell-secreted pain modulators such as interleukin-1 beta, interleukin-8, and interferon [24]. Depending on the extent of bone metastases, radiation therapy or radiopharmaceuticals can be used instead of narcotics to alleviate the pain with the objective of improving the quality of life.

Radiotherapy for focal painful metastases with delivery of 2000–3000 rads induces pain relief in 60–90% of cases [25, 26]. Controlling pain of multiple metastases using external beam radiotherapy is difficult. Hemibody irradiation using 800 rads to the lower half of the body and 600 rads to the upper half has resulted in a complete response in 30%, partial response in 50%, and no response in 20% of patients. Radiotherapy used for painful skeletal metastases often produces significant side effects such as nausea, vomiting, and diarrhea, as well as bone marrow toxicity in one-third of patients. Vomiting and diarrhea can be severe in 10% of cases and hematological side effects can be life threatening in approximately 9% of patients [27].

Bone-seeking radiopharmaceuticals emitting beta particles have been used to deliver local radiotherapy to metastases to decrease pain at their sites. Radiopharmaceuticals that are taken up at the sites of bone metastases will cause less toxicity than external radiation therapy. These radiopharmaceuticals control pain while causing only transient bone marrow depression, which is usually mild. The uptake of these radiopharmaceuticals by metastases is several folds (up to 15–20 times) that of normal bone. These agents are absorbed by hydroxyapatite crystals at the site of active new bone, similar to Tc-99m-MDP. They include phosphorus-32, strontium-89, rhenium-186 diphosphonate, and samarium-153 EDTMP. The list of radiopharmaceuticals for bone palliation has been increasing including Re-188, Lu-177, and others [28].

13.4.1 Radiopharmaceuticals

13.4.1.1 Strontium-89 Chloride (Sr-89 Chloride)

Systemic radionuclide therapy with Sr-89 chloride was first used to relieve pain from bone metastases in 1937 and regained popularity in the 1980s. It is a pure beta-emitter with a relatively long half-life of 50.5 days. It is a chemical analogue of calcium, and accordingly it concentrates avidly in areas of high osteoblastic activity. After intravenous injection, strontium quickly accumulates in the mineral bone matrix where active bone formation takes place. Therefore, there is preferential uptake in and around metastatic tumor deposits which has been confirmed by external measurements using the gamma-emitting radionuclide Sr-85 and by autoradiography. It was found that Sr-89 concentration is 2–20 times greater in bone metastases than in normal bone [29]. The biological half-

life of Sr-89 in bone lesions is about 90 days, compared to about 2 weeks in normal bone which can be explained by the immature nature of reactive bone compared to normal lamellar bone. This selective uptake and prolonged retention at sites of increased bone mineral turnover provide precise targeting of bone lesions. The radionuclide is typically administered as a single 150 MBq (4 mCi) intravenous dose. Overall, pain relief occurs in up to 80% of patients, of whom 10–40% became effectively pain free. The mean duration of palliation is 3–4 months [30, 31]. Furthermore, 89Sr-chloride may cause slowing of metastatic progression due to inhibition of expression of cell adhesion molecules (E-selectins) that participate in the metastatic process. The significant transient decrease in serum E-selectin concentration as observed after systemic radionuclide therapy in a study on 25 men with metastatic prostate carcinoma is an indication of such an observation [32] and may provide opportunities for clinical trials.

13.4.1.2 Samarium-153 Ethylenediaminetetra-methylene Phosphonate (Sm-153-EDTMP)

Samarium-153 is produced in the nuclear reactor by neutron activation of both natural Sm-203 and 98% enriched Sm-152 targets. It has a relatively short half-life of about 48 h. Coupling of the radionuclide to ethylenediaminetetramethylene phosphonate (EDTMP) leads to the high uptake of the radionuclide by bone. Gamma camera imaging is possible due to the 103-KeV gamma ray emitted during decay of Sm-153. The resulting images are similar to those obtained with Tc99m-MDP or other diphosphonates showing increased uptake at the site of metastases. The calculated lesion-to-normal bone ratio was reported to be 4.0 and to soft tissue ratio to be 6.0 [33].

Administration of 153Sm-EDTMP according to the supplier's recommendations at 37 MBq (1 mCi)/kg would deliver a bone marrow dose of 3.27–5.90 Gray (Gy), which would induce myelotoxicity as a side effect. Dosimetric calculation by urine collection and whole-body scintigraphy has been used to limit the bone marrow dose to 2 Gy by Cameron and associates [34]. This was achieved by anterior and posterior whole-body images obtained 10 min and 5 h after the intravenous injection of 740 MBq (20 mCi) of 153Sm-EDTMP with determination of bone activity by imaging and by counting urine collected for 5 h. The total administered activity of 153Sm-EDTMP predicted on a 2-Gy bone marrow dose was found to be 35–63% of the standard recommended dose of 37 MBq/kg. The authors reported pain relief in eight of the 10 patients treated using this dosimetric method [34].

13.4.1.3 Rhenium-186 Ethylene Hydroxy Diphosphonate (Re-186-EHDP)

Similar to Sm-153, Re-186 has been coupled to a bone-seeking phosphonate, ethylene hydroxy diphosphonate (EHDP). This radionuclide emits beta particles with a maximum energy of 1.07 MeV and gamma photons with an energy of 137 KeV which allows bone scanning. Re-186-EHDP undergoes renal excretion within 6 h after intravenous injection, as is the case with the common bone scanning agents. At 4 days, 14% of the radioactivity remains in the bone [35].

Several studies have shown encouraging clinical results of palliative therapy using 186Re-HEDP with an overall response rate of approximately 70% for painful osseous metastasis from prostate and breast cancer. Myelosuppression has been limited and reversible, which makes repetitive treatment safe [36, 37]. In a study of 31 patients with various cancers (10 prostate, 10 breast, 4 rectum, 5 lung, 2 nasopharynx) and bone metastases treated with a fixed dose of 1295 MBq (35 mCi) of Re-186 HEDP. When necessary, the same dose was repeated two to three times after an interval of 10–12 weeks. The mean response rate was 87.5% in patients with breast and prostate cancer, 75% in patients with rectal cancer, and 20% in patients with lung cancer. The overall response rate was 67.5% and the palliation period varied between 6 and 10 weeks. The maximal palliation effect was observed between the third and seventh weeks [37].

13.4.1.4 Tin-117 M- Diethylenetri- aminepentaacetic Acid (Sn-117m-DTPA)

Tin-117 m is a reactor-produced radionuclide, with a half-life of 13.6 days. Contrary to the other radionuclides mentioned above, this radionuclide emits internal conversion electrons. Tin-117 m is linked to diethylenetriaminepentaacetic acid (DTPA). More than 50% of the administered activity is absorbed by bone in patients with metastatic carcinoma with a bone-to-red marrow ratio of up to 9:1. Its 159 KeV photon energy allows correlative imaging with a similar uptake pattern as Tc99m-MDP [38].

In a preliminary study of 10 patients by Atkins et al. [39], none of the patients who received Sn-117 m-DTPA for palliation developed marrow toxicity. Another recent study on 47 patients treated with Sn-117-DTPA showed that the experimental mean absorbed dose to the femoral marrow was 0.043 cGy/KBq. In comparison to P-32-orthophosphate, Sn-117 m-DTPA yielded up to an eightfold therapeutic advantage over the energetic beta emitter P-32. Accordingly, it was suggested that internal conversion electron emitter Sn-117 m offers a large dosimetric advantage over the energetic beta-particle emitters allowing higher administered activity for alleviating bone pain, while minimizing marrow toxicity [40].

13.4.1.5 Phosphorus-32 Orthophosphate

This radionuclide is used uncommonly for the treatment of bone metastases. Dosimetric studies have demonstrated a relatively high dose to the bone marrow from the highly energetic beta particles of this radionuclide causing myelosuppression with pancytopenia. Increased incidence of acute leukemia has been reported although this was reported following P-32 therapy in patients with polycythemia vera.

13.4.1.6 Rhenium-188 Dimercaptosuccinic Acid Complex [re-188(V)DMSA]

Re-188(V)DMSA, a potential therapeutic analogue of the tumor imaging agent Tc99m(V) DMSA, is selectively taken up in bone metastases. In a study by Blower PJ et al. [41] on 10 patients with metastatic prostate cancer studied by

Tc99m(V)DMSA and 188Re(V)DMSA to compare their biodistribution, only minor differences between both radiopharmaceuticals were found. Accordingly, Tc99m(V)DMSA scans are predictive of 188Re(V)DMSA biodistribution and could be used to estimate tumor and renal dosimetry and assess the suitability of patients for Re-186(V) DMSA treatment [41]. This advantage makes this tracer a candidate for more trials as a potentially successful agent for bone metastases palliation.

13.4.1.7 Radium-223 (Ra-223) Dichloride

Ra-223 dichloride has both palliative and therapeutic effects approved for the treatment of castration-resistant prostate cancer with symptomatic bone metastases. This will be discussed in the Metastatic Prostate Carcinoma section.

13.4.2 Mechanism of Action

Metastatic bone pain is believed to be due to mechanical factors due to local bony destruction and to humoral factors resulting from secretion of certain mediators by tumor and peri-tumoral cells. Although the mechanism of action of these radiopharmaceuticals in relieving bone pain is not completely known, the therapeutic effect is thought to be achieved by delivering sufficient energy from the sites of reactive bone directly to the cells of metastases and/or to peri-tumor cytokine-secreting cells that may be responsible for the patient's pain. Pain relief by radiation was found to be independent of the radiosensitivity of the tumor and therefore the mechanism of action does not involve actual killing of the tumor cell. It is more likely that radiation interrupts processes that are maintained by humoral pain mediators in the microenvironment of the tumor [42]. This view is also supported by absence of a dose–response relationship [43].

13.4.3 Choice of Radiopharmaceutical

It has been demonstrated that myelosuppression is less severe using radionuclides with relatively shorter half-lives favoring the use of Sm-153, Re-186, Sn-117, and Sr-89. Other physical properties including radiolabeled conjugate biological uptake and clearance, product-specific activity, range and type of emissions, and resultant effects on tumor and normal tissue cellular survival should be all considered along with the clinical outcome to choose a radiopharmaceutical. The response rate of different radiopharmaceuticals currently in use appears not to differ significantly [44].

13.4.4 Clinical Use

Radiopharmaceutical therapy is indicated for the treatment of patients with painful widespread bone metastases. However, the patient with pain secondary to either spinal cord or peripheral nerve invasion by adjacent metastases will not benefit from such treatment. The contraindication in pregnancy is absolute, and relative contraindications include preexisting severe myelosuppression, urinary incontinence, severe insufficiency, and spinal cord compression or pathological fracture. A pre-therapy bone scan within 3 mos, neurological examination, and blood counts should be available before the patient is treated. Follow-up blood counts should be performed at least biweekly to evaluate myelotoxicity. The response to these radiopharmaceuticals is more or less similar, with an average success rate of 70–80% [45–51].

The difference in half-life of the radiopharmaceuticals and the extent of bone metastases have consequences for both the onset and the duration of pain relief. Relief rates using the newer agents are not significantly different and are comparable with those of external beam radiotherapy, but side effects are minimal and compare favorably with those of the older agent P-32.

Using radionuclides along with chemotherapy for palliation is being investigated and may prove useful. Palmedo et al. reported a case of a patient with disseminated bone metastases due to breast cancer and multifocal pain. Because of persisting pain after the first cycle of chemotherapy, 1295 MBq Re-186 HEDP was administered and pain relief was significant. Subsequently, the patient received combined chemotherapy along with Re-186 HEDP therapy and remained pain free. Follow-up Tc99m-MDP bone scan showed significant regression of osseous metastases. The authors speculated that the combination of Re-186 HEDP and chemotherapy resulted in significantly increased palliation of metastatic bone disease [52].

The side effects, which are mainly hematological, vary among the agents used, being more pronounced with P-32 than with the newer agents. Some agents have the advantage of emitting gamma energy suitable for scintigraphy such as samarium-153 EDTMD (ethylenediaminetetramethylene phosphonate). Tin-117 m-DTPA differs from the other radiopharmaceuticals in that it emits conversion electrons rather than beta particles. These conversion electrons have low energy and a shorter path in tissue and may then result in less marrow toxicity [49, 53].

13.5 Treatment of Neuroendocrine Tumors

Neuroendocrine tumors constitute a heterogeneous group of neoplasms originating from neuroendocrine cells that secrete biogenic amines and polypeptide hormones. Recently, the incidence of these tumors has gradually increased worldwide. The clinical behavior of neuroendocrine tumors is significantly variable; they may be hormonally active or nonfunctioning, ranging from very slow-growing tumors to highly aggressive and very malignant tumors. Surgery is currently the only available curative treatment for these tumors, but for patients who have inoperable primary, recurrent or metastatic disease, few therapeutic options are available. The goals of radionuclide therapy for neuroendocrine tumors are to control symptoms and pain, improve the quality of life, reduce medical requirements, and stabilize the disease. Additionally, in limited disease it is used to reduce tumor volume, reduce hormone secretion, and help complete remission.

Several neuroendocrine tumors are candidates for radionuclide therapy. I-131 has been used to treat neuroblastoma, pheochromocytoma, and paraganglioma. More recently octreotide and other analogues labeled with In-111, Y-90, and Lu-177 are being used [54–56] (see later).

I-131 metaiodobenzylguanidine (MIBG) is being used for the treatment of pheochromocytoma, malignant paraganglioma, neuroblastoma, medullary thyroid carcinoma, and symptomatic carcinoid tumors. The radiopharmaceutical resembles guanethidine and is concentrated by normal and abnormal sympathetic adrenergic tissue.

When I-131 MIBG is administered intravenously, it is transported by blood to be taken up by normal adrenergic tissue such as the adrenal medulla and sympathetic nervous system and by tumors of neuroectoderm-derived tissue. The uptake by these tumors is secondary to active uptake-1 mechanism and passive diffusion through the cell membrane, followed by active intracellular transport to the neurosecretory granules in the cytoplasm, where it is retained.

In normal adrenergic tissue such as the adrenal medulla, heart, and salivary glands, as well as in pheochromocytoma, 90% of MIBG is stored in the neurosecretory granules, while in neuroblastoma it was found that up to 60% is stored within the extragranular cells. A major part of the radiopharmaceutical is excreted unchanged in urine. Other than in the adrenergic tissues, uptake is normally noted in the liver, spleen, urinary bladder, bowel, lungs, nose, near the trapezium muscle in children, and in the uterus in some women [57, 58]. The radiation effect is due to emission of beta particles from the decaying I-131 with a mechanism similar to that in treating thyroid disorders. A long list of medications is known to block the uptake and/or retention of MIBG by the target tissues, while some reports have suggested that others such as calcium channel blockers may increase its uptake. The mechanism of interference of these drugs varies. Beta-blockers, for example, interfere with the uptake by inhibiting the uptake mechanism-1 and by depleting the neurosecretory granules, while reserpine exerts this action by depleting the granules and inhibiting the intracellular transport. More recently peptide therapy has been increasingly used to treat these tumors (shown later in the chapter).

13.5.1 Neuroblastoma

Therapeutic amounts of I-131 MIBG can be delivered to neuroblastoma with acceptable bone marrow toxicity [59–61]. Among patients with stages 3 and 4 neuroblastoma who had failed treatment with chemotherapy, I-131 MIBG induced partial remission in many children and complete remission in a small number of patients. The agent has also been used for early therapy at the time of diagnosis, with a success rate comparable to that of chemotherapy with fewer side effects [60]. Since some neuroblastomas express somatostatin receptors, peptide receptor radionuclide therapy particularly with 177Lu-DOTATATE is also beneficial.

13.5.2 Pheochromocytoma

Malignant pheochromocytoma and its metastases are known to be resistant to chemotherapy and external beam radiation therapy. I-131 MIBG has a limited role in the treatment of malignant pheochromocytoma, functioning paraganglioma, and medullary carcinoma of the thyroid. Palliative effects have been achieved in patients with pheochromocytoma [62]. Several reports from the USA and Europe have collectively shown a response of 62.5% among patients with pheochromocytoma [44]. Soft tissue metastases responded better than skeletal metastases.

13.5.3 Carcinoid Tumor

Carcinoid liver metastases are common and rarely can be resected. Treatment for symptomatic patients with unresectable disease includes chemotherapy, interferon-alpha, and the somatostatin analogue, octreotide. The response to these medical therapies is usually poor. Hepatic artery ligation and embolization are alternatives and have a better response rate. Preliminary experience also suggests that external beam radiotherapy can be useful. I-131 MIBG and radiolabeled octreotide have recently been tried.

I-131 MIBG is highly concentrated in more than 60% of carcinoid metastases. Carcinoid tumor cells stain positive for chromogranin A [63]. I-131 MIBG targets metabolically active lesions, reduces hormonal secretion, and improves symptoms [64, 65]. Data indicate a partial response in 20% of patients and a palliative effect in more than 50% of those with end-stage disease. I-131 MIBG causes temporary myelosuppression, which makes its use favorable compared with chemotherapy. It is also preferred to interferon alpha and octreotide, which require frequent subcutaneous injections.

Pathologically, I-131 MIBG produces gross cystic changes in liver metastases which probably are due to ischemic necrosis. Surgical deroofing and aspiration of cysts can lead to regeneration of normal liver tissue [64].

13.6 Radioimmunotherapy

Monoclonal antibodies are now contributing increasingly to cancer treatment, following early disappointments. I-131 anti-CD-20 and I-131 anti-CD-22 are good examples which are used for non-Hodgkin's lymphomas. These antibodies can be used alone to kill tumor cells or conjugated with drugs, cytotoxic agents, and radionuclides to improve their effects.

Radioimmunotherapy using monoclonal antibodies conjugated with isotopes allows the delivery of radiation to tumor tissue while sparing normal tissue. This radiation can be administered as a single large dose of radiolabeled monoclonal antibodies or, more commonly, in multiple fractions [66–68].

Although the way they work is not entirely clear, generally monoclonal antibodies can kill tumor cells through the following mechanisms [69]:

1. Activation of host immune system to lyse tumor cells, e.g., complement, antibody-dependent cellular cytotoxicity (ADCC).
2. Directing biologically active agents to tumor cells (e.g., drugs, toxins, cytokines, and isotopes).

3. Triggering or interfering with the function of physiologically important cell receptors.
4. Inducing indirect antitumor response by triggering the formation of autoantibodies or activation of cellular responses to tumor antigens to destroy tumor cells.
5. Killing tumor cells by apoptosis, which is simply an intrinsic "programmed" cell death characterized by chromatin condensation and DNA degeneration.

The use of radioimmunotherapy for treating lymphoma has been expanding in the last decade. It is currently being used for recurrent and relapsed disease of low-grade B cell and follicular and transformed lymphomas. Clinical trials are being conducted for aggressive B cell, mantle cell, and non-follicular indolent B cell types as well as chronic lymphocytic leukemia. Results of a study on the long-term impact of radioimmunotherapy using yttrium-90 (^{90}Y)–ibritumomab tiuxetan in advanced-stage follicular lymphoma in first remission showed a median duration of progression-free survival of 4.1 years after radioimmunotherapy and 1.1 years for controls [70].

13.7   Radionuclide Synovectomy

There may be a need for a definitive solution to the joint pain of many arthropathies, particularly rheumatoid arthritis, after failure of conventional medications. Therapeutic nuclear medicine offers an alternative to surgical synovectomy. Several radiopharmaceuticals can destroy the synovial membrane when injected intraarticularly (radionuclide synovectomy or radiosynoviorthesis) and the patients become pain free.

Yttrium-90 colloid, erbium-169 citrate colloid, rhenium-186 colloid, phosphorus-32 (P-32) colloid, and others are all used to treat synovial disease [71, 72]. Since these colloids vary in their physical characteristics and thus in their range of penetrability, they are used differently to achieve therapeutic effects and avoid injuring the surrounding tissue. Accordingly, some radiopharmaceuticals are used for the knee while others are used for small joints (Table 13.2). Yttrium-90 citrate or silicate is generally used for big joints such as the knee; rhenium-186 colloid is used for the shoulder, elbow, hip, and ankle; and erbium-169 citrate for the small joints in the hands and feet (Fig. 13.3).

Table 13.2 Physical properties and main uses of major radiopharmaceuticals for synovectomy

Isotope	Mode of decay	Physical half-life (days)	Main energy	Penetration range	Main use/adult dose
^{90}Y-silicate or citrate colloid with an average particle size of 10 nm	Emission of beta particles	2.7	2.24 MeV	3–5 mm in soft tissue, 2.8 mm in cartilage, max. 11 mm in soft tissues	Knee joint; 185 MBq
^{169}Er-citrate colloid with an average particle size of 10 nm	Emission of beta particles	9.4	0.4 MeV	Max 1 mm in soft tissue and 0.7 mm in cartilage	Small joints of hand and feet; 37 MBq
^{186}Re-sulfide colloid with an average particle size of 5–10 nm	Emission of beta particles and gamma rays (92.2%); electron capture (7.8%)	3.7	Gamma 137 KeV, beta 1.07 MeV	1.2 mm in soft tissues and 0.9 mm in cartilage	Shoulder, elbow, and wrist joints; 74 MBq
^{32}P-colloid with an average particle size of 5–20 nm	Emission of beta particles	14	1.7 MeV	Max 7.9 mm in soft tissue	Knee, elbows, and ankles; 37 MBq

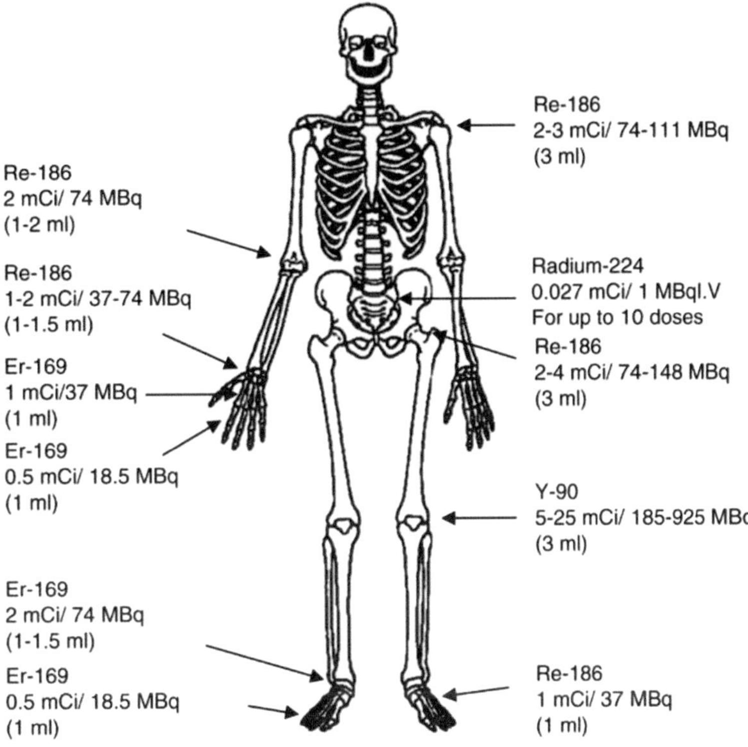

Fig. 13.3 Diagram illustrating the choice of radiopharmaceuticals for radiosynovectomy of different joints

13.7.1 Radiopharmaceuticals for Synovectomy

13.7.1.1 Yttrium-90 Colloid (^{90}Y)

This radionuclide is used predominantly for radionuclide synoviorthesis of the knee joint. It is also for malignant pleural and peritoneal effusions. The pharmacological characteristics of the silicate and citrate forms are the same. The average range in tissue is 3.6 mm and the maximum is 11 mm. After direct intra-articular administration, the colloid penetrates into the surface cells of the synovia. Small amounts of particles are transported through the lymphatics, mainly after active or passive movement of the joint, from the knee to the regional lymph nodes. The safety of this modality of management has been reported, and hence the patients' age should not be regarded as a limiting factor [73]. It is recommended that Y-90 synoviorthesis should be performed in very young patients, when the amount of synovium is still moderate. Once the degree of

synovitis has become severe, the expected results of radioactive synoviorthesis are worse [74].

13.7.1.2 Rhenium-186 Sulfide ([^{186}Re] Colloid)

This radiopharmaceutical is used particularly for radionuclide synoviorthesis of the hip, shoulder, elbow, wrist, or ankle joint. After intra-articular injection, it is absorbed by the superficial cells of the synovia. Beta radiation leads to coagulation necrosis and sloughing of these cells.

13.7.1.3 Erbium-169 Citrate [^{169}Er] Colloid

This is more suitable for the radionuclide synoviorthesis of metacarpophalangeal, metatarsophalangeal, and proximal interphalangeal joints. Beta radiation of the absorbed radiopharmaceutical in the synovia causes coagulation necrosis and sloughing of cells, as with other colloids used for other joints. ^{169}Er colloid has an affinity to chelates; therefore, the simultaneous administration of iodine contrast medium containing EDTA should be avoided.

Absolute contraindications for the use of the three therapeutic radiopharmaceutical colloids for synovectomy are pregnancy and continued breastfeeding.

13.7.1.4 Phosphorus-32 Chromic Sulfate (P-32)

^{32}P chromic phosphate has a 14-day half-life, is several times larger than ^{90}Y silicate, Re-186, Er-169, or ^{198}Au colloids, and emits only beta radiation. Its beta radiation has a soft tissue penetration midway between them at 2–3 mm. These physical advantages have led some investigators to use it for the treatment of rheumatoid arthritis and hemophilic arthritis [75, 76].

13.7.1.5 Radioactive Gold Au-198

Radioactive gold (Au-198) has a mean soft tissue penetration of only 1–2 mm. It has also been used also radiosynovectomy. It has a physical half-life of 197 days and a colloid particle size ranging from 20 to 70 μm.

13.7.1.6 Rhenium-188 Colloid

Rhenium-188 is a generator-produced beta-emitting radionuclide; the importance of 188Re for radionuclide therapy is increasing rapidly. Jeong [77] prepared 188Re-colloid and compared its properties with 188Re-colloid. They found that 188Re tin colloid is more advantageous over 188Re sulfur colloid since it showed higher labeling efficiency, allowed better control of the particle size, and lower residual activity in the injection syringes [8].

13.7.1.7 Dysprosium-165 (Dy-165)

This radionuclide has a short half-life of 2.3 h, energetic beta emission with a tissue penetration of 5.7 mm, and a very large particle size. Furthermore, it has a 3.6 abundance of gamma emission that can be used by the gamma camera to detect any possible leak. It showed a response rate of 65–70% with the best results in patients with early-stage joint disease [78].

13.7.1.8 Ho-166-Ferric Hydroxide

The first experience with Ho-166 was recently reported [79]. Knee joints of 22 patients were treated with a mean activity of 1.11 GBq (mCi). Ho-166 has a maximum beta energy of 1.85 MeV with a mean penetration in inflamed synovial layer of 2.2 mm and a maximum of 8.7 mm. Its particle size is 1.2–12 nm.

13.7.2 Mechanism of Action

Although the mechanism of action cannot be totally explained, the current belief is that after intra-articular administration the radioactive particles are absorbed by superficial cells of the synovium. Beta radiation leads to coagulation necrosis and sloughing of these cells.

13.7.3 Choice of Radiopharmaceutical

The choice of radiopharmaceutical depends on the physical characteristics and the size of the joint to be treated as well as the disease status. The therapeutic agents are particulate in nature and labeled with beta-emitting radionuclides. Radiation tissue penetration is proportional to the energy of the beta particles. For example, yttrium-90, with its highly energetic beta, has a mean soft tissue penetration of 3–4 mm, while rhenium-186 has a mean penetration of 1–2 mm, the beta of phosphorus-32 has a soft tissue penetration midway between them at 2–3 mm, and both radioactive gold and Re-186 have a mean soft tissue penetration of only 1–2 mm. Radiopharmaceuticals with shallow depth of penetration are not optimal for large joints such as the knee or for patients with extensively thickened synovium as in cases with rheumatoid arthritis and pigmented villonodular synovitis. Since the rate of exposure to the radiation is proportional to the severity of the post-therapy inflammatory reaction, a radionuclide with a moderately long half-life of days may be preferred to that with a half-life of a few hours. It appears that there is an inverse relationship between the size of radioactive particle used and the tendency for the radiocolloid to leak from the joint space which, in general, makes the choice of a relatively large radiocolloid more appropriate. A radionuclide that emits only beta radiation would have more advantages than those which emit both beta and gamma radiation in order to minimize whole-body radiation.

13.7.4 Clinical Use

Hemophiliac patients with chronic synovitis and hemarthropathy, rheumatoid arthritis, pigmented villonodular synovitis, psoriatic arthritis, ankylosing spondylitis, and collagenosis are candidates for this treatment modality. Furthermore, persistent effusion after joint prosthesis is a relative indication [80].

The absolute contraindications for the use of the therapeutic radiopharmaceutical colloids for synovectomy are pregnancy and continued breastfeeding. Fresh fracture, serious liver disease, myelosuppression, and acute infections are other contraindications. Relative contraindications include children or young adults, in which case therapy should only be administered if the estimated benefit outweighs the potential risks [81]. The presence of a Baker cyst in the knee joint is considered by some workers in the field as a contraindication. Ultrasonography is particularly important for the knee joint to exclude the presence of a Baker cyst which is an evagination of the medial dorsal part of the joint capsule in communication with the main joint. If there is inflammation in the knee joint, the effusion can be pumped into Baker cyst by enhanced motion. If a valve mechanism exists in the connection duct, this could have a deleterious effect after radiosynovectomy. The increased pressure in the cyst might lead to its rupture and the radioactive fluid getting into the surrounding tissue of the joint. The consequence could be possible necrosis of the muscles,

nerves, and blood vessels. Radiosynovectomy should be delayed for 4–6 weeks after arthroscopy [81].

Two or three-phase bone scans should be obtained before planning therapy to assess the degree of inflammation of the joint and soft tissue and in order to be able to decide if radiosynovectomy is possible and if the patient would benefit from this therapy. Scintigraphy is particularly important to evaluate the extent of abnormalities in the joint being treated and quantitation methods could be used before and after therapy. History of arthroscopy must be checked. Ultrasound or MRI is also helpful to assess the amount of effusion, joint space, and the status of the synovium to ensure homogenous distribution of the radiopharmaceutical. Complete blood cell count must be obtained before therapy as well as pregnancy test for women of childbearing age. Injection should be done using an aseptic technique. Radiosynovectomy can generally be repeated in 6 months.

The largest number of treated patients are those with rheumatoid arthritis and hemophilia. Good results are generally obtained among those patients as well as those with psoriatic arthropathy. On the other hand, in osteoarthritis with recurrent joint effusion, radiosynovectomy has not been as successful in relieving the symptoms. A good response is reported in 40–70% of patients [82]. In patients with advanced cartilage destruction or bone-on-bone interaction, the synovial membrane is likely to be practically nonexistent. Accordingly, patients with less radiological damage generally show better results than those with more severe damage. If there is initially a poor response or a relapse, more than half the patients may benefit from a reinjection [71, 83]; 2190 joints were treated with radiosynovectomy with a minimum of 1 year follow-up but without specifying the radiopharmaceutical used and the overall success rate was 73%. For rheumatoid arthritis it was 67%, whereas it was 56% for osteoarthritis, 91% for hemophilia and Willebrand's disease, and 77% for pigmented villonodular synovitis [83].

13.8 Treatment of Primary and Secondary Liver Malignancies

Blood supply to the normal liver depends on portal vein and to a much lesser extent on hepatic artery. Tumors on the other hand depend on their blood supply on arterial supply and are additionally hypervascular. This forms the basis of selective internal radiotherapy (SIRT) for hepatocellular carcinomas and metastases. This approach is considered a combination of embolization and radiation. Microscopic radioactive spheres of approximately 35 µm in size are administered through a catheter in the hepatic artery. These occlude the small branches of the hepatic artery, which reduces the blood supply to the metastatic tissue. Ho-166 microspheres, Re-188 microspheres, Re-188 lipiodol, and Y-90 microspheres are all being used [84–87]. This therapy is used as an adjunct therapy before and after surgery and it may be curative. It is recommended as an option of palliative therapy for large or multifocal hepatocellular carcinomas without major portal vein invasion or extrahepatic spread. It can also be used for recurrent unresectable HCC, as a bridging therapy before liver transplantation, as a tumor downstaging treatment, and as a curative treatment for patients with associated comorbidities who are not candidates for surgery. Combined I-131 lipiodol and chemotherapy are also being studied [85].

Currently, microspheres are labeled either with pure beta emitters (e.g., yttrium-90: Y-90) or with combined beta/gamma emitters such as rhenium-188. The decay of the radionuclide results in prolonged radiation of the tumor tissue, with a dosage of approximately 150–200 Gy. Because the radionuclides used are beta emitters, the energy is deposited only in a few millimeters around the microsphere; e.g., 90% of the energy is deposited within 5.3 mm in the case of Y-90 with preservation of the normal liver tissue [86, 87].

13.9 Peptide Receptor Radionuclide Therapy

Since cells express on their plasma membranes receptor proteins with high affinity for regulatory peptides such as somatostatin, peptide analogues

Table 13.3 Radiolabeled somatostatin analogues for treatment of neuroendocrine tumors

111In-DTPAOC (111indium-DTPAO] octreotide)
111In-DOTA-TATE (111indium-DOTA-TYR3-octreotate)
90Y-DOTATOC (90yttrium-DOTA-TYR3-octreotide)
90Y-DOTA-TATE (90yttrium-DOTA-TYR3-octreotate)
177Lu-DOTATOC (177lutetium-DOTA-TYR3-octreotide)
177Lu-DOTA-TATE (177lutetium-DOTA-TYR3-octreotate)

are used to image and treat receptor-positive tumors. The amount of these receptors changes with diseases. Overexpression of such receptors is the pathophysiologic basis of visualization and treatment of receptor-positive tumors [88]. Peptide receptor radionuclide therapy (PRRNT) is a molecularly targeted radiation therapy using systemic administration of a radiolabeled peptide designed to target with high affinity and specificity receptors overexpressed on tumors.

High level of expression of somatostatin receptors on several tumor cells is the molecular basis of the utilization of radiolabeled somatostatin analogues in diagnostic and therapeutic nuclear oncology. Several radiolabeled somatostatin analogues therapeutic radiopharmaceuticals (Table 13.3) have been used to treat patients with NETs in recent years. Since peptides can be produced easily and have rapid clearance, rapid tissue penetration, and low antigenicity, several labeled peptides have been developed over the last few years. These include somatostatin, cholecystokinin (CCK), gastrin, vasoactive intestinal peptide (VIP), bombesin, substance P, and neuropeptide Y (NPY) analogues [56, 89].

Candidate patients for PRRNT using radiolabeled somatostatin analogues are mainly those with sstr2-expressing NET of the gastroenteropancreatic and bronchial tracts but may also include patients with phaeochromocytoma, paraganglioma, neuroblastoma [56], or medullary thyroid carcinoma. Iodine-negative metastases of differentiated thyroid cancer may express somatostatin receptors and could benefit from Y-90 DOTA octreotide or lanreotide [82]. Detection of somatostatin-positive metastases before considering this treatment should be done using diagnostic sstr imaging with Ga-68 labeled somatostatin analogs or In-111 labeled octreotide or lanreotide. Some metastases respond to octreotide while others respond to lanreotide, and there is no apparent explanation. Combination of I-131 and Y-90 DOTA octreotide or lanreotide is being considered.

NETs have proven to be ideal neoplasms for PRRNT, as the majority of these malignancies overexpress somatostatin receptors. Appropriate candidates for PRRNT are patients presenting with well-differentiated or moderately differentiated neuroendocrine carcinomas, defined as NETs of grade 1 or 2 according to the WHO classification of 2010 [90–93]. A study (82) has shown that In-111 DTPA octreotide effect is dependent on tumor size in animal models bearing somatostatin pancreatic tumor expressing somatostatin receptor type2 (sst_2). Complete response was seen in 50% of tumors of 1 cm or less in diameter while the response was less pronounced with increasing tumor size. This study indicates that this therapy may be preferred to start as early as possible when tumors are small.

Combined [^{90}Y]DOTA-TATE and [^{177}Lu] DOTA-TATE therapy has been found feasible and effective therapeutic option in NET refractory to conventional therapy. In a study of 26 patients with metastatic neuroendocrine tumors treated with four therapeutic cycles of alternating [^{177}Lu]DOTA-TATE (5.55 GBq) and [^{90}Y]DOTA-TATE (2.6 GBq), a median progression-free survival longer than 24 months was achieved. Among patients with pretreatment carcinoid syndrome, 90% showed a symptomatic response or a reduction in tumor-associated pain [94]. Peptide receptor radionuclide therapy for somatostatin-positive neuroendocrine tumors has resulted in improved symptoms, prolonged survival, and an enhanced quality of life.

13.10 Treatment of Malignant Effusions

Radiopharmaceuticals can also be used in the treatment of malignant effusions. After intrapleural or intraperitoneal administration, Y-90 colloid is distributed in the effusion and penetrates the surface cells of tumors. The radionuclide destroys free tumor cells in malignant effusions and may have an additional radiation effect on metastases and mesothelioma by tumor penetrational intratumoral distribution.

13.11 Other Therapeutic Procedures

13.11.1 Treatment of Bone Tumors

13.11.1.1 Osteogenic Sarcoma

Targeted radionuclide therapy using 153Sm-EDTMP was reported to give substantial palliative effect in a case of relapsed primary osteogenic sarcoma in the first lumbar vertebra with progressive back pain after conventional treatment modalities had failed. The patient was bedridden and developed paraparesis and impaired bladder function. On a diagnostic bone scan, intense radioactivity was localized in the tumor. The patient was treated with 153Sm-EDTMP treatment twice, 8 weeks apart using 35 and 32 MBq/kg body weight, respectively. After a few days, the pain was significantly relieved and by the second radionuclide treatment the paresis subsided. For 6 months he was able to be up and about without any neurological signs or detectable metastases. Eventually, however, the patient redeveloped local pain and paraparesis, was reoperated, and died 4 months later. The investigators recommended further exploration using 153Sm-EDTMP as a boost technique, supplementary to conventional external radiotherapy given dramatic transient improvement observed in this case [95].

Another case was also reported which illustrated high-activity Sm-153-EDTMP therapy within a multimodal therapy concept to improve local control of an unresectable osteosarcoma with poor response to initial polychemotherapy. A 21-year-old woman with an extended, unresectable pelvic osteosarcoma and multiple pulmonary metastases was treated with high activity of Sm-153-EDTMP. Subsequently, external radiotherapy of the primary tumor site was performed and polychemotherapy continued, followed by autologous peripheral blood stem cell reinfusion. Within 48 h after Sm-153-EDTMP treatment, the patient had complete pain relief. Three weeks later the response was documented by a 3-phase Tc99m-MDP bone scan which showed a decrease in tracer uptake in the primary tumor and metastases. Whole-body F-18 FDG-PET also demonstrated an interval decrease in uptake. Further evaluation of feasibility and efficacy of this multimodal therapy combination of high-activity Sm-153-EDTMP therapy, external radiation, polychemotherapy, and stem cell support for unresectable osteosarcomas is warranted [96].

An animal study was conducted on 15 dogs with spontaneous osteogenic sarcoma and local pain. They were treated with Sm-153-EDTMP. The tumors were located in the extremities, scapula, maxilla, and frontal bone. The dogs were injected intravenously one to four times with 153Sm-EDTMP; 36–57 MBq/kg body weight. Three dogs had surgery in addition to the radionuclide treatment. Platelet and WBC counts showed a moderate and transient decrease with no other toxicity observed. The average tumor doses after a single injection were approximately 20 Gy. Seven dogs had metastases on autopsies. Even though none of the dogs was cured, nine of the dogs had obvious pain relief, and five of them seemed pain free: one for 13 months and one for 48 months [97].

13.11.1.2 Multiple Myeloma

Recent use of high-dose Ho-166-DOTMP (Ho-166-1, 4, 7, 10-tetraazcyclododecane-1, 4, 7, 10-tetramethylene-phosphonic acid) in patients with multiple myeloma has been reported [86]. Thirty-two patients were treated with 581–3987 mCi with an average of 2007 mCi (74.3GBq). Ho-166 has a half-life of 26.8 h and a beta emission of 1.85 Mev (51%) and 177 Mev (48%) as well as an 80.6 Kev (6.6%) gamma emission suitable for a gamma camera imaging. The beta particles have a mean range of 4 mm in soft tissue and can deliver high levels of radiation to the marrow and trabecular bone [98]. This radiopharmaceutical has selective bone uptake and rapid urinary excretion of the remaining activity. However, due to the high doses used,

catheterization and continuous irrigation of the urinary bladder after therapy has to be used to reduce radiation dose to bladder mucosa. This agent has the potential to treat patients with resistant multiple myeloma. However clinical studies with emphasis on the outcome in comparison with the currently used high dose of chemoradiotherapy with or without stem cell rescue are warranted to evaluate the impact on the poor survival of patients affected by the tumor. Also, more studies are needed to compare the adverse effects of this agent to the high incidence of systemic toxicities of the currently available radiopharmaceuticals [99–102]. Holmium-166 tetraphosphate (Ho-166 DOTMP), a high-energy beta emitter, is now used in treating bone and bone marrow-based tumors such as multiple myeloma [103]. The mechanism of action is through cell death by beta particles.

13.11.1.3 Metastatic Prostate Carcinoma

A study was conducted to explore the effects of Re-186-HEDP treatment on the progression of lumbar skeletal metastasis in an animal model using the Copenhagen rat model and to correlate the eventual treatment efficacy with the radionuclide tissue distribution. The 186Re-HEDP administration, given either 1 day or 8 days after surgical induction of lumbar metastasis was found to significantly increase the symptom-free survival of the animals. These results were confirmed by a significant decrease in the presence of histologically detectable tumor tissue. Biodistribution studies demonstrated the uptake of the major part of the radionuclide within bone tissue. The uptake of radioactivity within the lumbar vertebrae on a microscopic scale, as shown by phosphor screen autoradiography, was concentrated in areas of bone formation and turnover. These results show that radionuclide treatment with Re-186-HEDP is a potentially efficacious treatment option in prostate cancer disseminated to the skeleton [104]. A clinical trial on selected patients with advanced, androgen-independent, prostate carcinoma who received consolidation bone-targeted therapy comprised of Sr-89 with weekly doxorubicin after induction chemotherapy had a longer survival compared with patients who did not receive the bone-targeted therapy [105]. More recently Ra = 223 dichloride and *Lu-177 PSMA are* used.

The FDG-PET therapy response assessments in men with osseous metastatic prostate cancer are not always in agreement with composite clinical designations of response, stable disease, or progression [106]. Uptake and sensitivity vary in the same tumor type, for example, prostatic cancer. Generally, the FDG avidity is low in treatment naïve prostate cancer, increased in CRPC, and almost always present in docetaxel-refractory prostate cancer [107, 108]. All this indicates that the FDG is not ideal for response assessment of prostate cancer osseous metastases, especially in earlier disease states.

Ra-223 Dichloride Treatment

Ra-223 dichloride is a bone-seeking calcium analogue, an alpha-emitter, approved for the treatment of castration-resistant prostate cancer with symptomatic bone metastases. It has both therapeutic and palliative effects. Ra-223 has alpha, beta, and gamma emissions with total decay energy of 28 MeV (mean 5.78 MeV). Ra-223 is produced from an actinium-227 (Ac-227) generator. Half-life of Ra-223 is 11.43 days. Its range in tissue is 0.04–0.05 mm with a highly localized effect and minimal detrimental effects on healthy tissues near tumor. Maximum α-energies of 223Ra are 5.78, 6.88, 7.53 MeV. Maximum β-energies are 450 keV and 490 keV. Gamma energy peaks of Ra-223 are 82, 154, 269, 351, and 402 keV. Ra-223 dichloride selectively accumulates in the bone, specifically in areas of high bone turnover through forming complexes with the mineral hydroxyapatite [109]. The high linear energy transfer of the alpha radiation results in a high probability of DNA double-strand breaks in the adjacent cells [109]. Radionuclide therapy with Ra-223 is given as single or repeated intravenous administration. The treatment is usually given on an outpatient basis with respect to national legislation and regulations. Hospitalization is recommended in cases of fecal incontinence or seriously ill patients. Contraindications are listed in EANM guidelines [109]. Patients should have bone metastases seen on recent bone scan (not older than 3 mos) and no known visceral metastatic disease. Supplementation of calcium, phosphates, or vitamin D should be paused about 4 days before and after each injection of radium-223. The dose is 55 kBq/kg, given at 4-week intervals for six injections [109].Ra-223 localization in the bone/bone metastases is around 44%–77% at 4 h. Fecal excretion is the major elimination route which is approximately 60% to 75% of the administered activity and 5% is excreted in the urinary tract. Instructions are given for 7–10 days. The most common side effects are diarrhea, nausea, vomiting, and thrombocytopenia. Risk of hematological adverse reactions increases if patients received chemotherapy or external beam radiotherapy or if patients have advanced diffuse metastases in the bones. Pain relief is rapid but not expected in every patient. The ALSYMPCA study (ALpharadin in SYMPtomatic Prostate CAncer) is an international clinical study to evaluate the efficacy and safety of Ra-223 [110–112]. The ALSYMPCA study showed an overall survival benefit with ^{223}Ra treatment (in over 900 patients). Also, the frequency of skeletal-related events was reduced with Ra-223 treatment. Improved survival with ^{223}Ra was accompanied by significant quality-of-life benefits, including a higher percentage of patients with meaningful quality-of-life improvements and a slower decline in quality-of-life over time.

Lu-177 PSMA Ligand Treatment

Luteium-177 (Lu-177) PSMA ligand therapies have demonstrated promising results in a significant proportion of men with metastatic prostate cancer who have failed other therapies. Treatment with Lu-177 PSMA ligands is currently undergoing clinical validation. Lu-177 is a radiometal produced in a reactor. Lu-177 is a medium-energy beta emitter (490 keV) with a maximal tissue penetration of <2 mm which provides better irradiation of small tumors. It also emits low-energy gamma rays, 208 and 113 keV which allows for ex vivo imaging after treatment.Lu-177 has a physical half-life of 6.73 days. Current clinical knowledge is predominantly based on two low molecular weight PSMA ligands: PSMA 617 and PSMA-I&T [113]. Patients should have adequate uptake of PSMA ligands on pre-therapy imaging. Dose calculations are based on disease burden, patient weight, and renal function. Injected doses range from 3.7 to 9.3 GBq (100–250 mCi) per single injection with up to six injections, generally at minimum 6-week intervals [113]. Contraindications to this treatment are described in detail at EANM guidelines [113]. For kidney protection (to decrease reabsorption of radiotracer via the proximal renal tubules and thereby decrease the radiation dose to the kidneys some institutes give IV amino acid infusion (lysine and arginine) over 4 h, starting 30 min prior to the treatment. Lu-177 PSMA is given as outpatient treatment in some countries and inpatient in other countries with respect to national legislation and regulations. Lu-177 PSMA is excreted via kidneys in the first 48 h following injection. Prospective clinical trials confirmed high response rates, low toxicity, and reduction of pain in metastatic castration-resistant prostate cancer. In 30%–70% of men treated with Lu-177 PSMA, there was a > 50% reduction in serum PSA levels [114]. In another study, 80% of all men had a PSA response to PSMA therapy [115].

13.12 Combined Therapeutic Approach

The use of radionuclide therapy has been used alone. Recently, several trials have used a combined approach combining radionuclides with other treatment modalities [116, 117]. Sr89 in combination with doxorubicin has been used for bone metastases. This combination was found to be associated with a longer time interval for disease progression and longer overall survival when compared to those who only received doxorubicin [117, 118]. Combining low-dose cisplatin with the standard dose of Sr-89 chloride was found to improve pain palliation significantly [119].

CHOP was also used in combination with I-131–tositumomab and Y-90–ibritumomab and Rituxan–CHOP combinations for untreated non-Hodgkin's lymphoma [120, 121].

Combining I-131 MIBG and chemotherapy or myeloablative chemotherapy has been also used

Table 13.4 Effects and mechanisms of action of therapeutic radiopharmaceuticals

Therapeutic procedure/target	Probable mechanism
Hyperthyroid	Cell injury/death to reduce or ablate the thyroid gland
Thyroid cancer	Cell death to ablate residual thyroid tissue, tumor, and metastases
Synovectomy	Phagocytosis of radiolabeled colloid by synoviocytes which are distributed uniformly on the surface of the synovium, with subsequent destruction of the synovium by the beta particles
Radioimmunotherapy	Destruction of tumor cells through multiple mechanisms including cell lysis, formation of autoantibodies, and/or apoptosis
Painful bone metastases	Uptake of the radiopharmaceutical by metastases and/or surrounding bone, with radiation injury or death to the tumor cells or the surrounding cytokine-secreting cells
Peptide therapy	High expression of peptide receptors such as somatostatin and cholecystokinin by cells of specific tumors

in a limited number of patients [122, 123]. In a pilot study, Y-90 biotin was used as an adjunct to surgery and radiation therapy for malignant glioma [124]. The disease-free interval and overall survival were significantly longer among patients with this adjunct therapy than in control group. External beam radiotherapy has been used in combination with I-131 MIBG for neuroblastoma, and paraganglioma and with I-131 for a large thyroid metastasis. This combined method takes into consideration the nonuniform dose distribution on the basis of tumor function and the radionuclide therapy dose delivered [125]. Combined chemotherapy and I-131 lipiodol for the treatment of hepatocellular carcinoma are being studied as mentioned earlier.

Table 13.4 summarizes the probable mechanisms of action of the major radiopharmaceutical tracers currently used. More choices in radionuclide therapy are now available to physicians for local and systemic uses to palliation and definitive therapy. The areas of research in the field of therapeutic nuclear medicine are wide open for developing new therapeutic radiopharmaceuticals and clinical applications.

References

1. Demeter S, Leslie WD, Levin DP (2005) Radioactive iodine therapy for malignant and benign thyroid disease: a Canadian national survey of physician practice. Nucl Med Commun 26:613–621
2. McKenzie JM, Zakrija M, Sato A (1978) Humoral immunity in graves' disease. Clin Endocrinol Metab 7:31
3. Maxon HR, Thomas SR, Saenger EL et al (1977) Ionizing irradiation and induction of clinically significant disease in human thyroid. Am J Med 63:967
4. Sofa AM, Skillern PG (1975) Treatment of hyperthyroidism with a large initial dose of sodium iodide I-131. Arch Intern Med 135:673
5. Woeber KA (2000) Update on the management of hyperthyroidism and hypothyroidism. Arch Intern Med 160:1067–1071
6. Hamburger JI (1980) Evaluation of toxicity in solitary nontoxic autonomously functioning thyroid nodules. J Clin Endocrinol Metab 50:1089–1093
7. Peter HJ, Studer H, Forster T, Herber H (1982) The pathogenesis of "hot" and "cold" follicle in multinodular goiters. J Clin Endocrinol Metab 55:941–946
8. Ginsberg J (2003) Diagnosis and management of Grave's disease. CMAJ 168:575–585
9. Bartalena L, Marcocci C, Bogazzi F, Manetti L, Tanda ML, Dell'Unto E et al (1998) Relation between therapy for hyperthyroidism and the course of Grave's ophthalmopathy. N Engl J Med 338:73–78
10. Reid JR, Wheeler SF (2005) Hyperthyroidism: diagnosis and treatment. Am Fam Physician 72:623–630
11. Perros P, Kendall-taylor P, Neoh C, Frewin S, Dickinson J (2005) A prospective study of the effects of radioiodine therapy for hyperthyroidism in patients with minimally active Grave's ophthalmopathy. J Clin Endocrinol Metab 90:5321–5532
12. Maxon HR, Thomas SR, Chen IW (1981) The role of nuclear medicine in the treatment of hyperthyroidism and well differentiated thyroid adenocarcinoma. Clin Nucl Med 6:87–98
13. Sankar R, Sekhri T, Sripathy G, Walia RP, Jain SK (2005) Radioactive iodine therapy in Grave's hyperthyroidism: a prospective study from a tertiary referral center in North India. J Assoc Physicians India 53:603–606
14. Allahabadia A, Daykin J, Sheppard MC, Gough SC, Franklyn JA (2001) Radioiodine treatment of hyperthyroidism. Prognostic factors for outcome. J Clin Endocrinol Metab 86:3611–3617
15. Haugen BR, Alexander EK, Bible KC, Doherty GM, Mandel SJ et al (2016) 2015 American Thyroid Association management guidelines for adult patients with thyroid nodules and differentiated thyroid cancer: the American thyroid Association guidelines task force on thyroid nodules and differentiated thyroid cancer. Thyroid 26:1–13
16. Terrier P, Sheng ZM, Schlumberger M et al (1988) Structure and expression of c-myc and c-fos proto-oncogenes in thyroid carcinomas. Oncogene 2:403
17. Lemoine NR, Mayall ES, Wyllie FS et al (1988) Activated ras oncogenes in human the thyroid cancers. Cancer Res 48:44–59
18. Atay-Rosenthal S (1999) Controversies on treatment of well-differentiated thyroid carcinoma and factors influencing prognosis. In: Freeman L (ed) Nuclear medicine annual. Lippincott/Williams and Wilkins, Philadelphia, pp 303–334
19. Beierwaltes WH (1978) The treatment of thyroid carcinoma with radioiodine. Semin Nucl Med 8:79
20. Rosario PW, Barroso AL, Rezende LI, Padrao EL, Fagundes TA, Reis JS, Purisch S (2005) Outcome of ablation of thyroid remnants with 100 mCi (3.7 GBq) iodine −131 in patients with thyroid cancer. Ann Nucl Med 19:247–250
21. Kolfuerest S, Igerc I, Lind P (2005) Recombinant human thyrotropin is helpful in the follow up and I-131 therapy of patients with thyroid cancer: a report of the results and benefits using recombinant thyrotropin in clinical routine. Thyroid 15:371–376
22. Intenzo CM, Jabbour S, Dam HQ, Capuzzi DM (2005) Changing concepts in the management of differentiated thyroid cancer. Semin Nucl Med 35:257–265
23. Fujie S, Okumura Y, Sato S, Akaki S, Katsui K, Himei K, Takemoto M, Kanazawa S (2005) Diagnostic capabilities of I-131, Tl-201, and Tc99m MIBI scintigraphy for metastatic differentiated thyroid carcinoma after total thyroidectomy. Acta Med Okayama 59:99–107
24. Ferreira SH, Lorenzethi BB, Bristow AF et al (1988) Interleukin-1 beta as a potent hyperalgesic agent antagonized by a tripeptide analogue. Nature 334:698–700
25. Poulson HS, Nielsen OS, Klee M et al (1989) Palliative irradiation of bone metastases. Cancer Treat Rev 16:41–48
26. Tong D, Gillick L, Hendrickson FR (1982) Palliation of symptomatic osseous metastases. Cancer 50:893–899
27. Salazar OM, Rubin P, Hendrickson FR et al (1986) Single-dose half-body irradiation for palliation of multiple bone metastases from solid tumors. Final radiation therapy oncology group report. Cancer 58:29–36
28. Bauman G, Charette M, Reid R, Sathya J (2005) Radiopharmaceuticals for the palliation of painful bone metastasis-a systemic review. Radiother Oncol 75:258–270

29. Pauwels EKJ, Stokkel MPM (2001) Radiopharmaceuticals for bone lesions imaging and therapy in clinical practice. Q J Nucl Med 45:18–26

30. Giammarile F, Mognetti T, Resche I (2001) Bone pain palliation with strontium-89 in cancer patients with bone metastases. Q J Nucl Med 45:78–83

31. Patel BR, Flowers WM Jr (1997) Systemic radionuclide therapy with strontium chloride Sr 89 for painful skeletal metastases in prostate and breast cancer. South Med J 90:506–508

32. Papatheofanis FJ (2000) Decreased serum E-selectin concentration after 89Sr-chloride therapy for metastatic prostate cancer bone pain. J Nucl Med 41:1021–1024

33. Ramamoorthy N, Saraswathy P, Das MK, Mehra KS, Ananthakrishnan M (2002) Production logistics and radionuclidic purity aspects of 153Sm for radionuclide therapy. Nucl Med Commun 23:83–89

34. Cameron PJ, Klemp PF, Martindale AA, Turner JH (1999) Prospective 153Sm-EDTMP therapy dosimetry by whole-body scintigraphy. Nucl Med Commun 20:609–615

35. Maxon HR, Thomas S, Hertzberg VS, Schroder LE, Englaro EE, Samaratunga R et al (1992) Rhenium-186 hydroxyethylidene diphosphonate for the treatment of painful osseous metastases. Semin Nucl Med 22:33–40

36. Han SH, De Klerk JM, Zonnenberg BA, Tan S, Van Rijk PP (2001) 186Re-etidronate. Efficacy of palliative radionuclide therapy for painful bone metastases. Q J Nucl Med 45:84–90

37. Kucuk NO, Ibis E, Aras G, Baltaci S, Ozalp G, Beduk Y, Canakci N, Soylu A (2000) Palliative analgesic effect of Re-186 HEDP in various cancer patients with bone metastases. Ann Nucl Med 14:239–245

38. Atkins HL, Mausner LF, Srivastava SC, Meinken GE, Cabahug CJ, D'Alessandro T (1995) Tin-117 m (4+)-DTPA for palliation of pain from osseous metastases: a pilot study. J Nucl Med 36:725–929

39. Atkins HL, Mausner LF, Srivastava SC, Meinken GE, Straub RF, Cabahug CJ et al (1993) Biodistribution of Sn-117 m DTPA for palliative therapy of painful osseous metastases. Radiology 186:279–283

40. Bishayee A, Rao DV, Srivastava SC, Bouchet LG, Bolch WE, Howell RW (2000) Marrow-sparing effects of 117mSndiethylenetriaminepentaacetic acid for radionuclide therapy of bone cancer. J Nucl Med 41:2043–2050

41. Blower PJ, Kettle AG, O'Doherty MJ, Coakley AJ, Knapp FF Jr (2000) 99mTc(V)DMSA quantitatively predicts 188Re(V)DMSA distribution in patients with prostate cancer metastatic to bone. Eur J Nucl Med 27:1405–1409

42. Krishnamurthy GT, Krishnamurthy S (2000) Radionuclides for metastatic bone pain palliation: a need for rational re-evaluation in the new millennium [comment]. J Nucl Med 41:688–691

43. Hoskin PJ, Ford HT, Harmer CL (1989) Hemibody irradiation (HBI) for metastatic bone pain in two histologically distinct groups of patients. Clin Oncol (R Coll Radiol) 1:67–69

44. Fischer M (1998) I-131 therapy of neural crest tumors. Nucl Med Newslett (King Saud Univ) 5:9–10

45. Quilty PM, Kirk D, Bolger JJ et al (1994) A comparison of the palliative effects of strontium-89 and external beam radiotherapy in metastatic prostate cancer. Radiother Oncol 31:33–40

46. Silberstein EB, Elgazzar AH, Kapilivsky A (1992) Phosphorus-32 radiopharmaceuticals for the treatment of painful osseous metastases. Semin Nucl Med 17:17–27

47. Maxon HR, Thomas SR, Hertzberg VS et al (1982) Rhenium-186 hydroxyethylidene diphosphonate for the treatment of painful osseous metastases. Semin Nucl Med 22:30–40

48. Elgazzar AH, Maxon HR (1993) Radioisotope therapy for cancer related bone pain. Imaging Insights 2:1–6

49. Windsor PM (2001) Predictors of response to strontium-89 (Metastron) in skeletal metastases from prostate cancer: report of a single centre's 10-year experience. Clin Oncol (R Coll Radiol) 13:219–227

50. Sideras PA, Stavraka A, Gouliamos A, Limouris GS (2013) Radionuclide therapy of painful bone metastases–a comparative study between consecutive radionuclide infusions, combination with chemotherapy, and radionuclide infusions alone: an in vivo comparison of their effectiveness. Am J Hosp Palliat Care 30:745–751

51. Dickie GJ, Macfarlane D (1999) Strontium and samarium therapy for bone metastases from prostate carcinoma. AustralasRadiol 43:476–479

52. Sciuto R, Festa A, Pasqualoni R, Semprebene A, Rea S, Bergomi S, Maini CL (2001) Metastatic bone pain palliation with 89-Sr and 186-Re-HEDP in breast cancer patients. Breast Cancer Res Treat 66:101–109

53. Kvinnsland Y, Skretting A, Bruland OS (2001) Radionuclide therapy with bone-seeking compounds: Monte Carlo calculations of dose-volume histograms for bone marrow in trabecular bone. Physics Med Biol 46:1149–1161

54. Spetz J, Dalmo J, Nilsson O, Wängberg B, Ahlman H, Forssell-Aronsson E (2012) Specific binding and uptake of 131I-MIBG and 111In-octreotide in metastatic paraganglioma–tools for choice of radionuclide therapy. HormMetab Res 44:400–404

55. Bomanji JB, Papathanasiou ND (2012). 111In-DTPA0-octreotide (Octreoscan), 131I-MIBG and other agents for radionuclide therapy of NETs) Eur J Nucl Med Mol Imaging 39(Suppl 1):S113–S125

56. Zaknun JJ, Bodei L, Mueller-Brand J, Pavel ME, Baum RP, Hörsch D, O'Dorisio MS, O'Dorisiol TM, Howe JR, Cremonesi M, Kwekkeboom DJ (2013) The joint IAEA, EANM, and SNMMI practical guidance on peptide receptor radionuclide therapy (PRRNT) in neuroendocrine tumours. Eur J Nucl Med Mol Imaging 40:800–816E

57. Gelfand MJ, Elgazzar AH, Kriss VM et al (1994) Iodine-123 MIBG SPECT versus planar imaging in children with neural crest tumors. J Nucl Med 35:1753–1757

58. Paltiel HJ, Gelfand MJ, Elgazzar AH, Washburn LC et al (1994) Neural crest tumors: I-123 MIBG imaging. Radiology 190:117–121

59. Hoefnagel CA, deKraner J, Voute PA, Valdes Olmos RA (1991) Preoperative I-131 MIBG therapy in the management of neuroblastoma (abstract). J Nucl Med 32:921

60. Hoefnagel CA, deKraner J, Valdes Olmos RA, Voute PA (1994) I-131 MIBG as a first time treatment in high risk neuroblastoma patients. J Nucl Med 15:712–717

61. Mastrangelo R, Lasorell A, Troncone L et al (1991) I-131 metaiodobenzylguanidine in neuroblastoma patients. J Nucl Med 35:248–251

62. Sisson JC, Shapiro B, Beirwaltes WH et al (1984) Radiopharmaceutical treatment of malignant pheochromocytoma. J Nucl Med 25:197–206

63. Hoefnagel CA (1991) Radionuclide therapy revisited. Eur J Nucl Med 18:408–431

64. Prvulovich EM, Stein RC, Bomanji JB et al (1998) Iodine-131 MIBG therapy of a patient with carcinoid liver metastases. J Nucl Med 39:1743–1745

65. Taal BG, Hoefnagel CA, Vables Olmos RA, Boot H, Beijen JK (1996) Palliative effect of metaiodobenzylguanidine in metastatic carcinoid tumors. J Clin Oncol 14:1829–1839

66. Press OW, Eary JF, Applelbaum FR, Martin PJ, Badger CC, Nelp WB, Glenn S, Buchko GM, Fisher LD, Porter B et al (1993) Radiolabeled-antibody therapy of B-cell lymphoma with autologous bone marrow support. N Engl J Med 329:1219–1224

67. Press OW, Eary JF, Applbaum FR, Martin PJ, Nelp WB, Glenn S, Fisher DR et al (1995) Phase II trial of I-131-B1 (anti-CD20) antibody therapy with autologous stem cell transplantation for relapsed B cell lymphomas. Lancet 346:336–340

68. De Nardo GL, De Nardo SJ, O'Grady LF, Levy NB, Adams GP, Mills SL (1990) Fractionated radioimmunotherapy of B-cell malignancies with I-131-Lym-1. Cancer Res 50:1014–1016

69. DeNardo GL, O'Donnell RT, Oldham RK, DeNardo SJ (1998) A revolution in the treatment of non-Hodgkin's lymphoma. Cancer Biother Radiopharm 13:213–223

70. Morschhauser F, Radford J, Van Hoof A et al (2013). ^{90}Yttrium-Ibritumomab Tiuxetan consolidation of first remission in advanced-stage follicular non-Hodgkin lymphoma: updated results after a median follow-up of 7.3 years from the international, randomized, phase III first-line indolent trial) J Clin Oncol 31:1977–1983

71. Deutsch E, Brodack JW, Deutsch KF (1993) Radiation synovectomy revisited. Eur J Nucl Med 20:1113–1127

72. Gschwend N (1989) Synovectomy. In: Kelly WN, Harris ED, Ruddy S et al (eds) Textbook of rheumatology. Saunders, Philadelphia, pp 1934–1961

73. Heim M, Goshen E, Amit Y, Martinowitz U (2001) Synoviorthesis with radioactive Yttrium in haemophilia: Israel experience. Haemophilia 7(Suppl 2):36–39

74. Rodriguez-Merchan EC, Jimenez-Yuste V, Villar A, Quintana M, Lopez-Cabarcos C, Hernandez-Navarro F (2001) Yttrium-90 synoviorthesis for chronic haemophilic synovitis: Madrid experience. Haemophilia 7(Suppl 2):34–35

75. Onetti CM, Guyierrez F, Hiba E et al (1982) Synoviorthesis with P-32 colloid chromic phosphate in rheumatoid arthritis and hemophilia, clinical, histopathological and arthographic changes. J Rheumatol 9:229–238

76. Rivard GE, Givard M, Belanger R et al (1994) Synoviorthesis with colloidal P-32 chromic phosphate for the treatment of hemophilic arthropathy. J Bone Joint Surg Am 76:482–487

77. Jeong JM, Lee YJ, Kim YJ, Chang YS, Lee DS, Chung JK, Song YW, Lee MC (2000) Preparation of rhenium-188-tin colloid as a radiation synovectomy agent and comparison with rhenium-188-sulfur colloid. Appl RadiatIsot 52:851–855

78. Siegel ME, Siegel HJ, Luck JV Jr (1997) Radiosynovectomy's clinical applications and cost effectiveness: a review. Semin Nucl Med 28:364–371

79. Ofluoglu S, Schwameis E, Zehetagruber I, Havlic E, Wanivenhaus A, Schweeger I, Weiss K et al (2002) Radiation synovectomy with Ho-166-ferric hydroxide: a first experience. J Nucl Med 43:1489–1494

80. Fischer M, Modder G (2002) Radionuclide therapy of inflammatory joint disease. Nucl Med Commun 23:829–831

81. Hauss F (1992) Radiosynoviorthese in der Orthopadie. Aktule Rheumatol 17:64–66

82. Asavatanabodee P et al (1997) Yttrium-90 radiochemical synovectomy in chronic knee synovitis: a one year retrospective review of 133 treatment interventions. J Rheumatol 24:639–642

83. Kresnik E, Mikososch P, Gallowitsch HJ, Jesenko R, Just H, Kogler D, Gasser J, Heinisch M, Unterweger O, Kumnig G, Gomez I, Lind P (2002) Clinical outcome of radio synoviorthesis: a meta-analysis including 2190 treated joints. Nucl Med Commun 23:683–688

84. Sundram FX, Jiomg JM, Zanzonico P, Bernal P, Chau T, Onkhuudai P, Divgi C, Knapp FF Jr, Padhy AK (2002) Trans-arterial rhenium-188 lipiodol in the treatment of inoperable hepatocellular carcinoma–results of a multi-Centre phase-1 study. World J Nucl Med 1:5–11

85. Uccelli L, Pasquali M, Boschi A, Giganti M, Duatti A (2011) Automated preparation of re-188 lipiodol for the treatment of hepatocellular carcinoma. Nucl Med Biol 38:207–213

86. Nijsen JF, van het Schip AD, Hennink WE, Rook DW, van Rijk PP, deKlerk JM (2002) Advances in nuclear oncology: microspheres for internal radionuclide therapy of liver tumours. Curr Med Chem 9:73–82

87. Van de Wiele C, Maes A, Brugman E, D'Asseler Y, De Spiegeleer B, Mees G, Stellamans K (2012) SIRT of liver metastases: physiological and pathophysiological considerations. Eur J Nucl Med Mol Imaging 39(10):1646–1655

88. Jong M, Kwekkeboom D, Volkema R, Krenning ER (2003) Radiolabelled peptides for tumor therapy: current status and future directions. Eur J Nucl Med 30:463–469

89. Rindi G (2010) The ENETS guidelines: the new TNM classification system. Tumori 96:806–809

90. Gulenchyn KY, Yaoy X, Asa SL, Singh S, Lawjj C (2012) Radionuclide therapy in neuroendocrine tumours: a systematic review. Clin Oncol 24:294–308

91. Sansovini M, Severi S, Ambrosetti A, Monti M, Nanni O et al (2013) Treatment with the radiolabelled somatostatin analog 177Lu-DOTATATE for advanced pancreatic neuroendocrine tumors. Neuroendocrinology 97:347–354

92. Pfeifer AK, Gregersen T, Grønbæk H, Hansen CP, Müller-Brand J et al (2011) Peptide receptor radionuclide therapy with 90 Y-DOTATOC and 177 Lu-DOTATOC in advanced neuroendocrine tumors: results from a Danish cohort treated in Switzerland. Neuroendocrinology 93:189–196

93. Kwekkeboom DJ, Krenning EP, Lebtahi R et al (2009) ENETS consensus guidelines for the standards of care in neuroendocrine tumours: peptide receptor radionuclide therapy with radiolabeled somatostatin analogs. Neuroendocrinology 90:220–226

94. Seregni E, Maccauro M, Chiesa C, Mariani L, Pascali C, Mazzaferro V, De Braud F, Buzzoni R, Milione M, Lorenzoni A, Bogni A, Coliva A, Vullo SL, Bombardieri E (2014) Treatment with tandem [90Y]DOTA-TATE and [177Lu]DOTA-TATE of neuroendocrine tumours refractory to conventional therapy. Eur J Nucl Med Mol Imaging 41:223–230

95. Bruland OS, Skretting A, Solheim OP, Aas M (1996) Targeted radiotherapy of osteosarcoma using 153 Sm-EDTMP. A new promising approach. Acta Oncologica 35:381–384

96. Franzius C, Bielack S, Sciuk J, Vollet B, Jurgens H, Schober O (1999) High-activity samarium-153-EDTMP therapy in unresectable osteosarcoma. Nucl Med 38:337–340

97. Aas M, Moe L, Gamlem H, Skretting A, Ottesen N, Bruland OS (1999) Internal radionuclide therapy of primary osteosarcoma in dogs, using 153Sm-ethylene-diamino-tetramethylene-phosphonate (EDTMP). Clin Cancer Res 5(10 Suppl):3148s–3152s

98. Boyouth Je Macey DJ, Kasi LP et al (1995) Pharmacokinetics, dosimetry and toxicity of holmium-166 DOTMP for bone marrow ablation multiple myeloma. J Nucl Med 36:730–737

99. Rajendran JG, Eary JF, Bensinger W, Durack LD, Vernon C, Fritzberg A (2002) High-dose 166Ho-DOTMP in myeloablative treatment of multiple myeloma: pharmacokinetics, biodistribution, and absorbed dose estimation. J Nucl Med 43:1383–1390

100. Alexanan R, Dimopoulos M (1994) The treatment of multiple myeloma. N Engl J Med 330:484–489

101. Barlogie B, Alexanian R, Dick KA et al (1987) High dose chemotherapy and autologous bone marrow transplantation for resistant myeloma. Blood 70:869–872

102. Hoefnagel CA (1988) Radionuclide cancer therapy. Ann Nucl Med 12:61–70

103. Srivastava S, Dadachova E (2001) Recent advances in radionuclide therapy. Semin Nucl Med 31:330–341

104. Geldof AA, van den Tillaar PL, Newling DW, Teule GJ (1997) Radionuclide therapy for prostate cancer lumbar metastasis prolongs symptom-free survival in a rat model. Urology 49:795–801

105. Logothetis C, Tu SM, Navone M (2003) Targeting prostate cancer bone metastases. Cancer 97:785–788

106. Yu EY, Muzi M, Hackenbracht JA et al (2011) C11-acetate and F-18 FDG PET for men with prostate cancer bone metastases: relative findings and response to therapy. Clin Nucl Med 36:192–198

107. Jadvar H (2013) Imaging evaluation of prostate cancer with 18 F- fluorodeoxyglucose PET/CT: utility and limitations. Eur J Nucl Med Mol Imaging 40(Suppl 1):S5–S10

108. Meirelles GS, Schoder H, Ravizzini GC et al (2010) Prognostic value of baseline [18F] fluorodeoxyglucose positron emission tomography and 99mTc-MDP bone scan in progressing metastatic prostate cancer. Clin Cancer Res 16:6093–6099

109. Poeppel TD, Handkiewicz-Junak D, Andreeff M, Becherer A, Bockisch A et al (2018) EANM guideline for radionuclide therapy with radium-223 of metastatic castration-resistant prostate cancer. Eur J Nucl Med Mol Imaging 45:824–845

110. Sartor O, Hoskin P, Coleman RE, Nilsson S, Vogelzang NJ et al (2016) Chemotherapy following radium-223dichloride treatment in ALSYMPCA. Prostate 76:905–916

111. Hoskin P, Sartor O, O'Sullivan JM, Johannessen DC, Helle SI, Logue J et al (2014) Efficacy and safety of radium-223 dichloride in patients with castration-resistant prostate cancer and symptomatic bone metastases, with or without previous docetaxel use: prespecified subgroup analysis from the randomised, double-blind, phase 3 ALSYMPCA trial. Lancet Oncol 15:1397–1406

112. Sartor O, Coleman RE, Nilsson S, Heinrich D, Helle SI, O'Sullivan JM et al (2017) (2017) an exploratory analysis of alkaline phosphatase, lactate dehydrogenase, and prostate-specific antigen dynamics in the

phase 3 ALSYMPCA trial with radium-223. Ann Oncol 28:1090–1097

113. Kratochwil C, Fendler WP, Eiber M, Baum R, Bozkurt MF et al (2019) EANM procedure guidelines for radionuclide therapy with ¹⁷⁷Lu-labelled PSMA-ligands (¹⁷⁷Lu-PSMA-RLT). Eur J Nucl Med Mol Imaging 46:2536–2544

114. Baum RP, Kulkarni HR, Schuchardt C et al (2016) 177Lu-labeled prostate-specific membrane antigen radioligand therapy of metastatic castration-resistant prostate cancer: safety and efficacy. J Nucl Med 57:1006–1013

115. Oudard STROPIC (2011) Phase III trial of cabazitaxel for the treatment of metastatic castration-resistant prostate cancer. Future Oncol 7:497–506

116. Valdes Olmos RA, Hoefnagel CA (2004) Radionuclide therapy in oncology: the drawing of its concomitant use with other modalities? Euro J Nucl Med Mol Imaging 31:929–931

117. Bodey RK, Flux GD, Evans PM (2003) Combining dosimetry for targeted radionuclide and external beam therapies using the biologically effective dose. Cancer Biother Radiopharam 18:89–97

118. Logothetis C, Tu S, Navone N (2003) Targeting prostate cancer bone metastases. Cancer 07:758–788

119. Sciuto R, Festa A, Rea S et al (2002) Effects of low dose cisplatin on Sr-89 therapy for painful bone metastases from prostate cancer: a randomized clinical trial. J Nucl Med 43:79–86

120. Horning SJ (2003) Future directions in radioimmunotherapy for B-cell lymphoma. Semin Oncol 30(suppl 17):29–34

121. Press OW, Unger JM, Braziel RM et al (2003) A phase 2 trial of CHOP chemotherapy followed by tositumomab/iodine I-131 tositumomab for previously untreated non-Hodgkin's lymphoma: Southwest Oncology Group Protocol S9911. Blood 102:1606–1612

122. Mastrangelo S, Tornesello A, Diociaiuti L et al (2001) Treatment of advanced neuroblastoma; feasibility and therapeutic potential chemotherapeutic potential of a novel approach combining I-131-MIBG and multiple drug chemotherapy. Br J Cancer 84:460–464

123. Yanik GA, Levine JE, Matthay KK et al (2002) Pilot study of iodine−131-metaiodobenzyl guanidine in combination with myeloablative chemotherapy and autologous stem-cell support for the treatment of neuroblastoma. J Clin Oncol 20:2142–2149

124. Grana C, Chinol M, Robertson C et al (2002) Pretargeted adjunct radioimmunotherapy with yttrium-90-biotin in malignant glioma patients: a pilot study. Br J Cancer 86:207–212

125. Bodey RK, Evans PM, Flux GD (2005) Targeted radionuclide therapy. Spatial aspects of combined modality radiotherapy. Radiother Oncol 77:301–309

Glossary

Abscess A collection of pus in tissues, organs, or confined spaces, usually caused by bacterial infection.

Absorbed dose Amount of energy absorbed per unit mass of target material.

ALARA "As low as reasonably achievable." A concept recommended by the US National Regulatory Commission for safe radiation practice.

Amplitude image A computer-generated image representing the analysis of a process whereby each pixel in the heart is evaluated with respect to movement changes over time. The amplitude image shows the magnitude of blood ejected from each pixel within the ventricular chamber.

Anion Negatively charged ion.

Ankylosing spondylitis The most common type of spondyloarthropathy with chronic inflammatory changes leading to stiffening and fusion (ankylosis) of the spine and sacroiliac joints with a strong genetic predisposition associated with HLA B27. Other joints such as hips, knees, and shoulders are involved in approximately 30% of patients.

Antibody A protein formed by the body to defend it against infection and other diseases.

Antisense oligonucleotides Synthetic single-strand DNA (or RNA) molecules designed to bind with high affinity to the complementary sequences of mRNA. Several antisense oligodeoxynucleotide pharmaceuticals have been developed as therapeutic agents that act to block protein synthesis by inactivating mRNA. This is the basis of antisense imaging.

Apophysis An accessory secondary ossification center that develops late and forms a protrusion from the growing bone where tendons and ligaments insert or originate.

Apoptosis A type (programmed) of cell death implicated in both normal and pathological tissue, designed to eliminate unwanted host cells in an active process of cellular self-destruction effected by a dedicated set of gene products.

Atrophy A decrease in size and function of the cell.

Attenuation The reduction of radiation intensity during its passage through matter due to absorption, scatter, or both.

Avulsion Complete separation of tendons or ligaments, with or without a portion of bone and/or cartilage.

Behçet's syndrome An uncommon disorder characterized by recurrent oral and genital ulceration, uveitis, retinal vasculitis, cutaneous pustules, erythema nodosum, cutaneous pathergy, and synovitis. The disease is more common in Mediterranean countries and Japan than in the United States.

Biological half-life Time required for half of the radioactivity to be eliminated from the body or an organ.

Brodie's abscess An intraosseous abscess in the cortex that becomes walled off by reactive bone.

Bronchial circulation Part of the high-pressure systemic circulation that supplies oxygenated blood to the lung tissue itself.

Budd-Chiari syndrome An uncommon condition usually caused by thrombosis of

© The Editor(s) (if applicable) and The Author(s), under exclusive license to Springer Nature Switzerland AG 2023
A. H. Elgazzar, *Synopsis of Pathophysiology in Nuclear Medicine*,
https://doi.org/10.1007/978-3-031-20646-7

the hepatic veins such as associated with polycythemia vera, following oral contraceptive use or renal cell carcinoma with tumor involving veins. Sulfur colloid liver scan typically shows decreased uptake in the right lobe with increased uptake in the caudate lobe representing hypertrophy of that lobe.

Bystander effect The directly irradiated cells communicate with adjacent cells and spread the effect of radiation to a larger number of cells.

Calcinosis cutis A term used to describe a group of disorders in which calcium deposits form in the skin, subcutaneous tissue, and connective tissue sheaths around the muscles but not within the muscles.

Calciphylaxis A condition of soft tissue calcification affecting mainly patients with chronic renal failure. The calcification involves the media of small- and medium-sized cutaneous arterioles with extensive intimal hyperplasia and fibrosis. There is also subcutaneous calcification and necrosis which may lead to sepsis, the main cause of morbidity which may be significant.

Cation Positively charged ion.

Chemotaxis Directional migration of leukocytes at varying rates of speed in interstitial tissue toward a chemotactic stimulus in the inflammatory focus. Through chemoreceptors at multiple locations on their plasma membranes, the cells are able to detect where the highest concentrations are of chemotactic factors and to migrate in their direction.

Costochondritis (Tietze's syndrome) This is a common painful condition affecting the costochondral junction usually in young patients and is self-limited. The etiology remains unknown although trauma and infection are proposed. It can affect any rib but the first and second ribs are most commonly involved.

Chronic obstructive airway disease Chronic bronchitis, emphysema, and bronchial asthma are collectively known as obstructive airway disease.

Colloid A substance that will not easily diffuse through membranes when dissolved in a liquid.

Complex regional pain syndrome type I (reflex sympathetic dystrophy) A pain syndrome that usually develops after an initiating noxious event with no identifiable major nerve injury, is not limited to the distribution of a single peripheral nerve, and is disproportional to the inciting event or expected healing response.

Connective tissue Body tissue that provides and maintains form in the body. It serves to connect and bind the cells and organs and gives support to the body. Unlike the other tissue types of the body that are formed mainly by cells, the major constituent of connective tissue is its extracellular matrix, composed of protein fibers, an amorphous ground substance, and tissue fluid in addition to cells such as fibroblasts, fat cells, and bone cells.

Conn's syndrome Primary aldosteronism with increased production of aldosterone by abnormal zona glomerulosa (adenoma or hyperplasia) leading to hypertension through the increased reabsorption of sodium and water from the distal tubules. A benign adenoma accounts for 75% of cases of this syndrome.

CPPD Calcium pyrophosphate dihydrate deposition disease, also called pseudogout and chondrocalcinosis, a type of crystal deposition arthropathy with such crystals deposited in cartilage, synovium, tendons, and ligaments.

Cushing's syndrome A disease caused by abnormal stimulation of zona fasciculata of adrenal gland leading to excessive secretion of cortisol. The stimulation of the zona fasciculata may be stimulated by excess ACTH from the pituitary gland, or less commonly the ectopic production of ACTH (as in small cell lung cancer and neural crest tumors) or corticotropin-releasing factor (CRF) (as in bronchial carcinoid and prostate cancer). The disease may also be due to autonomous adrenal cortisol production due to adrenal adenoma or hyperfunctioning adrenal carcinoma.

Detector sensitivity The ratio between the output and the input variable being measured.

Dose rate Dose rate expresses the time for which dose is administered.

Dosimetry A process of calculating the level of radiation exposure from a radioactive source.

Dystrophic calcification A type of soft tissue calcification that occurs in the setting of normal serum calcium and phosphate levels and occurs in damaged, inflamed, neoplastic, or necrotic tissue.

Ectopic hyperparathyroidism Parathyroid disease due to abnormalities in ectopically located glands.

Effective half-life Time required to reduce radioactivity by half by a combination of physical and biological elimination processes.

Endocarditis Inflammation of endocardium, which may be infective or non-infective

Endochondral ossification Most of the skeleton is formed by this type of ossification where a preexisting cartilage forms first and then undergoes ossification.

Enteropathic arthropathies Arthropathies associated with inflammatory bowel diseases including ulcerative colitis, Crohn's disease, Whipple's disease, intestinal bypass surgery, and celiac disease.

Entheses The sites of insertion of tendons, ligaments, and articular capsule to bone.

Enthesopathies A pathological process affecting entheses particularly trauma and or inflammation resulting in regional periosteal reaction with osteoblastic bone activity.

Epididymis A comma-shaped structure lying on the testicle on its posterolateral surface.

Epididymitis An inflammatory condition affecting the epididymis usually in adults secondary to infection or following trauma. Bacteria usually reach the epididymis from the prostate, seminal vesicles, and urethra or uncommonly hematogenously.

Erythropoiesis The formation of mature red blood cells in the bone marrow starting with the first stem cell progeny committed to erythroid differentiation and ending with the release of red cells into the circulation.

Eutopic hyperparathyroidism Parathyroid disease with typical location of glands.

Exudate An inflammatory extravascular fluid with a high protein content, much cellular debris, and a specific gravity above 1.020. This is the hallmark of acute inflammation, which may also be called exudative inflammation. It indicates significant alteration in the normal permeability of small blood vessels in the region of injury.

Fibrous dysplasia A benign bone disorder characterized by the presence of the fibrous

tissue in lesions of trabeculae of nonlamellar bone (woven bone), which remains essentially unchanged.

First-pass radionuclide angiography Examination of the initial transit of a radionuclide bolus through the different major vascular compartments can provide information about the function of each chamber.

Flare pattern on bone scan An initial apparent deterioration of primary or some or all metastatic lesions on the bone scan, followed by improvement usually accompanying successful treatment.

Fracture A break in the continuity of a bone.

Fracture delayed union Fracture union is delayed beyond the expected time (usually 9 months).

Fracture nonunion Complete cessation of repair process of a fracture.

Ganglioneuroma A benign tumor found in older children and young adults that is most commonly present in the adrenal medulla and the posterior mediastinum. The tumor consists of mature ganglion cells and is well encapsulated; it is frequently calcified and rarely hormone active.

Gas exchange airways Consists of the more distal bronchioles (respiratory) and the alveoli that are lined by nonciliated mucus membrane.

Gene therapy A method designed to manipulate the expression of genes in order to inhibit tumor growth.

Gout A metabolic disorder that results in hyperuricemia and leads to deposition of monosodium urate monohydrate crystals in various sites in the body, especially the joint cartilage.

Heterotopic ossification A specific type of soft tissue calcification that may or may not follow trauma and is due to a complex pathogenetic mechanism believed to be due to transformation of certain primitive cells of mesenchymal origin in the connective tissue septa within muscles, into bone-forming cells.

Hibernated myocardium Hibernation occurs in the myocardium that has undergone a down-regulation of contractile function, thus reducing cellular demand for energy, in response to chronic ischemia. It requires the restoration of blood flow in order to improve function.

Homeostasis The term describing maintenance of static, or constant, conditions in the internal environment by means of positive and negative feedback of information.

Hydrocephalus Conditions that produce imbalance between the rate of production and absorption of the cerebrospinal fluid, leading to dilatation of the ventricular system. They may result from obstruction to the flow and absorption of CSF or rarely from overproduction of CSF.

Hyperplasia An increase in cell number.

Hypertrophic cardiomyopathy An idiopathic process that affects mainly the LV myocardium, but the right ventricle may also be involved. Other causes of myocardial hypertrophy such as systemic hypertension and aortic valve stenosis must first be excluded.

Hypertrophic osteoarthropathy A form of periostitis that may be painful and may be associated with clubbing of fingers and toes, sweating, and thickening of skin. It may be primary or follows a variety of pathological conditions predominantly intrathoracic and is characterized by periosteal new bone formation.

Hypertrophy An increase in cell size which can lead to enlargement of an organ or part of it.

Immigrant cells The cells that travel transiently through blood or lymph and enter connective tissue as needed. These cells include erythrocytes (red blood cells), granulocytes, monocytes, lymphocytes, plasma cells, and platelets.

Impingement syndromes A group of painful conditions caused by friction of joint tissue which include bone impingement, soft tissue impingement, and entrapment neuropathy depending on the type of tissue involved.

Inflammation A complex nonspecific tissue reaction to injury by living agents such as bacteria and viruses leading to infection or nonliving agents including chemical, physical, immunological, or radiation injurious agents.

Inflammatory bowel disease (IBD) An idiopathic disease, probably involving an immune reaction of the body to its own intestinal tract. The two major types of IBD are ulcerative colitis and Crohn's disease.

Information density The count number per square centimeter within an image.

Intensity A term describing the energy or number of particles passing through an area unit per unit of time.

Intramembranous ossification Occurs through the transformation of mesenchymal cells into osteoblasts seen in flat bones of the skull, part of the mandible, and part of the clavicle.

Involucrum A layer of new bone formation around the site of skeletal infection formed secondary to the body response to infection.

Ionizing radiation A radiation that causes ionization (production of ion pair) when passing through a material.

Isotope dilution Diluting a radiotracer (or tracer) of known activity (or mass) in an unknown volume. By measuring the degree to which the radiotracer was diluted by the unknown volume, one can determine the total volume (or mass) of the unknown volume.

Jod-Basedow The condition of iodine-induced hyperthyroidism, which characteristically occurs in persons with nodular thyroid glands after iodine supplementation in endemic goiter areas. Iodine-containing medical products, including amiodarone, radiographic dyes, and kelp, may also cause Jod-Basedow.

Juxtaglomerular apparatus The afferent arteriole has specialized smooth muscle cells called juxtaglomerular (JG) cells that form this system and store renin and stretch receptors which respond to changes in arteriolar pressure. The system releases renin when stimulated.

Lactase deficiency A common cause of malabsorption that is found in 15% of Caucasian, 50% of blacks, and about 90% of Asians. Often, patients may have partial lactase deficiency that causes symptoms but not full-blown malabsorption syndrome. Treatment is to avoid lactose-containing dairy products (milk, ice cream, and cheese) and use lactose enzymes to aid in digestion.

Lisfranc injury Fracture or fracture dislocation of tarsometatarsal joints.

List mode An acquisition method for cardiac blood pool studies in patients with arrhythmias. Following acquisition of cardiac-gated blood pool study, each individual beat can be reviewed to eliminate atrial or ventricular premature beats that exceed a determined R-R interval duration (arrhythmia rejection). The acceptable beats can then be framed in the most appropriate timing interval for the type of analysis needed.

Lower respiratory airways Trachea, bronchi, bronchioles, and alveolar ducts connected by the larynx.

Maffucci syndrome A nonhereditary disorder characterized by multiple enchondromas and multiple bony hemangiomas.

Malunion Healing of a bone fracture in a non-anatomical orientation.

Marine-Lenhart syndrome Graves' disease with incidentally functioning nodule(s) which is responsive to thyroid-stimulating hormone. It is not responsive to thyroid-stimulating immunoglobulins. It appears as cold but after successful treatment with radioiodine, it will show uptake on follow-up thyroid scan since TSH level starts to rise.

Mast cells The secretory cells that mediate immediate hypersensitivity reactions. These cells are distributed along blood vessels in connective tissue. Stimulation of these cells by a variety of stimuli such as mechanical trauma, heat, X-rays, and toxins induces secretion of their granule contents, mainly histamine.

Megaloblastosis A morphological abnormality that occurs predominantly in the erythroid precursor cells in the bone marrow and in other replicating cells in human subjects due to deficiency of vitamin B12 and folate or metabolic abnormalities involving these vitamins.

MEN (multiple endocrine neoplasia) An autosomal dominant syndrome that involves hyperfunctioning of two or more endocrine organs. Primary hyperparathyroidism, pancreatic endocrine tumors, and anterior pituitary gland neoplasms characterize type 1 MEN. Medullary thyroid carcinoma, pheochromocytoma, and hyperparathyroidism caused by parathyroid gland hyperplasia characterize type MEN 2A. MEN 2B is defined by medullary thyroid tumor and pheochromocytoma.

Metachondromatosis A hereditary (autosomal dominant) disorder characterized by the presence of multiple enchondromas and osteochondromas.

Metaplasia An alteration of cell differentiation.

Metastatic calcification The type of soft tissue calcification that involves viable undamaged normal tissue as a result of hypercalcemia and/or hyperphosphatemia associated with increased calcium phosphate product locally or systematically.

Monoclonal antibody An antibody derived from a single clone of cells and hence binds only to one unique epitope.

Moyamoya disease A noninflammatory, non-atherosclerotic, nonamyloid vasculopathy characterized by chronic progressive stenosis or occlusion of the terminal internal carotid arteries. It occurs mainly under the age of ten with a smaller peak during the fourth decade. It presents with transient ischemic attacks and occasionally headache and seizures. Intracranial hemorrhage is the serious complication.

Murine antibody An antibody produced by mouse.

Mutation Any inherited change in the genetic material involving irreversible alterations in the sequence of DNA nucleotides.

Myositis ossificans progressive The congenital and rare form of heterotopic ossification.

Necrosis Cellular death resulting from the progressive degradative action of enzymes on the lethally injured cells, ultimately leading to the processes of cellular swelling, dissolution, and rupture. The morphological appearance of necrosis is the result of denaturation of proteins and enzymatic digestion (autolysis or heterolysis) of the cell.

Nephron The functional unit of the kidney. It consists of a glomerulus and a tubule. Urine is formed as a result of glomerular filtration, tubular reabsorption, and tubular secretion.

Neuroblastoma A malignant tumor of the sympathetic nervous system of childhood. It accounts for up to 10% of childhood cancers and 15% of cancer deaths among children. Seventy-five percent of neuroblastoma patients are younger than 4 years. The tumor has the potential to mature into pheochromocytoma or ganglioneuroma.

Nonuniformity A term describing variations of intensity of an image.

Ollier disease A nonhereditary disorder characterized by multiple enchondromas with a predilection for unilateral distribution.

Osteochondritis dissecans Transchondral fracture with fragmentation and separation of portions of cartilage or cartilage and bone which is most prevalent in adolescents.

Osteomalacia Abnormal mineralization of bone with a decrease in bone density secondary to lack of both calcium and phosphorus with no decrease in the amount of osteoid (bone formation).

Osteomyelitis A term applied to skeletal infection when it involves the bone marrow.

Osteopetrosis A rare inherited metabolic bone disease characterized by a generalized increase in skeletal mass due to a congenital defect in the development or function of the osteoclasts leading to defective bone resorption.

Osteoporosis Reduction of bone tissue amount increasing the likelihood of fractures.

Oxalosis Deposition of calcium oxalate crystals that leads to arthropathy.

Pair production When a photon with energy greater than 1.02 MeV is converted into an electron and a positron, the process is called pair production. It occurs when the high-energetic photon passes through a strong electric field.

Paraganglioma Pheochromocytoma arising at sites other than adrenal medulla (extra-adrenal).

Parkinson's disease A neurological disorder characterized by tremor, rigidity, akinesia, bradykinesia, and postural instability.

Pathological fracture A fracture at a site of preexisting abnormalities that weakens bone.

Phase image A computer-generated image representing evaluation of each pixel in the heart with respect to count changes over time. This helps identify abnormal timing of ventricular contraction.

Pheochromocytoma A rare tumor arising from chromaffin cells of the adrenal medulla. It commonly produces excessive amounts of norepinephrine, attributable to autonomous functioning of the tumor, although large tumors secrete both norepinephrine and epinephrine and in some cases also dopamine. Releasing the catecholamine into the circulation causes hypertension and other signs.

Physical half-life Time required for half of a radioactivity to decay.

Plantar fasciitis (calcaneal periostitis) An inflammatory condition that can occur as an isolated entity such as secondary to occupation or may accompany spondyloarthropathies.

Pneumocytis Jiroveci (carnii) An opportunistic pathogen currently classified as a fungus. It causes an infection leading to significant morbidity and mortality in human immunodeficiency virus and nonhuman immunodeficiency virus-associated immunosuppressed patients although it also occurs in non-immunocompromised patients.

Podagra A term describing affection of the metatarsophalangeal joint of the great toe in gout and the most typical finding of gouty arthritis.

Primary hyperparathyroidism Hyperparathyroidism caused by neoplastic or hyperplastic parathyroid glands or when nonparathyroid tumors such as bronchogenic or renal cell carcinomas secrete ectopically parathyroid hormone or a biologically similar product.

Pseudoarthrosis A gap between the fracture bone ends containing a space filled with fluid. Also termed false joint.

Pulmonary circulation A low-pressure, low-resistance system through which oxygen enters and carbon dioxide is removed.

Radiolabeling The process of attaching radioactive isotope.

Reactive arthritis (Reiter's disease) A syndrome characterized by a combination of nongonococcal urethritis, arthritis, and conjunctivitis.

Renal osteodystrophy A metabolic condition of bone associated with chronic renal failure.

Resolution Ability to separate or discriminate very close quantities by a detector.

Rheumatoid arthritis An autoimmune disease causing inflammation of connective tissue mainly in the joints with synovial inflammatory response triggered by immune complexes in the blood and synovial tissue through activation of plasma protein complement. This inflammation spreads from the synovial membrane to the articular cartilage, joint capsule, and the surrounding tendons and ligaments leading to pain, loss of function, and joint deformity.

SAPHO syndrome A syndrome characterized by synovitis, acne, palmoplantar pustulosis, hyperostosis, and osteitis. The small and large joints of the feet, ankles, knees, hips, sacroiliac joints, and shoulders are affected by the synovitis.

Sarcoidosis A multisystem granulomatous disorder, occurring most commonly in young adults, more commonly in blacks and in temperate areas with an unknown etiology, but it is believed to be due to exaggerated cellular immune response on the part of helper/inducer T lymphocytes to exogenous or autoantigens.

Scattered radiation This term describes radiation that during its passage through a substance deviates in direction with possible loss of energy.

Secondary hyperparathyroidism Hyperparathyroidism due to compensatory hyperplasia of parathyroids in response to hypocalcemia.

Septic tenosynovitis An inflammatory condition affecting generally the flexor tendons of the hands and feet of diabetic patients and resulting from penetrating injuries or spread of infection from a contiguous focus of infection.

Sequestrum Segmental bone necrosis that develops when normal blood supply to the bone is interrupted by the edema and ischemia produced by the inflammation.

Shin splints Periosteal elevation with reactive bone formation secondary to extreme tension on muscles or muscle groups inserting on bones.

Slipped capital femoral epiphysis Displacement of the proximal femoral epiphysis or simply femoral head from the femoral neck at the site of the growth plate during the growth condition.

Spondyloarthropathies A group of seronegative arthropathies formerly called rheumatoid variants that share common clinical and radiographic features with characteristic involvement of the sacroiliac joints, spine, and, to various degrees, the peripheral joints, which are linked to HLA B27 histocompatibility antigen and include ankylosing spondylitis, psoriatic arthritis, reactive arthritis (Reiter's disease), and enteropathic spondylitis.

Spondylolysis A loss of continuity of bone of the neuroarch of the vertebra due to stress or trauma.

Spondylolisthesis Forward (rarely backward) movement of one vertebra on another usually as a result of fracture of the neuroarch.

Spontaneous intracranial hypotension (SIH) An increasingly recognized condition due to CSF leak without apparent prior cause. It can cause postural headache, which in this case is secondary to low CSF pressure.

Sprains Tears to tendons.

Stem cells Undifferentiated cells in adults known also as pluripotent cells, precursor cells that are not totally committed to a specific function.

Strains Tears to ligaments.

Stress fracture A pathological condition of bone due to repeated episodes of stress; each is less forceful than that needed to cause acute fracture of the bony cortex.

Stunned myocardium Continued dysfunction due to ischemia-induced oxidative stress.

Synovial joints Specialized joints found mainly in the appendicular skeleton and which allow free motion.

Tertiary hyperparathyroidism The condition of patients who develop hypercalcemia following long-standing secondary hyperparathyroidism due to the development of autonomous parathyroid hyperplasia, which may not regress after correction of the underlying condition, as with renal transplantation.

Thyrotropin-releasing hormone (TRH) A tripeptide originating from the hypothalamic median eminence, which stimulates the secretion and synthesis of thyroid-stimulating hormone from the anterior pituitary.

Toddler's fracture Fracture in preschool children which is typically a nondisplaced spiral fracture of the mid-tibia but also involves other fractures including the fibula, calcaneus, talus, metatarsal, and cuboid bones in this age group.

Transient synovitis A joint inflammation of unknown origin and self-limited course affecting most frequently boys between 5 and 10 years of age. It was known as toxic synovitis and affects preferentially the hip or knee and subsides without antibiotics.

T-score A parameter used to express bone mineral density by relating an individual's bone density to the mean BMD of healthy young adults, matched for gender and ethnic group.

Tumor grading Grading is a scheme that attempts to determine the degree of malignancy and is based on the evaluation of certain parameters such as degree of tumor cellularity, resemblance of tumor cells to their normal forebears morphologically and functionally, cellular pleomorphism or anaplasia, mitotic activity (number and abnormality), and necrosis.

Tumoral calcinosis A type of soft tissue calcification characterized by large, calcified, periarticular soft tissue masses of calcium phosphate near the large joints such as the hip, the shoulder, and the elbow, in addition to the wrist, feet, and hands.

Uniformity correction Addition or subtraction of counts to the image in order to correct for flood field irregularities.

Upper respiratory airways Nasopharynx and oropharynx.

Ventilation The process by which air flows in and out of the gas exchange airways.

Ventricular ejection fraction The stroke volume divided by the end-diastolic volume.

Whipple's disease A systemic bacterial illness usually affecting middle-age men causing malabsorption and presenting diarrhea, arthritis, fever, weight loss, swollen lymph nodes, and skin pigmentation. It is diagnosed mainly by a small bowel biopsy through an endoscope, and the treatment is antibiotics for 1 year or longer.

Wolff-Chaikoff effect An intrathyroid autoregulatory mechanism other than the hypothalamus-pituitary-thyroid axis mechanism. When intrathyroid iodine concentrations are significantly increased, the rate of thyroid hormone synthesis is decreased, with a reduction in iodothyronine synthesis and a decrease in the DIT/MIT ratio.

Woven bone Immature nonlamellar bone that is later normally converted to lamellar bone.

Z-score A parameter used to express bone mineral density by comparing the bone density value of an individual to the mean value expected for his/her age-matched peer.